Bull's Handbook of Sports Injuries

Second Edition

NOTICE

Medicine is an ever-changing science. As new research and clinical experience broaden our knowledge, changes in treatment and drug therapy are required. The authors and the publisher of this work have checked with sources believed to be reliable in their efforts to provide information that is complete and generally in accord with the standards accepted at the time of publication. However, in view of the possibility of human error or changes in medical sciences, neither the authors nor the publisher nor any other party who has been involved in the preparation or publication of this work warrants that the information contained herein is in every respect accurate or complete, and they disclaim all responsibility for any errors or omissions or for the results obtained from use of the information contained in this work. Readers are encouraged to confirm the information contained herein with other sources. For example and in particular, readers are advised to check the product information sheet included in the package of each drug they plan to administer to be certain that the information contained in this work is accurate and that changes have not been made in the recommended dose or in the contraindications for administration. This recommendation is of particular importance in connection with new or infrequently used drugs.

Bull's Handbook of Sports Injuries

Second Edition

William O. Roberts, MD, MS, FACSM
Associate Professor of Family Practice
University of Minnesota School of Medicine
St. Paul, Minnesota

McGraw-Hill
Medical Publishing Division

*New York   Chicago   San Francisco   Lisbon   London
Madrid   Mexico City   Milan   New Delhi   San Juan
Seoul   Singapore   Sydney   Toronto*

Bull's Handbook of Sports Injuries, Second Edition

Copyright © 2004, 1999 by The McGraw-Hill Companies, Inc. All rights
reserved. Printed in the United States of America. Except as permitted
under the United States Copyright Act of 1976, no part of this publication
may be reproduced or distributed in any form or by any means, or stored
in a data base or retrieval system without the prior written permission of
the publisher.

The views expressed in this work are those of the individual authors and
do not reflect the official policy or position of the Departments of the
Navy, Army or Air Force, the Department of Defense, or the U.S.
Government.

1 2 3 4 5 6 7 8 9 0 DOC/DOC 0 9 8 7 6 5 4

ISBN 0-07-140291-8

This book was set in Times Roman by The GTS Companies/York,
PA Campus
The editors were Darlene Cooke, Lisa Silverman, and Marsha Loeb.
The production supervisor was Richard Ruzycka.
Project management was provided by Jennsin Publishing Services.
The index was prepared by Jerry Ralya.
RR Donnelley was printer and binder.
This book was printed on acid-free paper.

Cataloging-in-Publication data is on file for this title at the Library of
Congress.

Contents

Contributors

Barry Bartlett, MD
Macmaster University, Hamilton, Ontario, Canada
Lacrosse

Wilma F. Bergfeld, MD
Professor, Departments of Dermatology and Pathology, Cleveland Clinic
Foundation Cleveland, Ohio
Dermatology Issues in Athletes

Joshua M. Berlin, MD
Senior Resident, Department of Dermatology, Cleveland Clinic
Foundation, Cleveland, Ohio
Dermatology Issues in Athletes

Mark Bouchard, MD, FACSM
Assistant Director, Maine Medical Center Sports Medicine Fellowship,
Portland, Maine
Gymnastic Injuries and Prevention

R. Charles Bull, MD, BSc (MED), FRCS(C)
Director, York University Sports Injuries Clinic, Toronto, Ontario, Canada
Lacrosse

Janus D. Butcher, MD, FACSM
Saint Mary's Duluth Clinic for Orthopedics and Sports Medicine, Duluth,
Minnesota; Head Physician, Cross-Country Ski Team, United States Ski
and Snowboard Association
Cross-Country Ski Injuries

T. Jeff Chandler, EdD, CSCS*D, FACSM
Editor-in-Chief, *Strength and Conditioning Journal;* Chair of
Exercise Science, Sport, and Recreation, Marshall University,
Huntington, West Virginia
Muscle Training and Conditioning

Michael Clarfield, MD, CCFP, DSP
Team Physician, Toronto Maple Leafs; Team Physician, National Tennis
Team; Company Physician, National Ballet of Canada; Director, The
Sports Medicine Specialists (Toronto); Assistant Professor, University of
Toronto, Toronto, Ontario, Canada
High Performance and the Treatment of the Elite Athlete

Richard G. Clarnette, MBBS, FRACS
Wakefield Orthopaedic Clinic, Adelaide, South Australia, Australia
Baseball Injuries

Doreen Cress, CAT (C)
Mississauga, Ontario, Canada
Lacrosse

Christopher T. Daley, MD, FRCS(C)
Carolina Orthopaedic Specialists, Valdese, North Carolina
Soft Tissue Injuries: Overuse Syndromes

William W. Dexter, MD, FACSM
Maine Medical Center, Director, Sports Medicine Program, Assistant
Director, Family Practice Residency Program, Portland, Maine
*Chest and Abdomen; Ear, Nose, and Throat Injuries; Strength Training
and Weight Lifting*

Steven R. Elias, MD, PhD
Medical Director, Schwan's USA Cup Soccer Tournament; Columbia Park
Medical Group, Fridley, Minnesota
Soccer Injuries

Ken Fern, MD
Clinical Spine Fellow, University of Toronto, Toronto, Ontario, Canada
Neck, Spinal Cord, and Back

Jonathan T. Finnoff, DO
Alpine Orthopaedic Specialists, North Logan, Utah
Cycling

Michael H. Ford, MD
Assistant Professor, Orthopaedic and Arthritic Institute, Sunnybrook and
Women's College Health Science Center, Toronto, Ontario, Canada
Neck, Spinal Cord, and Back

Lorie Forwell, MSc(PT)
Head Team Physician, Utah State University, North Logan, Utah
Swimming

Peter J. Fowler, MD
Fowler Kennedy Sport Medicine Clinic, University of Western Ontario,
London, Ontario, Canada
Swimming

Peter G. Gerbino, MD, FACSM
Division of Sports Medicine, Department of Orthopaedic Surgery,
Children's Hospital, Harvard Medical School, Boston, Massachusetts
Knee Injuries; Stress Fractures

Chris Hand, MD
Surgeon Commander, C J Hand FRCS (Tr&Orth), Royal Navy Consultant,
Queen Alexandra Hospital and Royal Hospital Haslar, Portsmouth, Hants,
United Kingdom
Baseball Injuries

Duncan K. Hodge, MD
Department of Orthopaedic Surgery, University of California, San
Francisco, San Francisco, California
Sideline Management of Common Dislocations

Mark R. Hutchinson, MD, FACSM
Associate Professor of Orthopaedics and Sports Medicine,
Director of Sports Medicine Services, University of Illinois at Chicago,
Chicago, Illinois
Chronic Exertional Compartment Syndrome

Mary Lloyd Ireland, MD, FACSM
Medical Director, Kentucky Sports Medicine Clinic, Lexington,
Kentucky
Chronic Exertional Compartment Syndrome

Neeru A. Jayanthi, MD
Sports Medicine Fellow, Department of Family Medicine, Indiana
University Methodist Sports Medicine Center, Indianapolis, Indiana
Knee Bracing

Don Johnson, MD, FRCS(C)
Director, Sports Medicine Clinic, Carleton University; Assistant
Professor, Orthopaedic Surgery, University of Ottawa, Ottawa, Ontario,
Canada
Computers in Sports Medicine; Football Injuries

Paul Johnson, MD
University of Alberta, Edmonton, Alberta, Canada
Football Injuries

Robert Kennedy, MD
The Sports Medicine Institute, Saint Joseph Regional Medical Center,
South Bend, Indiana
Foot and Ankle

Tae Kyun Kim, MD, PhD
Division of Sports Medicine and Shoulder Surgery, Department of
Orthopaedic Surgery, The Johns Hopkins University, Baltimore,
Maryland
Evaluation and Treatment of Shoulder Injuries

Jim Macintyre, MD, MPE, FACSM, DSM
Adjunct Assistant Professor, Department of Family and Preventive
Medicine; Adjunct Associate Professor of Ballet, University of Utah,
Salt Lake City, Utah
Dance Injuries

Derek Mackesy, MD
Institute for Preventive Sports Medicine, Ann Arbor, Michigan
Role of the Physician, Trainer, and Coach

Paul H. Marks, MD, BASc, FRCS(C)
Assistant Professor, Department of Surgery, University of Toronto;
Head Team Physician and Orthopaedic Surgeon, Toronto Raptors
Basketball Club and Varsity Blues Intercollegiate Athletics, Toronto,
Ontario, Canada
Basketball Injuries

Ronica Martinez, MD
Sports Medicine Fellow, Department of Family Medicine, Kaiser
Permanente Medical Center, Fontana, California
Return to Play: Making the Correct Decision

Shauna Martiniuk, MD
Lecturer, University of Toronto; Staff Emergency Physician, Mt. Sinai
Hospital, Toronto, Ontario, Canada
Ice Hockey

Edward G. McFarland, MD, FACSM
Division of Sports Medicine and Shoulder Surgery, Department of
Orthopaedic Surgery, The Johns Hopkins University, Baltimore,
Maryland
Evaluation and Treatment of Shoulder Injuries

Douglas B. McKeag, MD, FACSM
AUL Professor and Chair, Department of Family Medicine, Indiana
University School of Medicine; Director, Indiana University Center for
Sports Medicine, Indianapolis, Indiana
Knee Bracing

Borna Meisami, MD, FRCS(C)
Department of Orthopaedics, Toronto Western Hospital, Toronto,
Ontario, Canada
Baseball Injuries

Anthony Miniaci, MD, FRCS(C)
Sports Health Unit, Cleveland Clinic Foundation, Cleveland, Ohio
Baseball Injuries

James L. Moeller, MD, FACSM
Sports Medicine Associates, PLC, Auburn Hills, Michigan; Chief, Division
of Sports Medicine, William Beaumont Hospital, Troy, Michigan
Figure Skating

Lloyd Nesbitt, DPM
Private Practice, Toronto, Ontario, Canada
Orthotics

Hyung Bin Park, MD
Assistant Professor, Department of Orthopaedic Surgery, College of
Medicine, Gyeong Sang National University, Jinju, South Korea
Evaluation and Treatment of Shoulder Injuries

Robert C. Pashby, MD
Department of Ophthalmology, University of Toronto, Hospital for Sick Children, Mt. Sinai Hospital, Toronto, Ontario, Canada
Eye Injuries and Eye Protection

Thomas J. Pashby, MD
Department of Ophthalmology, Emeritus, University of Toronto, Hospital for Sick Children, Scarborough Centenary Hospital, Toronto, Ontario, Canada
Eye Injuries and Eye Protection

Andrew Pipe, CM, MC, FACSM, Dip Sport Med
Chair, Canadian Centre for Ethics in Sport; Team Physician, Canadian Men's National Basketball Team; Chair, FINA Doping Control Review Board; Associate Professor and Director, Prevention and Rehabilitation Centre, University of Ottawa Heart Institute, Ottawa, Ontario, Canada
Drugs and Ergogenic Aids in Sport

Robert Quinn, MD
Dominican Rehabilitation Center of Santa Cruz, Santa Cruz, California
Track and Field Injuries

Douglas W. Richards, MD, DSM
Medical Director, David L. MacIntosh Sports Medicine Clinic; Assistant Professor, Department of Family and Community Medicine, University of Toronto; Team Physician, Toronto Raptors Basketball Club, National Women's Basketball Canada, and Varsity Blues Intercollegiate Athletics, Bloor Medical Centre, Toronto, Ontario, Canada
Basketball Injuries

Glen Richardson
Orthopaedic and Sport Medicine Clinic of Nova Scotia, Dalhousie University, Halifax, Nova Scotia, Canada
The Athlete's Arthritic Knee

Sami F. Rifat, MD, FACSM
Sports Medicine Associates, PLC, Auburn Hills, Michigan
Figure Skating

Debra W. Roberts, PT
PTKids, Mahtomedi, Minnesota
Rehabilitation and Physical Therapy

William O. Roberts, MD, MS, FACSM
Associate Professor of Family Medicine, University of Minnesota School of Medicine, Phalen Village Clinic, St. Paul, Minnesota
Heat and Cold Injuries; Endurance Training; Rehabilitation and Physical Therapy; Track and Field Injuries; Endurance Training; Lacrosse

Mark Roettger, DDS
Assistant Professor, University of Minnesota School of Dentistry; Private Practice, Stillwater, Minnesota
Dental Injuries

Aaron Rubin, MD, FACSM, FAAFP
Program Director, Kaiser Permanente Sports Medicine Fellowship; Team
Physician, University of California, Riverside and Rubidoux High School,
Fontana, California
Emergency Sideline Care and Airway Management

Marc R. Safran, MD, FACSM
Co-Director, Sports Medicine; Associate Professor, Department of
Orthopaedic Surgery, University of California, San Francisco,
San Francisco, California
Sideline Management of Common Dislocations; Racquet Sports

Robert Sallis, MD, FAAFP, FACSM
Co-Director, Kaiser Permanente Sports Medicine Fellowship Program;
Team Physician, Pamona College, Los Osos High School
Return to Play: Making the Correct Decision

Michael L. Schwartz, MD
Professor of Surgery, University of Toronto, Toronto, Ontario, Canada
Head Injuries and Concussions

Ato Sekyi-Out, MD, FRCS(C)
William Osler Health Centre, Brampton, Ontario, Canada
Basketball Injuries

Stephen M. Simons, MD, FACSM
The Sports Medicine Institute, Saint Joseph Regional Medical Center,
South Bend, Indiana
Foot and Ankle Injuries

Mark Snowise, MD
Suburban Internal Medicine, Lee, Massachusetts
Ear, Nose, and Throat Injuries

William D. Stanish, MD, FRCS(C), FACS
Director, Orthopaedic and Sport Medicine Clinic of Nova Scotia,
Dalhousie University, Halifax, Nova Scotia, Canada
The Athlete's Arthritic Knee; Soft Tissue Injuries: Overuse Syndromes

Charles H. Tator, MD, PhD, FRCS
The Toronto Hospital, Western Division, Toronto, Ontario, Canada
Head Injuries and Concussions

David Thorson, MD
MinnHealth Family Physicians, White Bear Lake, Minnesota
Alpine Skiing and Snowboard Injuries

L. Tyler Wadsworth, MD
Sports Medicine Consultants, PC, St. Louis, Missouri
Golf Injuries

Laurie Weiser, MD
Maine Medical Center, Sports Medicine, Family Practice Residency
Program, Portland, Maine
Strength Training and Weight Lifting

C. Stewart Wright, MD
Assistant Professor, Orthopaedic and Arthritic Institute, Toronto,
Ontario, Canada
Wrist and Hand Injuries

Gilbert Yee, MD, Med, FRCS(C)
Scarborough General Hospital, Scarborough, Ontario, Canada
Basketball Injuries

Atsushi Yokota, MD, PhD
Osaka Medical College, Department of Orthopaedic Surgery, Osaka, Japan
Evaluation and Treatment of Shoulder Injuries

Preface

Sports medicine is a passion and hobby that increases my effectiveness as a primary care physician. The spirit of the George Sheehan essay entitled, "Every patient is an athlete" is the foundation of my approach to patients. The first edition of *Bull's Handbook of Sports Injuries* captures the essence of exercise and activity medicine applied to athletes of all walks and abilities in a "folksy" style that is easy to read and apply to daily office and sideline encounters. Doctor Bull intended the book "to improve sport safety and highlight issues to improve the sports medicine team." My goal in the second edition of the book is to enhance the practical aspects injury prevention and care and maintain the down-to-earth, team-oriented approach initiated by Dr Bull. Not an easy task considering the breadth of the initial edition.

The second edition features the return of several authors whose work has heavily influenced my education and practice in the office and in the public health arena. Doctors Tator, Stanish, Pashby, Fowler, Pipe, and Nesbitt have made an impact on the health and safety of athletes worldwide, and I am grateful for their contributions to the second edition along with the other authors from the original book who updated their chapters. There are several new authors, both established or up and coming practitioners in the sports medicine world, who stepped in to replace the original authors who were unable to contribute again or to write on new topics added to the second edition.

The book is organized in three sections: Sports Medicine Issues, Injury and Illness, and Sport-Specific Issues. The first section deals with general issues and essential background information needed to care for athletes and active people. The second section addresses problems associated with specific joints and activity issues related to injury and illness in athletes. The final section is devoted to the problems associated with specific sports and activities that are common to the office practice of most sports medicine physicians and providers. You may find a different twist on a common topic when addressed from the perspective of a particular sport. Many of the chapters are organized in the following format to make it easy to find important facts that you need:

Quick Look
Introduction
Epidemiology
Pathophysiology
Injuries
Evaluation
Management
Confounding Conditions
Prevention
Sideline Tips
Summary

Each chapter is a strong mix of evidence-based and expert opinion evaluation and care protocols seasoned by the sideline and office experience of the authors. The Quick Look section at the chapter beginning is designed to put important information at the tip of your fingers with the supporting details in the text.

From the simple advice for ankle sprains to the more complex evaluation of the low back in dancers and Nordic skiers, the book is filled with practical facts that you can use for all your patients. As highlighted in the Golf chapter, the adage "Practice makes perfect" is often more realistically stated as "Practice makes permanent." Advising a patient to take lessons in golf, skiing, or any sport may be the single most "preventative" sports medicine advice that we can give our athletes. In addition, the full set of Team Physician Consensus Conference Statements is included in the Appendix. I hope you find the second edition of *Bull's Handbook of Sports Injuries* a useful reference in your office or on the sidelines.

Acknowledgments

Darlene Cooke from McGraw-Hill took the time to convince me that I could take on the revision of this book and most of the time I thank her for that. Her advice and council were integral to completing the second edition and I wish her the best in a challenging time. The book would not have been possible without the support of the McGraw-Hill team past and present and I would like to acknowledge the efforts of Lisa Silverman and Marcia Loeb who managed to keep me on task.

I would also like to thank all the authors for their time and contributions to this edition. The chapter contents were a great review for the ABFP Sports Medicine Sub-Specialty Board Examination. The second edition would not be possible without the foundation and vision developed for the first edition by Charles Bull and I owe him a debt of gratitude for his efforts writing and editing the first edition of this book.

The American College of Sports Medicine (ACSM) gave permission for us to reprint the Team Physician Consensus Conference Statements in the book and I hope the statements will augment the usefulness of this edition. The ACSM education and network has advanced and enhanced my sports medicine experience.

I would also like to thank my family who as a group put up with the time demands of the writing and review process, and individually advanced my education as a sports physician, coach, spouse, and father. Finally special thanks to Debra Roberts, my life partner, who indulges my sports medicine pursuits and contributed her physical therapy experience and expertise to this book and my career. She has been described as a saint by many for putting up with me and truly deserves the title.

Bull's Handbook of Sports Injuries

Second Edition

I | ISSUES

1 | Role of the Physician, Trainer, and Coach

Derek Mackesy

THE SPORTS MEDICINE TEAM

The skills and strength needed for survival and war were transformed into games of skill during times of peace. Historians claim that the first sports physician was Herodicus. During the fifth century BC, he treated athletes and other injured Athenians with therapeutic exercises and diet. His most famous pupil was Hippocrates, who later wrote of the value of exercise in both the treatment of injuries as well as the prevention of illnesses.

As civilization progressed and athletic contests became more organized, more highly trained and skilled athletes competed in teams and as individuals. Retaining fitness and recovering from injuries proved increasingly important as the sophistication and popularity of sport grew. The need for physicians, trainers, and therapists knowledgeable in the formal care and rehabilitation of athletes progressed simultaneously. Injury prevention through regulation, equipment, and playing rules, as well as pertinent research, became extremely important in the realm of athletic medicine.

The success of an individual athlete or collective team is not only measured in wins and losses, but also in how effective the sports medicine team has been in preventing and effectively treating the injuries that invariably occur. The care of the athlete is a team effort in which members of the sports medicine team support each other for the benefit of the athlete and the team. Depending on the level of participation, the medical support team might consist of a single individual (i.e., athletic trainer, physiotherapist, paramedic, or physician). In such situations, the individual practitioner must develop a network of support personnel who can assist when and where additional professional management is needed.

Professional, national, university and, to a certain extent, high school teams often have a medical support team consisting of a number of different sports medicine personnel. Both clinical and nonclinical support may be utilized. The individual responsible for assembling the team must ensure that all members of the medical support team have high professional standards and work well together in a team situation. Availability and communication are the hallmarks of a successful sports medicine team. Individuals who may be part of the sports medicine team include the following:

1. Primary care sports medicine physician
2. Orthopedic surgeon
3. Coach
4. Athletic trainer
5. Physiotherapist
6. Sports psychologist
7. Nutritionist
8. Dentist
9. Internist
10. Equipment manager
11. Strength coach
12. Fitness advisor
13. Other sport-specific specialists

3

Specific areas of responsibility for the diagnosis and treatment of injuries need to be defined to avoid conflict between various members of the team. One member of the team should be responsible for availability, event coverage, and any problems that may be encountered on a day-to-day basis.

TEAM PHYSICIAN

The team physician has a vital position that entails multifaceted responsibilities to the athlete, the team, and the medical profession. Team physicians are expected by parents, coaches, and management to make decisions about athletes' health, qualifications to join the team, and ability to participate safely. These decisions are often made in a setting of intense time pressure, which may affect the success of the team and the future of the athlete. These health and safety decisions influence the athlete's mental, economic, and physical well-being.

Protecting the health, safety, and well-being of the participating athlete begins at the preseason assessment. A comprehensive history and examination should be done prior to the start of organized training. A review of past injuries, current medication and supplements, allergies, and a full physical examination must be conducted. Ancillary fitness testing, blood and urine analysis, and sports-specific tests are discretionary and dependent on medical necessity and budgetary constraints.

Each athlete should have an up-to-date chart detailing current injury status, treatment plan, and current medication and supplements. Confidentiality is essential and the team physician must be sensitive to the extent of information that is provided to the coaching staff and management. Release of medical information to the public and media should be cleared with the athlete (and parents) and the team administration.

The team physician must be readily available for his or her team. A well-organized coverage system with other members of the medical team should provide for care during games, practices, and travel. The team physician should be available to the athletes on the sidelines, in the training room, and in the office. It is essential to maintain good medical records for patient care and medical-legal purposes. It becomes particularly important when more than one member of the medical team is involved in the treatment of the patient. The team physician also has responsibilities to the coach, to the management, and to the ethics of the medical profession.

As an integral part of any sporting team, the team physician cannot simply do his or her job from the stands. During participation, he or she should be as close to the action as possible. By watching the play in a vigilant manner, the team physician can note the injuries as they may happen in an attempt to understand the mechanism. He or she should be "more than just a privileged spectator." The suggested contents for a medical bag for a team physician are listed in Table 1-1.

ATHLETIC TRAINER

Athletic training is the "front line" discipline in sports medicine, usually working under the supervision of a team physician. Its practitioners are the most closely involved with the day-to-day care of the modern athlete. Today's athletic trainer must have a working knowledge of virtually every aspect of sports medicine to successfully prevent, treat, and rehabilitate athletic injuries and illness. An athetic trainer must be familiar with basic medical procedures to understand the implications of medical treatment and communicate well with physicians and coaches.

A well-trained certified athletic trainer is a valuable member of the primary sports medicine team that usually consists of the coach, the athletic trainer, and the team physician. An athletic trainer's responsibilities include the following:

1. Preventing, evaluating, and managing injuries and illness
2. Communicating with the team physician and coaches
3. Managing the training room
4. Educating athletes and coaches for nutrition, hydration, and environment issues
5. Research

Injury Prevention and Management

The preventative approach within sports medicine has yielded significant reduction in injury rates for all sports. Recommendations for protective eyewear during racquet sports and ice hockey, heat and cold activity modifications, rule changes, and protective equipment innovations have led to significant diminution in sports-related injuries and associated health-care costs.

The health of each athlete must be continually monitored before, during, and after the competitive season. A complete history and physical is essential prior to the start of each professional sport's season and many teams require a post-season evaluation as well. At the community and high school level of competition, periodic examinations with annual "interval" health questionaires are common practice.

Athletic trainers should know how to create effective conditioning programs to assist the athlete in gaining and maintaining maximum performance, although this is usually a coaching function. The athletic trainer must also monitor playing surfaces, environmental conditions, and hazardous structures that may inadvertently cause injury.

The day-to-day burden of the athletic trainer is early recognition and evaluation of athletically related injuries. He or she must have a thorough knowledge of the sports medicine sciences, as well as confidence in his or her ability to respond skillfully in an emergency situation.

The athletic trainer is often the first provider of treatment to the injured athlete, usually executing the direct instructions or agreed upon protocols of a supervising physician. After evaluating an injury and rendering first aid (when no physician is present), the athletic trainer must decide on the appropriate treatment and determine whether medical attention is necessary. With direction from the physician, the athletic trainer organizes a treatment regimen, using a variety of therapeutic methods, supportive procedures, or other techniques to aid in recovery.

Injury rehabilitation is often one of the most challenging of the profession. The athletic trainer should establish the goals and criteria for recovery from injury, and should be able to assess by objective measurement when the goals have been achieved to assist in the athlete's to return to participation.

Communication

The athletic trainer requires a constant and timely flow of oral, written, and electronic communication to facilitate evaluation, treatment, and return

TABLE 1-1 Suggested Contents of Team Physician's Bag

Equipment	Medication
Diagnostic Tools	Injection
Stethoscope	Atropine, 0.4 mg/mL, four 1-mL vials
Otoscope/ophthalmoscope (Check batteries: if recharge-	Betamethasone, 6 mg/mL, one 5-mL multidose vial
able, periodically discharge and recharge fully)	Epinephrine (1:1000) 1 mg/mL, four 1-mL, ampules
Sphygmomanometer (aneroid)	and/or 0.3-mg autoinjector
Clinical thermometer	Meperidine 100 mg/cc, two 1-mL ampoules
Reflex hammer	Morphine sulfate 15 mg/cc, two 1-mL ampoules
Safety pins	Lidocaine (1% without epinephrine), one 20-mL vial
Tongue depressors	Bupivacaine hydrochloride (0.5%) one 50-mL vial
Latex examination gloves	Glucagon, one 1-mg vial with diluent
Tape measure	Promethazine 50 mg/mL, two 1-mL ampoules
Mini-Maglite	Diazepam 5 mg/mL, two 2-mL ampoules
Resuscitation Tools	Naloxone 0.4 mg/mL, one 1-mL vial
Oral airways	Sodium bicarbonate (8.4%) one 50-mL vial
Pocket resuscitation mask	Sodium chloride (0.9%) two 30-mL vials
Oral screw	Inhalation
Tongue forceps	Albuterol inhaler
Laryngoscope	Oxymetazoline (0.05% nasal spray), one 15-mL bottle
Ambu bag	Oral
Endotracheal tubes, one 6.5 mm, one 7.5 mm	Amoxicillin capsules, 250 mg
Surgical Tools	Diphenhydramine capsules, 25 mg or 50 mg
Bandage scissors (large, sturdy, sharp)	Erythromycin capsules, 250 mg
Syringes	Ibuprofen tablets, 600 mg

Needles, three each: 18 gauge × 1.5 inch
        three each: 25 gauge × 1.5 inch
Steri-Strips, two packets, 1/8 inch, 1/4 inch
Sterile latex gloves
Minor surgical set:
Scalpel handles, three: (BT3) with
Detachable blades (10, 11 and 15)
Iris scissors
Thumb forceps
Splinter forceps
Nylon suture, two each: 4-0, 5-0, and 6-0
Drape
Disposable suture set:
Needle holder
Hemostat
Scissors
Drape
Suture removal scissors
Rubber tourniquet

Antacid tablets
Sublingual nitroglycerin tablets, 0.4 mg
Chlorzoxazone caplets, 500 mg
Acetaminophen caplets, 500 mg
Acetaminophen tablets with codeine, 30 mg
Loperamide capsules, 2 mg
Propoxyphene napsylate tablets with acetaminophen,
    650 mg
Dextrometorphan liquid, 100-mL bottle
Topical
Proparacaine (0.5%) (eye anesthetic)
Polymyxin-neomycin-garamycin ophthalmic solution
Colymycin-hydrocortisone otic solution
Nitrofurazone cream
Mupirocin ointment
Corticosteroid cream
Ketoconazole cream (2%)

decisions. When communicating with the athlete's parents, physicians, coaches, students, and other professionals, the athletic trainer must be precise, intelligent, and professional.

Management of the Athletic Training Room

The purchase of supplies and equipment for the training room, sidelines, and travel bags, and maintaining appropriate records on all the athletes is an essential duty of the athletic trainer. Athletic trainers cannot dispense medications to athletes without direct physician supervision and physicians may not lawfully delegate prescriptive drug dispensing acts to trainers.

Education and Research

Athletic trainers often instruct athletes in all aspects of the injury, including the nature, condition, and procedures to be followed for rapid recovery. They provide information about their profession to coaches, parents, and the community. They also provide ongoing instruction to assistant trainers, students, and volunteer personnel. The athletic trainer may counsel the athlete on emotional problems, substance abuse, or personal problems. At the first sign of serious psychosocial difficulties with an athlete, the athletic trainer must make proper professional referrals.

Professional Certification

Both the National Athletic Trainers' Association and the Canadian Athletic Therapists' Association provide certification examinations that evaluate clinical competence. Certification ensures that proper educational preparation and clinical experience has been obtained prior to passing a written and practical examination.

It is the trainer's responsibility to maintain his or her active certification status as well as work toward improvement of personal knowledge and skills within the profession.

COACH

The coach is directly responsible for teaching individual sport-specific skills, physical conditioning, and strategy necessary for competitive team participation. As a member of the sports medicine team, he or she should impart a proper game philosophy, respect for the rules of play, and an overall safety awareness. Coaches must show concern for safety by meeting with team members to inform them of potential injuries, and outline an approach to prevention. The "win at all cost" attitude can be extremely dangerous for athletes, who often feel an obligation to fulfill the coaches' expectations. Coaches are responsible for orchestrating effective and safe conditioning programs that ensure the endurance, strength, flexibility, and agility necessary for the particular sport.

The coach must also provide, or delegate to a competent aide, emergency care of athletic injuries and application of first aid in the absence of the trainer or team physician. At least one member of the coaching staff should have CPR training and basic first aid knowledge.

Unfortunately, some coaches distrust the medical team and paramedical practitioners, and often feel that the main role of the sports medicine clinician is to prevent the athlete from practicing or playing. The coach must

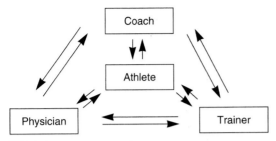

FIG 1-1   The sports medicine team.

understand that the team physician and athletic trainer are part of team aiming to maximize the performance and health of the athlete (Fig. 1-1).

It is imperative that the coach is involved in the health care decision-making process. Some coaches overestimate their medical knowledge and demand that an injured player be put back into the game against the advice of the physician or athletic trainer. Involving the coach in the decision-making process and explaining the rationale behind any recommendations increase the chance of the athlete's and coach's compliance with your recommendation. A knowledgeable and ethical coach, when told that one of his players has to miss the remainder of the game, would say, "Take good care of him. We'll be alright."

When good rapport with the coach has been established, all parties benefit. The coach will have a better understanding of what the medical team can provide the team and will be more likely to seek help for minor problems that, when managed properly, will prevent subsequent major problems. Conversely, the clinician will benefit from an increased understanding of the demands of a specific sport and may have an opportunity to institute preventative measures, which will ultimately improve team performance and reduce health-care costs.

Although game officials enforce rules during competition, coaches are responsible for teaching game regulations and insisting that they be followed. Often, injuries result from blatant violations of rules that are designed to keep a sport safe. Coaches must discipline players who place teammates and opponents at risk for injury with intentional disregard for the rules of play and sportsmanship. A team should play to win, but always within the rules of the sport.

ATHLETE

The health and performance of the athlete are the main focus of the sports medicine team. Many people contribute to the athlete's optimal performance and provide specific treatment should the athlete become injured (Fig. 1-2). It behooves the athlete to be cognizant of the professional expertise provided by the sports medicine team and its support system.

Injury prevention strategies, such as appropriate warmups, stretching, and use of protective equipment, are necessary for the athlete to perform well. The athlete must know to report injuries early and to follow the instructions of the medical team. It is essential that players report any other treatments being received for their injuries. Athletes must play an active role in their own physical conditioning during the off-season, preseason, and in-season programs.

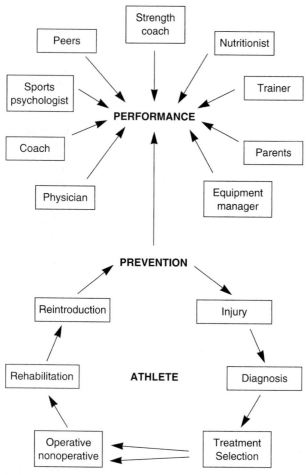

FIG 1-2   The health and performance of the athlete are the main focus of the sports medicine team.

Athletes should refrain from the ingestion of alcohol or drugs. One would hope that today's athlete is aware of the detrimental effects that narcotics, hallucinogenic drugs, anabolic steroids, and alcohol have on the body, but studies show that athletes abuse these substances at rates similar to the general population. Team members must inform the medical staff of any medication they plan to take. Seemingly benign over-the-counter medications can render a drug test positive or interfere with homeostasis during activity.

Athletes are also responsible for the proper care, fit, and maintenance of equipment. Examination of personal equipment should be routine before and after each practice and game, and concerns should be addressed by the athletic trainer.

The sports medicine team must earn and gain the confidence and respect of the athlete so that all health issues can be discussed openly and honestly without fear of condemnation or reprisal.

AVOIDING DANGEROUS PITFALLS

1. The team physician should be chosen based on training and qualifications to treat the majority of maladies that a particular team may encounter, *not* because he or she has an interest in sports or is a friend of the coach or manager.
2. The team physician is *not* just a privileged spectator, but an integral member of the sports medicine team who must be available and who should lead by example.
3. The team physician must *not* allow an athlete to compete in his or her chosen sport without having a complete history and medical examination.
4. Do *not* hesitate to obtain a second opinion in a case where the diagnosis is not clear.
5. Do *not* hesitate to elicit consultation from an appropriate member of the sports medicine team. Do *not* be pressured to provide care beyond your personal sense of expertise and skill.
6. The athlete's physical and emotional welfare always come first, *not* the outcome of the game. The team physician must *not* be a party to win-at-all cost mentality.
7. Do *not* wait for a catastrophic on-field event to take place to see if the appropriate emergency response plan works. Practice to ensure that it will work.
8. The use of radiographic imaging techniques is *not* to be neglected when diagnosing and treating sports-related injuries.
9. The competent team physician does *not* belittle the benefits rendered by teaching, continuing medical education, and sports-related research.
10. A physician should *not* agree to provide care for an athletic team without first carefully reviewing his or her professional liability insurance. As in all medical practice, it is essential to maintain accurate records.
11. Do *no* harm! Do everything within your professional capacity to identify, treat, and prevent injuries to members of your team.

REFERENCES

Arnheim DD. *Modern Principles of Athletic Training*. St. Louis: Times Mirror/Mosby; 1989.

Brukner P, Khan K. *Clinical Sports Medicine*. Roseville, New South Wales: McGraw-Hill; 1993.

Duff JF. *Youth Sports Injuries*. New York: Macmillan; 1992.

Mellion MB. *Sports Medicine Secrets*. Philadelphia: Hanley and Belfus; 1993.

Mellion MB, Walsh WM, Shelton GL. *The Team Physician's Handbook*. Philadelphia: Hanley and Belfus; 1990.

Snider RK. *Essentials of Musculoskeletal Care*. Rosemont, Ill: American Academy of Orthopaedic Surgeons; 1997.

SPORTS MEDICINE RESOURCES

American Academy of Family Physicians Sports Committee
8880 Ward Parkway
Kansas City, MO 64114
(816) 333-9700

The American Academy of Orthopaedic Surgeons Sports Medicine
Committee
6300 North River Road
Rosemont, IL 60018
(708) 823-7186

American Academy of Pediatric Sports Medicine
1729 Glastonberry Road
Potomac, MD 20854
(301) 424-7440

American College of Sports Medicine
P.O. Box 1440
Indianapolis, IN 46206-1440
(317) 637-9200

American Medical Society for Sports Medicine
11639 Earnshaw
Overland Park, KS 66210
(913) 327-1415

American Orthopedic Society for Sports Medicine
2250 East Devon Avenue
Suite 115
Des Plaines, IL 60018
(708) 803-8701

Canadian Academy of Sport Medicine
1600 James Naismith Drive
Gloucester, ON, Canada K1B 5N4
(613) 748-5851

Canadian Athletic Therapists Association
4825 Richard Road, S.W.
Calgary, AB, Canada T3E 6K6
(403) 240-7228

Disabled Sports USA
451 Hungerford Drive
Suite 110
Rockville, MD 20850
(301) 217-0960

National Athletic Trainers' Association
2952 Stemmons Freeway
Suite 200
Dallas, Texas 75247
(214) 637-6282

Sport Physical Therapy Section of the American Physical Therapy
Association
220 Grand View Drive
Suite 150
Fort Mitchell, KY 41017
(606) 341-6654

Sports Physiotherapy Canada
1600 James Naismith Drive
Gloucester, ON, Canada K1B 5N4
(613) 748-5794

| # Rehabilitation and Physical Therapy for the Injured Athlete

William O. Roberts and Debra W. Roberts

QUICK LOOK

Soft tissue and joint injury is common in sports, so developing an understanding of etiology, patient care, and physical therapy utilization is essential to the practice of sports medicine and care of active people.

- Describe the general consequences of soft tissue and joint injury
- Direct an immediate management plan for acute injury
- Coordinate an extended management plan for injury
- Develop a return to practice and competition protocol for athletes following injury
- Describe the science of physical therapy modalities and interventions

INTRODUCTION

Soft tissue injury is a common occurrence in sports activity from acute trauma and repetitive forces in a dose–response relationship to volume of activity. The more exposure that an athlete has to training and competition, the greater the risk of injury. The common types of soft tissue injury include sprains, strains, and contusions. The goals of soft tissue injury care are to restore normal function to the greatest possible degree in the shortest possible time, to minimize tissue damage following injury, and to minimize deconditioning of cardiovascular and musculoskeletal systems during recovery from injury.

The disability duration varies with the severity of initial injury and severity determines loss of time from activity. Time lost varies from a short-duration nuisance injury to several months. Disability from quadriceps contusions ranges from of 2–60 days based on injury severity determined by the ability to flex at the knee after injury (Ryan, 1991).

- Mild (knee flexion >90°), average 13 days lost
- Moderate (knee flexion 45–90°), average 19 days lost
- Severe (knee flexion <45°), average 21 days lost

Rehabilitation is essential for optimizing the return to activity after injury and should not be delayed until after the injury has healed. Normal forces can induce injury if the athlete is allowed to return to activity too early while inflammation, which reduces tensile strength in the affected tissue, persists. Optimally, an injury should be fully healed for full return, or at a minimum, healed enough to withstand normal sport forces in a protective or supportive brace. Injuries become recurrent and chronic from inadequate treatment of the original injury, and return to training and competition before full recovery has occurred (Agre, 1985). Using a functional brace until the injury is fully rehabilitated decreases the risk of re-injury.

Athletes need realistic healing times to plan for return to competition. Use a reasonable time range for return to activity that accounts for healing times for the various tissues. The complete healing time for ligament sprains and muscle strains is 10–12 weeks; muscle contusion is 1–10 weeks; and bone fracture is 6–8 weeks. There are longer healing times for some fractures, like navicular fractures, and shorter healing times in growing children and adolescents. An athlete with a soft tissue injury who is pain free and able to use a functional brace may sometimes return to practice and competition within days.

Cost-effective care is also an issue with athlete rehabilitation. The use of office protocols along with the prudent use of physical therapy services can help with cost reductions. In the care of low back pain, considering all patients, the cost of physical therapy is minor compared to the combined cost of narcotic and NSAID prescription medications. With physical therapy, too little too late is expensive, and too much too soon is expensive. The use of physical therapy for hot packing, ultrasound, and massage (HUM therapy) without utilizing the examination, manual therapy, and management skills of the physical therapist is inappropriate.

CYCLE OF TISSUE INJURY

Tissue overload, both from acute and chronic repetitive causes, can result in tissue injury and functional biomechanical deficits that include inflexibility, weakness, and muscle imbalance. If treatment focuses only on the voluntary muscle response, as with weight-training programs, the soft tissue continues to be at risk and the athlete may be unable to manage the high-speed and high-risk maneuvers encountered during competitive play. Proprioceptive abilities need to be challenged early in injury rehabilitation and the use of return progression will retrain muscle responses to activity.

INJURED SOFT TISSUE

Strain injury of the muscle-tendon-bone unit by overload injury or indirect trauma accounts for 30–50% of sports-related injury. The common mechanisms are macrotrauma and repetitive microtrauma. Macrotrauma is an excessive single-tensile force with soft tissue failure most commonly occurring at the muscle-tendon interface, although the failure can occur at the tendon bone interface, the mid muscle, or the mid tendon. Soft tissue injury occurs in the failure range on a stress-strain curve and follows Hooke's law for material strength, just as ropes and steel connectors do. The tissue failure or tear can occur at the microscopic or the macroscopic level. Repetitive microtrauma or overuse injury is the result of excessive repetitive-tensile forces in the plastic range on a stress-strain curve that causes tissue deformation. An inflammatory response may not occur. This tissue injury is a *tendonosis* or *tendinopathy*, rather than a true *tendinitis*. Healing a muscle-tendon-bone injury requires a balance between resting the injured tendon, stressing the tendon in the planes of functional motion, and preventing atrophy of the surrounding muscles.

Sprain or ligament injuries are also caused by overload injury or indirect trauma via macrotrauma and microtrauma mechanisms. Ligament healing with conservative therapy is uniformly effective in grade I and grade II sprains. Re-injury to the ligament is prevented with bracing and support that does not allow the joint to stress the ligament outside the normal range of motion. The treatment of grade III ligament injuries in high-level athletes is controversial and in some cases, may have better outcome with surgical repair, although the majority may be treated with conservative management.

Muscle can also be injured by direct muscle trauma from high-velocity compressive forces that result in contusion with tissue and blood vessel disruption, due to muscle tissue crush, and hematoma, due to localized hemorrhage into potential space. The general pathophysiology includes injury *shock*, which shuts down normal muscle function, muscle tissue disruption, localized bleeding into tissue, and an initial reparative inflammatory response.

The inflammatory response to injury starts with hemorrhage and infiltration of cellular elements that produce pain, effusion, and edema. Chemical mediators include vasoactive substances (histamines, anaphylatoxins, kinins, and prostaglandins) that increase vasodilatation and vascular permeability, chemotactic factors that increase cell motility to direct cell movement to the inflammatory focus, and degradive enzymes that catalyze hydrolysis of tissue components. The initial inflammation phases are reparative, but continued inflammation responses can be destructive. The goal of athlete injury rehabilitation is to curtail the late inflammatory responses to reduce pain, effusion, and immobility.

During soft tissue healing, collagen deposition combined with fibroblasts form the cellular fibrin matrix to bridge the repair. Connective tissue develops the structure most suited to resist and react to forces, and following Wolff's law; early tensile loading promotes collagen growth and proper alignment. Functional stresses (tensile loads) improve healing and outcome; no stress usually results in disorganized scar formation and less ligament strength.

ACUTE SOFT TISSUE INJURY CARE

The care of soft tissue injury can be divided into three phases labeled immediate, early, and late management. The initial care or immediate management uses the acronym PRICE, which stands for protect, relative rest, ice, compression, and elevation. Early management encompasses early mobilization, range of motion, protected function, stretching, strengthening, alternate activities for cardiovascular and uninjured area conditioning, and neuromuscular reeducation. The final, or late, phase of management is to develop a protocol for return to activity that includes return progressions, return to practice, and finally, return to competition.

GENERAL PRINCIPLES OF INJURY REHABILITATION

The key to effective injury rehabilitation is to establish an accurate diagnosis so that the correct therapy can be instituted early in the course of healing. In the early stages of healing, the effort should minimize local effects of acute injury. Immediate steps to limit tissue damage by minimizing bleeding, edema, and free radical damage set the stage for optimal healing times. Over the course of the injury, the plan should also minimize scarring of tissue, adhesions to adjacent tissue, and calcification of the soft tissues. The major complications of soft tissue injury are myositis ossificans traumatica and acute compartment syndromes.

With any injury, it is critical to allow time for proper healing through relative rest of the injured part to avoid stress and strain on the injury before the tissue strength is ready for the load. This can often be accomplished with functional bracing or supportive taping (Lohrer, 1999). Taping increases the proprioceptive amplification ratio and helps retrain the body to use the ability to locate a joint in space during activity. Fatigue decreases the ratio and increases injury risk. Full immobilization causes *cast disease*, with a 20% loss of muscle strength the first week and a 20% loss of remaining strength each additional week. Atrophy is particularly rapid if muscles are splinted in a shortened position.

Pain control after an injury is important for both comfort and healing. Protective splinting will put the injured part at rest, support it for pain relief, and may decrease the need for medications. Ice packing for tissue cooling provides acute pain relief and may be used early in an injury prior to stretching with supervision. Pain medications are used for comfort and to relieve spasm in the acutely injured area. Acute pain management with medications is safe and often underused. The management of acute pain differs from chronic pain. Pain medications should not be used as a means to return an athlete to play. Analgesic pain medications are either narcotic or non-narcotic, such as acetaminophen or non-steroidal anti-inflammatories. Local anesthetics, either topical or injected, can provide great relief from acute pain and allow earlier, supervised, range of motion. Transcutaneous electric nerve stimulation (TENS) is useful for both acute and chronic pain control and may allow the rehabilitation program to progress with less discomfort. Acupuncture, acupressure, and other such techniques may also relieve pain.

After a short rest period, early mobilization is important for the best outcome in soft tissue injury. When a splint is necessary, position the muscle at its greatest length. The athlete should begin passive range of motion as soon as the pain allows, advancing to active range of motion, and beginning isometric and isotonic contractions as soon as motion can be tolerated. Stretching can be passive, active, or active assisted. Proprioceptive neuromuscular facilitation stretching is a contract-relax sequence that is done with a partner and consists of a contraction against resistance, muscle relaxation, and then a stretch with the partner's assistance. How much to stretch is difficult to quantify. Pain-free tension on muscle produces no stretch, and post-exercise pain usually means too much stretch, so education of the injured athlete is very important.

Strengthening an injured part along with core strengthening will decrease the chance of re-injury after return to competition. Strength training of targeted muscles may be effective in the rehabilitation of many overuse injuries. The methods and types of strengthening used in rehabilitation of injury are the same as those used in strength training for athletes and include isometric, isotonic, and isokinetic techniques. Injury may require modification of weight-lifting techniques with functional progressions for multi-joint exercises. Adaptations for normal training may be used in the rehabilitation sequence, such as low-weight, high-repetition rather than high-weight, low-repetition sets. Strengthening after injury should emphasize closed kinetic chain activities with the limb in contact with a surface, rather than open chain activities, where the limb is not in contact with a surface. For example, the foot is in contact with the floor doing a partial squat for VMO strengthening, which requires use of the core muscles to stabilize the hip and trunk for maximum benefit. Water-based activities are ideal for rehabilitation (Prins, 1999) Water exercise promotes activity following injury and the early resumption of rehabilitation can expedite the recovery process while maintaining cardiovascular fitness. The physical properties of water provide resistance throughout the joint range of motion and the water's buoyancy can be used to decrease the stress on the injured joint. Neuromuscular and proprioceptive retraining is especially important because it focuses on the underlying neuromuscular imbalances and the movements that are at a subconscious or involuntary level.

Balance is a critical function in most sports activities and balance training will decrease the risk for re-injury after return to activity. Athletes can be tested on exercise balls or on unstable surfaces for lower extremity testing. The same activities can be used for balance training and proprioceptive retraining following ligament injuries.

Modalities can play an important role in injury rehabilitation. In the acute phase, ice (therapeutic cold) is the only modality proven to make a difference in outcome over time. Tissue cooling causes vasoconstriction, which diminishes capillary and arteriolar blood flow to decrease swelling, limit inflammation, and decrease pain and spasm. Ice is generally used for 48 hours or until the swelling is down. A bag of ice is applied to the injured part alternating 15–20 minutes on and 15–20 minutes off. In some cases, a damp cloth can be inserted between the ice bag and the skin for safety and comfort. Ice massage with an ice block placed directly on the skin and moved over the painful area for 5–10 minutes until the area is numb is equally effective. Precautions for icing include major nerves and poor circulation in the area of injury. Compression augments the tissue cooling effects of ice to limit swelling. Applying a splint to keep a muscle in tension can be used to provide compression. For example, use a hinged knee brace locked at 120° for 24 hours to keep a contused quadriceps muscle group at full length. Elevation decreases hydrostatic pressure, limits swelling, and decreases healing time. Interventions that are not recommended in acute phase contusion or hematoma injury care include aspiration, steroid injection, and local heat application (Young, 1993) Heat will increase swelling in acutely damaged tissue and slow the healing time.

In the post-acute phase (subacute and chronic), other modalities are useful for pain control and improved tissue flexibility. Heat, either deep or superficial, will increase blood flow, loosen tissue for stretching, and decrease pain. Ultrasound can enhance soft tissue extensibility, provide deep heat, and be used for local steroid phonophoresis. Treatment with pulsed ultrasound can promote the satellite cell proliferation phase of myoregeneration (Rantanen, 1999). Massage can break down tissue adhesions and promote removal of tissue waste products. Electrotherapeutic modalities can decrease pain, spasm, and swelling; and can also be used in the acute injury phase. These modalities include electrical stimulation, electrical stimulation for tissue repair, high-voltage pulsed current, transcutaneous electrical nerve stimulation (TENS), and neuromuscular electrical stimulation (NMES). NMES can be used for strengthening an innervated muscle after joint injury if the joint must be immobilized or if the athlete is having difficulty activating the muscle due to disuse or pain. Iontophoresis, using electric current for local steroid or anesthetic administration, to a depth of about 1 cm may be of some benefit in inflamed tissues. Range-of-motion exercises alone are ineffective in targeting many of the small movements of the bones surrounding the injury site. Manual therapy techniques, including joint mobilization, are used to restore normal joint play (mobility) and to relieve pain. This is an under used intervention.

ROLE OF PHYSICAL THERAPY

The practical application of physical therapy in athletes is to reduce swelling, relieve pain, mobilize soft tissue and joints to increase flexibility, and develop supervised or instructed strengthening and rehabilitative programs. Physical therapy is provided by licensed or registered physical therapists and can include manual therapy techniques, electrotherapeutic modalities, the fabrication and application of orthotics, protective and supportive splints and braces, protective taping and cushioning, perceptual training and balance, coordination and agility training risk reduction, and neuromuscular reeducation. In a comparison of active training (injured muscle group strengthening, postural retraining, trunk strengthening, and balance work) versus physical therapy (transverse friction massage, transcutaneous nerve stimulation, laser therapy, and stretching the injured muscle group) in athletes with groin pain, and those in the active group had better outcomes, with full return to previous levels of activity, after a 12-week program (Holmich, 1999). However, most physical therapists dealing with athletes use an active training philosophy that includes strengthening and rarely limit the therapy to the areas tested in this protocol.

In an observational study of physical therapy supervision in ankle sprains, unsupervised patients had reduced ankle strength and postural control at 6 weeks compared to the supervised group, but the variables normalized at 4 months independent of supervised rehabilitation (Holme, 1999). However, the findings demonstrated that supervised rehabilitation reduced the number of re-injuries and may play a role in injury prevention.

Evidence-based clinical practice guidelines were published in a 2001 issue of *Physical Therapy* with the therapeutic effectiveness of each intervention assigned letter ratings. Grade A was defined as having a clinical importance more than 15% and statistical *P*-value less than 0.05. Grade C was defined as clinical importance about 15% and *P* was not significant. Mobilization and manipulation were not included in the evaluation sets. In the care of low back pain (LBP), grade A interventions included continuing normal activities for acute LBP and therapeutic exercises for subacute and chronic LBP. Grade C interventions included therapeutic exercise, mechanical traction, ultrasound, and TENS. For patellofemoral knee pain, there were insufficient data to classify exercise and no data to grade massage, thermotherapy, TENS, electric stimulation, electromyographic biofeedback, or combined rehabilitation modalities. In the treatment of shoulder pain, grade A was assigned to therapeutic ultrasound for calcific tendinitis and grade C to therapeutic ultrasound for capsulitis, bursitis, and tendinitis. Looking at the scope of physical therapy interventions, outcome data for many of the commonly used interventions need to be documented. Outcomes from supervised exercise programs seem to produce the most favorable and long-lasting outcomes.

The American Physical Therapy Association developed the *Guide to Physical Therapist Practice* (2001) with the goals of improving the understanding physical therapy practice to enhance the quality of care, improve patient satisfaction, promote appropriate utilization, increase efficiency of practice, reduce unwarranted variation in services, and promote cost reduction through prevention and wellness initiatives. The philosophy and practical advice can be applied to the care of athletes.

Maintain Athletic Fitness After Injury

A quick and safe return to competition after an injury depends on sport readiness. An athlete must remain fit during the rehabilitation process to return to the field of play as soon as the injury healing is complete. Early participation within a safe range of skill-directed activities should help maintain strength and cardiovascular fitness. Sport-specific closed kinetic chain strengthening, balance, and proprioceptive activities can speed the return progression. Core strengthening programs utilizing closed kinetic chain exercises are an integral part of accelerated rehabilitation programs and increase the effectiveness of rehabilitation. The goal of the supervised and directed rehabilitation is to allow more normal physiologic activations and biomechanical motions that pertain to the sport. Closed kinetic chain activities induce facilitation patterns that allow muscles to be activated in normal sequences and isolated to recover normal strength.

Sport-specific strength training away from the injury site should emphasize stabilization exercises for hypermobile joints and postural correction. Proprioception has an important role in the afferent-efferent neuromuscular control arc that is critical for athletes in competition. The control arc is disrupted with joint and soft tissue injury and restoring proprioception allows the body to maintain stability and orientation during the static and dynamic activities so critical to safe athletic participation. Kinesthetic and neuromuscular retraining activities promote the return of kinesthetic sense, which is disrupted in ligament injury and necessary for balance and optimum athletic function. The Feldenkrais method uses manual and verbal directed movement patterns that retain the inherent motor patterns lost through injury or dysfunction. These programmed movements expand the neuromuscular capabilities and motor control of the whole body. They increase functional abilities, balance, and body awareness. It is also important to develop alternate activities for endurance and cardiovascular fitness that are as sport specific as possible to maintain the muscle anaerobic pathways and aerobic systems.

Return to Normal Athletic Function

The return to competition is a complex process that should begin as soon as the injured unit will tolerate movement to optimize motor relearning and aerobic fitness. The relearning process will vary in length of time dependent on the severity of the injury and the skill of the athlete. The return progressions start with basic skill activities related to the sport so that the neurophysiologic learning process is repeated to re-learn the neuromuscular patterns *(engrams)* necessary to safely participate in the sport of the injured athlete. An athlete needs normal strength to avoid substitution patterns while relearning the skills, as substitution patterns will develop abnormal engrams with increased risk of injury and decreased effectiveness on the field of play. The athlete can progress to higher skill level activities as both functional capacity and ability return. During the rehabilitation, it is important for an athlete to attend team meetings and chalk talks to remain connected to the team.

The return to practice should be initiated as soon as skills and function return to a level that non-contact team activities can be done safely. It may be possible to participate in safe training activities, like free throw practice shooting in basketball or similar skills in other sports, that allow the athlete to maintain engrams and remain part of the team long before conditioning drills and live contact activity is considered safe.

The final return to competition should be based on tissue healing. The athlete should be pain free with normal range of motion and normal strength (strength, power, and endurance) equal to uninjured counter-part, have full functional capacity with general body strength conditioning and cardiovascular fitness, and no joint instability. Protective equipment and padding must meet rule requirements to protect other players and the injury. And finally, the athlete and parents, if the athlete is a minor, should be given informed consent regarding the risks of future injury and disability based upon previously sustained injury before allowing the athlete to return to full competition.

SUMMARY

General injury evaluation and care for an injured athlete requires an accurate diagnosis. The care plan can be divided into immediate care (PRICE), early management to activate the athlete during healing, and return progressions that lead to full competition. For the safest and quickest return to competition, the rehabilitation plan should:

- Control the inflammatory process
- Control pain
- Restore joint range of motion and soft tissue extensibility
- Improve muscular strength
- Improve muscular endurance
- Develop specific, sport-related biomechanical skill patterns
- Maintain or improve general cardiovascular endurance
- Establish maintenance programs
- Promote safe return to activity

REFERENCES

Agre JA. Hamstring injuries. *Sports Med.* 2:21–33, 1985.

American Physical Therapy Association. *Guide to Physical Therapist Practice*. 2nd ed. Alexandria, Va: Author; 2001.

Aronen JG, Chronister RD. Quadriceps contusions: Hastening the return to play. *Phys Sportsmed.* 20: 130–136, 1992.

Bell GW. Aquatic sports massage therapy. *Clin Sports Med.* 18:427–435, ix, 1999.

Crossman J. Psychological rehabilitation from sports injuries. *Sports Med.* 23:333–339, 1997.

Danchik JJ, Yochum TR, Aspegren, DD. Myositis ossificans traumatica. *J Manip Physio Ther.* 16:605–614, 1993.

El Hawary R, Stanish WD, Curwin SL. Rehabilitation of tendon injuries in sport. *Sports Med.* 24:347–358, 1997.

Ellen MI, Young JL, Sarni JL. Musculoskeletal rehabilitation and sports medicine: Knee and lower extremity injuries. *Arch Phys Med Rehab.* 80(suppl 1):59–67, 1999.

Ellen MI, J Smith J. Musculoskeletal rehabilitation and sports medicine: Shoulder and upper extremity injuries. *Arch Phys Med Rehab.* 80(suppl 1):50–58, 1999.

Fees M, Decker T, Snyder-Mackler L, Axe MJ. Upper extremity weight-training modifications for the injured athlete. A clinical perspective. *Am J Sports Med.* 26:732–742, 1998.

Geraci MC. Rehabilitation of pelvis, hip, and thigh injuries in sports. *Phys Med Rehab Clin N Am.* 5:157–173, 1994.

Hergenroeder AC. Prevention of sports injuries. *Pediatrics.* 101:1057–1063, 1998.

Herring SA. Rehabilitation of muscle injuries. *Med Sci Sports Exerc.* 22:453–456, 1990.

Hoffman MD. Principles of musculoskeletal sports injury rehabilitation. *Wisc Med J.* 96:38–48, 1997.

Holme E, Magnusson SP, Becher K, Bieler T, Aagaard P, Kjaer M. The effect of supervised rehabilitation on strength, postural sway, position sense and re-injury risk after acute ankle ligament sprain. *Scand J Med Sci Sports.* 9:104–109, 1999.

Holmich P. Effectiveness of active physical training as treatment for longstanding adductor-related groin pain in athletes: Randomized trial. *Lancet.* 353:439–443, 1999.

Jobe FW, Pink M. The athlete's shoulder. *J Hand Ther.* 7:107–110, 1994.

Karlsson J, Swärd L, Kälebo P, Thomée R. Chronic groin injuries in athletes. *Sports Med.* 17:141–148, 1994.

Keeves RK, Laskowski ER, Smith J. Upper extremity weight-training modifications for the injured athlete: A clinical perspective [comment]. *Am J Sports Med.* 27:545–546, 1999.

Kenal KA, Knapp LD. Rehabilitation of injuries in competitive swimmers. *Sports Med.* 22:337–347, 1996.

Kibler WB. Diagnosis, treatment and rehabilitation principles in complete tendon ruptures in sports. *Scan J Med Sci Sports.* 7:119–129, 1997.

Kibler WB. Closed kinetic chain rehabilitation for sports injuries. *Phys Med Rehab Clinics N Am.* 11: 369–384, 2000.

Laskowski ER, Newcomer-Aney K, Smith J. Proprioception. *Phys Med Rehab Clinics N Am.* 11:323–340, 2000.

Laubach WJ, Brewer BW, Van Raalte JL, Petitpas AJ. Attributions for recovery and adherence to sport injury rehabilitation. *Aust J Sci Med Sport.* 28:30–34, 1996.

Locke S. Exercise-related chronic lower leg pain. *Aust Fam Phys.* 28:569–573, 1999.

Lohrer H, Alt W, Gollhofer A. Neuromuscular properties and functional aspects of taped ankles. *Am J Sports Med.* 27:69–75, 1999.

Martinek V, Friederich NF. To brace or not to brace? How effective are knee braces in rehabilitation? *Orthopade.* 28:565–570, 1999.

Nigg BM, Nurse MA, Stefanyshyn DJ. Shoe inserts and orthotics for sport and physical activities. *Med Sci Sports Exerc.* 31(suppl 7):421–428, 1999.

Petruska AJ. Upper extremity weight-training modifications for the injured athlete: A clinical perspective [comment]. *Am J Sports Med.* 27:391–393, 1999.

Philadelphia Panel Evidence-Based Clinical Practice Guidelines on Selected Rehabilitation Interventions for Low Back Pain. *Phys Ther.* 81:1641–1674, 2001.

Philadelphia Panel Evidence-Based Clinical Practice Guidelines on Selected Rehabilitation Interventions for Knee Pain. *Phys Ther* 81:1675–1700, 2001.

Philadelphia Panel Evidence-Based Clinical Practice Guidelines on Selected Rehabilitation Interventions for Neck Pain. *Phys Ther.* 81:1701–1717, 2001.

Philadelphia Panel Evidence-Based Clinical Practice Guidelines on Selected Rehabilitation Interventions for Shoulder Pain. *Phys Ther.* 81:1719–1730, 2001.

Philadelphia Panel Evidence-Based Clinical Practice Guidelines on Selected Rehabilitation Interventions: Overview and Methodology. *Phys Ther.* 81:1629–1640, 2001.

Press JM, O'Connor A. Cost containment in sports rehabilitation. *Phys Med Rehab Clin N Am.* 11:721–728, 2000.

Prins J, Cutner D. Aquatic therapy in the rehabilitation of athletic injuries. *Clin Sports Med.* 18:447–461, ix, 1999.

Rantanen J, Thorsson O, Wollmer P, Hurme T, Kalimo H. Effects of therapeutic ultrasound on the regeneration of skeletal myofibers after experimental muscle injury. *Am J Sports Med.* 27:54–59, 1999.

Renstrom P. Swedish research in sports traumatology. *Clin Orthop Rel Res.* 191:144–158, 1984.

Roberds I, DiGuiseppi C. Injury prevention. *Arch Dis Child.* 81:200–201, 1999.

Roi GS, Respizzi S, Dworzak F. Partial rupture of the pectoralis major muscle in athletes. *Int J Sports Med.* 11:85–87, 1990.

Ryan JB, Wheeler JH, Hopinson WH, Arciero RA, Kolakowski KR. Quadriceps contusions. *Am J Sports Med.* 19:299–304, 1991.

Saal JA. Rehabilitation of the injured athlete. In: DeLisa JA, ed. *Rehabilitation Medicine: Principles and Practice.* 2nd ed. Philadelphia: Lippincott; 1993;1113–1164.

Safran MR, Zachazewski JE, Benedetti RS, Bartolozzi AR, Mandelbaum R. Lateral ankle sprains: a comprehensive review part 2: Treatment and rehabilitation with an emphasis on the athlete. *Med Sci Sports Exerc.* 31(suppl 7):438–447, 1999.

Smyth M. After an injury. What next? *Aust Fam Physician.* 28:555–560, 1999.

Spring H, Pirlet A, Tritschler T, van de Velde R. Physiotherapy for the recreational athlete. *Therapeutische Umschau.* 58:509–514, 2001.

Thein JM, Brody LT. Aquatic-based rehabilitation and training for the elite athlete. *J Orthop Sports Phys Ther.* 27:32–41, 1998.

Tyrdal S, Pettersen OJ. The effect of strength training on 'handball goalie's elbow'—A prospective uncontrolled clinical trial. *Scand J Med Sci Sports.* 8:33–41, 1998.

Vanderthommen M, Crielaard JM. Muscle electric stimulation in sports medicine. *Revue Medicale de Liege.* 56:391–395, 2001.

Wilson RW, Gieck JH, Gansneder BM, Perrin DH, Saliba EN, McCue III FC. Reliability and responsiveness of disablement measures following acute ankle sprains among athletes. *J Orthop Sports Phys Ther.* 27:348–355, 1998.

Young JL, Laskowski ER, Rock, MG. Thigh injuries in athletes. *Mayo Clin Proc.* 68:1099–1106, 1993.

3

High Performance and the Treatment of the Elite Athlete

Mike Clarfield

> John Brown injured his leg badly in the game last night. He will be having an MRI tomorrow. The MRI can tell us if he can play the game next week.

A sports medicine physician is trained to treat athletes. Elite althletes are fine-tuned machines demanding the most from their bodies and the most from medical care providers. The most challenging aspect for a sports medicine physician treating elite athletes is the demands the athletes place on themselves and on the physician. The gratifying part is that their performance, which the physician helps to optimize, will be seen by thousands of people. Although the athlete derives most of the fame, medical people involved with elite athletes also receive notice by association. Treating the elite athlete can, therefore, be very stressful. On the other hand, it can be fun to participate in high-exposure events.

It takes years of experience to develop the expertise to understand the elite athlete's body and mental state and it is important to be in touch with both factors to treat them effectively. Athletes must have full confidence that the physician understands the nature of their injuries in relation to their sport or activity to trust in the prescribed treatment and health advice. When treating elite athletes, it is important to understand that their goals are paramount. Then, and only then, can you develop a relationship of mutual trust with an elite athlete.

Elite athletes, whether professional players, Olympic athletes, or prima ballerinas, place high physical and mental demands on themselves. Nonetheless, different athletes may have varied approaches to their bodies. It is important to understand the inherent differences in different sport activities to understand how to treat the injuries. The recovery and expectations may be quite different for athletes in various sports, and a physician must adjust treatment appropriately.

Elite athletes are the most demanding patients; to accept the challenge and reap the benefits of treating elite athletes, a physician must be prepared to develop relationships with these individuals without losing objectivity during evaluation and treatment. The physician must also step out of the spotlight to maintain confidentiality for the athletes and not try to act as a spokesperson for the press.

INJURIES OF THE ELITE ATHLETE

Elite athletes do sustain injuries, and they will depend on a physician to understand the injuries so that they can return to participation as soon and as safely as possible. The athlete will demand a return to the activity at the same, if not at a higher, preinjury level. When an athlete pushes to the limits, there is a fine line between high performance and the point at which the body breaks down and becomes injured. The goal of the sports medicine physician is to proactively prepare athletes to reduce and avoid injuries. When an athlete does get injured, it is important that the athlete be rehabilitated to the level where he or she can go back to the activity with the least risk of injury and maintain a high performance.

The injuries sustained by the elite athlete are no different than injuries sustained by any other person. It is simply that the competition demands and time pressure on elite athletes that makes treating these injuries different. With experience, the difference is more understandable.

It is important to attend some of the elite athlete's competitions or performances to better understand what the athlete does and the level of the competition. This allows the physician to treat the athlete with more confidence. Over time, the athlete will become more comfortable with the physician and will develop a relationship that will facilitate treatment. Gaining an elite athlete's respect through good medical care will facilitate the physician-patient relationship.

Perhaps the most challenging aspect in dealing with an elite athlete is dealing with acute injuries. Most athletic injuries occur during an event as opposed to practice. This is particularly true for acute traumatic injuries. Once an acute injury has occurred, the physician is called into action. The medical personnel at an event must be prepared for all emergencies. Not only must he or she be capable of treating an acute injury, but, he or she must do so while being watched by the thousands of spectators at the event and watching on television. The field treatment will almost always be captured on film. The medical personnel covering elite athlete events should practice and train for emergencies before they actually happen so that the on-field care will be efficient and smooth.

In any acute injury that is life-threatening, be it a head, cervical spine, or airway or organ injury, the ABCs of acute medical care are paramount. The athlete must be stabilized on the field before he or she is evacuated. If there is a risk of spinal injury the athlete must be properly back boarded before being taken off the playing area. Once off the field of play and in the privacy of a medical room, the medical care will be more efficient. The medical room must be equipped to deal with emergencies; again, practice of the emergency protocols ensures that these athletes get the best care available. Protocols must be in place to transport the athlete safely and efficiently to the hospital where more intensive medical care is available.

Sometimes luck is on your side. In a professional hockey game I was attending several years ago, one of our players suffered a ruptured spleen. Fortuitously, when we paged the general surgeon who happened to be in the stands attending the game. He was available to assist with the immediate care and helped save this player's life.

Fortunately, there are not many life-threatening injuries in athletics, but there are many acute injuries. Certain sports have a predisposition to particular injuries. The doctor must be aware of the common injuries in a given sport and the mechanics that cause injury. A classic lateral inversion sprain is very common in a sport such as basketball or volleyball. In sports, when an athlete wears a more rigid boot, such as in skating, hockey, or skiing, lateral inversion sprains are rare, but rotational syndesmodic injury is common. The physician must be aware of this to assess and treat the injury appropriately. Following an injury, the athlete, coach, and team management immediately want to know the prognosis and receive an estimate of return to play. This is, perhaps, the most stressful and challenging part of dealing with elite athletes. Athletes are often injured during competition and can be evaluated on site to determine an immediate or delayed return to play recommendation. The great satisfaction in treating athletes is assisting with the athlete's and team's safe performance. Obviously, the team physician wants the team or athlete to do well, but the team physician must be able to disassociate from the excitement and the pressure from the team to win at all costs. The physician–patient relationship must be maintained, and the physician must remain the athlete's advocate for safety by considering the athlete's short-term career and long-term life expectations. Athletes must be protected from returning to play with injuries that have long-term or life-threatening consequences. In a very short time, usually without the aid of any other investigations, the side line physician must decide if the athlete can safely continue to participate.

Even if the athlete does return, you must watch carefully to make sure that the athlete is performing up to the level of expectation. If he or she does not, then the physician may have to withdraw the athlete for re-evaluation and reconsider the initial decision. The player will rarely mention deficiencies if the urge to play is high.

Once the decision is made that the athlete cannot play, then a definitive diagnosis must be made and the appropriate treatment plan initiated. Often, further investigations, such as MRI, must be done to make the diagnosis definitive and classify the injury severity. With the elite athlete, these investigations must be obtained expediently to allow the athlete to deal appropriatly with the injury. These investigations should only be used as adjunct to your own clinical impression, although the media will sometimes think an MRI reveals the diagnosis and dictates the return to play. When dealing with elite athletes, the physician soon learns that these fine-tuned bodies respond to injuries in a somewhat different manner than other patients seen in the office.

Communication is of paramount importance in dealing with an elite athlete. Everyone must be kept abreast of the athlete's injury and progress, but the athlete's consent must be obtained to give this information to the coach or management. Again, physician–patient confidentiality must be maintained. The general time line concerning when the athlete can expect to return to certain levels of activity and eventually, play, should be presented to the coaching staff to allow planning for the return to competition. The athlete, physician, and therapist must all work together to help the athlete return as soon and as safely as possible.

By following the preceding guidelines and maintaining the patient–physician relationship, a physician will soon gain the patient's respect. As in any situation, it is tough to gain respect and very easy to lose it. Therefore, it is important to maintain professionalism at all times. Once the respect of the players and/or the management is lost, you will not be dealing with elite athletes much longer. The treatment of the elite athlete's injuries is not any different than the treatment of any other person. The difference lies in the intensity of the treatment.

Whereas a recreational athlete may receive therapy a few times a week for an injury, the elite athlete may receive therapy three times a day to treat the same injury. Not only that, the difference in recovery is quite incredible if the injury is treated immediately and thoroughly, as opposed to being left for even 24 to 48 hours. Many secondary problems are avoided with immediate treatment. Functional rehabilitation is the key to allowing the injury to heal and to maintaining "playing shape" to prevent further injury.

There are more mitigating factors concerning an elite athlete's return to play than there are with weekend or high-level recreational athletes. The return to play decision involves more people and more stress on the athlete when he or she returns. The ultimate decision of when the athlete returns to play is the athlete's. Medical personnel are there only to advise and provide guidance, although the athlete usually follows the medical personnel's guidelines.

There are two extremes of injured athletes; the athlete who wants to return to play too soon and the athlete who wants to delay return as long as possible. Elite athletes have many advisors, some good and some bad, who will influence the athlete's decision. Most athletes have a lot of pride and want to return as soon as they can. They want to prove to themselves they can go back to their own form. They want to show support to their team. An athlete does not feel comfortable watching his or her team or opponents compete from the sidelines. Nonetheless, there are other factors that may effect the decision. One of the most important factors is the athlete's contract. The athlete may have to return to play as soon as possible to prove that he or she can play to renegotiate a new contract. On the other hand, if a contract dispute with management exists, then the athlete may want to delay return, as he or she may not feel that the team is supportive. An athlete may have bonus clauses in the contract that can have financial implications that cannot be attained without playing. Often, an athlete has a lot of fear going back to play, which can amplify with time away from playing. There is a fear the injury may inhibit the ability to play. The athlete may feel that he or she has lost some of the skills or speed needed to participate at the previous level. The athlete may have been performing poorly before the injury, which will only escalate this fear. An injured athlete should focus on recovery, mentally as well as physically. It is important for the physician to be aware of all these other factors and try to deal with them appropriately. There may be additional social factors that the physician may not be aware of, such as marital problems. The physician must keep all channels of communication open and explore all possibilities to give the athlete every opportunity to express feelings and cope with the decision of returning to play. In most cases, this happens very smoothly, and the athlete returns within the appropriate time lines.

Elite athletes depend on their bodies to perform as a financial means to an end. It is for this reason that many athletes request a second opinion. If the athlete is concerned or the injury is complicated, it may be prudent to encourage a second opinion. Facilitate the second opinion by sending along all clinical notes and investigations that have been done. The second opinion will help the athlete deal with the injury, knowing that more than one physician has been consulted. This will often appease other people involved in the athlete's decision. Sometimes a second opinion is necessary, as there may be a limited number of physicians who have dealt with a unique or specific injury. There are a limited number of physicians who see the volume of certain injuries to develop the skills to assess and treat at an optimum level. Elite athletes have unique injuries and want to see a physician who has the most experience dealing with the injuries. As a physician who treats elite athletes, it is important to ignore your ego and allow the athlete to seek a second opinion. This in fact may make your job somewhat easier, as it takes some of the pressure off of the physician. In the rare case where there is a discrepancy or the injury is very unusual, a third opinion may even be required.

MEDICAL LEGAL ISSUES

Medical legal issues must always be a concern when treating elite athletes. Because athletes may have contracts worth millions of dollars, there may be legal consequences if an athlete is or felt to be mistreated. It is now virtually impossible to obtain enough insurance to cover some of the multimillion dollar lawsuits that have come forward. Most teams will not cover a physician for malpractice. The legislation varies from country to country and from state/province to state/province. Therefore, it is important that you know the situation in the locale where you are practicing.

Although lawsuits involving elite athletes are not common, it is important to treat within the standards of care that applies to all patients. The athlete cannot be placed at risk with an early or untreated return to sport. Eventually, it is the athlete's decision to return; therefore all the risks must be explained. Proper communication between the athlete and the physician will ensure that everyone understands the problem fully.

At an event, it is more of a challenge to maintain proper clinical notes and document the care rendered. Nonetheless, it is of paramount importance to maintain clinical notes to ensure that all care is documented clearly and legibly. If an athlete decides to return to play against your advice and consent, it should be well documented and if possible a release should be signed.

Up until 2003, Canadian physicians were fully covered under the Canadian Medical Protective Association (CMPA). Since then the CMPA will not cover physicians treating professional athletes. Thus, physicians in Canada now require supplemental insurance when treating professional athletes. It is crucial to communicate with the CMPA to determine what they will in fact cover or not cover you for.

It is important to check if your insurance covers you in different jurisdictions. Your policy may stipulate that they will only cover lawsuits that have jurisdiction in the particular state/province or country that you live in. This is important when some of the athletes come from countries different from those which they are playing in. It may also be a factor when you travel with athletes to other sites/provinces or countries where you normally practice. Not only may you not be licensed in that locale, but your insurance may not cover you there either. It at all possible a release signed by your athlete to only bring a lawsuit against you in a certain jurisdiction may help to eliminate this issue. By the same token, physicians must be extra careful when treating foreign athletes not known to them.

Any lawsuit against a physician by a professional athlete will attract media attention and the details will be carefully scrutinized by the public. While any lawsuit against a physician is not great, a lawsuit with a lot of media attention is obviously a lot worse. This can expose the physician to an extensive financial and personal burden.

MEDIA

Sports journalists make their career writing about elite athletes and events. Therefore, anything that happens to an elite athlete will be portrayed in the media. Because injuries or medical problems greatly affect the athlete's career, the media want to know exactly what is going on with the athlete. The media will often approach the physician to find out the exact nature of the medical problem and the implications for the athlete.

As stated previously, the most important thing is to maintain physician–patient confidentiality. If you are going to talk to the media, it is important that the athlete knows exactly what will be said and that the athlete has given permission to do so. Athletes are like any other patient; a physician cannot freely disclose medical problems. If, for some reason, the athlete does not want the injury disclosed, the physician must respect his or her wishes. For a physician involved in team sports, it is important to communicate with the management and follow the team protocol for releasing information to the media. Often the information does not go through the medical personnel but through a press release from the front office. If a release of medical information is going through the front office, it is important that the physician review the press release so that there is no confusion about the diagnosis or misrepresentation of medical opinion.

It is important to learn how to deal with the media. The media are by nature always looking for an angle or controversy, and medical issues are no exception. Although media personnel can be good friends, they can also work against the team physician. If there is a message the physician wants to send through the media, he or she must learn to allow the media to receive the appropriate information. The media can then be used to an advantage to deliver a message to the public.

DRUGS

Prescription medications are frequently used to treat illnesses and injuries sustained by the elite athlete. Special care must be given so that the drugs prescribed will not adversely affect the athlete's performance. Side effects of the medication must be weighed against the potential benefits of the medication. It is important to document all medications given to the athlete, as with any patient. Medications must be explained to the individual athlete so that he or she understands what is being taken. If you are going to give an athlete an injection, such as cortisone, the procedure and the implications must be fully explained.

When treating athletes competing at an international level, the physician may have to consult an approved medication list to ensure that the athlete is not taking a banned substance. This includes over-the-counter medications. Medical personnel treating athletes should have a list of banned substances readily available or check the anti-doping web site for the most current listings. Although athletes are generally aware of the need to check medications, it is prudent to be proactive and advise an athlete to check the medications with the sport governing body.

Athletes at the elite level may take performance-enhancing drugs. To an athlete competing in international events, such as the Olympics, these are banned substances. Most professional sports either do not test at all or do random testing for performance-enhancing drugs, such as anabolic steroids. It is important that medical personnel train elite athletes to be aware of what drugs the athletes may be ingesting and their implications. The physician must be aware of possible side effects of the medications and be available to counsel these athletes about the pros and cons of taking performance-enhancing drugs. An elite athlete may approach a physician to help him or her monitor the use of performance-enhancing substances. This places the physician in a significant ethical dilemma. On the one hand, the physician would seem to condone these actions by monitoring banned substances. On the other hand, if the physician knows the situation, the athlete may well take the substances anyway and not respect or have confidence in the physician to come to him or her if the athlete develops complications. This is one of the toughest ethical dilemmas the physician has in dealing with elite athletes.

Elite athletes have also been known to take mind-altering recreational drugs. This may include alcohol as well as any other drug available on the black market. Medical personnel should keep their eyes open for evidence of a problem with any of these drugs. The physician must be to deal with drug use on a professional and nonconfrontational level to help the athlete. Many professional sports now have set protocols to help an athlete with a substance abuse problem.

If an athlete has a problem with substance abuse, it may affect the ability to perform at the elite level and may be life-threatening. If the physician suspects that there is a problem, he or she must confront the problem and deal with it in the best interests of that individual.

PERSONAL PROBLEMS

Elite athletes are human and some athletes have the same problems of substance abuse, promiscuity, and infidelity that exist in society. Certainly, athletes today are much more educated about all of these issues. Nonetheless, the team physician may be called on to deal with such issues. The physician must deal with these problems discreetly and without judgment. Medical personnel dealing with elite athletes will hear and see more than is known by the general public. Maintaining confidentiality is crucial.

Athletes' personal problems may affect performance as well as how they respond to an injury. Medical personnel must be aware of this and deal with it appropriately. On the other hand, the physician or medical personnel may not even be aware of personal problems that may be affecting the athlete's recovery. Often, it is months later that you gain clarity. At times, medical personnel must be part physician and part psychologist.

IMPORTANCE OF THE TEAM PHYSICIAN

The physician treating elite athletes has a very important part in the athlete's success. Athletes rely on their physician and medical personnel to keep them healthy and performing at the highest level. They trust the medical personnel to do the utmost for them. They demand the most from themselves and thus demand the most from those working with them. Treating the elite athlete requires a great deal of time, patience, and commitment. Although your role is crucial to the athlete, it is important to maintain professionalism. It is important not to take too much credit when they perform badly and not to take too much credit when they perform well. The athletes are truly the great stars, especially judged by their financial rewards. To maintain their respect and confidence in you as a trained medical person, it is vital to maintain professionalism. If you can do this, the satisfaction of treating elite athletes makes all that time and dedication worthwhile. The longer you treat these athletes, the more you learn to respect and understand what drives them to perform at such a high level.

4 | Drugs and Ergogenic Aids in Sport

Andrew Pipe

RESPONSIBILITIES OF THE SPORT MEDICINE PRACTITIONER

The deaths, in the 1960s, of the European cyclists Knut Jenssen and Tommy Simpson stunned the sport world and catalyzed the development of modern approaches to doping control. Sadly, the problems posed by doping grow more complex and represent a significant challenge for sport organizations, sport medicine practitioners, and governments. All sports medicine professionals should be aware of the problems posed by drug use in sport. Fundamental concerns about the well-being of the athletes entrusted to our care and a consideration of the side effects of many drugs abused in sport have led to regulations against their use. The degree to which the integrity of sport is eroded by the perception that athletic achievements are now the product of biochemistry or pharmacology rather than the result of talent, dedication, and training is also cause for concern. The discipline of sport medicine is itself tarnished by the perception that sport medicine professionals are practitioners of a murky, sinister science in which victory is pursued at all costs and by all means. The provision or prescription of banned drugs is antithetical to the practice of good medicine, a violation of professional ethics, and subverts the principals upon which sporting competition is based.

For more than three decades, sports medicine organizations and sport authorities have sought to address the problems posed by doping through the development of rules and regulations concerning the appropriate and inappropriate uses of drugs and other substances in sport. At times, such rules have proven frustrating for those with responsibilities for the care of athletes with specific medical conditions. On other occasions, the rules seem to have been applied or interpreted with a remarkable degree of inconsistency. Sport organizations have, in the past, differed markedly in the way in which anti-doping rules were developed, applied, and interpreted.

The World Antidoping Agency (WADA) was established in 2000 and as a consequence it is hoped that a new international consensus will develop around a universally accepted anti-doping code. Sport leaders, governments, and anti-doping organizations met in Copenhagen in 2003 to adopt a World Antidoping Code (Code). The Code will provide for standardized approaches to the development and application of anti-doping programs and ensure consistency in all of their elements. The Code provides for uniform procedures, testing methodologies, results management, and sanctions. Responsibility for the preparation and distribution of the "List of Prohibited Substances," previously the responsibility of the IOC Medical Commission, now rests with WADA, who now assumes responsibility for the preparation, review, and circulation of the banned list (List), that will be developed in accordance with a set of principles enshrined as a standard of the World Code. (Similar standards will govern many other elements of doping control practice.) An annual, and systematic, review of the list will be undertaken by WADA with specific opportunity for consultation and comment. It is important that sport medicine professionals, with their special expertise and perspectives, take the opportunity to participate in such consultations, and that they remain fully aware of any changes that may occur in the list as a result of these processes. The WADA Code provides for the granting of *Therapeutic Use Exemptions* (TUEs) in cases where there are clear and appropriately documented indications for the use of an otherwise banned medication.

All sports medicine practitioners will support anti-doping rules that are cogent, fair, grounded in science, and that have been developed in accordance with an understanding of sport and the special circumstances of athletes. To the extent that anti-doping regulations, or their application, do not meet these criteria, sport medicine professionals must advocate their change.

A familiarity with the relevant rules regarding doping is essential for any sport medicine practitioner. Athletes assume that health professionals working in sport are familiar with the rules and that they will not provide medications or other compounds that might cause them to run afoul of the regulations. It may be argued that athletes must ultimately be responsible for all that they consume (including medications and supplements). It can equally be argued that those who profess special expertise in the care of the athletic patient have an equal responsibility to ensure that such patients do not receive care that would result in violations of anti-doping regulations. This latter argument is all the more compelling when dealing with young athletes or in considering the relative degree of sophistication that might be necessary for an athlete to distinguish between banned or permitted medications. All practitioners should become familiar with the WADA Code, List, and the processes for applying, when appropriate, for TUEs.

As doping methodologies become more sophisticated, it becomes clearer that many could not occur without the active involvement or connivance of misguided physicians or scientists. Undoubtedly, the anti-doping strategies of the future will focus largely on identifying such individuals and removing them from sport.

THE LIST OF PROHIBITED SUBSTANCES AND METHODS

It would be impossible in these pages to attempt a comprehensive discussion of the banned list and its implications for the sport medicine professional. What follows is an attempt to review the general categories and provide specific, practical advice for the practitioner.

Stimulants

Notwithstanding the problems posed by the ingestion of medicinal mushrooms, herbal preparations, and the various tonics that were reported in association with the early Olympic games, the contemporary concern with doping in sport began earlier in the 20th century when it became clear that amphetamines were being used in cycling races. The sudden deaths during competition of riders who had taken amphetamines spurred the development of rules against such use and were instrumental in the development of the IOC Medical Commission. An understandable concern for the protection of athletes' safety and health was coupled with a desire to ensure that competitors not be cheated by those whose performance was artificially accentuated. Sadly, the perverted ingenuity of some competitors and their handlers, then as now, seemed to know no bounds and it soon became clear that it was necessary to forbid the use of a variety of stimulating compounds. The list has grown significantly. Included within this list have been widespread compounds as caffeine and the sympathomimetics. The latter products are found all over the world in an almost endless list of over-the-counter cough, cold, sinus, and allergy medications and pose special problems for athletes and their medical advisors. Great care must be taken to ensure that athletes do not inadvertently consume such compounds at a time when competition is imminent. Cases of *inadvertent doping* occur frequently and can cause considerable pain for athletes and their physicians. Perhaps more importantly, the degree to which athletes are sanctioned in such circumstances erodes the confidence of athletes in anti-doping measurers and undermines support for programs that seek to bring doping to a minimum. The situation is made somewhat easier by the use of urinary thresholds which, it has been argued, permit some degree of distinction between the inadvertent medicinal use of such products and deliberate attempts to dope. Nevertheless, there is a body of evidence that suggests that most sympathomimetics are incapable of enhancing performance.

The exception is *ephedrine*, which when combined with caffeine has demonstrated an ability to increase endurance performance. In the meantime, vigilance is required of practitioners and athletes alike. Physicians should know that the use of nasal decongestants containing *xylometazoline* is permitted. These agents are commonly available in North America. When in any doubt about the status of any product or medication it is important that practitioners verify the same by contacting an appropriate authority. (In Canada, contact the Canadian Centre for Ethics in Sport: 1-800-672-7775; web site: www.cces.ca. In the United States, contact the United States Anti-Doping Agency: 1-800-233-0393; web site: www.usantidoping.org.)

Caffeine has also been a controlled stimulant. A threshold was established for the detection of this compound and a urinary concentration of less than 12 μg/mL will not be reported as a positive. Athletes and physicians should be advised, however, that it is possible, given individual circumstances and patterns of caffeine use, for athletes to approach this level in the course of the ingestion of caffeine-containing beverages and foods.

A sad reality of modern sport has been the degree to which certain patterns of drug use have become more common within certain sport subcultures. A number of deaths have, for instance, been associated with cocaine use in basketball and result, in part, from cocaine's capacity to produce marked coronary vasoconstriction. Its use is banned in sport. Such phenomena underscore the sport physician's responsibility to provide clear, nonjudgmental advice to athletes about the use of recreational drugs and other health-related behaviors in addition to the obvious need to address the issue of the ethics and safety of the use of performance-enhancing products.

The beta-agonist medications *salbutamol, salmeterol, formoterol,* and *terbutaline* now so commonly used in the treatment of asthma and the prevention of exercise-induced bronchospasm have been considered stimulants for anti-doping purposes.

Narcotics

Narcotics have been banned in sport in order that such products are not used to eliminate the pain and discomfort associated with injury or overexertion. In this way, an athlete's health might be safeguarded. Commonly used and more benign narcotics such as the analgesic *codeine* and the cough suppressant *dextromethorphan* are permitted.

Anabolic Agents

A product of the German chemical industry, anabolic steroids were first developed in the hope that they might have military application. In the late 1950s their use became apparent in the athletic community and by the 1960s they had been introduced to North America. Sharing the basic structure of the fundamental male hormone testosterone, all synthetic anabolic agents possess both anabolic and androgenic capabilities. Modifications of anabolic products influence the anabolicity and androgenicity of a particular compound and determine whether it can be ingested orally. Although the use of these compounds exploded in the athletic community in the 1970s and 1980s, scientists and sport medicine practitioners were reluctant to attest to their effectiveness because of the lack of evidence for such in the scientific literature. That evidence was not available largely because ethical considerations precluded the administration of the large quantities of a variety of anabolic agents typical of the doses used by many athletic users. Clear evidence about the effectiveness of anabolic steroids in improving performance did not become available until 1996 when Bhasin and colleagues demonstrated an increase in muscle size and strength following the administration of anabolic steroids (Bhasin et al., 1996).

All anabolic agents are also androgenic, given that they are all essentially modifications of the male sex hormone testosterone. Consequently, the administration of exogenous anabolics can lead to the development of masculine features in the female and an accentuation of the normal effects of anabolic activity in the male. (Table 4-1). It is important to understand that there is as yet no body of information reflecting long-term experience with those known to have administered large quantities of anabolic-androgenic agents. It may take decades before the consequences of such self-administration become clear. The tragic revelations of widespread, systematic use of anabolic steroids throughout the sport system of the former German Democratic Republic (East Germany) and recently the Soviet Union represent the first glimpses of the implications of the sustained use of these products in athletes (Franke and Bererdork, 1997). It is known that the use of anabolics may cause problems in a variety of organ systems of certain

TABLE 4-1 Side Effects of Anabolic Steroids
Premature closure of the epiphyses in adolescents
Distortion of lipid profiles
Disruption of liver enzyme activity
Cholestasis
Jaundice
Peliosis hepatitis
Gynecomastia
Acne
Virilization of females:
   Male-pattern baldness
   Deepening of the voice
   Development of facial hair
   Clitoral hypertrophy
Accentuation of secondary sexual characteristics in males
Testicular atrophy
Reduction in sperm count
Changes in mood states

unfortunate users. Such problems may involve the cardiovascular, hepatic, hematologic, endocrine, and reproductive systems (Bagatelli and Bremner, 1996). Case reports are appearing with increasing frequency describing the more lurid complications associated with steroid use in sport (Menkis et al., 1991; Yoshida et al., 1994). It is probably correct to assume that such complications are underreported.

The sports clinician may at times be approached by athletes, or their coaches, with a request that anabolic use be monitored in order that the athlete's health might be safeguarded. Physicians contemplating such a strategy should remind themselves that to participate in such practices is to become ensnared in doping activity (Pipe, 1993). Such conduct, in the first instance, is not in keeping with the ethical practice of sport medicine; second, it exposes the physician to a range of problems, vulnerabilities, and legal liabilities that should be self-evident.

The extent to which anabolic use is common in sport is not clear. No reliable data exist. Sadly there is evidence that the use of anabolics has spread to nonathletic youth who administer such drugs in attempts to develop a certain muscular appearance (Melia and Pipe, 1996).

In many nations year-round, out-of-competition testing of athletes, seen as the only appropriate way to deter and detect anabolic use, has been implemented (Bahr and Tjorhmon, 1998). Sport physicians must be familiar with the procedures and protocols in use in the environments in which they practice.

Diuretics

Diuretics are banned in sport because they have been used to accelerate the excretion of other banned drugs or to facilitate weight loss in sports in which competition is arranged by weight categories (e.g., rowing, wrestling, judo, and other combative sports). Most health professionals will understand the electrolyte disturbances that can accompany the use of diuretics; such hazards may be accentuated when other bizarre strategies are applied in attempts to lose weight. Despite such knowledge, the use of diuretics (and laxatives) has been commonplace in wrestling in North America. A number of deaths of collegiate wrestlers in late 1997 may serve to focus more attention on the practice of *making weight* and the associated abuse of diuretics and other drugs. There is, in the author's view, a profound responsibility for sport medicine professionals to speak out about such practices and to ensure that athletes for whom they have responsibility are not involved in such practices.

Peptide Hormones, Mimetics, and Analogs

In this category are included a variety of hormones that have been used in attempts to produce anabolic effects. They include human chorionic gonadotrophin, corticotrophin, human growth hormone (HGH), and the respective releasing factors for such products. Such compounds are not commonly used in the treatment of athletes and their provision in the absence of a documented clinical indication for their use betrays a sinister intent on the part of a physician and/or athlete. HGH is now available as a genetically engineered product and it is speculated that many physicians are under considerable pressure to provide this product to ensure optimal height; others abuse this compound in an attempt to derive an anabolic benefit (Dean, 2002).

Erythropoietin (EPO), the hormone that stimulates the production of red blood cells, is also now relatively widely available as a product of genetic engineering. Among the unscrupulous, its use has superseded the practice of *blood doping* (see below), a tactic in which the red blood cell mass is artificially increased to accentuate the blood's oxygen-carrying capacity and as a consequence, aerobic performance (Ekblom and Berglund, 1991).

There are growing concerns that an associated increase in blood viscosity may induce a hypercoagulable state or otherwise potentiate the risk of cardiovascular or cerebrovascular collapse in those using EPO. A number of deaths are alleged to have occurred in cycling attributable to EPO use (Ramator, 1990). Officials in all sports in which aerobic capacity is fundamental to success are understandably concerned about the use of this product. There are evolving means to detect its use with urine or blood tests. In some sports (notably cycling, track and field, and cross-country skiing) blood tests are being applied in an attempt to identify athletes with levels of hemoglobin or a hematocrit greater than an arbitrarily developed threshold and to detect the presence of EPO or its analogs in the blood. Athletes with hematocrits that are above threshold are then denied permission to compete on the basis of a concern for their health and the blood is then tested for the markers of EPO use. This approach is not without shortcomings and will undoubtedly spawn controversy in the future. It has been widely speculated, and it is now becoming clearer, that many athletes and their handlers are measuring their own hemoglobin levels in the hours before a race and making adjustments, via the use of IV fluids, to ensure that they pass the screening tests. Widespread, frequent, and out-of-competition blood testing to permit the development of an athlete's hematologic profile would seem to be the only approach likely to be effective in the long term to address this burgeoning problem. It is not an exaggeration to say that the use of rEPO and similar products is already jeopardizing the credibility and therefore the long-term viability of many endurance sports.

PROHIBITED METHODS

Enhancement of Oxygen Transfer

It was noted several years ago that the reinfusion, after a certain period of time, of previously withdrawn red blood cells would increase the red cell mass, thereby increasing aerobic performance. This led to the practice of *blood doping* athletes in a variety of sports. These approaches often involved physicians and exercise scientists who cast their ethical and clinical responsibilities to the wind. In 1984, members of the US cycling team at the Los Angeles Olympics practiced blood doping using unmatched blood under the supervision of a physician and with the encouragement of a prominent exercise physiologist! Predictably some athletes became ill and required hospitalization; others won gold medals. Following the discovery of this incident, the IOC developed rules specifically prohibiting this practice, which has been superceded to a great extent by the use of EPO products.

Agents with Anti-Estrogenic Activity

Because the use of anabolic-androgenic steroids can result, paradoxically, in increased levels of circulating estrogens, many male athletes have used drugs that reduce estrogen levels to prevent the development of estrogen effects (principally gynecomastia). As a consequence, such drugs are banned in male athletes. There is, however, disquieting evidence that female athletes may be using such products to reduce levels of circulating estrogen and thereby permit their natural androgens to exert greater effect (Seehusen and Glorioso, 2002).

Pharmacologic, Chemical, and Physical Manipulation

Attempts to manipulate physiology or tamper with urine samples to reduce the likelihood of the detection of doping practices are banned by the WADA Code. By way of example, the use of probenecid to reduce the excretion of anabolics, or the substitution of clean urine via catheterization or other techniques are specifically prohibited.

Gene Doping

The advent of gene transfer technologies poses a number of potential scientific and ethical quandaries for sport physicians. Will the introduction of genes that enhance bone healing and strength be considered performance enhancement? Would the introduction of genes that can dramatically increase the strength or type of muscle tissue be considered in the same way? Given that these new therapies are almost upon us, sport authorities have already introduced regulations that would ban their use unless there was a distinct therapeutic indication.

CLASSES OF PROHIBITED SUBSTANCES IN CERTAIN SPORTS

The rules of certain international federations ban the use of specific substances. Thus *alcohol* is banned in several target sports; the *cannabinoids* may be banned by federations and are prohibited during an Olympic Games; *local anesthetics* are permitted; the systemic use of *glucocorticosteroids* is forbidden, but local and other forms of use are permitted; and *beta-blockers* are prohibited in some sports. It is important for sport medicine professionals to be familiar with the list of restricted substances and the various notification requirements. Failure to adhere to these rules could, unfortunately, lead to problems for athletes and their medical advisers. Confusion surrounds this category; many practitioners are unaware of the notification requirements just as they have been ignorant of their ability to obtain TUEs for athletes who require otherwise banned medications.

Implications for the Health Professional

All health professionals involved in sport have a responsibility to be familiar with the rules relating to doping. More importantly, they have a responsibility to ensure that their own practices reflect a commitment to drug-free sport. In this respect, there is a need to ensure that athletes, their coaches, and other members of the sporting entourage understand their roles in addressing this unfortunate issue. All need clear, reliable information and sport scientists and physicians are its logical source. It is most likely that the list of banned substances will undergo changes in the years ahead; the necessity for vigilance in this area is obvious. Special care must be taken to ensure that athletes and others understand the problems that can develop in association with the use of supplements, nostrums, herbal preparations, and nutritional supplements. Physicians have particular obligations to ensure that in treating or advising athletes they do not produce a situation in which athletes run afoul of anti-doping regulations. Finally, all should serve as advocates not only for drug-free sport, but also for the development of appropriate, realistic, and relevant regulations and their intelligent administration.

ERGOGENIC AIDS

Athletes and their advisors have for centuries sought access to foods or compounds that might dramatically accentuate their athletic performance (Mottram, 1988). Hundreds of such products have been used in the past and a preoccupation with the pursuit of a nutritional holy grail continues apace! Surprisingly, in this supposedly sophisticated and scientific age, athletes and their coaches frequently fall prey to the exhortations of those whose accomplishments are in marketing rather than in maximizing performance. The list of products that have been touted as capable of enhancing athletic performance seems endless and cannot possibly be dealt with here. More than a decade ago, the retail sales of dietary supplements in the United States generated $3.3 billion in sales (Cowart, 1992). In 1999, it was estimated that the annual sales of supplement products in the United States totaled $12 billion (*Consumer Reports*, 1999).

Not only single preparations are suggested as the route to increased sporting success. Each year it seems that another diet guru appears on the scene whose approach (and heavily marketed book and/or products) makes extravagant promises of new levels of energy, endurance, and accomplishment. Sadly, among many athletes and their coaches, nutrition has become a religious movement rather than a scientific discipline. Ironically, in the pursuit of the ergogenic panacea, many proven, well-documented approaches to performance enhancement are often ignored. The value of a well-balanced diet, designed with the particular needs of an athlete's specific sport, is the foundation of any successful athletic performance yet often derided by those who seek more exotic approaches to nutrition. There is abundant evidence that in the presence of such a diet protein requirements are easily met; the specific needs of female athletes may merit the use of supplementary iron. For many female athletes a simple reduction of training load and an increase in caloric intake may enhance performance and accentuate health. Simple attention to adequate rest, the provision of appropriate hydration, and the ongoing replacement of energy stores can be profoundly ergogenic for all athletes. The training cultures of many sports have come to emphasize prodigious training loads that may often be counterproductive in terms of health, performance, and nutritional status. Success, it has been said, consists of doing ordinary things extraordinarily well. Nevertheless, there are certain techniques or approaches that are capable of enhancing performance. What follows is a brief discussion of the most significant of these.

Mental Preparation

The recognition that psychological factors can significantly constrain or increase performance has led to the development of *sport psychology* (Weinberg, 1995). Mental skills including visualization, other forms of mental rehearsal, self-arousal techniques, focusing, and disassociation strategies have all become part of the repertoire of many successful athletes and might be described as *psychoergogenics*. They are beyond the scope of this discussion, but are an important element in the scientific preparation of the modern athlete.

Nutritional Strategies

As noted, the provision of an appropriately designed diet is central to the optimization of performance. The provision of a diet high in complex carbohydrates in the period before endurance events lasting more than 1 hour is now commonplace; it serves to ensure an optimal supply of muscle glycogen and is commonly known as *carbohydrate loading*. Evidence continues to accumulate of the value of replacing small amounts of carbohydrate during the course of an athletic event.

The beneficial effects of fluid replacement during competition are also clear. It is not that long ago, however, that coaching techniques in some sports stressed fluid restriction!

Female athletes, particularly those in endurance sports or sports in which there is an unfortunate preoccupation with body size or image, are at specific risk of developing iron deficiency. The optimization of iron intake and hemoglobin levels will have an obvious effect on performance.

NUTRITIONAL SUPPLEMENTATION

A number of specific products have been used in the belief that they can enhance performance. It is not possible to discuss them all, nor any in detail, in this brief review. Additional information may be found elsewhere (Armsey and Green, 1997; Clarkson, 1996; Williams, 1998). The sport medicine practitioner has a special responsibility to try to ensure that athletes understand the problems that may surround the use of certain supplements: problems that may follow from the lack of evidence of their efficacy; that there are no regulations concerning their preparation, purity, labeling, or marketing; and concerns relating to their safety. Sir William Osler once observed that "It is the responsibility of the physician to persuade the public not to take medicines." His advice was intended for a population fascinated by nostrums and snake-oil; it may be equally appropriate for those intent on the pursuit of a nutritional panacea. Athletes too often place their faith in nutritional supplements of dubious or no value. As a consequence of the passage in 1994 of legislation favorable to the nutritional supplement manufacturers (Dietary Supplement and Health Education Act), it is no longer possible to have any confidence in the labeling, content, or quality of any nutritional supplement produced or distributed in the United States. Given that supplement products are aggressively marketed to, and used by, members of the athletic community there are obvious implications for sport medicine professionals. Not only may supplement products contain varying levels of products of questionable value, it is also the case that some products may be contaminated with steroid precursors, stimulants, or other compounds that can cause an athlete to fail doping control tests.

Branched Chain Amino Acids

These constituents of protein-rich foods are touted as being helpful in overcoming the central nervous system component of fatigue. There are theoretical grounds to support this contention, but research findings in this regard are inconclusive.

Beta-Hydroxy-Beta-Methylbutyrate

It is speculated that beta-hydroxy-beta-methylbutyrate (HMB), a metabolite of the amino acid leucine, is capable of decreasing protein breakdown thereby exerting an anabolic effect of sorts. Animal research has shown increased lean muscle mass and decreased levels of body fat in association with HMB supplementation. Limited human research conducted by the developers of this product has supported the animal findings. The safety of this compound is unknown at this point. (It is very important to distinguish this product from gamma-hydroxybutyrate [GHB], which, it is claimed, facilitates sleep and weight control.) GHB has been marketed particularly to body builders and it has been implicitly suggested that it can affect growth hormone release. Its actual effects in this regard are unknown. What is clear is that its use was associated with many cases of poisoning in the United States in 1990. No deaths resulted, but hospitalization and respiratory support was required for several unfortunate individuals (Centers for Disease Control, 1991).

Caffeine

Caffeine is present in an abundance of commonly ingested food and beverages. Caffeine's use has been controlled in sport; urinary levels of more than 12 μg/mL being considered as doping. It is known to improve performance in a variety of tasks, particularly in those accustomed to regular caffeine intake (Graham and Spriet, 1996). Athletes should understand that a small increase in normal caffeine intake might cause the development of *caffeinism*, in which anxiety, nervousness, and irritability will all contribute to a diminished performance. This is particularly true of those unaccustomed to regular caffeine ingestion.

Carnitine (L-Carnitine)

Formed in the body from several amino acids, carnitine is suggested to enhance aerobic power by facilitating the use of fatty acids in energy production, thereby sparing glycogen (the principal energy source in aerobic activity) consumption. It is also theorized that carnitine might enhance the delivery of pyruvate (produced by the breakdown of glucose) to the mitochondria and accentuate energy production. There is little evidence to support either view (Vuchovich, Costill, and Fink, 1994).

Choline (Lecithin)

Perhaps a more popular supplement several years ago, choline was promoted as having the ability to maintain adequate levels of acetylcholine, a neurotransmitter, during periods of prolonged aerobic exercise. The research evidence to support this view is inconclusive (Spector et al., 1995). Dietary choline is found in egg yolks, organ meats, spinach, and wheat germ.

Chromium

An essential mineral, chromium is claimed to enhance the development of lean muscle mass and to reduce body fat. Interest in this mineral increased when it became apparent that exercise causes chromium loss. It is suggested that chromium supplementation improves insulin sensitivity and promotes the transfer of amino acids into the muscle cell, thereby stimulating protein synthesis. Recent, well-designed investigations have failed to support the contention that chromium supplementation improves lean body mass or strength (Clancy et al., 1994). In addition, concerns exist about the potential hazard of excess chromium intake above that recommended as a daily requirement (Wasser and Feldman, 1997).

Creatine

Creatine is a compound that exists normally in the body and is found in the normal diet in animal protein. Creatine is normally found in muscle where it is combined with phosphate to form creatine phosphate. Creatine phosphate is responsible for providing and replenishing muscle energy in situations involving the rapid production of maximal effort. Many laboratory investigations have confirmed that the addition of supplemental creatine increased performance in repetitive tasks of maximal effort (Greenhaff et al., 1994; Maughan, 1995). Whether this translates into increased performance capacity in the course of an actual athletic event is more difficult to prove. Several other investigators have shown no evidence of increased performance in athletic situations. More studies are necessary to resolve these contradictory findings. At this point one can say that the evidence does exist to support the use of creatine in enhancing repeated explosive muscular activity and thus it may assist in accentuating training intensity. That has not prevented the development of a thriving market in the sale of this supplement to athletes at every level of ability in a variety of sports.

Ephedra

The ephedrines (ephedrine, pseudoephedrine, etc.) occur naturally in a number of plants and are a common ingredient of traditional medicines (e.g., ma huang or Chinese ephedra). Refined ephedrines once played a role in the treatment of asthma and are now frequently found in nasal decongestants and cough and cold medications. As noted, they have frequently been the cause of so-called inadvertent doping. More recently, the nutritional supplement industry has aggressively marketed ephedrine-containing products to athletes as performance enhancers and to those seeking assistance with weight loss. Tragically, there is little evidence to support any significant effect in either area. What has become clear is that there are specific dangers associated with the use of these products and a number of deaths, some highly publicized, are felt to have resulted from the use of such supplements (Haller and Benowits, 2000; Samenuk et al., 2002). Complicating the issue is the fact that no regulation of any nutritional supplement is required in the United States since the passage of the Dietary Supplement and Health Education Act of 1994. Consequently, doses of these products vary enormously, their quality is always in question, and their presence may go unnoted by consumers unaware of the guises in which these products may appear.

Ginseng

The allure of ginseng as a supplement is perhaps explained by the traditional use of this product in oriental medicine and the degree of formal and informal marketing surrounding its use. Although there is little doubt that the ginsenosides (the constituents of ginseng) are biologically active, there is no clear evidence that they are capable of enhancing performance (Bahrke and Morgan, 1994). Many of the commercial preparations of ginseng are blends of a variety of ginsenosides of differing quality and potency; this makes the evaluation of their properties more difficult. As with all so-called natural supplements, there are no regulations to control the ingredients, purity, or accuracy of the labeling of these products. It is known that some of these supplements have been deliberately or inadvertently contaminated with other pharmacologically active substances. Athletes must be aware of such unfortunate realities and, to the extent possible, assure themselves of the quality and purity of any products they may be considering purchasing or consuming.

FINAL THOUGHTS

Sport is a powerful, and normally positive, cultural force in our community and in the modern world. Unfortunately, there are those who would cheat to secure sporting success. There are others who would exploit athletes and their trust by manipulating their training practices or programs. The artificial enhancement of athletic training or athletic accomplishments by pharmacologic means is both irresponsible and unethical. Health professionals involved in sport have a central responsibility to care for athletes in the most complete sense and to protect and preserve the integrity of any sporting experience. This may seem a naive or hopelessly optimistic perspective. Nevertheless, the true magic of sport is that it is a place where seemingly naive or hopelessly optimistic aspirations can often become reality!

REFERENCES

Armsey TD, Green GA. Nutrition supplements: Science vs. hype. *Phys Sports Med.* 1997;25.

Bagatelli CJ, Bremner WJ. Androgens in men—Uses and abuses. *N Engl J Med.* 1996;334;707–714.

Bahr R, Tjornhom M. Prevalence of doping in sports: Doping control in Norway, 1977–1995. *Clin J Sport Med.* 1998;8:32–37.

Bahrke MS, Morgan WP. Evaluation of the ergogenic properties of ginseng. *Sports Med.* 1994;18:229–248.

Bhasin S, Storer TW, Berman N, et al. The effects of supraphysiologic doses of testosterone on muscle size and strength in normal men. *N Engl J Med.* 1996;335:1–7.

Centers for Disease Control. Multistate outbreak of poisonings associated with illicit use of GHB. *JAMA.* 1991;265:447–448.

Clancy SP, Clarkson PM, DeCheke ME, et al. Effects of chromium picolinate supplementation on body composition, strength, and urinary chromium loss in football players. *Int J Sport Nutr.* 1994;4:142–153.

Clarkson PM. Nutrition for improved sports performance: Current issues on ergogenic aids. *Sports Med.* 1996;21:293–401.

Cowart VS. Dietary supplements: Alternatives to anabolic steroids? *Phys Sports Med.* 1992;20:189–198.

Dean H. Does exogenous growth hormone improve athletic performance? *Clin J Sport Med.* 2002;12:250–253.

Ekblom B, Berglund B. Effect of erythropoietin administration on maximal aerobic power. *Scan J Med Sci Sports.* 1991;1:88–93.

Franke WW, Bererdork B. Hormonal doping and androgenization of athletes: A secret program of the German Democratic government? *Clin Chem.* 1997;43:1262–1279.

Graham TE, Spriet LL. Caffeine and exercise performance. *Sports Sci Exch.* 1996;9:1–5.

Greenhaff PL, Bodin K, Soderland K, et al. the effect of oral creatine supplementation on skeletal muscle phosphocreatine resynthesis. *Am J Physiol.* 1994;266:E725–E730.

Haller CA, Benowitz NL. Adverse cardiovascular and central nervous system events associated with dietary supplements containing ephedra alkaloids. *N Engl J Med.* 2000;343:1833–1838.

Herbal treatments: The promises and pitfalls. *Consumer Reports* 1999;64:44–48.

Maughan RJ. Creatine supplementation and exercise performance. *Int J Sport Nutr.* 1995;5:994–1001.

Melia P, Pipe A, Greenberg L. The use of anabolic-androgenic steroids by Canadian students. *Clin J Sport Med.* 1996;6:9–14.

Menkis AH, Daniel JK, McKenzie N, et al. Cardiac transplantation after myocardial infarction in a 24 year-old bodybuilder using anabolic steroids. *Clin J Sport Med.* 1991;1:138–140.

Mottram DR. Drugs and their use in sport. In: Mottram DR, ed. *Drugs in Sport.* Champaign, IL: Human Kinetics, 1988;1–31.

Pipe AL. Sport, science and society: Ethics in sports medicine. *Med Sci Sports Exerc.* 1993;25:888–900.

Ramotar J. Cyclists' deaths linked to erythropoietin? *Phys Sports Med.* 1990;18:48–49.

Samenuk D, Link MS, Homound MK, et al. Adverse cardiovascular and effects temporally associated with ma huang, an herbal source of ephedrine. *Mayo Clin Proc.* 2002;77:12–16.

Seehusen DA, Glorioso JE. Tamoxifen as an ergogenic agent in women body builders. *Clin J Sport Med.* 2002;12:313–314.

Spector SA, Jackman MR, Sabounjian LA, et al. Effect of choline supplementation in trained cyclists. *Med Sci Sports Exerc.* 1995;27:668–673.

Vuchovich MD, Costill DL, Fink WJ. Carnitine supplementation: Effect on muscle carnitine and glycogen content during exercise. *Med Sci Sports Exerc.* 1994;26:1122–1129.

Wasser WG, Feldman NS. Chronic renal failure after ingestion of over-the-counter chromium picolinate. [Letter] *Ann Intern Med.* 1997;126:410.

Weinberg RS, Gould D. *Foundations of Sport and Exercise Psychology.* Champaign, IL: Human Kinetics; 1995.

Williams MH. *The Ergogenics Edge: Pushing the Limits of Human Performance.* Champaign, IL: Human Kinetics; 1998.

Yoshida EM, Karim MA, Shaikn JF, et al. At what price glory? Severe cholestasis and acute renal failure in an athlete abusing stanozolol. *Can Med Assoc J.* 1994;151:791–793.

5 | Emergency Sideline Care and Airway Management

Aaron Rubin

QUICK REFERENCE

Emergency Sideline Care and Airway Management

- Be comfortable at the venue and with the equipment
- Appropriate dress for the venue and conditions
- Have a disaster plan
- Check the venue for dangers and emergency access
- Check communications equipment
- Decision process for immediate or delayed return to play versus transport for definitive care
- First-priority injuries: Airway, breathing, circulation, disability (cervical spine, head, limb at risk) myocardial infarction, hyperthermia, hypothermia, acute asthma, penetrating injury, and severe burns
- Second-priority injuries: Suspected fractures, dislocations, minor head injury, dental injury, lacerations, abrasions and moderate burns
- Third-priority injuries: Small laceration, abrasions, sprains, strains, contusions, mild heat illness, and cramps

One of the major functions of the team physician is the emergent treatment of the injured athlete. At times, this extends to spectators, officials, and others at sporting venues. Proper training, preparation, planning, and understanding of the type of injury and illness that could befall the athlete and others are essential for effectively performing this duty.

FIELD PROTOCOL

Most physicians are comfortable in the relatively controlled setting of their office, the emergency department, or the athletic training room. The team physician needs to gain a level of comfort at the sports venue as well. This begins by proper dress for the elements. It would be difficult to pay attention to an injured athlete in the cold, wet, mud if there are personal concerns about being cold, wet, and muddy. Appropriate clothing, including foot-wear for prolonged standing in the elements, is essential for changing weather conditions. Weather can change rapidly, and the team physician should be prepared for the worst possible conditions.

One should consider some type of visible identification as well. This can be time saving if responding to untoward medical events on the opponents' sideline or in the stands. An identification badge, or embroidered name and identification on a jacket or shirt, can be utilized.

The team physician should be familiar with the venue. A "walk around" should be performed before every event to determine if there are any potential problems present for the athletes, such as immobile objects near the field or court, holes in the turf, or other dangerous possibilities. Communication, especially cell phones, should be checked to see if they function.

The team physician should meet the paramedics, athletic trainers, game officials, security, and others involved with care of the athletes on both sidelines. To accomplish this, the team physician must arrive at the venue well before the start time of the event.

MEDICAL ORGANIZATION

The size of the medical staff is determined by the size of the event, potential for injury, and number of the participants and spectators. Planning for the event must include plans for care of spectators. The team physician should not be distracted from the care of the athletes by minor injuries or illness in the stands, but cannot ignore serious conditions affecting spectators if no alternative is present.

The team physician should be on or near the field or court and in close communication with the athletic trainer. In general, the athletic trainer will evaluate and attend to the athlete on the field. Arrangements should be made for when the physician will go onto the field. This could be a signal from the athletic trainer based on the apparent severity of the injury. If needed, paramedics should be called onto the field by the physician.

Individuals must be assigned to direct rescue personnel into the venue, control crowds, open gates and doors, and work with family members. Having a person designated to get family members from the stands and stay with them during the initial moments of an incident can help in gaining pertinent medical information and keep the family members from coming onto the field and potentially interfering with initial care.

EQUIPMENT

Equipment and medical supplies are also largely dictated by the number of spectators and athletic participants. It is not possible to have supplies for every contingency at a given venue. Equipment needs are also influenced by the ability to receive outside help and transport individuals to definitive medical care. There have been multiple lists created to help choose basic medical equipment (Table 5-1).

These supplies can be divided into three basic groups related to the usual responsible party for the equipment: the emergency medical services, the athletic trainer, and the team physician.

True emergencies involve immediate threat to life or limb. The care of these injuries and conditions often require supplies that are carried by an emergency response squad. Airway equipment, defibrillator, advanced cardiac life support drugs, intravenous fluids, cervical spine immobilization, acute allergy and asthma medications, emergent splinting material, record keeping and organization for mass casualty incidents, communication equipment, and transportation are some of the general supplies in this category.

The athletic trainer's kit includes many of the items needed to care for the most common problems of the athlete. This includes bandages, tape, bracing and splinting material, over-the-counter medications, wound care items, and other items.

The team physician's bag will vary depending on the sport and type of athlete. Some considerations beyond the athletic trainer's kit may include splinting, suturing, and medications.

COMMUNICATION

The ability to easily and concisely communicate with other members of the sports medicine team and ancillary persons is essential. Cell phones are ubiquitous, but must be able to connect to a cell site to function. Cell phones

TABLE 5-1 Emergency Sideline Supplies

Team physician	Emergency medical services	Athletic trainer
Pocket Gear	Medications	Air or cardboard splints
Bandage shears	Activated charcoal	Hard cervical collar
Exam gloves	Adenosine	Oropharyngeal airway
Pocket mask	Epinephrine 1:1000 10 mL	Blanket
Penlight	Epinephrine 1:1000 1 mL	Crutches
Knife/multitool		Ice chest and ice
4 × 4 sponges	Epinephrine 1:10,000 10 mL	Plastic bags
Pen/paper		6" ace wraps
Airway	Albuterol inhalation 2.5 mg	4" ace wraps
Cellular phone		Facemask removal device
Sideline Instruments	Aspirin, chewable 81 mg	Adhesive tape (1½")
BP Cuff (various sizes)	Atropine 0.4 mg/cc	Under wrap
Oto/ophthalmscope	Atropine 1 mg/mL	Elastikon 3"
Thermometer	Calcium chloride	Lightplast 2" and 3'
Glucose monitor	Dextrose 50%	Heel and lace pads
Pulse oximeter	Diphenhydramine inj.	Plastic ice wrap
Needle forceps	Furosemide inj.'	Band Aids—various sizes
Hemostat	Glucagon	
Scissors	Dopamine	Tape adherent (Tuf- skin)
Disposable cautery	Magnesium sulfate	Steri-strips 1/8"
Headlamp	Naloxone	Cotton-tipped applicators
Batteries (to fit above)	Nitroglycerine tab or spray	Tongue blades
Eye Tray	Normal saline inj 10 mL	Skin lubricant
Cobalt blue light	Pitocin	Peroxide
Flourescein strips	Phenylephrine HCl	Antibiotic ointment
Irrigating solution	Procainamide	3 × 3" gauze pads
Tetracaine 0.5% topical ophthalmic	Terbutaline	4 × 4" gauze pads
Neurologic/Orthopedic	Verapamil inj.	Telfa pads
Air splints	Lidocaine	Heat balm
"Sam" splint	Lidocaine	Bandage scissors
Cast padding	Viscous Lidocaine	Tape cutter (aka Shark)
Readi splints (fiberglass)	**Controlled Substances**	Forceps or tweezers
4 × 35 inch	Midazolam 5 mg/mL	Nail clipper
3 × 15 inch	Morphine SO$_4$	Triangular bandage
3 × 12 inch	**IV Fluids**	Penlight
Knee immobilizer	Normal saline 250 mL	Mirror
Elastic bandages (3, 4, 6 inch)	Normal saline 1000 mL	Blood pressure cuff
Finger splints (aluminum)	**Solutions**	Stethoscope
Triangular bandages	Normal saline irrigation 1000 mL	Multifunction tool
Wound Care	**Equipment**	Crutches
Gauze pads	Antiseptic swabs	Tape
Bandages	Syringes TB, 3, 5, 10, 20, 60 mL	Rigid backboard
Saline irrigation	Hypo needles 18, 20, 22, 25 g	Cervical collars (sizes)
Povidone-iodine swabs	IV catheters 14, 16, 18, 20, 22, 24 g	Facemask removal device
Lidocaine 1% injection plain		Pen
		Eyewash
		Contact lens care kit

—cont.

TABLE 5-1 Emergency Sideline Supplies (*Continued*)

Team physician	Emergency medical services	Athletic trainer
Lidocaine 1% injection with epinephrine	Intraosseous needles	Thermometer
	3-way stopcock	Lip balm
	Solution administration set	Foam and felt
Disposable suture tray		Moleskin
	Buretrol administration set	Mouthpieces
Sutures (4-0 nylon, 6-0 nylon, 4-0 absorbable)		Ibuprofen
	IV extension tube	Acetaminophen
Sterile gloves	Conductive defib pads	Antacid tablets
Sterile fields	EKG pads	
Steri-strips, assorted	Rigid cervical collars, pediatric/adult	
Tincture of benzoin ampules	Sterile burn sheets	
Topical antibiotic unit dose	Meconium aspirator	
	OB kit	
Syringes, needles, assorted	Endotracheal tubes cuffed 6.0, 7.0, 8.0	
Sharps disposal container	ET tubes uncuffed 2.0, 3.0, 4.0, 5.0	
Biohazard bag	Adult Pertrach device	
Roll gauze (3, 4, 6 inch)	Pediatric Pertrach device	
Nonadherent bandages	Naso/orogastric tubes, 10, 12, 14, 16, 18 g	
Bio-occlusive dressing	Suction catheters 6, 8, 12 french	
Exam gloves	Yankauers tonsil tip	
Medications (Non-ACLS)	Small volume nebulizer	
Albuterol inhaler with aerochamber	Malleable stylet adult and pediatric	
Epinepherine 1:1000 (Epi-Pen)	Water-soluble lubricating jelly	
Diphenhydramine 25 mg injection	Oropharyngeal airways (infant, child, and adult)	
Diphenhydramine 25 mg capsules	Nasopharyngeal airways (infant, child, and adult)	
Antacid tablets	Vaseline gauze	
	Nasal cannulas (adult and pediatric)	
	Adult non-O_2 rebreather mask	
	Adult simple O_2 mask	
	Pediatric O_2 mask	
	Anti-nausea tablets/injection	
	Anti-diarrhea tablets (Loperamide 2 mg)	
	Ibuprofen 200 mg	
	Acetaminophen 325 mg	
	Anesthetic ear drops	
	Aspirin 81 mg	

TABLE 5-1 Emergency Sideline Supplies (*Continued*)

Emergency medical services		
Aspirin 325 mg	Saline locks	Head immobilization
Nitroglycerin 0.4 mg	One-way flutter valve	devices
	Ankle and wrist	Long backboard with
Travel Medications	restraints	straps
Penicillin 250 mg	Pneumatic or rigid	Pediatric
Cephalexin 250 mg	splints	immobilization board
Ciprofloxacin 250 mg	Sterile bandages	Short extrication
Azithromycin 250 mg	compression	device
	Gauze pads (4 × 4)	Traction splint
Miscellaneous	Roller bandage 2,	Triage tags (START
Bag or case	3, 4, 6 inch	system)
Blanket or space	Bandage shears	Suction device
blanket	10 × 30 universal	Suction device (wall
Prescription pad	dressing	mounted)
Information sheets for	Emesis basin	Laryngoscope handle
injured (head injury,	Bedpan or	with batteries
ankle sprain, knee	fracture pan	Laryngeal blades #1,
injury, wound, etc)	Urinal	2, 3, 4 curved and
Injury recording		straight
system	**Equipment**	Magill forceps,
Micro tape recorder	Ambulance cot	pediatric and adult
Rain jacket/pancho	and collapsible	In-ambulance O_2
Appropriate clothing	stretcher	source
Protective goggles/	Straps to secure	Ventilation bags
mask/gown/gloves	patient to cot	(ambu bags)
	Sheets, pillows, cases,	with connections,
ACLS/ATLS	blankets	adult and pediatiric
Medication if no EMS	Portable O_2 with	End-tidal CO_2 device
readily available	regulator	Stethoscope
(see EMS list)	Glucose monitoring	Blood pressure cuffs
Consider automated	device	(infant, pediatric,
external defibrillator	Communications	adult, large, thigh)
Oxygen	radios 800 MHz	Pressure infusion bag
Bag valve mask	Defibrillator/monitor/	Flashlight
Combi-tube	pacemaker	
Crichothryrotomy kit		

should be checked each time at the venue and telephone numbers of key personnel exchanged. Emergency calls from cell phones (9-1-1) are handled differently in different jurisdictions and the physician must be aware of potential delays in obtaining a response.

Family radios are useful if used over short distances. There is no privacy on these radios and care should be exercised when transmitting information.

If the event or venue covers a large area, the physician may consider amateur radio (HAM radio). If available and properly trained, police or fire radios are usually extremely reliable, though also lack privacy.

DECISION PROCESS

The sideline physician must make decisions regarding the health of the athlete. A straightforward approach is to decide if the injured athlete falls into one of three categories. These include a minor injury that can allow for almost **immediate return** to play, an injury that requires time or treatment to allow a **delayed return,** or an injury that will **not allow return** to play. Those not able to return to play are further divided into those that need immediate transport to emergency facilities, those needing to be further evaluated in short time or after the contest, and those that can safely be further evaluated later.

To determine the need for further treatment or evaluation, the physician must have a plan for approaching injuries. Once the injury is prioritized, the decision process becomes more evident.

First-priority injuries are those that threaten life or limb or carry a likelihood of permanent or prolonged disability. These injuries can be categorized by ABCD (Airway, Breathing, Circulation, Disability). Conditions include loss of airway, breathing, or circulation. The first priority would also include potential disability caused by cervical spine injury, lumbar spine injury, severe head injury, or extremities at risk. Medical conditions that are first priority include suspicion of acute myocardial infarction, heat stroke, hypothermia, acute asthma, evolving cerebrovascular attack, serious eye trauma, significant burns, and severe blunt or penetrating abdominal or thoracic injury.

Second-priority injuries are those that require immediate treatment and evaluation to decrease pain and disability. These include suspected fractures, dislocations, minor head injury, dental injury, and lacerations, abrasions, or moderate burns requiring care.

Fortunately, third-priority injuries are the most commonly encountered. These include small lacerations, abrasions, sprains, strains, contusions, exercise (heat) exhaustion, and exercise-induced cramps.

DISASTER PLAN

The disaster plan for each venue and event should be predetermined. The plan needs to include who responds initially and in subsequent support roles, communications, access to the venue, and security concerns. Generally, the athletic trainer will be the first responder to the downed athlete on the field, with the physician available as soon as necessary. If the injury appears significant based on mechanism of injury or appearance of the athlete from the sideline, both may choose to respond.

Persons should be designated to call the emergency medical service (EMS), direct them upon arrival and open any gates or doors to gain access, provide security, and as much privacy as possible to the injured athlete, inform and stay with the parents or friends, and assist EMS in preparing the athlete for transport.

Someone should also be designated to act as a liaison to the media and provide consistent, accurate, and appropriate information. The physician and other medical staff should not disclose any information to the press without the expressed consent of the athlete. This type of medicine is practiced in the public eye and may be videotaped or otherwise recorded.

SPECIALIZED TRAINING

Ideally, the team physician should have specialized training in sports medicine to properly prepare to handle potential emergencies that can arise. While it is not possible for there to be such trained physicians at all athletic events, there are many physicians willing to volunteer or work as team physicians. They should consider additional training in basic cardiac life support (BLS), advanced cardiac life support (ACLS) (American Heart Association—www.americanheart.org), and basic trauma life support (BTLS) (Basic Life Support International, Inc.—1-800-495-BTLS). Advanced trauma life support (ATLS) involves mostly in-hospital care, but can be initiated on the field by the team physician. In addition to basic emergency care, the team physician should be well versed in the care of athletic injuries.

The team physician should be aware of emergency response in the area that he or she is practicing. The physician should be prepared for a mass casualty event in case of a natural disaster (earthquake leading to stands collapse) or manmade (shooting with multiple casualties in the stands and panicked exiting of spectators) or terrorist attack. Very often, the team physician will be the first to the scene and must be able to provide appropriate care and calm the situation. To do such, the physician must be aware of triage techniques and the incident command system (ICS).

A mass casualty incident (MCI) is defined as an incident where casualties outnumber the number of caregivers. Triage involves determining the victims in need of immediate care, those that could survive with delayed care and, most difficult, those victims that will require too much attention from limited resources to survive or are obviously dead. One method of rapid triage is the simple triage and rapid treatment (START) method (Fig. 5-1), which allows for evaluation of multiple injured in a rapid fashion. More treatment can be provided if there are enough resources to evaluate and care for multiple victims. The ICS is designed to organize multiple responders to an MCI. This allows for a single commander to organize multiple responders. The team physician will most likely act in the medical team as opposed to overall command of the incident (Fig. 5-2). In most athletic settings, the triage of casualties separates those who need more intensive care from those who will most likely recover with minimal intervention.

SPECIFIC INJURIES

Definitive treatments of specific injuries are covered in the individual chapter. For an overall outline, a physician should consider the mnemonic **ABCDEF,** which stands for **A**irway, **B**reathing, **C**irculation, **D**isability, **E**xposure and Examination, **F**inal disposition.

Airway management in the unconscious athlete must also address possible cervical spine injury. The tongue falling back in the throat is the most common cause of airway obstruction. Blood, vomitus, mouth guard, teeth, food, gum, and direct injury to the neck are other causes of compromised airway. Medical conditions, such as anaphylaxis, seizures, hypoglycemia, and status asthmaticus, can also lead to airway obstruction.

The airway can most often be obtained by proper positioning of the athlete. Most often, the athlete must be in a supine position to manage the airway. Special exception may occur in cases of motor sports, with the delay in getting total access to the athlete-driver, water sports where airway may need to be obtained before removal from the water, and other circumstances that may make it difficult to place the player flat on the back. Special airway devices discussed as follows will help in these situations.

The jaw-thrust or chin-lift maneuvers can be used to lift the tongue out of the airway. Jaw lift without head tilt is performed by placing the third, fourth,

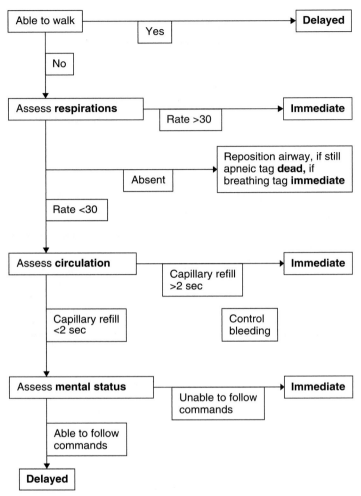

FIG 5-1 Simple Triage and Rapid Treatment (START). (*Adapted from Ontario [CA] Fire Department Office of Preparedness.*)

and fifth fingers of each hand under the angle of the athlete's mandible and lifting upward to elevate the tongue out of the airway. The chin lift is performed in a similar manner, but by lifting with fingers beneath the chin.

The airway cay be maintained by use of a nasopharyngeal or oropharyngeal airway. These do not protect the airway from aspiration. Oral or nasal tracheal intubation can be performed by the properly trained individual with proper equipment.

Alternative airway devices include the esophageal-tracheal combitube (ETC) and laryngeal mask airway (LMA). The LMA is a device that is blindly inserted into the pharynx which, when properly seated, seals the larynx and provides a stable airway. It requires less instruction and equipment to utilize.

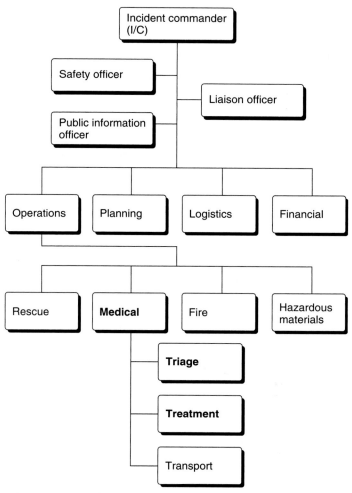

FIG 5-2 Diagram of the Incident Command System with an emphasis on the Operations/Medical branch. (*Source: From Sports Injuries and Emergencies: A Quick-Response Manual.*)

The ETC is also blindly inserted to provide a protected airway. Two cuffs are inflated to obstruct the hypopharynx and esophagus. If the tube has been inserted into the esophagus, as occurs over 98% of the time, the air is forced between the cuffs and into the trachea. If, by chance, the tube was inserted into the trachea, the athlete can be ventilated by a second portal directly into the lungs. It also requires less training and equipment to use and can be used in athletes not in the supine position. A cricothyroidotomy kit may be necessary for laryngeal crush injuries that can occur in hockey, softball, and baseball.

An additional concern in the athlete is the ability to access the head and face in the helmeted athlete. The team physician should be aware of safety equipment and practice removal of the facemask in sports such as football and hockey and complete helmet removal in motor sports. In football, the helmet should generally not be removed due to the difficulty of maintaining a neutral cervical spine in an athlete wearing shoulder pads. There are various tools available to remove facemasks in football players.

Breathing may resume spontaneously once the airway is open. If not, respirations must be provided to the victim. Mouth-to-mouth resuscitation provides adequate ventilation, but should be conducted using a barrier device such as a face shield or pocket mask to provide protection to the rescuer. A bag-valve-mask (BVM) can be used if the person is properly trained. Supplemental oxygen can be provided by BVM to give a high flow of oxygen.

Circulatory support involves chest compressions if the victim is pulseless. Support of circulation also involves establishment of intravenous lines for fluid support, control of hemorrhage, and medication to support blood pressure once fluid status is known.

Disability must be minimized. The highest concern is to prevent paralysis, permanent brain damage, and loss of use of limbs. Cervical spine injury must be suspected in any unconscious athlete or any with neck pain, numbness, tingling, or weakness. Cervical spine immobilization and transport to an appropriate emergency department is required (see Chapter 16).

Head injury requires early diagnosis to prevent the athlete from too early return to activity and to provide rapid transport to an appropriate neurosurgical facility for emergent treatment (see Chapter 11).

Any pulseless extremity is at risk for ischemic loss of tissue. Special attention should be paid to any suspected knee dislocation, as these injuries need immediate orthopedic evaluation and studies to prove that no arterial damage has occurred.

Myocardial infarction is more likely to occur in spectators and older athletes. Early use of aspirin, oxygen, and pain control are important. The most likely cause of early death is ventricular fibrillation, which can be treated with early defibrillation with a standard defibrillator or automated external defibrillator (AED). Rapid transport to an appropriate facility for definitive treatment is mandatory.

Heat stroke is a medical emergency that requires rapid cooling measures to decrease the mortality risk. Immediate rectal temperature measurement and ice tub immersion is the preferred treatment. If a rectal temperature cannot be obtained and heat stroke is suspected, apply ice packs to the neck, axilla, and groin for first aid, and then transport for definitive medical care and monitoring.

Hypothermia is best treated in the hospital with careful warming and attention to treatment of the extremities to diminish the effects of frostbite. If there is any risk of refreezing the tissue, it is better to delay the treatment than to treat on site.

EXPOSURE AND EXAMINATION

Once life-threatening and disability-causing injuries have been excluded, the attention must be turned to more minor maladies. Proper exposure and examination are necessary, with attention paid to preserving the athlete's privacy and modesty.

Musculoskeletal examinations are outlined in other chapters. Special attention for the sideline physician is the need to apply proper splints to remove the athlete from the field without worsening the injury or causing undue pain. Air, vacuum, cardboard, prepackaged fiberglass, and SAM splints are commercially available to provide proper immobilization to remove the athlete from the contest and provide comfort during transport to appropriate facilities.

Skin injuries must be cleaned and closed or covered to prevent contamination and infection. Bleeding must be controlled before return to competition. Closure of lacerations is appropriate if the care provider is properly trained and equipped. Adequate informed consent and assurance that tetanus status is up to date are important.

Athletes with eye injuries should be tested for visual acuity. Serious eye injuries need immediate transport to the emergency department for evaluation and treatment to prevent disability.

Tooth loss or fracture is best treated by a dentist soon after the injury. An avulsed tooth should be replaced or transported in the athlete's mouth or in a saline-moistened gauze pad to a dentist. Preplanning is important, as there are few emergency dentists available, and having the location of an emergency dental clinic or team dentist can be extremely helpful (see Chapter 14).

This leads to the final disposition for the athlete. The team physician must have plans for immediate transfer to medical facilities when needed and advice for routine care when appropriate.

REFERENCES

Advanced Trauma Life Support Program for Doctors. Chicago: American College of Surgeons;1997;1–504.

Cantwell JD. Automatic external defibrillators in the sports arena: The right place, the right time. *Phys Sports Med*. 1998;26:33.

Cummins RO, ed. *ACLS Provider Manual*. Dallas: American Heart Association; 2001.

Chameides L, Hazinski MF, eds. *Pediatric Advanced Life Support*. Dallas: American Heart Association; 1997.

Doerges V, Sauer C, Ocker H, et al. Airway management during cardiopulmonary resuscitation—A comparative study of bag-valve-mask, laryngeal mask airway and Combitube in a bench model. *Resuscitation*. 1999;41:63–69.

Emory JE, ed. *Basic Trauma Life Support*. 4th ed. Upper Saddle River, NJ: Brady/Prentice Hall Health, 2000.

The American Heart Association in collaboration with the International Liaison Committee on Resuscitation. Guidelines 2000 for Cardiopulmonary Resuscitation and Emergency Cardiac Care. Part 6: Advanced cardiovascular life support: Section 3: Adjuncts for oxygenation, ventilation and airway control. *Circulation* 2000;102(suppl I):95–104.

Jaworski C. Advances in emergent airway management. *Curr Sports Med Rep*. 2002;1:133–140.

Norris RL, Peterson J. Airway management for the sports physician. Part 1: Basic techniques. *Phys Sports Med*. 2001;29:23–29.

Norris RL, Peterson J. Airway management for the sports physician. Part 2: Advanced techniques. *Phys Sports Med*. 2001;29:15–28.

Rubin AL, ed. *Sports Injuries and Emergencies: A Quick Reference Manual*. New York: McGraw-Hill; 2003.

Rubin AL. Automated external defibrillators: Selection and use. *Phys Sports Med*. 2000;28:112–114.

Rubin AL, Sallis RE. Management of on-the-field emergencies. In: Safran MR, McKeag DB, Van Camp SP, eds. *Manual of Sports Medicine*. Philadelphia: Lippincott-Raven; 1998.

Tintinalli JE, Kelen GD, Stapczynski JS, eds. *Emergency Medicine: A Comprehensive Study Guide*. New York: McGraw-Hill; 2000.

6 | Sideline Management of Common Dislocations

Marc R. Safran and Duncan K. Hodge

QUICK LOOK

- Many dislocations can be safely and appropriately reduced in experienced hands on the field, optimizing comfort and minimizing the morbidity of late treatment.
- Treating physician or athletic trainer must be aware of possible complications of injury and from treatment, including neurovascular injury or fracture.
- Neurovascular status must be properly documented before and after intervention.
- Formal radiographic confirmation should be obtained at earliest convenience following joint reduction.
- On-site joint reduction should be easily obtained and not forced.
- The treating clinician should attempt one reduction only; repeated attempts are not recommended.
- Some dislocations are not reducible without surgical intervention.

Joint dislocation is a common injury in many of today's sports, causing significant morbidity and time away from training and competition. For this reason, it is important for sports medicine physicians, trainers, and coaches to be familiar with these injuries and their treatment. The spectrum of injury can be from benign to serious depending on the joint involved, with the added possibility of certain complications, such as fracture and neurovascular compromise. Prompt diagnosis is necessary to triage these injuries appropriately for treatment in the emergency room, or in some situations, in the hands of experienced personnel, for reduction on the sidelines.

Although somewhat controversial, many experienced team physicians support the premise that closed reduction of most dislocations can be attempted on the field if fracture is not suspected. There are many advantages of early joint relocation including avoidance of significant muscle spasm. Reducing a dislocation before the onset of muscle spasms makes the maneuver easier and also relieves pain and suffering. Muscle spasms can significantly complicate closed reduction, and in fact, sometimes obviate open reduction. In addition to it being easier to reduce the dislocation before muscle spasms and swelling set in, other advantages include preservation of skin viability, decompression of neurovascular tension, and ease of splinting and transportation. Opponents to on-the-field reductions argue that without radiographs, there is a risk that the joint is not dislocated, but actually fractured. Thus, the clinician risks manipulating a fracture or fracture-dislocation, which may result in further displacement, laceration of neurovascular structures, or joint damage by motion of an intra-articular fracture. Other arguments against on-the-field or sideline reduction include limited anesthesia and limited help and possible medico-legal sequelae.

It is the experience of the senior author that fractures associated with dislocations more commonly occur in the skeletally immature and older athletic populations. This factor should be considered when deciding when and whether to attempt reduction on the field without radiographs. Finally, the comfort of the athlete should be taken into consideration. The person attempting the on-the-filed reduction should have formal training and an understanding of the anatomy, mechanism of injury, method of reduction, and possible complications. If an examiner is confident that they can reduce a simple dislocation, this will provide quick relief for the athlete in question. On the other hand, several failed attempts at reduction will cause pain in the injured athlete and further muscle spasm, complicating the possibility of successful relocation.

After weighing the risks and benefits, if the examiner is going to attempt a reduction, it is of paramount importance to document neurovascular status *before and after* the reduction trial. Closed reduction in an initially neurologically intact athlete, although not frequent, can result in compromise of neurovascular structures. In terms of general aftercare, adequate immobilization is necessary for any joint dislocation to allow soft tissue healing. In addition, all reductions should be followed up with timely radiographic examination to confirm complete and concentric reduction as well as to rule out fracture. Further, acute aftercare should include ice, local compression, rest, immobilization (if indicated), and elevation.

Of note, if a fracture is suspected, there is generally no need for reduction on the field unless the limb is in jeopardy. These injuries should be splinted and the patient transported to the nearest hospital or treating facility. If a fracture is open, the injury should be covered and the patient should be immediately transported for emergent surgical intervention.

SHOULDER DISLOCATION

Epidemiology

The shoulder is the most commonly dislocated major joint in athletes. The traumatic disruption of the glenohumeral articulation in sports is typically unidirectional and more specifically, anterior in nature. A common scenario is a unidirectional, anterior dislocation of the shoulder occurring after a football player is tackled. Posterior and even inferior dislocation can also occur, but are seen much less frequently (>90% of dislocations are anterior) and thus will not be discussed in depth here.

Pathophysiology

In anterior dislocation of the shoulder, the head of humerus is displaced anteriorly with respect to glenoid, and is most commonly inferior to the coracoid process (also known as anterior-inferior, or subcoracoid dislocation). The mechanism of this injury is usually caused by a combination of abduction, extension, and a posteriorly directed force applied to the arm (or an anteriorly directed force to the back of the shoulder). These forces drive the humeral head anteriorly, stretching the shoulder capsule and often detaching the labrum from the glenoid, commonly known as the Bankart lesion.

Evaluation

Anterior dislocation usually presents with the athlete holding the injured arm in slight abduction and external rotation. The patient is usually unable and unwilling to abduct the arm further or internally rotate it completely. A fullness, which is the humeral head, can often be palpated anteriorly and sometimes inferiorly in the axilla. Posteriorly, the acromion is prominent, and a sulcus below it may be evident.

Management

Traumatic shoulder dislocation is an extremely painful injury, secondary to soft tissue injury and more pronounced following the onset of muscle spasm.

For this reason, anterior dislocation can often be reduced more easily on the field soon after it occurs before significant spasm sets in. Reduction usually can be achieved on the sidelines without any anesthesia. Relaxation and cooperation of the athlete is paramount to successful reduction, and often achieved by encouragement of the clinician performing the reduction.

Reduction

There are many techniques for reduction of the shoulder on the sidelines. The technique described here is the one preferred by the senior author. After assessing the neurologic status of the axillary nerve by checking the sensation over the lateral arm, the reduction is as follows. With the athlete supine, the arm or the dislocated shoulder is gently and slowly elevated to full elevation. This can be done with the clinician supporting the arm under the elbow and at the wrist. When in the full elevation position, gentle traction is applied to the arm upward and outward. With this traction applied, the thumb of clinician's other hand is used to push the humeral head over the glenoid rim onto the glenoid surface, reducing the shoulder (Fig. 6-1).

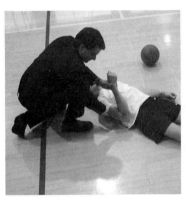

A

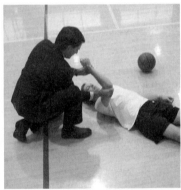

B

C

FIG 6-1 Reduction of anterior shoulder dislocation. (A) The shoulder is gently brought into full forward elevation. (B) Traction is applied longitudinally (upward) and outward with one hand while the other reduces the humerus head by pushing the humeral head into the glenoid fossa (C).

Aftercare

Following reduction, the athlete's arm should be immobilized in a sling or immobilizer. Radiographs are necessary after reduction to document adequate reduction and rule out fractures. Rehabilitation consists of active assisted range-of-motion exercises and strengthening of the rotator cuff and periscapular muscles.

Return to Sport

The injured athlete may return to training and competition when full motion and strength equivalent to the uninjured side is achieved.

Complications

Recurrence is the most common complication following acute shoulder dislocation, particularly in younger athletes. The recurrence rate may be as high as 80–90% in athletes below the age of 20 years at the time of their first dislocation, and decreases sharply in those sustaining such a dislocation during the fourth or fifth decades of life (Hovelius 1999). The most common neurologic complication is injury to the axillary nerve, which has been reported to occur in 10–25% of acute dislocations. This is usually a traction neuropathy that should completely resolve over time. Rotator cuff tears are more common in those over the age of 40 years at the time of the initial dislocation. Fractures of the greater tuberosity and glenoid are well-known complications of shoulder dislocation.

ELBOW DISLOCATION

Epidemiology

The elbow is the second most commonly dislocated major joint in adults and the most common in children. Contact sports are the most common activity to sustain the injury, though falls from height with high jumping or pole vaulting have been described.

Pathophysiology

Elbow dislocations usually occur secondary to a fall on an outstretched hand, and occasionally occur as a traction injury in wrestling. The classification of the dislocation is based on the displacement of the proximal ulna in relation to the distal humerus. Ninety percent of these dislocations involve posterior or posterolateral displacement of the forearm relative to the distal humerus. Anterior dislocations are less common, resulting from a direct blow to the posterior elbow. Pure medial and lateral dislocations have also been reported, but are rare and related to higher energy mechanisms.

Evaluation

Pain, soft tissue swelling, deformity, and lack of range of motion about the elbow are the clear presenting signs. Close inspection and careful palpation should be done to elucidate the direction of displacement to assist reduction. In the case of posterior dislocation, the upper extremity is generally found somewhat shortened and slightly flexed at the elbow. The olecranon is prominent posteriorly with some dimpling proximal to the olecranon, while there is fullness in the antecubital fossa. Bony crepitus on examination signals concomitant fracture, and in this scenario, radiographic examination would be advisable before a reduction attempt.

Management

Reduction

After the neurovascular examination is completed, reduction is performed as follows. For reduction of posterior dislocations, the examiner stabilizes the distal humerus with one hand, and then applies longitudinal traction to the proximal forearm with gentle anterior force until a pronounced clunk into flexion is achieved (Fig. 6-2). Flexion of the elbow should be avoided until reduction is achieved to avoid damage to the brachial artery. Following reduction, stability through range of motion of the elbow is verified, taking care with increasing extension, which can cause redislocation in unstable injuries. Stability of collateral ligaments of the elbow should also be assessed with gentle varus and valgus stress testing in addition to repeating the neurovascular examination.

Aftercare

Postreduction x-rays should be obtained to verify concentric reduction and rule out interposed soft tissues or bony fragments and fractures. The elbow should be placed in a long arm splint or bivalved cast in 90° of flexion for 5–10 days.

Upon reevaluation, early range of motion is tantamount in regaining acceptable elbow joint mobility. Studies have shown that strict elbow immobilization for more than 3 weeks is associated with ultimate poor range of motion (Cohen et al., 1998). In stable reductions, early active range of motion may begin as soon as symptoms permit. For unstable injuries, immobilization in a fracture brace allows early range of motion with an extension block that is gradually decreased after 3 weeks. Follow-up x-rays should be taken to document maintenance of reduction, as unstable injuries have a tendency to sublux or redislocate, despite immobilization.

Return to Sport

Criteria for return to sport include stability through a functional range of motion, and strength and stamina sufficient to withstand the demands of the athlete's sport and position. Full recovery can require 6–18 months. Taping of the elbow in slight flexion, a custom-padded elbow strap, or a hinged brace may be used to allow protection from hyperextension upon the athlete's return to practice and competition.

Complications

Long-term loss of extension is the most common sequelae to complicate a reduced elbow dislocation. Compared to other joints, recurrent instability in simple elbow dislocations is extremely rare, occurring in less than 1–2% of cases (Cohen et al., 1998). Associated fractures of the coronoid process, olecranon, or radial head are common in elbow dislocation. Posterior and posterolateral dislocations may also have associated fractures of the medial

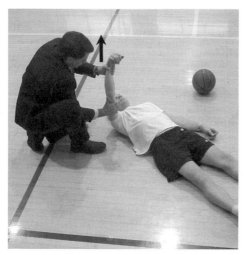

A

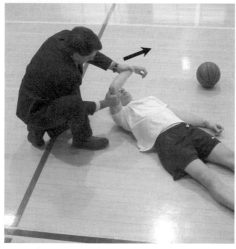

B

FIG 6-2 Reduction of elbow dislocation (posterior). (A) Medial-lateral displacement is first corrected. (B) Longitudinal traction is applied to the forearm while the other hand stabilizes the distal humerus and provides gentle anterior force with a thumb at the olecranon. Once a pronounced "clunk" is achieved, the elbow is brought into flexion.

epicondyle. There is a significant incidence of neurovascular injury in the elbow, with up to 20% of cases with associated compromise to the brachial artery, ulnar, median, radial, or anterior interosseus nerves. Wrist and shoulder injury can also occur concomitantly, in up to 10–15% of cases, and should be ruled out in any case of elbow dislocation.

KNEE DISLOCATION

Epidemiology

Although knee dislocation is usually encountered after a high-velocity traumatic injury, such as a motor vehicle accident, it can occur from lower energy mechanisms and therefore may be encountered on the field or court. To dislocate the knee, usually three ligaments must be torn (usually both cruciates and one collateral). There is a significant concern for vascular injury to the popliteal vessels in such dislocations, and therefore a thorough and objective evaluation by means of Doppler pressure measurements with comparison to the contralateral side and/or angiography is required. Knee dislocations may spontaneously reduce; therefore any knee injury involving three ligaments should be considered as a potential dislocation and treated accordingly. For those dislocations that do not spontaneously reduce, a reduction should be attempted at the sidelines to prevent neurovascular compromise of the extremity. A non-reducible knee dislocation constitutes a surgical emergency if there is neurovascular compromise.

Pathophysiology

Classification of knee dislocation is based on the displacement of the tibia in relation to the femur. The most common type of dislocation is anterior, which usually occurs due to hyperextension along with an anterior force against the distal thigh.

Posterior dislocation occurs from a direct blow to the anterior, proximal tibia, which forces it posteriorly in relation to the distal femur. Again, the cruciates fail with this force, and collateral ligament injury is present. Vascular injury, specifically stretching or tearing of the popliteal artery, is the most common in anterior and posterior dislocations.

Medial and lateral dislocations occur secondary to extreme varus or valgus stress to the knee, which involve injury first to the collaterals, followed by cruciate injury. An example of rotatory instability is injury to the posterior cruciate ligament (PCL) and posterolateral corner caused by a posteriorly directed force applied to the anteromedial tibia of a hyperextended knee. Injury to the common peroneal nerve is most common in this type of dislocation. Other rotatory combinations of injury can occur.

Evaluation

Complete sustained dislocation of the knee is a straightforward diagnosis, with joint deformity, pain, swelling, and lack of range of motion the obvious presenting signs. A grossly unstable knee involving multiple ligaments should be a presumed occult dislocation until proven otherwise. Stability of anterior cruciate ligament (ACL), PCL, and collateral ligaments should be tested by the usual clinical examinations. Even in the event of normal appearing circulation and pulses, if a knee dislocation is thought to have occurred, objective examination by Doppler pressure measurement of ankle brachial indexes must be performed. Any abnormality warrants an arteriogram, and if vascular injury is confirmed, emergent repair by a vascular surgeon. A tear of the intimal layer of the popliteal artery may occur with a knee dislocation resulting in normal pulses initially but later the artery may occlude, thus serial examinations are important, especially if no angiogram is obtained.

Management

Although knowledge of the direction of injury can help reduction, it is often not necessary to successfully reduce the knee. Gentle axial traction of the distal extremity is often enough to reduce the tibia back under the femur. In the case of posterior dislocation, flexion of the knee with anterior pull on the leg may be necessary for the proximal tibia to clear the femoral condyles (Fig. 6-3). Uncommonly, a knee dislocation (buttonholed posterolateral) cannot be reduced without surgery. All dislocations, complete or presumed, should be placed in a knee immobilizer and transferred to the nearest emergency room for further evaluation.

Return to Sport

Return to sport depends of course on the injury, likely surgical reconstruction of ligaments, and associated injury to other structures. Due to the great extent of damage that can occur with this type of injury, some athletes will never return to sport. For those who do recover, training may resume only when there is full and pain-free range of motion, good strength, and full functional use has been achieved–usually at least a year from surgical reconstruction.

Complications

Popliteal artery disruption occurs in 20–40% of all knee dislocations (highest with posterior knee dislocation). Studies have reported a lower incidence of vascular injury for knee dislocation by a lower-energy mechanism (Shelbourne, 1991). There is a significant risk of amputation in those with knee dislocations complicated by vascular injury. Neurologic injury, especially of the peroneal nerve, has a poor prognosis for complete recovery. Gross fracture or osteochondral injuries are quite common with this injury mechanism.

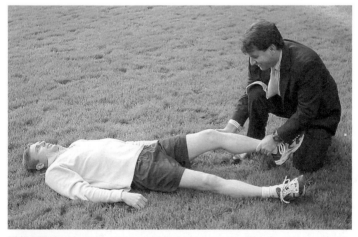

FIG 6-3 Reduction of knee dislocation (posterior): Gentle axial traction is applied distal to a partially flexed knee. Anterior push on the proximal tibia may assist clearance for a posterior dislocation as the tibia passes beyond the femoral condyles.

PATELLAR DISLOCATION

Epidemiology

Although patellar dislocations can occur after a prodromal period of sub-luxation, acute injury after a single traumatic event is more common in athletes. The patella is displaced outside the trochlea to the lateral side of the knee.

Pathophysiology

Patellar dislocation can occur as a non-contact injury or due to a direct blow to the medial patella. In the former case, a pivoting, jumping, or twisting motion from a flexed and valgus positioned knee causes failure of the medial retinaculum and vastus medialis obliquus (VMO).

Evaluation

The athlete will usually describe a history of a popping sensation in the knee, followed by the joint "giving out." Acute and often tense hemarthrosis is frequently encountered on physical examination. Focal tenderness will be appreciated over the medial retinaculum and sometimes at the superior aspect of the adductor tubercle. Integrity of the ligamentous structures of the knee should be examined through stability testing.

Management

Reduction

Spontaneous reduction is frequently the case when the knee is brought into extension. Otherwise, during extension, the examiner may provide medially directed pressure on the laterally displaced patella to bring it back into position in the trochlea (Fig. 6-4).

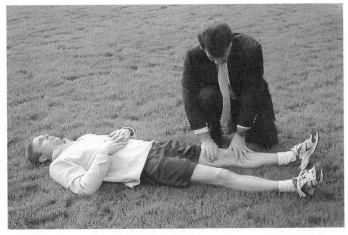

FIG 6-4 Reduction of patellar dislocation: Medially directed pressure is applied to the laterally displaced patella with the knee in full extension.

Aftercare

Immobilization in a knee immobilizer or rehabilitation brace locked in extension is required. In addition, it is advisable to use a pad laterally on the knee to medialize the patella in a reduced position during the time of immobilization. Early active range of motion exercises with the patella taped or braced medially will help regain joint mobility. A postreduction radiograph will demonstrate any osteochondral avulsion fractures that commonly accompany this injury.

Return to Sport

Athletes may return to training and competition in 6–8 weeks with a knee sleeve with lateral buttress if there is no effusion, full range of motion, and strength at least 80% of the contralateral (normal) side.

Complications

Osteochondral fractures complicate up to 30% of patellar dislocations. The loose bodies produced usually require arthroscopic removal (Hutchinson, 1995). Recurrent instability demonstrated by repeated patellar dislocation is an indication for surgical realignment of the extensor mechanism. Concomitant injury of the ACL, medial collateral ligament (MCL), or both is possible with this injury pattern.

FINGER DISLOCATIONS

Epidemiology

Dislocation of the finger joints is seen quite commonly, usually when a ball or an opponent hyperextend the finger. Sports that place severe mechanical strain on the digits, such as rock climbing or wrestling, also can cause dislocation via direct failure of stabilizing structures. Of the digits, the little finger is the most commonly dislocated, primarily due to its lateral prominence in the abducted position, and subsequent tendency to get caught on jerseys or other opponents in contact sports.

Pathophysiology

The proximal interphalangeal (PIP) joint is most commonly dislocated, via a hyperextension injury that dislocates the middle phalanx dorsally in relation to the proximal. In a simple dislocation, the volar plate avulses at its attachment at the base of the middle phalanx. Collateral ligaments and joint capsule may also be disrupted in this injury mechanism.

Volar dislocation of the PIP joint is less common and for this reason may actually be overlooked. The mechanism of injury classically involves a violent force applied to a flexed PIP joint, resulting in proximal rupture of a collateral ligament and subsequent tearing of the insertion of the extensor tendon's central slip.

In contrast to the simple dislocations described, the PIP joint can also be subject to complex dislocation or rotatory subluxation. In this type of dislocation, the condyle of the proximal phalanx buttonholes through a longitudinal rent in the extensor hood between the central slip and lateral band.

The metacarpalphalangeal (MP) joint is less commonly dislocated in the fingers, primarily due to its recessed position in the web spaces of the hand.

However, the MP joint of the thumb, less protected by the soft tissues and more vulnerable in abduction, is subject to frequent injury. As in the PIP joint, MP joint dislocation occurs most commonly in the dorsal direction. But here, the more attenuated volar plate is not anchored by check ligaments, and can become interposed in the joint to prevent reduction (complex dislocation). Volar dislocation of the MP joint is quite rare.

Evaluation

As with most dislocations, the injured athlete will complain of pain and demonstrate tenderness to palpation and decreased range of motion at the affected joint. Dorsal PIP dislocations can be recognized visibly by excessive prominence of the middle phalanx, and by particular tenderness to palpation at the volar aspect of the joint. Volar PIP dislocations are often more subtle, but show some evidence of malrotation on close clinical inspection.

Simple dorsal dislocation of the MP joint presents with the proximal phalanx in approximately 60–80° of hyperextension in relation to the metacarpal. However, complex dorsal dislocations demonstrate only a moderate extension deformity of the MP joint. Volar displacement of the metacarpal head produces palmar prominence and dorsal hollowing.

Management

Reduction

For dorsal PIP dislocation, the reduction maneuver involves traction, mild hyperextension, and the direct pressure on the base of the middle phalanx. In the case of a volar PIP dislocation, hyperextension, traction, and then gentle flexion will usually allow reduction. Closed reduction of a complex or rotatory PIP dislocation is rarely successful and usually requires open treatment.

Simple dorsal MP joint dislocations must be carefully reduced so as not to produce an irreducible complex dislocation. In contrast to the analogous PIP injury, neither hyperextension nor traction should be used. Instead, the examiner should first flex the wrist and then apply steady pressure in a distal and volar direction over the dorsal base of the proximal phalanx. Complex dorsal dislocation and volar MP joint dislocation are usually irreducible in closed fashion, and often require open reduction.

Aftercare

For dorsal PIP dislocations, immobilization consists of *extension block splinting* for 3 weeks. The finger is splinted with the PIP joint in 20–30° of flexion to allow adequate healing of the volar plate. Following discontinuation of the splint, an active flexion program should begin along with a period of buddy taping (approximately 2 weeks or until asymptomatic) for continued protection of the joint. Volar PIP dislocations are splinted in extension for approximately 6 weeks.

As complex or rotatory dislocations are generally reduced by open means, they usually require immobilization for approximately 4 weeks for proper healing of repaired collateral ligaments and central slip.

Simple dorsal MP joint dislocations are immobilized for approximately 2 weeks. In the case of thumb dislocation, a plaster thumb spica splint will provide the best immobilization. Follow a similar time course as the analogous injury in the PIP. Complex dorsal and volar MP joints are immobilized for a similar period of time following open reduction.

Return to Sport

Following brief initial periods of immobilization, athletes have been known to return to competition while wearing low-profile or silicone splints. But, return to sport without immobilization is only advisable when the affected joint is pain free and fully stable through a full range of motion.

Complications

Without adequate early motion of reduced dislocations, joint stiffness is a common sequela. Inadequate splinting and healing of finger dislocations can result in residual instability and recurrent dislocations. In the case of dorsal PIP dislocation, inadequate healing of the volar plate may manifest as a swan neck deformity.

OTHER JOINTS OF INTEREST

Hip Dislocation

Although an uncommon injury in sports, hip dislocation is a true orthopedic emergency and therefore merits mention. The high-energy mechanism required to dislocate the hip joint usually occurs by violent impact to the knee while the hip is flexed. On the field, this might take the form of a football or rugby tackle, or as a hockey check on the ice. The femoral head almost always dislocates posteriorly. Since the blood supply to the femoral head enters through the joint capsule, it can be disrupted in this injury. Emergent reduction of the hip joint is necessary to restore blood supply and prevent the development of avascular necrosis (AVN) of the femoral head. A study by Dreinhofer et al found that among simple posterior dislocations, 19% were complicated by AVN and 26% were complicated by osteoarthritis (Dreinhofer, 1994). The risk of AVN increases if reduction is delayed more than 6 hours or multiple closed reduction attempts are made. Sciatic nerve injury may also be present (in 10% of posterior dislocations), so careful neurologic examination is tantamount.

The patient will likely be found with the hip flexed and internally rotated. If reduction in the controlled setting of an emergency room cannot be ensured within a 6-hour window, closed reduction should be attempted in the field. With the patient supine on the ground with hip flexed and knee bent at 90°, the examiner applies upward traction to the injured lower extremity while an assistant applies counterforce against the pelvis on the ground (Fig. 6-5). The examiner may provide gentle rotation to assist the reduction. Concentric reduction must be verified by plain radiographs, and possibly by CT scan. Post-reduction treatment varies with regard to immobilization and traction. Weight-bearing status also remains a controversial point, but if a simple posterior dislocation is reduced in a timely fashion, with no increased risk of AVN, partial weight bearing can begin as soon as possible and advanced as tolerated. Rehabilitation, strengthening, and range-of-motion exercises are recommended for 6 weeks. Athletes may return to full activity and sport once full strength and range of motion are regained. Note that hip dislocations may be irreducible in a closed fashion and many require open reduction or may be unstable due to associated fractures of the acetabular wall.

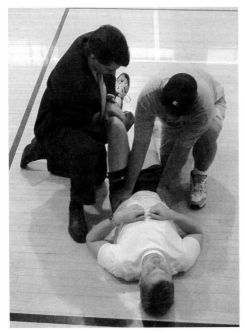

FIG 6-5 Reduction of hip dislocation: While an assistant applies counterforce to the pelvis, upward traction is applied to the lower extremity (flexed 90° at the hip and knee). Gentle internal and external rotation at the hip can assist reduction.

Ankle and Subtalar Dislocation

Dislocation of the ankle without fracture is quite rare. When it does occur, the tibiotalar joint is displaced in the medial, lateral, posteromedial, or posterior direction (in order of decreasing frequency). The mechanism is thought to be due to an axial load applied to the ankle in a plantar flexed position. Neurovascular injury is not commonly reported. Reduction is achieved through axial traction and gentle correction of the direction of deformity. The athlete should be immobilized in a short-leg splint or cast for 6 weeks, the first 2 weeks of which should be non-weight bearing.

Subtalar dislocation secondary to sport injury is well described, particularly in basketball. The dislocation primarily occurs in the medial direction, though lateral is also possible. Subtalar dislocation can be difficult to reduce due to tendon interposition, has a higher incidence of osteochondral injury, and has a poorer overall prognosis following injury. Following closed reduction, short-leg cast immobilization for 4–6 weeks followed by a short-leg walking cast for an additional 4 weeks is recommended.

CONCLUSION

Prompt diagnosis of dislocation on the playing field can allow knowledgeable examiners to triage injuries appropriately and speed initial treatment. When concomitant fracture can be excluded on physical examination, neurovascular status is noted, and benefits outweigh the risks, closed reduction can often be attempted on the sidelines. It is recommended that a reduction should not be attempted on the sidelines if a fracture is suspected. The attempt at reduction should be easy, and if the initial attempt to reduce the dislocation is not successful, then aborting any further attempts on the sideline and transportation to a facility with radiographic capability and anesthetics is recommended. Successfully reduced joints should be reexamined for neurovascular status, immobilized appropriately, and verified radiographically at the nearest hospital. Joint specific aftercare and rehabilitation allow for timely return to sport once pain-free range of motion and full strength are regained.

REFERENCES

Brukner P, Khan K. *Clinical Sports Medicine*, 2nd ed. Sydney: McGraw-Hill; 2001.

Cohen MS, Hastings H, Hastings H 2nd. Acute elbow dislocation: Evaluation and management. *J Am Acad Orthop Surg*. 1998;6:15–23.

Dreinhofer KE, Schwarzkopf SR, Haas NP, et al. Isolated traumatic dislocation of the hip: Long-term results in 50 patients. *J Bone Joint Surg Br*. 1994;76:6–12.

Fu FH, Stone DA. *Sports Injuries: Mechanisms, Prevention, Treatment*. Baltimore: Williams & Wilkins; 1994.

Good L. The dislocated knee. *J Am Acad Orthop Surg*. 1995;3:284–292.

Gustilo RB, Kyle RF, Templeman DC. *Fractures and Dislocations*, vol 1. St. Louis: Mosby; 1993.

Harries M, Williams C, Stanish W, Micheli L. *Oxford Textbook of Sports Medicine*. New York: Oxford University Press; 1994.

Hovelius L. The natural history of primary anterior dislocation of the shoulder in the young. *J Orthop Sci*. 1999;4:307–317.

Hutchinson MR, Ireland ML. Patella dislocation: Recognizing the injury and its complications. *Phys Sports Med*. 1995;23:53–60.

Melone C. Complex joint injuries of the hand. In: Petrone FA, ed. *AAOS Symposium on the Upper Extremity Injuries in Athletes*. St. Louis: Mosby; 1986;142–169.

Melone C. Joint injuries of the fingers and thumb. *Emerg Med Clin North Am*. 1985;3:319–331.

Neviaser RJ, Neviaser TJ, Neviaser JS. Anterior dislocation of the shoulder and rotator cuff rupture. *Clin Orthop*. 1993;Jun:103–106.

O'Donoghue DH. *Treatment of Injuries to Athletes*, 4th ed. Philadelphia: Saunders; 1984.

Perrin DH. *The Injured Athlete*, 3rd ed. Philadelphia: Lippincott-Raven; 1999.

Safran MR, McKeag DB, Van Camp SP. *Manual of Sports Medicine*. Philadelphia: Lippincott-Raven; 1999.

Shelbourne KD, Porter DA, Clingman JA, et al. Low-velocity knee dislocation. *Orthop Rev*. 1991;20:995–1004.

7 | Return to Play: Making the Correct Decision

Robert Sallis and Ronica Martinez

Deciding when to return an athlete to play is an essential role for the physician who cares for active or athletic patients. Whether the patient is a professional athlete, a weekend warrior, or an amateur exerciser, the health care provider must be prepared to help the patient decide if and when they should return to his or her sport or activity. An organized approach to making return to play decisions is essential to ensure the safety of sports and exercise participants. We believe that such an approach can and should be used with all active patients, not just the competitive athlete.

Unfortunately, most return to play decisions will be based on consensus opinion and personal experience, since there are few evidenced-based recommendations available. The 2002 Team Physician Consensus Statement on Return to Play Issues provides an important framework that can be used for making return to play decisions (Table 7-1). This statement was developed through the collaborative effort of six professional organizations concerned with clinical sports medicine issues, to help guide team physicians in making return to play decisions. These guidelines are also quite applicable to other active and athletic patients trying to return to sports or exercise after an injury or illness.

In this chapter, we define the term, return to play, and identify the critical path for making these decisions. We discuss the approach for deciding on return to play (RTP) with both musculoskeletal and medical conditions and identify important outside factors that may impact on the RTP decision (such as psychological and medical-legal issues). We also explore the RTP process as defined in the Team Physician Consensus Statement and discuss its use to safely return the active or athletic patient to competition. Finally, we discuss some commonly encountered conditions that may pose challenging RTP decisions.

RETURN TO PLAY CRITICAL PATH

Return to play can be defined as the process of deciding when an injured or ill athlete may safely return to competition without putting themselves or others at risk for injury or illness. A critical path exists from the time of injury to the point of returning the patient to the desired activity. This path involves a continuum from the sidelines to the training room to the office or hospital. This continuum should be as seamless as possible and involve good communication between players, coaches, and the medical staff. Such communication is essential to foster trust and understanding among all the parties involved.

The return to play decision really begins on the sidelines or on-site at the event where the injury or illness occurs. Sideline or event physicians must use clinical judgment (usually without the availability of diagnostic tests) in deciding about return to play. Sometimes, the decision is quite obvious, other times, it is not. Preventing players from returning to play without a good reason will likely discourage open communication between the team physician and other players and coaches, rendering the team physician ineffective.

TABLE 7-1 The Team Physician and Return-To-Play Issues
Consensus Statement

Summary
The objective of this Consensus Statement is to provide physicians who are responsible for the healthcare of teams with a decision process for determining when to return an injured or ill athlete to practice or competition. This statement is not intended as a standard of care, and should not be interpreted as such. This statement is only a guide, and as such is of a general nature consistent with the reasonable and objective practice of the healthcare professional. Individual decisions regarding returning an injured or ill athlete to play will depend on the specific facts and circumstances presented to the physician.

Adequate insurance should be in place to help protect the athlete, the sponsoring organization, and the physician.

This statement was developed by the collaborative effort of six major professional associations concerned with clinical sports medicine issues; they have committed to forming an ongoing project-based alliance to "bring together sports medicine organizations to best serve active people and athletes." The organizations are: American Academy of Family Physicians, American Academy of Orthopaedic Surgeons, American College of Sports Medicine, American Medical Society for Sports Medicine, American Orthopaedic Society for Sports Medicine; and the American Osteopathic Academy of Sports Medicine.

Definition
Return-To-Play is the process of deciding when an injured or ill athlete may safely return to practice or competition.

Goal
The goal is to return an injured or ill athlete to practice or competition without putting the individual or others at undue risk for injury or illness.

To accomplish this goal, the team physician should have knowledge of and be involved with:

- Establishing a Return-To-Play Process
- Evaluating Injured or Ill Athletes
- Treating Injured or Ill Athletes
- Rehabilitating Injured or Ill Athletes
- Returning an Injured or Ill Athlete to Play

Establishing a return-to-play process
Establishing a process for returning an athlete to play is an essential first step in deciding when an injured or ill athlete may safely return to practice or competition.

It is essential for the team physician to coordinate:

- Establishing a chain of command regarding decisions to return an injured or ill athlete to practice or competition
- Communicating the Return-To-Play process to player, family, certified athletic trainers, coaches, administrators and other healthcare providers
- Establishing a system for documentation
- Establishing protocols to release information regarding an athlete's ability to return to practice or competition following an injury or illness

It is essential that the Return-To-Play process address the:

- Safety of the athlete
- Potential risk to the safety of other participants
- Functional capabilities of the athlete
- Functional requirements of the athlete's sport
- Federal, state, local, school and governing body regulations related to returning an injured or ill athlete to practice or competition

TABLE 7-1 The Team Physician and Return-To-Play Issues
Consensus Statement (*Continued*)

Evaluating injured or ill athletes

Evaluation of an injured or ill athlete establishes a diagnosis, directs treatment and is the basis for deciding when an athlete may safely return to practice or competition. Repeated evaluations throughout the continuum of injury or illness management optimize medical care.

It is essential the evaluation of an injured or ill athlete include:

- A condition-specific medical history
- A condition-specific physical examination
- Appropriate medical tests and consultations
- Psychosocial assessment
- Documentation
- Communication with the player, family, certified athletic trainer, coaches and other healthcare providers

In addition, it is desirable that:

- The team physician coordinate evaluation of the injured or ill athlete

Treating injured or ill athletes

Treatment of an injured or ill athlete promotes the safe and timely return to practice or competition.

It is essential that treatment of the injured or ill athlete:

- Begin in a timely manner (see *Sideline Preparedness for the Team Physician: A Consensus Statement,* (2000)
- Follow an individualized plan, which may include consultations and referrals
- Include a rehabilitation plan
- Include equipment modification, bracing, and orthoses as necessary
- Address psychosocial issues
- Provide a realistic prognosis as to the safe and timely return to practice or competition
- Include continued communication with the player, family, certified athletic trainer, coaches and other healthcare providers

- Include documentation

In addition, it is desirable that:

- The team physician coordinate the initial and ongoing treatment for the injured or ill athlete

Rehabilitating injured or ill athletes

Comprehensive treatment includes proper rehabilitation of an injured or ill athlete, which optimizes the safe and timely return to practice or competition. The team physician should be involved in a network that integrates expertise regarding rehabilitation. This network should include certified athletic trainers, physical therapists, medical specialists and other healthcare providers.

It is essential that the rehabilitation network:

- Coordinate the development of a rehabilitation plan that is designed to:
- Restore function of the injured part
- Restore and promote musculoskeletal and cardiovascular function, as well as overall well-being of the injured or ill athlete
- Provide sport-specific assessment and training, which can serve as a basis for sport-specific conditioning (see *The Team Physician and Conditioning of Athletes for Sports: A Consensus Statement,* (2001)
- Provide for continued equipment modification, bracing and orthoses
- Continue communication with the player, family, rehabilitation network and coaches concerning the athlete's progress
- Include documentation

In addition, it is desirable that:

- The team physician coordinate the rehabilitation program for the injured or ill athlete

Returning an injured or ill athlete to play

The decision for safe and timely return of an injured or ill athlete to

TABLE 7-1 The Team Physician and Return-To-Play Issues
Consensus Statement (*Continued*)

practice or competition is the desired result of the process of evaluation, treatment and rehabilitation.

It is essential for Return-To-Play that the team physician confirm the following criteria:

- The status of anatomical and functional healing
- The status of recovery from acute illness and associated sequelae
- The status of chronic injury or illness
- That the athlete pose no undue risk to the safety of other participants
- Restoration of sport-specific skills
- Psychosocial readiness
- Ability to perform safely with equipment modification, bracing and orthoses
- Compliance with applicable federal, state, local, school and governing body regulations

Prior to Return-To-Play, these criteria should be confirmed at a satisfactory level.

Conclusion

Using the information in this document allows the team physician to make an informed decision as to whether an injured or ill athlete may safely return to practice or competition.

The Return-To-Play process should be under the direction of the team physician whenever possible. While it is desirable that the team physician coordinate evaluating, treating and rehabilitating the injured or ill athlete, it is essential that the team physician ultimately be responsible for the Return-To-Play decision.

Individual decisions regarding returning an injured or ill athlete to play will depend on the specific facts and circumstances presented to the team physician.

Available Resources

On-going education pertinent to the team physician is essential. Information regarding team physician-specific educational opportunities can be obtained from the six participating organizations:

American Academy of Family Physicians (AAFP)
11400 Tomahawk Creek Pkwy, Leawood KS 66211
800-274-2237 • www.aafp.org

American Academy of Orthopaedic Surgeons (AAOS)
6300 N River Rd, Rosemont IL 60018
800-346-AAOS • www.aaos.org

American College of Sports Medicine (ACSM)
401 W Michigan St, Indianapolis IN 46202
317-637-9200 • www.acsm.org

American Medical Society for Sports Medicine (AMSSM)
11639 Earnshaw, Overland Park KS 66210
913-327-1415 • www.amssm.org

American Orthopaedic Society for Sports Medicine (AOSSM)
6300 N River Rd Suite 200, Rosemont IL 60018
847-292-4900 • www.sportsmed.org

American Osteopathic Academy of Sports Medicine (AOASM)
7611 Elmwood Ave Suite 201, Middleton WI 53562
608-831-4400 • www.aoasm.org

Expert Panel:
Stanley A. Herring, M.D., Chair, Seattle, Washington; John A. Bergfeld, M.D., Cleveland, Ohio; Joel Boyd, M.D., Edina, Minnesota; Timothy Duffey, D.O., Columbus, Ohio; Karl B. Fields, M.D., Greensboro, North Carolina; William A. Grana, M.D., Tucson, Arizona; Peter Indelicato, M.D., Gainesville, Florida; W. Ben Kibler, M.D., Lexington, Kentucky; Robert Pallay, M.D., Hillsborough, New Jersey; Margot Putukian, M.D., University Park, Pennsylvania; and Robert E. Sallis, M.D., Alta Loma, California.
    Please refer to the Suggested Readings for further information.
(*Source: From Herring et al., 2002.*)

The objective of the sideline evaluation is to quickly sort each injury or illness into one of three categories. These include:

1. Life or limb threatening—the goal is to immediately stabilize and transport the patient.
2. Serious—the athlete should be withheld from competition and appropriate arrangements made for follow-up and treatment.
3. Minor—the goal should be to help the athlete to return to play.

From the sidelines or site of competition, the path then moves to the training room, the office, and even the hospital if needed. The first priority is to establish or confirm a working diagnosis. Arrangements should be made for consultation, diagnostic imaging, and laboratory evaluation as needed. Next, should be the development of a treatment plan along with decisions about rehabilitation or treatment modalities that may be helpful. Once the athlete is ready to return to competition, equipment modifications or bracing should be suggested where appropriate. With athletes who cannot play or practice, it is essential to give a plan to maintain fitness, as well as rehabilitation for injury (modified rest). Rarely should complete rest be the plan. Throughout this process, it is critical to communicate with the player (and parents), coaches, and trainers.

The critical path to return to play is essentially the same, whether the athlete has a musculoskeletal or medical problem. In the athlete with a musculoskeletal problem, the path begins with diagnosis and appropriate initial treatment. This includes an acute management phase (RICE), followed by rehabilitation as pain allows. Early range-of-motion exercises as tolerated can speed recovery from many conditions. Finally, a functional progression of activity should be followed prior to allowing return to play. An example of such a progression could include sequential sessions of walking, jogging, running, sprinting, and then cutting. Activity would advance in intensity as soon as the patient was able to perform without pain.

Similarly, the path for return to play with a medical problem also begins with diagnosis and appropriate treatment. Next, an assessment must be made regarding potential risks to the athlete of participation. Additionally, the physician should also assess risks to other participants (primarily where the condition is infectious). Where the risk is low, a similar progression of activity should be followed leading to a return to play.

GENERAL PRINCIPLES FOR RETURN TO PLAY DECISION

There are some important general principles that should be followed when deciding on return to play. First and foremost, the physician should always put the welfare of the athlete first. In doing so, do not assume every athlete actually wants to return to play. It may be appropriate to ask them, as an occasional athlete will use injury to discontinue a sport or sport season.

It is also critical to try to maintain cardiovascular fitness and strength during the recovery period. Part of every treatment and rehabilitation program should be a plan to maintain fitness and strength as much as possible. Failure to do so will only further delay an athlete's return to his or her pre-injury or illness level.

Finally, the physician must also take into consideration the demands of the sport and the player's position in light of the injury or illness. As an example, a shoulder problem would require much more scrutiny in deciding return to play in a baseball player than in a soccer player.

OTHER CONSIDERATIONS

There are common pitfalls to be avoided when making return to play decisions. First, *do not be a coach.* Do not let game situations affect judgment. Whether the team is ahead or behind or whether the player is a star or a reserve, should not affect your decision. Second, *do not be a fan.* Do not let your partiality to the team or players affect judgment. And third, *do not consider the importance of the player to the game, but do consider the importance of the game to the player* when you make a return to play decision. (Never say, "this is only a high school football game.")

Keep in mind the psychological issues that commonly impact the return to play decision. Players must remain a part of the team as much as possible. They should maintain a daily activity routine that is similar to their teammates while recovering from an illness or injury. It is common to see depression, anger, or acting out among injured or ill players. It is again important not to underestimate the importance of the sport to the player.

Lastly, there are a variety of medical-legal issues that can also affect the return to play decision. It is important to remember that a physician can make recommendations regarding return to play, but the ultimate decision rests with the athlete (and parents, in the case of a minor) and the school. The American's with Disabilities Act and Rehabilitation Act of 1973 prohibit discrimination against people with disabilities. These laws have been used to force an athlete's participation despite objections from physicians and team staff. In addition, experience has shown that waivers are of limited value, especially where minors are concerned (Mitten, 1996).

RETURN TO PLAY PROCESS—THE ESSENTIAL COMPONENTS

The 2002 Team Physician Consensus Statement on Return to Play Issues divided the return to play process into four phases (Herring et al., 2000). These included:

1. Evaluating injured or ill athletes.
2. Treating injured or ill athletes.
3. Rehabilitating an injured or ill athlete.
4. Returning an injured or ill athlete to play.

The consensus statement (see Table 7-1) presents details of the essential components of each of these phases.

SPECIFIC CONDITIONS

Again, realizing that there are very few evidence-based guidelines, the following is a review of return to play recommendations for some commonly encountered conditions.

Illness

Upper Respiratory Infection and Febrile Illness

Probably the most common illness encountered by an athlete is an upper respiratory infection (URI) and febrile illness. A "neck check" approach is a simplistic guide. For symptoms above the neck (congestion, rhinorrhea, or sore throat), the athlete can usually practice or compete at a lower intensity level. If symptoms are below the neck (cough, chest congestion, fever, chills, myalgias) or if there are any systemic symptoms, it is recommended that the athlete abstain (McGrew, 2002; O'Kane, 2002). The team physician must take into account whether clearance must be made for practice or competition and decide accordingly. The athlete must take into account the risk of spreading the illness to teammates and coaches.

Hepatitis

The American Medical Society for Sports Medicine (AMSSM) position statement recommends that an athlete's return to practice or competition status must be guided by his or her clinical condition. He or she must have normal liver function tests and there should be no clinical evidence of hepatomegaly (Committee on Sports Medicine and Fitness, 1999; McGrew, 2002).

Human Immunodeficiency Virus

Multiple organizations (including the American Academy of Pediatrics, NCAA, NFL, and World Health Organization) agree that an athlete with HIV infection is permitted to participate in competitive sports at all levels. The team physician should evaluate an athlete interested in contact sports (such as wrestling, football, and boxing), on an individual basis (Committee on Sports Medicine and Fitness, 1999). The physician must make a medical judgment as to whether the athlete poses a significant risk of communicating the disease to others in competition. If it is felt that there is a risk for disease spread, a reasonable accommodation should be made to allow competition.

The team physician must pay special attention to confidentiality and legal issues regarding blood-borne pathogens. Except for reporting as required by law, the patient must give consent for clinicians to share information about HIV status with sports organizations or school officials (Committee on Sports Medicine and Fitness, 1999).

Mononucleosis

The recommendations for infectious mononucleosis and return to play are similar to viral infection and fever. Most experts agree with a relative restriction (avoidance of resistance training and contact activity) during the first 3 weeks after diagnosis and/or onset of symptoms (since splenic rupture usually occurs during the first 3 weeks of the illness). An athlete must have normal liver function tests, improving symptoms, and a normal spleen size by clinical examination (MacKnight, 2002; McGrew, 2002). The team physician must make sure that the athlete's strength is adequate to safely participate in his or her sport or activity, keeping in mind that it may take months for the athlete to get back to pre-illness strength and conditioning (McGrew, 2002). If the athlete does have evidence of an enlarged spleen, the recommendation by the AAP is to avoid all contact activity; however, there are no clear guidelines. Sonogram may be useful to document normalization of an enlarged spleen.

Contagious Skin Conditions

Herpes Gladiatorum

Herpes gladiatorum is the clinical diagnosis given when herpes simplex virus affects wrestlers. Athletes should not participate in contact sports if there is evidence of vesicular lesions or ulcers on any exposed skin. If the lesions are scabbed and dry, it may be reasonable to allow competition. Some physicians recommend return to competition only after 120 hours (5 days) of oral treatment with acyclovir 400 mg tid (Dienst, 1997; National Federation of State High School Associations, 2002).

Fungal Infections

NCAA guidelines stipulate that an athlete must have received at least 3 days of topical treatment for skin lesions, and 2 weeks of systemic treatment for scalp lesions, to participate. Those players with extensive or active lesions should be excluded from contact sports. Lesions should be covered with a gas-permeable dressing and stretch tape (Bergfeld, 1984; Dienst, 1997; National Federation of State High School Associations, 2002).

Impetigo

Return to practice or competition for impetigo is similar to herpes simplex virus. The athlete should not return to contact sports if lesions are weeping or have a moist crust (Bergfeld, 1984; Dienst, 1997; National Federation of State High School Associations, 2002). It is reasonable to allow return to play after at least 5 days of antibiotics if the lesions are dry and crusted (National Federation of State High School Associations, 2002).

Injuries

Concussions

Concussion management is among the most controversial subjects with regard to return to play. While multiple grading systems and guidelines for return to play exist, none are evidenced based. Despite this, guidelines can be useful to help guide return to play decisions after concussion (Kushner, 2001). Among the most commonly used concussion guidelines are those issued by the American Academy of Neurology (AAN), which are outlined as follows.

AAN Guidelines for RTP After Concussion

1. *Grade 1 Concussion* [no loss of consciousness (LOC), symptoms lasting less than 15 minutes]
   A. *First one:* remove from contest. Observe every 5 minutes for the development of amnesia or postconcussive symptoms, both at rest and with exertion. May return if no amnesia or other symptoms appear after 20 minutes.
   B. *Second one:* if in the same game, should eliminate player from that game. Should sit out 1-week symptom free.

2. *Grade 2 Concussion* (no LOC, symptoms lasting more than 15 minutes).
   A. *First one:* remove from contest with no return that day. Observe for signs of evolving intracranial pathology. May return to play after 1-week symptom free.
   B. *Second one:* hold player out for 2 weeks symptom free.

3. *Grade 3 Concussion* (any LOC)
   A. If player is unconscious, assume cervical spine fracture and place on spine board. Transport to nearest hospital for evaluation. Strongly

consider CT scan or MRI. Admit to hospital if signs of pathology detected.
B. *First one:* if brief *(seconds)*, hold player out for 1-week symptom free. If *prolonged (minutes)*, hold player out for 2 weeks.
C. *Second one:* hold player out for 1-month symptom free at minimum (may be longer).

Transient Brachial Plexopathy (Cervical Burners)

Prior to return to play after a cervical burner, there must be a complete resolution of symptoms, along with an intact neurologic examination (including normal strength and sensation in the upper extremities). There should also be full cervical spine range of motion, and normal atlanto-axial compression (Spurling) test. Athletes with neck pain, radiating arm pain, or loss of neck motion should be removed from play until further evaluation (McAlindon, 2002; Proctor, 2000; Shannon, 2002). Athletes with recurrent burners or persistent symptoms need radiographic evaluation of the neck including flexion and extension views. Neck strengthening exercises, equipment modifications, and changes in blocking and tackling technique may help prevent recurrences (Sallis, 1992).

Acromioclavicular Joint Separations

Athletes can return to play after a type 1 or 2 injury when full range of motion is pain-free and muscle strength is adequate (Hutchinson, 1996). Type 3 injuries involve a complete acromioclavicular (AC) dislocation. The majority of these can be treated conservatively, but can take as long as 10–12 weeks to allow the athlete to return to practice and competition (Hutchinson, 1996). All AC separations should be treated on an individual basis, with a goal for pain-free range of motion and good muscle strength.

Shoulder Dislocation

In the acute phase, the shoulder should be immobilized for 1–3 weeks until resolution of pain. Passive range-of-motion (ROM) exercises should then be started as tolerated, followed by aggressive physical therapy. Return to play is considered only when there is full ROM and strength (typically 3 months or more) (Safran, 2002). Some expert opinion is moving toward early return to play when there is no pain, smooth ROM below 90 degrees, and strong muscle activation for deltoid and rotator cuff with a brace to limit abduction. A graduated sports-specific activity program should precede return to play. Surgery may be considered in younger at risk athletes.

Anterior Cruciate Ligament Tears and Reconstruction

There is tremendous variability in the return to play recommendations after ACL surgery. Typically, rehabilitation progresses in three stages:

1. Stage 1 (about 6–8 weeks duration) consists of controlling pain and regaining range of motion. Crutches are typically used for 5–10 days, followed by progressive weight bearing.
2. Stage 2 (about 3–5 months duration) primarily involves regaining full muscle strength. Use of cycling and treadmill are helpful, along with specific therapy exercises.
3. Stage 3 (about 2–7 months duration) consists of a graduated return to activity.
4. Most patients return to activity between 6 and 12 months after surgery.

Ankle Sprains

There is no specific time-line for deciding RTP after an ankle sprain, as decisions must be individualized. Prior to returning an athlete to competition, he or she must undergo proper rehabilitation to achieve full and pain-free range of motion, proper strengthening for activity, proprioceptive training, and sports-specific exercises (Hockenbury, 2001; Sallis, 1997). If all of these are satisfactory, consideration to return to competition can be made. Bracing or an orthosis may be helpful.

CONCLUSION

Deciding on return to play is an important responsibility of any provider who cares for active or athletic patients. Clinical judgment is essential in making these decisions, especially when on the sidelines. Unfortunately, there are very few evidence-based guidelines to help with the return to play decision. The decision path should begin on the field and continue on to the training room, the office, and/or hospital when needed. Following a step-wise approach, including evaluation, treatment, and rehabilitation, will help ensure a safe return from injury or illness.

REFERENCES

Allen CR, Kang JD. Transient quadriparesis in the athlete. *Clin Sports Med.* 2002;21:15–27.

Aubry M, Cantu R, et al. Summary and agreement statement of First International Conference on Concussion in Sport. Vienna, 2001.

Bergfeld WF. Dermatologic problems in athletes. *Primary Care.* 1984;11:151–160.

Committee on Sports Medicine and Fitness. Human immunodeficiency virus and other blood-borne viral pathogens in the athletic setting. *Pediatrics* 1999;104.

Dienst WL, Dightman L, et al. Pinning down skin infections: Diagnosis, treatment, and prevention in wrestlers. *Physician Sports Med.* 1997;25.

Evans NA, Chew HF, Stanish WD. The natural history and tailored treatment of ACL injury. *Physician Sports Med.* 2001;29.

Herring SA, Bergfeld JA, Boyd J, et al. The team physician and return-to-play issues: A consensus statement. *Med Sci Sport Exerc.* 2002;34:1212–1214.

Hockenbury RT, Sammarco GJ. Evaluation and treatment of ankle sprains. *Physician Sports Med.* 2001;29.

Hutchinson MR, Ahuja GS. Diagnosing and treating clavicular injuries. *Physician Sports Med.* 1996;24.

Johnson RJ. Acromioclavicular joint injuries, identifying and treating 'separated shoulder' and other conditions. *Physician Sports Med.* 2001;29.

Kushner DS. Concussion in Sports: Minimizing the Risk for Complications. *Am Fam Physician.* 2001;64:1007–1014.

MacKnight JM. Infectious mononucleosis, ensuring a safe return to sport. *Physician Sports Med.* 2002;30.

Mast EE, Goodman RA. Prevention of infectious disease transmission in sports. *Sports Med.* 1997;24:1–7.

McAlindon RJ. On field evaluation and management of head and neck injured athletes. *Clin Sports Med.* 2002;21:1–14.

McGrew CA, Martinez R. What recommendations should be made concerning exercising with a fever and or acute infection. In: MacAulley D, Best T, eds. *Evidence Based Sports Medicine.* 1st ed. London: British Medical Journal; 2002;83–96.

Mitten MJ. When is disqualification from sports justified? Medical judgement vs patients' rights. *Physician Sports Med.* 1996;24.

Moeller JL. Contraindications to athletic participation: Cardiac, respiratory, and central nervous system conditions. *Physician Sports Med.* 1996;24.

Moeller JL. Contraindications to athletic participation: Spinal, systemic, dermatologic, paired-organ, and other issues. *Physician Sports Med.* 1996;24.

National Federation of State High School Associations. *Physician release for wrestlers to participate with skin lesions.* June 2002.

O'Kane JW. Upper respiratory infection, helpful steps for physicians. *Physician Sports Med.* 2002;30.

Proctor MR, Cantu RC. Head and neck injuries in young athletes. *Clin Sports Med.* 2000;19:693–715.

Safran MR, Dorey FJ, Sachs RA. How should you treat an athlete with a first time dislocation of the shoulder. In: MacAulley D, Best T, eds. *Evidence Based Sports Medicine.* 1st ed. London: British Medical Journal; 2002;318–350.

Sallis RE, Jones K, Knopp W. Burners: Offensive strategy for an underreported injury. *Physician Sports Med.* 1992;64.

Sallis RE, Massisino F. *ACSM'S Essentials of Sports Medicine.* St. Louis: Mosby; 1997.

Shannon B, Klimkiewicz JJ. Cervical burners in the athlete. *Clin Sports Med.* 2002;21:29–35.

Stacey A, Atkins B. Infectious disease in rugby players—Incidence, treatment and prevention. *Sports Med.* 2000;9:211–220.

Vaccaro AR, Watkins B, et al. Review- Cervical spine injuries in athletes: Current return-to-play criteria. *Orthopedics.* 2001;24:699–703.

SUGGESTED READINGS

AAFP, AAP, AMSSM, AOSSM, AOASM. *Preparticipation Physical Evaluation,* 2nd ed. The Physician and Sportsmedicine; Minneapolis; McGraw-Hill Healthcare; 1997.

Adams BB. Transmission of cutaneous infections in athletes. *Br J Sports Med.* 2000;34:413–414.

American College of Sports Medicine, American College of Cardiology, 26th Bethesda Conference, Recommendations for competition in athletes with cardiovascular abnormalities. *Med Sci Sports Exerc.* 1994;26:5223–5283.

American Medical Society for Sports Medicine, American Academy of Sports Medicine. Human Immunodeficiency Virus and Other Blood-Borne Pathogens in Sports, Joint Position Statement. *Clin J Sports Med.* 1995;5:199–204.

Cantu RC. Return-to-play guidelines after a head injury. *Clin J Sports Med.* 1998;17:45–60.

Cantu RC. Stingers, transient quadriplegia and cervical spinal stenosis; return-to-play criteria. *Med Sci Sports Exerc.* 1997;29(7 Suppl): S233–235.

Committee on Sports Medicine and Fitness. Cardiac dysrhythmias and sports. *Pediatrics.* 1995;95:786–789.

Goodman R, Thacker S, Soloman S, et al. Infectious disease in competitive sports. *JAMA* 1994;271:862–866.

Herring SA. Rehabilitation of muscle injuries. *Med Sci Sports Exerc.* 1990;22:453–456.

Kibler WB, Herring SA, Press JM. *Functional Rehabilitation of Sports and Musculoskeletal Injuries.* Aspen; Gaithersburg, Md: 1998.

Kibler WB, Livingston BP. Closed-chain rehabilitation for upper and lower extremities. *J Am Acad Orthop Surg.* 2001;9:412–421.

Maron BJ. Cardiovascular risks to young persons on the athletic field. *Ann Intern Med.* 1998;129:379–386.

Mellion, MB, Walsh WM, Madden C, Putukian, M, Shelton GI eds. *Team Physician's Handbook,* 3rd ed. Philadelphia: Hanley & Belfus, 2002.

Mitten MJ, Mitten RJ. Legal considerations in treating the injured athlete. *J Orthop Sports Phys Ther.* 1995;21:38–43.

8 | Computers in Sports Medicine

Don Johnson

How can rehabilitation team members improve communication in clinical sports medicine? By the use of computers. The modern practice of sports medicine will gradually evolve to the computerization of the patient record, outcome studies, and the on-field documentation of the athlete's injury. The days of the sideline "jock doc" with a trusty little bag of zinc oxide tape and T3s will be replaced with a modern sports medicine trained physician and with a handheld computer. The accurate and timely documentation of athletic injuries will be more detailed and important in the future. The new physician must know how to communicate with the patient and their family, the referring physician, and with other physicians for educational purposes.

COMMUNICATION

Communication with the Patient

The old paternalistic days of the sports doc simply saying "We will fix you and make you better" is no longer acceptable as informed consent. After an Internet search about his or her options for treatment, the patient is often as well informed as the treating physician. Accordingly, the physician must keep his or her knowledge of sports medicine injuries and treatment up to date.

The patient will understand explanations much better if he or she can review handouts, video tapes, or web sites with the relevant information about the condition. The physician should refer the patient to specific Internet sites for patient information. A good place to start is http://www. orthogate.com. Go to the OWL, orthopedic web listing, and look under the category of patient information sites. The information sites are all approved by an orthopedic surgeon before listing. This will assure that the patient is reading sanctioned medical information.

Another way to achieve this goal is to establish a clinic web site with suitable patient information that you have authored. An example of this is found at www.carletonsportsmed.com under patient information. The information can be changed and easily updated when required. The decision aid for anterior cruciate ligament (ACL) injury provides the patient with the necessary information to make a choice from the options for ACL treatment.

Patients may also use www.google.com to search the Internet for information. Some of the sites, such as Bobs bum knees (http://factotem.org/cgi-bin/kneebbs.pl), provide a message board for patients to chat about their ACL injury. This type of information from other patients that have had an ACL injury can be invaluable and may fill a gap that the medical staff members are unable to provide.

Communication about the Patient

The documentation of the patient's problem and treatment must be more detailed than in the past. This is especially true for the sideline work that is required of the sports physician. Even if this is a Friday night high school football game involving your son, you must document the results of your examination and treatment on the sidelines. There should also be universal

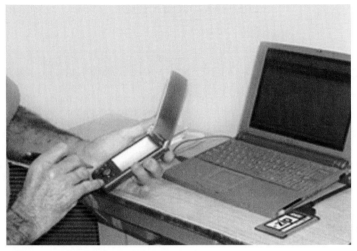

FIG 8-1   The electronic documentation of the patient record on a handheld PDA.

access to the athlete's medical history and demographics. The easiest and quickest way to do this is to carry the information on a handheld device (Fig. 8-1), input any new information at the time of examination, and later sync this to your office computer. This becomes part of the patient chart, and can be reviewed when the patient returns for follow up the next week.

Yes, this will increase your office expenditures. You need to have a handheld computer and software that is present on both the office computer and the handheld. If you just want to use handheld offsite electronically, the information you gather may be printed from the office computer and put into the traditional paper patient chart. Eventually, sports medicine physicians will want to move toward an electronic system for the office. Will there be any return on the investment? The main return is the peace of mind that you have documented your off-site treatment in a timely and adequate fashion.

What is required? A handheld PDA, such as the Compaq iPAC, that runs Windows Pocket PC is needed. One version of software is Team Physician from Aristar (www.aristar.com). This software can be upgraded to the full musculoskeletal module for use in the office. The patient can be registered and the entire patient file recorded electronically. An electronic tablet, such as the viewpad by Viewsonic, makes the in-office application much more user friendly. The tablet is about the same size as a normal 11 × 8.5 sheet of paper, providing more electronic real estate to work on. The data are entered on the touch screen using pull-down menus. The viewpad may be synched with the office computer in the same fashion as the handheld PDA. This system is very quick and efficient, after the short learning curve.

The results of the examination and on-field treatment can be sent to the trainer, team, or referring physician. Everyone will appreciate this detailed and timely transfer of information.

Communication with the Physician

The information about the patient may be communicated to the athlete's physician by the usual referral letter. The letter can be generated electronically from the information entered via the handheld computer. To get further input from the treatment team members, the information can be presented in a PowerPoint presentation at sports medicine rounds. Most of the university-based sports medicine clinics have weekly rounds to discuss sports medicine topics. A modern version of the rounds process is electronic mailing lists. The information can be posted to a site where other sports medicine physicians can give opinions on suitable treatment for the patient. An example of a sports medicine mailing list can be found on the www.orthogate.com site.

Information can be posted to a web site to inform other physicians about sports medicine topics. An example of this is found at www.carleton-sportsmed.com under physician education. The information is topical and can be easily updated as required.

Using an electronic record makes the acquisition of data much more reliable and easy for use to carry out clinical research. The International Knee Documentation Committee (IKDC) form for outcome of ACL reconstruction is now available electronically. The patient can fill in the subjective evaluation form online, or at the office on a touch screen. The physicians follow-up examination is entered either on a computer or handheld device and added to the data collected preoperatively. These data reside on the electronic office server computer, but can be accessed by satellite laptops in the examination rooms. The data can be output into a research access database for analysis.

From these data, publications and research papers can be generated concerning the outcome of treatment for ACL injuries and surgery. Rounds, sports medicine symposiums, and international meetings will benefit from research data that are collected in this fashion.

This type of data collection can be done among several physicians and surgeons and the results pooled to improve the data collection. With the use of handheld devices, the information can be collected at remote sites and taken back to the main server. Multiple sports clinics and physicians can collaborate and share data.

The information gathered can be shared with other physicians in the form of scientific papers, symposiums, and instructional courses. These methods all help to educate other sports medicine physicians about a particular patient's problem.

- The Internet can be searched with MEDLINE to obtain the latest peer-reviewed literature concerning the patient's condition. All the relevant information is only a few clicks away when using PubMed. http://www.ncbi.nlm.nih.gov/entrez/query.fcgi?CMD=Limits&DB=Pub Med

The physician can receive the monthly table of contents via e-mail from scientific journals, such as *The American Journal of Sports Medicine* and *The Journal of Arthroscopy*. Any subscriber can read articles of interest each month online.

Finally, online continuing medical education sites are available to review the latest concepts in the problem that you have encountered with a patient. The American Academy of Orthopedic Surgeons (www.aaos.org) developed a service called Orthopedic Knowledge Online to provide the latest information on all orthopedic topics. The site has text, images, and video to illustrate the individual topics.

Communication, and the resulting information overload, is a part of daily life. To be successful, physicians just need to know how to manage it.

9 | Muscle Training and Conditioning

T. Jeff Chandler

DEFINITION AND IMPORTANCE OF MUSCULAR CONDITIONING

Muscular conditioning implies the growth and development of muscle tissue as well as improvements in the force and power output of the muscle. Strength is the ability of a muscle to produce force, and power is how rapidly the athlete can develop force, or force output per unit of time. Optimal levels of strength and power are important for athletes to both improve performance and decrease injury risk. Additionally, there are health benefits associated with resistance training that include decreasing resting blood pressure (BP), decreasing exercise heart rate (HR) and BP, causing positive changes in blood lipids, improving glucose tolerance, improving body composition, improving bone mineral density, reducing anxiety or depression, reducing the risk of musculoskeletal injury, and improving the ability to perform activities of daily living (Conley, 2001).

PHYSIOLOGIC ADAPTATIONS TO RESISTANCE TRAINING

Muscle Size

Appropriate loading of a muscle causes *muscular hypertrophy,* which is the enlargement of the diameter of the individual muscle fiber. The force a muscle is capable of producing is strongly related to the cross-sectional area of the given muscle. When a muscle is loaded appropriately, it will adapt by synthesizing a greater volume of contractile proteins, actin and myosin. Increases in the cross-sectional area of human muscle tissue due to training is believed to be primarily due to hypertrophy. *Hyperplasia*, an increase in the number of muscle cells or muscle fibers, is controversial in humans. Hyperplasia has been demonstrated in animal studies; however, there is conflicting published research as to its existence in humans (Gollnick, 1973; Gonyea, 1980).

Neural Adaptations

Resistance training affects the neuromuscular system by improving the ability of the body to recruit additional motor units and to increase the rate of firing of the motor unit. The neural component of muscle force production is the primary reason for the initial increases in strength in an untrained individual. This neural component also includes improved coordination of muscle firing patterns, basically allowing the prime movers to contract and the opposing muscle groups to relax at the appropriate time, to maximize force production. As a resistance trainer increases in experience, there may be an improvement in the synchronization of motor unit recruitment as well as an overriding of the Golgi tendon organ protective mechanism in muscle tissue, which will allow for greater force production (Harris, 2000).

Biochemical Changes

With high-intensity training, there can be a significant increase in muscle glycogen, creatine phosphate, and adenosine triphosphate substrate stores.

There also may be an increase in the quantity and activity of the glycolytic enzymes, including myokinase and creatine kinase (MacDougall, 1977). Participation in repetitive, continuous low-intensity, high-volume training (endurance training) may improve the oxidative capacity of the muscle. Improvements in the oxidative capacity of the muscle occur primarily in the type I fibers, which have oxidative capacities that are already developed; however, there can be some modification of the type IIa fibers' moderately developed oxidative capacity (Kraemer, 2000).

PRINCIPLES OF RESISTANCE TRAINING

Loading

To achieve muscle growth and increases in muscle strength, the muscle has to be loaded by some external mechanism. Optimal loading, sometimes referred to as the principle of overload, refers to a load greater than one the muscle is accustomed to handling. Loading can be achieved through various modes: a weighted implement, manual resistance, resistive machinery, or elastic resistance. Simply moving body weight can provide a resistance-training load for some muscles in many athletes.

To achieve significant gains in strength and potential muscle growth, an optimal level of loading is required. In resistance training, loading is sometimes expressed as a percentage of the greatest load an individual can lift through a given movement, a *one-repetition maximum* (1RM). For example, this could be how much an athlete can bench press for one repetition. Training loads can be calculated as a percentage of this value. Depending on the goal of the training session, the load may be applied during one repetition of the movement or over a number of repetitions. If using a one-repetition maximum lift is contraindicated or not desired, one-repetition maximums can be estimated based on the number of repetitions completed with a lesser resistance. Also, the program can be based on a percentage of another value, say a 10RM, which would be the amount of weight that could be lifted for 10 but not 11 repetitions.

Adaptation

There are specific adaptations to resistance training loads, and these adaptations will be specific to the load, intensity, and volume of training chosen. To achieve continued improvement over time, loads must be cyclical and progressive in nature. Periodized programs allow the planning of this cyclical, progressive loading throughout the training year.

Progression

Gains in hypertrophy, strength, and power will not continue unless the load is increased progressively over time. Generally, all loads are lifted an assigned number of times, or repetitions. An individual must perform the desired number of repetitions based on the goals of the training session.

Individual Differences

Individuals will respond differently to the same training program. What works for one individual in a specific situation may not work for another individual. When developing resistance-training programs, there may be more than one method of achieving a specific goal. Some athletes respond well to higher frequencies and intensities of resistance training, and some athletes fail to respond. It is always important to monitor the response of the individual athlete to the training program.

Reversibility

Adaptations to resistance training are reversible. If an athlete does not continue to resistance train at the same level of intensity, the improvements made as a result of the training will not last. Detraining is the loss of the physiologic benefits of training. Aerobic detraining is generally more rapid because it is based on decreases in aerobic enzyme concentrations. Muscle strength is more resistant to rapid detraining. With detraining, the athlete tends to revert to the untrained state (Kraemer, 2000).

Variability

Variability includes variation in load, tempo, and exercise selection. Without such variability, an athlete may experience training plateaus, and perhaps, overtraining.

Variation in load should occur in a periodized manner depending on the goals of the training session. To increase maximal strength, the athlete should work with a program that focuses on a hypertrophy phase followed by a strength phase. To increase power, the athlete should focus on a program that progresses from a hypertrophy phase to a strength phase to a power phase.

The tempo of an exercise is essentially the movement velocity, and tempo can be divided into a concentric and eccentric phase. The tempo of an exercise will be dependent on the specific goals of the activity.

Variation in exercise selection obviously involves selecting a variety of exercises. Using the same exercises day after day may promote staleness, overtraining, and overuse injuries. Whenever possible, the athlete should choose a variety of exercises as long as those exercises meet the desired goals of the training session.

Desired Goals of Training

Resistance-training programs can be designed to meet specific goals of the individual athlete and the needs of the sport. Sport-specific programs are designed to improve performance qualities specific to performance in that sport.

The endurance athlete or the athlete who is required to produce repeated, submaximal muscle contractions during an event likely would develop the strength endurance capabilities of the muscle. Combining resistance training with aerobic conditioning may promote a more rapid decrease body fat percentage, but also may interfere with maximal strength and power gains (Kraemer, 1995).

In sports where size and body mass are important, the goal of specific phases of training may be to increase muscle size. Specific resistance-training protocols are most likely to promote muscle hypertrophy. There are a number of sports that require that an individual increase his or her size or body mass, which is accomplished primarily through muscle hypertrophy. Strength gains expressed independent of body mass are referred to as *absolute strength*. A one-repetition maximum lift is an example of a test of absolute strength. Relative strength is strength expressed per unit of body mass or perhaps lean muscle mass. An example of a measure of relative strength would be to take absolute strength and divide it by body mass or lean muscle mass. This measure equates the larger individual with the smaller individual. For example, males are generally stronger than females on measures of absolute strength, but females are very close or equal to males on measures of relative strength expressed per unit of lean muscle mass.

Strength-to-mass ratio is the ratio of strength to body mass. Some athletes may be concerned with the strength-to-mass ratio. This is often true in sports where body weight classifications are used, such as boxing and wrestling. With this athlete, the goal is to increase strength without the associated increase in body mass.

Power development is an outcome of the appropriate type of resistance training. Power is speed-strength, or the ability to generate force in the shortest possible period of time. An athlete with a high power output is able to generate very large forces over short time periods. The vertical jump is a common test of lower body power. The more rapidly the muscles contract, the higher the vertical jump. Power is desirable for any sport or activity that requires that force be generated rapidly, which includes most competitive sports.

VARIABLES OF RESISTANCE-TRAINING EXERCISE PRESCRIPTION

Intensity: Load

Intensity is often represented by the percentage of the individual's one-repetition maximum (1RM). It is generally agreed on that increases in strength require the use of loads or intensities that represent between 60 and 100% of the 1RM (Polquin, 1990).

A load that represents 100% of the 1RM will require an individual to recruit as many motor units as possible to develop the required force. The act of producing maximal force is referred to as a *maximal voluntary contraction* (MVC). As resistance decreases below the MVC, fewer motor units are required to lift the load. To express maximal strength, it is necessary to stimulate maximal motor unit recruitment.

Resistance training results in both physiologic and neural adaptations. One of these physiologic adaptations is hypertrophy. As stated previously, the force a muscle is able to exert is related to its cross-sectional area. Muscular hypertrophy results in increases in lean muscle mass. Bodybuilders who tend to train at an intensity that represents between 60 and 80% of the 1RM with a greater volume of training exhibit greater hypertrophy gains. Powerlifters tend to use intensities of 80% and greater and lower volumes of training (Gollnick, 1973; Schmidbleicher, 1991). Powerlifters have exhibited greater hypertrophy gains in their fast-twitch type IIb muscle fibers (Gollnick, 1973; Schmidbleicher, 1991). To achieve increases in strength-endurance, intensities of below 60% of the 1RM are generally prescribed.

As the resistance decreases below the 1RM, the number of repetitions an individual will be able to perform will increase. This associated relationship is referred to as the *1RM continuum* (Table 9-1). The 1RM continuum is affected by the level of training experience of the individual, the gender

TABLE 9-1 The Relationship Between Maximum Number of Repetitions and Training Effect

Maximum number of reps	% of 1RM Maximum	Training effect
1	100.0	Strength/power
2	94.3	
3	90.6	
4	88.1	
5	85.6	
6	83.1	
7	80.7	Strength
8	78.6	
9	76.5	
10	74.4	Hypertrophy
11	72.3	
12	70.3	
13	68.8	
14	67.5	
15	66.2	Endurance
16	65.0	
17	63.8	
18	62.7	
19	61.6	
20	60.6	

of the individual, the muscle group trained, and individual differences. For any given exercise, there is no specific number of repetitions associated with a certain percentage of the 1RM. Intensity of exercise should be assigned based on the number of goal repetitions rather than a specific percentage of the 1RM. This method of assigning intensity is also best for the novice because it is not easy to determine the 1RM with someone who has never lifted before. Since the number of repetitions performed has a general relationship to the percentage intensity of the given load, there will still be a clear indication of the intensity of the workload performed (see Table 9-1).

Volume: Sets and Repetitions

The combination of the number of sets and the number of repetitions performed are referred to as the volume of training. The volume of the training stimulus is similar to the duration of an aerobic training program. Total workload is strongly related to many of the effects of a resistance training program. While novices have shown improvements using a single set of a specific number of repetitions, continued improvement will relate more strongly to the total workload. The number of repetitions and, thus the intensity of the exercise, are determined by the goal of the specific phase of the training program. The number of times this training stimulus may be applied or the number of sets of repetitions that should be performed is subject to an inverse relationship with the number of repetitions performed. The number of repetitions performed and the amount of resistance used depend on the goals of that particular phase of training.

Frequency

How often an athlete must train to achieve results depends on both goals and experience. The novice can achieve improvements with just two training sessions of a body part per week. For the more advanced athlete, there is likely little difference between three training sessions a week and five training sessions per week. However, in an athletic situation, even minute differences may be the difference between first and second place, and may be important. Some investigators believe that the increased frequency may lead to tissue breakdown, increased injury risk, and increased risk of overtraining. The goal should be to train the muscle at as high a frequency as possible while at the same time, avoiding these and other possible negative side effects. It is generally recommended that similar muscle groups be trained two to three times per week. Recovery time between training sessions is important for tissue repair and energy repletion.

Rest

The rest between each training stimulus during a training session depends on the goals of the program. As the goal of training shifts from strength endurance, to muscular hypertrophy, to strength, and to power development, the length of time of rest must increase. In strength-endurance training, the goal is to work the muscle for a longer period of time with a lower resistance to improve the physiologic endurance properties of the muscle. Rest, therefore, is of limited importance and should be short. In hypertrophy training, the rest period lengthens to some degree so that the heavier loads may be used.

In strength and power training, one goal is to train the neural recruitment patterns of the muscle, attempting to achieve full motor unit recruitment for maximal force output. Neural system training combined with high force output training requires that energy stores within the muscle be completely replenished between sets. It takes approximately 3 minutes for ATP stores to be 100% replenished within the muscle after exhaustive anaerobic exercise (Harris, 2000). The nervous system also needs time to recover. Therefore, the rest between sets in strength and power training is generally in the 3- to 5-minute range.

Rest between exercises is dependent on the order of the exercise prescription. If the next exercise to be performed uses a different muscle group, then the length of rest can be shorter. If the same muscle is trained in the next set, the length of rest between exercises is similar to the times between exercise sets.

Tempo

The speed and timing of the eccentric/concentric actions during an exercise is referred to as the *tempo* of the movement. Tempo can be expressed by the length of the concentric and eccentric actions, and the length of the pause, if any, between the two actions. Most athletic situations require rapid development of muscle force. The specificity of training principle would dictate that the tempo be based on a sport-specific characterization of the sport. Since strength, by definition, is not measured with respect to time, it is likely that the tempo in the hypertrophy and strength phases will be slower. As the athlete progresses to a power phase, which by definition is measured per unit of time, the movement velocity will progress toward explosive sport-specific velocities. Purposefully slow movements move away from the force velocity curve, and may not produce improvements in force or velocity (Fig. 9-1).

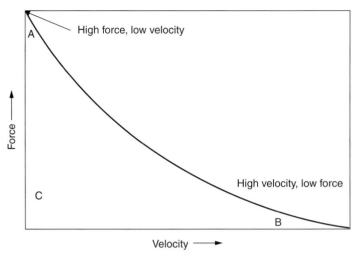

FIG 9-1   The concentric force/velocity curve. **A** represents a high force, low velocity movement, such as a 1RM max on a squat. **B** represents a low force, high velocity movement, such as throwing a baseball at maximal velocity. **C** represents training intentionally slow, moving away from the force velocity curve. To shift the force velocity curve up and to the right (i.e., to improve power), training must be as close as possible to the curve.

TRAINING MODES

Type of Load

All resistance-training programs involve the use of external loads. The nature of these loads is really determined by their relationship to the mechanical strength curve of the muscle to be trained and the degree to which they may need to be balanced (stable or unstable loads). There are several types of loads.

Unstable Loads

Free Weights. Free weights are any load that is free standing and must be balanced by the body while being manipulated through an exercise pathway. The amount of resistance offered by the free weight does not change, so the load lifted is limited by the weakest point in the range of motion. In most human motions, this point is found either at the beginning or at the end of the range of motion. Free weights can be used to mimic the requirements of most sports more realistically than most machines, as well as requiring that the load be balanced.

Elastic Resistance. Elastic resistance equipment uses the elastic properties of materials such as rubber to create a load. It is an easy and modifiable way of achieving resistance. However, with elastic resistance, the load is not physiologic in that it increases throughout the entire range of motion. This type of resistance does not replicate a human strength curve. The elastic resistance is often greatest at the end of the range of motion, which may be the weakest angle. In addition, a number of elastic bands must be available for different exercises. Depending on how the elastic bands are used, the exercise may or may not develop synergistic support and stabilization. As the elastic is used over time, the amount of resistance offered may decrease.

The Body. Using body weight or some part of body weight can be an effective method of resistance training in many instances. The resistance acts similarly to the use of free weights. The athlete is limited, however, by their initial strength level. For example, a young athlete who cannot perform a pushup will not be able to train using that exercise. Some exercises may be modified so that they are easier or harder within certain limitations. For example, pushups can be performed from the knees or with the feet on a chair depending on the goal of the exercise and the athlete's strength level. In advanced athletes with good strength, body weight exercises often become an endurance exercise rather than a strength exercise. For example, the athlete who can do 10 pushups maximally is training for strength, and the athlete who can do 100 pushups is training for endurance.

Stable Loads

Fixed Resistance. A fixed-resistance load is similar to a free weight in that it does not adjust for the changes in force production caused by the human strength curve. The load is fixed, however, in some form of equipment frame using weight stacks, pulleys, and fixed bearing joints. This type of machine is often referred to as *selectorized equipment* because weight stacks with pins used to "select" the load. The fact that the load is stabilized eliminates the requirement for the load to be balanced and tends to decrease the requirement for synergistic support and stabilization. This type of load may be acceptable to beginner programming, where an individual may be intimidated by the loading of a free weight or the requirement to balance the load.

Variable Resistance. This form of loading is similar in set-up to the fixed-resistance load. It differs from the fixed-resistance equipment in its method of load application. Variable-resistance equipment attempts to adjust the load through a range of motion so that it adjusts to the mechanical strength curve of the human body. The load is adjusted through the range of motion by the use of a cam that has been built to match the "average" mechanical strength curve. Variable-resistance equipment attempts to resolve the "perceived" problem of free weights allowing a resistance no greater than the resistance that can be performed through the weakest angle. Although cam machines may allow muscle to be exercised at nearer maximal intensity at each angle through a range of motion, this resistance pattern is not specific to many sports or activities. Another problem with variable-resistance equipment is that it is often built for the average-sized individual, and the desired variable-resistance effect occurs only on individuals of "average" size.

Isokinetic Resistance. Isokinetic resistance requires the use of complex machinery fitted with transmission-like gears that are able to limit the speed of contraction of a muscle through a specific range of motion. To make the speed constant, the device constantly adjusts the resistance based on the force applied. An assumption must be made that the athlete is performing with maximal effort, since by slowing down intentionally, the machine will offer less resistance. The resistance will only allow the limb to achieve a specific speed through a range of motion. If the athlete pushes harder to try to move the limb faster, the machine will offer more resistance to keep the speed of movement constant. No matter how hard the individual pushes, the limb will only move at the set speed. Isokinetic resistance supposedly strengthens muscle maximally at each angle through a range of motion.

There are a number of disadvantages to isokinetic resistance training. Isokinetic resistance is not functional to most sports or activities, and is therefore not an ideal form of training for many sports. It requires expensive machinery that can only train small numbers of athletes at a given time. Some isokinetic devices include an eccentric component, some do not. The use of isokinetic exercise equipment is relegated primarily to rehabilitation of athletic injuries.

Hydraulic Resistance. Hydraulic resistance uses liquids or gases housed in cylinder-like chambers to produce resistance similar to that found when moving a limb through water. Hydraulic resistance is similar to isokinetics in that the resistance reacts to the initiation of greater forces by producing greater resistance forces. Due to the nature of fluid resistance, an exact isokinetic effect is not obtained. In addition, hydraulic resistance does not provide eccentric load, requiring that every motion performed there be a push and pull manner. This allows for balanced development of agonist and antagonist; however, the muscles do not receive the benefits of eccentric training. A lack of eccentric loading may decrease muscle soreness, but will limit the carryover value of the training activity to the sport.

Choice of Exercise

There are a number of exercises that may target a similar group of muscles or specific muscle. These exercises may, in appropriate situations, be exchanged throughout the duration of a resistance-training program to achieve variety as long as they meet the specific goals of that exercise session. Exercises should be chosen based on the specificity of the exercise to the sport, the goal of the program, and the experience of the participant. Exercise options include using mode variations, changing the angle of the exercise, and utilizing both single-limb and double-limb movements.

PRINCIPLES OF PROGRAM DESIGN

Strength-Endurance Training

Strength-endurance development requires the application of low to moderate-intensity loads, generally below 60% of the 1RM over a high volume of training (usually two to three sets of above 20 repetitions). The desired effect of strength endurance training is to improve the short-term endurance of the muscle. This type of training may be of benefit to the endurance athlete in whom muscular endurance may be a factor. Increasing the number of sets (two to three), decreasing the length of rest time between sets (45 to 30 seconds), and using large muscle group exercises (squats, presses), will achieve improvements in the muscle's short-term endurance capacity. Increasing the strength of the muscle will also improve the short-term endurance capacity of the muscle.

Absolute Strength Training (Hypertrophy)

If absolute strength is the goal of the athlete, it is best to use loads that represent approximately 60 to 80% of the 1RM. Rest periods can vary but generally should be in the range of 3 to 5 minutes to allow complete ATP recovery. In an athlete focusing on hypertrophic strength development, it is not uncommon to use three to four sets of an exercise of between 6 and 20 repetitions and the use of a large number of exercises (as many as four to six) for one muscle group.

Relative Strength Training

Relative strength refers to the development of strength expressed as a function of body weight. Increasing the strength-to-mass ratio requires that larger intensities of training (80% of the 1RM and above) be applied using a lower volume of training (four to five sets of one to six repetitions). The use of heavy loads improves the neural activation of motor units, leading to significant increases in strength without significant increases in muscle mass. In a periodized concept of training, the athlete may move through a hypertrophy phase into a strength phase of training. The increased hypertrophy, in this case, would increase the potential for basic strength gains.

Training with high intensities requires that longer rest periods be used between each set of an exercise. It is not uncommon to use rest periods of between 3 and 5 minutes. This long rest period allows for regeneration of ATP and neural recovery so that the second bout of exercise may be performed at maximal intensity. Movement velocity or tempo should be submaximal. This allows for variety, since power exercises will be performed at maximal velocity. It also allows for recruitment of stabilizing and assistance muscle groups.

Power Training

Power development requires that the velocity of contraction increase, or the force of contraction be increased without increasing the time. Power training affects motor unit activation and firing rate to produce explosive force. In addition, it allows the muscle spindle to fire, increasing force output through the stretch reflex. A significant strength base is necessary prior to attempting the exercises involved in power development such as weightlifting lifts and plyometrics.

The intensity and volume of training may be varied with power training, but the athlete should be progressing to sport-specific loads and velocities. If the athlete is required to accelerate a light object explosively, throw a baseball for example, then training should move to this end of the force velocity curve (see Fig. 9-1). It is important that the movement velocity be explosive in nature. Rest times between sets again are in the 3 to 5-minute range to allow complete recovery between sets (Table 9-2).

TABLE 9-2 Loading Parameters in Relation to the Desired Training Effect

Variables	Endurance	Hypertrophy	Strength	Power
Intensity	<60%	60–80%	80–100%	60–100%
Sets	2–4	2–6	5–12	1–12
Repetitions	>20	6–20	1–5	1–12
Rest	10–60 s	10–240 s	180–300 s	120–600 s
Tempo	Moderate	Varied	Slow/moderate explosive	

PERIODIZATION OF TRAINING

Periodization refers to the manipulation of training variables over specific periods of time for the purpose of promoting maximal performance at the appropriate time and decreasing the risk of overtraining (Stone, 1987). A periodized conditioning plan usually covers a year, particularly in seasonal sports. The same principles may be applied to other time periods as well. Even though the sport of football is a yearly seasonal sport, the freshman athlete entering a university program is essentially on a 5-year plan. The goal is to maximize performance over that time period.

The concept of periodization involves the manipulation of volume and intensity of training through specific periods or seasons of the year. A *needs analysis* is performed to determine the type of training that would be most beneficial to the athlete. The needs analysis essentially has two parts. First, the demands of the sport are evaluated to make decisions about the desired performance capabilities of the athlete. Second, the athlete is evaluated to determine individual deficiencies related to the desired performance profile. The athlete must choose times during the year when maximal performance is desired.

Cycles

The periodized conditioning program is divided into cycles. In most cases, a training year makes up a macrocycle, a period of months (perhaps a season) makes up a mesocycle, and a period of several days or a week makes up a microcycle. Each cycle has a specific training goal, and the training variables are manipulated to achieve that goal. The following are some common training phases to employ.

General Preparatory Phase

The general preparatory phase is an introductory phase of training; usually, it uses parameters of training that are characteristic of the strength endurance format of training, low-intensity/high-volume resistance training. Depending on the needs of the sport and the fitness profile of the athlete, it may be coupled with interval training or other forms of training to initiate the individual to the training program. This type of phase may be employed with the novice or may be used as a reintroduction to a long-term training program for a high-performance athlete. It represents a reasonable method of introducing or reintroducing resistance training to an athlete. This phase usually will last 5 to 8 weeks.

Specific Preparatory Phase

The specific preparatory phase of training defines the goals of an individual more specifically with respect to the training program. Usually, the intensity of the training increases, with moderate to high volumes of training. Exercises must become more specific to the requirements of the individual's goals or the sport for which the athlete may be preparing. This phase should last between 6 and 8 weeks but may be somewhat longer or shorter as necessary.

Precompetition Phase

The *precompetition phase* is marked by an increase in intensity and a decrease in the volume of resistance training. In most sports, the time spent in practicing the sport has increased, and the overall volume of resistance training must decrease. Exercises are more sports specific and less time is spent on training assistance muscle groups. The length of each phase varies due to several factors, including the time schedule relative to competitions. The phase should be long enough for the athlete to adapt to the training program prescribed, and not so long as to allow staleness and plateauing.

Competitive Phase

In longer-season sports, it may be necessary to address a competitive phase, sometimes referred to as a maintenance phase that will maintain strength levels as much as possible throughout the length of the competitive season. The use of moderate intensities and moderate to low volumes of training usually occur during this time.

Peaking Phase

In most sports, the major competitions the athlete should peak for are evident. However, this is not always the case, particularly in sports with a long competitive season, such as football. Prior to a major competition, the athlete who desires to peak physiologically should further decrease the volume of training to promote full rest and recovery for competition.

Cyclic Progression

If the macrocycle is defined as a 1-year period of time, the training cycles are planned at the mesocycle level, and eventually, the microcycle level. The macrocycle can be broken down into a series of mesocycles, with each mesocycle broken down into a series of microcycles that are cyclically manipulated to prevent overtraining as well as to prevent boredom and provide motivation.

The basic concept of cyclic progression is that if a program does not change over time, adaptation to the exercise stimulus will cease. A program with limited variation may cause strength improvements to plateau, and the athlete is more likely to become bored with the program. Since intensity is a major factor in the improvement of strength, the manipulation of intensity is very important at promoting maximal strength gains. One technique of manipulating training intensity is known as staired progression.

Staired Progression

Staired progression (Fig. 9-2) is a method of manipulating training intensity within the framework of a training phase over a series of microcycles. Staired progression attempts to initiate a physiologic state known as *supercompensation* within the muscle tissue of the body. When an athlete is introduced to a new training stimulus or load at the beginning of a microcycle that is higher than the previous load, fatigue will occur. If the same load is maintained over the period of this same microcycle during following training sessions, the body will begin to adapt to this new training intensity. This new level is referred to as a new *ceiling of adaptation* (Bompa, 1993).

At the beginning of a microcycle, the individual may feel both physiologically and psychologically capable of handling a greater load. The inten-

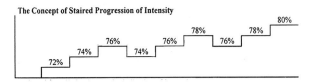

FIG 9-2 The concept of staired progression of intensity. (*Reprinted with permission from Bompa T. Periodization of Strength. Don Mills, Ontario, Veritas, 1993.*)

sity should then be increased to challenge the body to adapt even further. This progression of intensity may continue through a period of two to four microcycles, at which point, an unloading period should be initiated (Bompa, 1993). The unloading period represents an opportunity for the body to regenerate after a series of intensive training microcycles. The unloading period should not return to initial levels of intensities; rather, it should be reduced to the level of intensity reached at the midpoint of the staired progression phase (see Fig. 9-2). The unloading period allows for tissue regeneration and protein synthesis as well as the replenishment of energy stores that will have been depleted over the period of staired progression. This replenishment of energy stores during the unloading phase may exceed the previous levels attained before the training stimulus was initiated. The energy replenishment above the initial levels is commonly referred to as *supercompensation*, and it may leave the individual in a heightened state of preparedness for another successive series of increasing training intensities (Zatsiorsky, 1995).

MANIPULATING INTENSITY AND VOLUME

Exercise prescription for the intensity and volume of resistance training can be manipulated in a number of ways. The simplest is a fixed format, indicating that the repetitions are associated with a specific intensity, and that they remain constant over the desired number of sets. An example would be six sets of five repetitions at 85% intensity. Another way of prescribing the volume and intensity is to describe them as unfixed and giving ranges for the repetitions and intensities. An example is three sets of 10 to 12 reps at 70 to 74%. Over a period of three to five sets using the same load, the athlete should not be able to maintain the same number of repetitions over multiple sets. The unfixed method takes into consideration that the first set may be performed to 12 repetitions, and the last set may be performed to 10 repetitions. This takes into consideration the variability of the repetition continuum, describing the associated intensity as a range rather than a specific number (Fig. 9-3).

Other methods of manipulating the volume and intensity include pyramid presentation or split-set presentation. An example of the pyramid style (which allows the athlete to cover a greater range of intensities in one workout) would be 1 × 10 at 75%, 1 × 8 at 78%, and 2 × 6 at 83%. The split style would look as follows: 2 × 10 at 75%, 2 × 6 at 83%, and 1 × 12 at 70%. There are a number of ways that the pyramid or split style can be applied, and there are very few rules associated with their application.

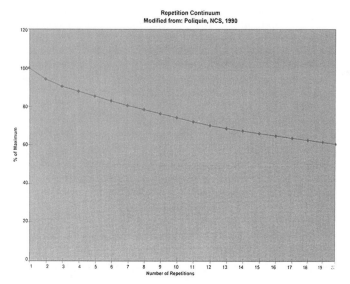

FIG 9-3   Relationship between maximum number of repetitions and training effect. (*Modified from Poliquin C. Loading Parameters of Strength Development. NCCP National Coaches Seminar, Level 4/5, January 1990.*)

SPECIAL CONSIDERATIONS IN RESISTANCE TRAINING

Core Development

All conditioning programs should address the need for core strength. The muscles of the low back and abdominals must be well prepared to provide support for the use of the limbs in strength movements. For some individuals, this may mean developing core strength first before any other training begins or before any significant strength training begins.

Balanced Exercise Prescription

Resistance-training programs should be planned to decrease the chances that a muscle strength imbalance will occur. Training imbalances can lead to postural imbalances and increased injury risk. A safe rule is that for every exercise assigned for the agonist, there must be an exercise assigned for the antagonist.

Technique

It is important that the exercises are performed with proper technique. Improper technique can lead to increased injury risk and reduced effectiveness of the exercise. Assigned exercises should be performed through a functional and sport-specific range of motion. Athletes must continually be monitored to prevent the development of exercise patterns using incorrect form.

TYPES OF RESISTANCE EXERCISES

In conventional resistance training, there are seven major motion patterns that occur. These are the press motion, the pull motion, the squat motion, the lunge motion, flexion/extension motion, adduction/abduction motion, and rotation. These motion patterns can be combined to provide variation. Variation also can be attained by changing the angle of the motion, the start or finish position of the motion, or the position of unaffected joints above or below the joint of motion, or by using dumbbells, barbells, or other modes of training. It is imperative that the athlete clearly understands these motion patterns, the muscles involved, and the effects of the exercise modifications. The development of exercises requires that the developer understand the concept of motion patterns and functional anatomy; once this is so, the athlete may be free to create any exercise that may affect any muscle. The following known exercises follow the motion patterns reflected in the previous discussion.

- *The press motion:* Bench press, decline press, incline press, military press, behind the neck press, the dip, the push press, etc.
- *The pull motion:* Upright row, pull-down, the chin-up, the clean, etc.
- *The squat motion:* Leg press, squats, hack squats, dead lifts, power cleans, etc.
- *The lunge motion:* The lunge, the split squat, the step-back lunge, the step-up, etc.
- *Flexion/extension motion:* The bicep curl, the triceps extension, the kick back, the push down, the crunch, the curl up, back hyperextensions, hip extension, hip flexion, leg extensions, leg curls, etc.
- *Abduction/adduction:* The fly, the lateral abduction, lateral adduction, lateral pulldown, lateral leg lifts, etc.
- *Rotation:* Shoulder rotation, hip rotation, rotary crunches, rotary extensions, etc.

When designing resistance-training programs, it is important to understand the concept of motion patterns so that the program achieves balance while being as efficient and as effective as possible. For example, to design a program that improves upper body strength, it is important to identify those muscles that need to be trained and the motion patterns that affect those muscles. Once this is known, then exercises should be chosen to develop strength in a balanced fashion, leaving room for variation using various angles and training modes.

TYPES OF DAILY PROGRAM ORGANIZATION

Aside from the overall periodization effect of a training program, there are particular methods of program organization at the daily workout level. Daily program design relies heavily on the training age of the participant, the type of training goals, and the time available for training. Several methods of daily program design are possible.

Full Body Routine

This style of organizing the daily workout is most often used with the novice or those individuals with time constraints, either due to lifestyle or other training requirements. This type of program involves breaking the body into muscle groups that are trained during the program. The body can be divided into an upper body, core, and lower body. Within these divisions, further division include: (upper body) press motion, press motion above the head, pull motion, pull motion from above the head; (core) flexion motion, extension motion, rotation motion; and (lower body) squat motion, lunge motion, ankle plantarflexion/dorsiflexion motion.

The full body program should be repeated no more than four times a week with 1 day's rest between sessions. Depending on the level of training of the athlete, it generally would take three training days per week to make significant gains, and two days per week to maintain strength levels. The following program is an example of the full body program.

UPPER BODY

Motion	Exercise
Press	Bench press
Pull	Cable row
Press above head	Dumbbell military press
Pull above head	Cable pulldown

CORE

Motion	Exercise
Flexion	Crunch
Extension	Back hyperextensions
Rotation	Rotary crunch

LOWER BODY

Motion	Exercise
Squat	Leg press
Lunge	Split squats
Ankle dorsiflexion/plantarflexion	Heel raises/toe lifts

The total number of exercises rarely should exceed 10, so it becomes extremely important that the program be both efficient and effective. Each of the major muscle groups and their synergists receive equal stimulus throughout the program, with few isolated single joint exercises included. Specific flexion/extension exercises and adduction/abduction exercises generally cannot be performed in the full body style program or it will become too long. These muscle groups are effectively trained in the combined press/pull/squat motions.

Upper and Lower Two-On, One-Off Split Routine

This type of program is best suited to the intermediate to advanced-level participant or the athlete. It is defined by the separation of the body into two-component training days. The first training day involves training of the upper body, and the second training day involves training of the lower body. Core group training can be structured in parts or grouped into a separate training session. The upper body and lower body programs should be broken down as follows: upper body, press motion, overhead press motion, pull motion, overhead pull motion, shoulder abduction/adduction (various planes), elbow flexion/extension core training flexion/extension; lower body, squat motion, hip flexion/extension, hip abduction/adduction, knee flexion/extension, ankle plantarflexion/dorsiflexion, core rotation. Each upper body and lower body split is followed by 1 day off, and then the cycle must begin again. This ensures that adequate rest is observed without the loss of potential training effects. A sample program is as follows.

UPPER BODY DAY

Motions	*Exercises*
Press	Bench press
	Incline dumbbell press
Shoulder abduction/adduction	Side lateral raise
	Lateral pulldown
Overhead press	Military press
Pull	Barbell bent over row
Overhead pull	Close grip front pulldown
Elbow flexion/extension	Incline dumbbell curls
	Triceps push downs
Core flexion/extension	Reverse crunch
	Back hyperextension

LOWER BODY DAY

Motion	*Exercise*
Squat	Squats
Hip flexion/extension abduction/adduction	Four-way hip
Knee flexion/extension	Leg extension/Leg curls
Ankle plantarflexion/dorsiflexion	Heel raises/toe lifts
The core rotation motion	Crossover cable crunch
	Rotary crunches

Each session includes approximately 10 exercises and should meet the goals of the cycle of training.

Multiple Split Routines

Multiple split routines are designed for the advanced resistance trainee. The desire to create greater muscle growth requires training with higher loads. This type of program seeks to maximize training volume but still allow adequate recovery. Quite often, similar movement patterns are combined to concentrate large volumes of training on specific body parts or muscle groups. Multiple splits might appear as follows.

Three Day On, One Day Off Split
DAY 1

Motion	*Exercise*
Upper body press motion	Bench press
	Incline dumbbell press
Upper body overhead press	Military press
Shoulder adduction	Cable crossovers
Shoulder abduction	Side lateral raise
Elbow extensions	Dips
	Dumbbell kick backs
Core extension	Back hyperextensions

DAY 2

Motion	*Exercise*
Upper body pull	Wide grip cable row
	Dumbbell row
Upper body overhead pull	Front pulldown

Close grip chin-up
Elbow flexion

Core flexion

Barbell curls
Preacher curls
Crunches

DAY 3
Motion

Lower body squat

Lower body lunge
Hip adduction/abduction, flexion/extension
Knee flexion/extension

Ankle plantarflexion/dorsiflexion
Core rotation

Exercise

Squats
Hack squats
Step-forward lunge
Four-way hip
Leg extensions
Leg curl
Heel raises/toe raises
Rotary crunches

With this style of training, the number of exercises may vary from day to day between as low as five exercises and as high as 10 exercises, depending on the desired volume of training. The multiple split may take many shapes and forms. Some conditioning specialists advocate the use of agonist/antagonist type training on the same day. They point to the fact that an inhibitory mechanism that is present during exercise and involves the limitation of force production due to an antagonistic inhibitory mechanism will be limited if the antagonist is fatigued prior to an agonistic exercise. Still other specialists feel that it is most efficient to train all those muscles involved in common motions on the same day, as was done in the preceding example. Modification of this area is certainly not limited to these two methods. Just make sure that the program developed is suited to the needs of the athlete and the sport.

Training for Fitness or Sport Performance

A differentiation must be made between the daily routine in sports preparation and fitness training. Generally, when a person trains for fitness or to improve appearance, he or she should work within the framework of a balanced training program that affects all the major muscle groups of the body during a training microcycle or week.

When training for sport performance, the daily routine of the training program is affected by the phase of training. For example, if the clinician were training a volleyball athlete for the season, the off-season would be broken down into several periods and phases. During the general preparatory phase, the athlete may work on overall muscular development using a multijoint program. During the specific preparatory phase, the time available to resistance train may be more limited, and the program must reflect the muscular development goals specific to that sport. A powerlifter, for example, should not spend more than 45 minutes to 1 hour on any one specific preparation session. The exercises he or she performs must be specific to the goals of powerlifting and must leave room for high-intensity training. A powerlifter may only be assigned three exercises to perform during the course of 45 minutes. This is necessary so that rest time between sets and intensity level remain where they must be to achieve maximal strength gains.

CONCLUSION

There are many ways to construct and implement a successful resistance-training program. There are several basic elements that must be included for the program to be efficient and effective. The most important of these ingredients are intensity and variety. For resistance training to cause maximal improvement in performance, each phase of training must have a specific purpose, and the program must be designed scientifically to meet that purpose. The concepts of designing a resistance-training program must continually be updated based on new research developments.

REFERENCES

Bompa T. *Periodization of Strength.* Don Mills, Ontario, Canada: Veritas Publishing; 1993.

Conley MH, Rozanek R. NSCA Position Statement: Health aspects of resistance exercise and training. *Str Cond J.* 2001;23:9–23.

Gollnick P, Armstrong R, Saltin B, et al. Effects of training on the enzyme activity and fiber composition of human skeletal muscle. *J Appl Physiol.* 1973;34:107–111.

Gonyea WJ. The role of exercise in inducing skeletal muscle fiber number. *J Appl Physiol.* 1980;48:421–426.

Harris RT and Dudley G. Neuromuscular anatomy and adaptations to conditioning. In: Baechle TR, Earle RW, eds. *Essentials of Strength Training and Conditioning.* Champlaign, Ill: Human Kinetics; 2000:19–20.

Kraemer WJ. Physiological adaptations to anaerobic and aerobic endurance training programs. In: Baechle TR, Earle RW, eds. *Essentials of Strength Training and Conditioning.* Champaign, Ill: Human Kinetics; 2000.

Kraemer WJ, Patton J, Gordon SE, et al. Compatibility of high intensity strength and endurance training on hormonal and skeletal muscle adaptations. *J Appl Physiol.* 1995;78:976–989.

MacDougall D, Ward GR, Sale DG, Sutton JR. Biochemical adaptation of human skeletal muscle to heavy resistance exercise and immobilization. *J Appl Physiol.* 1977;43:700–703.

Polquin C. Loading parameters of strength development. NCPP National Coaches Seminar, Level 4/5, 1990.

Schmidtbleicher D, Haralanbie G. Changes in contractile proteins of muscle after strength training in man. *Eur J Appl Physiol.* 1991;46:221–228.

Stone MH, O'Bryant HS. *Weight Training, A Scientific Approach.* Minneapolis: Burgess; 1987.

Zatsiorsky V. *Science and Practice of Strength Training.* Champaign, Ill: Human Kinetics; 1995.

10 Endurance Training

William O. Roberts

Endurance training generally refers to improvements in the cardiorespiratory and muscular systems that allow increases in prolonged exercise. Endurance training benefits long distance running, biking, Nordic skiing, soccer, and other long duration, continuous activity events, but may also improve performance in activities that have a more anaerobic pattern like soccer, football, and basketball. The general approach to endurance training is similar to that of muscle strengthening with periodization of the training program to meet competition needs, and training cycles that emphasize frequency, intensity, volume, and rest. Intense, high-volume training programs are imbedded into smaller cycles that improve performance over a preseason and competitive season with a final peak for the play-offs or championships. The competitive cycle should be followed with a less intense recovery or transition period that will meld into the next preparatory cycle. Sport-specific training provides the most benefit for competition; cross-training can be useful in the recovery cycle and during injury rehabilitation.

Children and adolescents are training at high levels and competing in greater numbers in many endurance sports. Less is known about training and related physiology in these age groups compared to adults, but it is obvious from competitions involving these young athletes that training improves performance. Research into endurance training and physiology is confounded in these athletes by the velocity of physical growth. Growth hormone is sensitive to exercise in this age group. Adolescents demonstrate reduced anaerobic power compared to adults, probably owing to differences in muscle structure and function that have yet to be elucidated. In contrast, aerobic training effects increase substantially in the adolescent years, at least in boys. This is due to the significant growth of the cardiorespiratory and musculoskeletal systems, and possibly to the hormonal changes that occur in adolescence. There is even less research on endurance training in adolescent girls. Observing girls in running competitions shows that young adolescents and pre-adolescents can often outperform their older peers and they may be advantaged in the adolescent years by less body mass and a higher percentage of lean body mass in early adolescence. There is no conclusive evidence that high-intensity training impairs growth, development, or maturation. However, there is concern that intense training and high-volume training can and will increase the number of overuse injuries in this age group. Nutrition is critical to the growing adolescent and even more so in the young athlete training at high intensity.

Women are also participating in endurance training and competitions in record numbers, and are closing the gap in the time differentials for many of the endurance events. It is difficult to extrapolate the findings from male athletes to female athletes because of the inherent differences in body composition and hormone levels. Discussions of the *female athlete triad* have focused on the risk of endurance activity in the absence of proper nutrition. There is no reason to believe that women cannot train safely following the same regimen as men if increases in volume and intensity go hand in hand with increases in the fuels needed to keep the body functioning at optimum levels.

The principles of endurance training can be applied to all patients in the arena of *training for health.* Daily aerobic activity benefits everyone and is

109

an inexpensive alternative to the diseases of inactivity like obesity, diabetes mellitus type 2, hypertension, and atherosclerotic vascular disease. Cardiac rehabilitation for patients who have had a myocardial infarction or other insult to the heart implements endurance training for improvements in lifestyle and function. Regular aerobic activity also reduces the maladies associated with aging.

DEFINITION OF ENDURANCE

Endurance is the ability to resist fatigue during exercise that results from a combination of muscle and cardiovascular adaptations that allow improvements in performance, especially in longer-duration activities. *Muscle endurance* focuses on the ability of the muscle to continue activity for the duration of an event at peak performance in any distance or duration. In contrast, *cardiovascular endurance* refers to the ability of the entire system supported by the heart and lungs to perform repetitive activity over time. The cardiovascular component of endurance is most commonly attributed to the term, but is only a part of the overall endurance performance of an individual athlete.

Sprints in running or swimming depend more on muscle endurance; the long-distance events require the addition of full cardiovascular adaptation to continue sustained effort. Although the sprints, especially if repeated several times in a given day, require good muscle endurance, the need for a fully endurance-trained cardiovascular system is not as essential. The distance competitor needs to maximally develop both systems to be competitive.

Endurance capacity or *potential* is measured by the amount of oxygen the body can process per unit mass per unit time and termed the *maximal oxygen uptake* (VO_{2max}). Oxygen consumption is linked to genetics, and athletes are born with the high potential engine that powers their activity. Athletes who have innately high VO_{2max} are more likely to be successful in long-duration events than those who are in the mid to low ranges of the scale. Sports like Nordic skiing and rowing that utilize nearly the entire muscle system of the upper and lower extremities require the highest oxygen consumptions. Athletes from burst-type activities like hockey and football are often in the mid ranges of VO_{2max}. The different forms of creatine kinase isoenzyme subunits of phosphocreatine are important in energy metabolism and performance. The genetic expression of the various forms may contribute to the variations in endurance performance between athletes and determine the level of competition at which an athlete can successfully compete.

TRAINING THE AEROBIC SYSTEM

Muscles utilize oxygen combined with glycogen to fuel the system. Oxygen utilization at the muscle level is improved with training resulting in higher VO_{2max}. As the utilization of oxygen improves, the supply of oxygen to the muscle must be increased to meet the demands of activity. These changes occur in the cardiovascular and respiratory systems, although a healthy respiratory system is seldom a limiting factor.

Cardiovascular Changes

The greatest changes induced by endurance training affect the cardiovascular system and its function during exercise. The exercise-induced changes affect heart size, stroke volume, heart rate, cardiac output, blood flow, blood pressure, and blood volume. The goal of training from a cardiovascular perspective is to maximize and optimize the transport of oxygen and fuel to the muscle, and removal of waste product and excess heat from the muscle. The heart is a muscle pump and responds to endurance training overload with an increase in interior size and wall thickness to produce a stronger pump and greater blood volume with each stroke. This hypertrophy from exercise is a normal response to training as opposed to the hypertrophy found in illness or pump failure. The heart wall also thickens in response to resistance training, but the ventricular volume does not increase.

The *stroke volume* increases with endurance training in part due to the larger ventricular volume induced by activity, but also due to more complete filling after training and more efficient emptying during ventricular contraction. Stated in another way, in response to prolonged exercise the ventricle increases in size, fills with more blood than the actual increase in ventricular volume, and empties more completely with contraction of the ventricle. Stroke volumes increase progressively as the state of training improves from sedentary to highly trained.

The *maximum heart rate* does not increase with training and may decrease slightly. Maximum heart rate does decrease linearly about 1 beat per minute with each year of age. The maximum heart rate is calculated with the formula $HR_{max} = 220 - age$ (in years). The heart rate does, however, change with sustained training in two ways: the resting heart rate drops and the heart rate during exercise at any given load is lower. Endurance training increases parasympathetic activity and decreases sympathetic activity in the heart at rest. The first morning resting heart rate is often in the 35–45 beats per minute range in highly trained athletes. This would be a pathologically low bradycardia in an untrained individual. Long-term endurance training also decreases submaximal heart rate during exercise by reducing sympathetic activity to the heart. Heart rate recovery time from exercise also decreases as aerobic training is advanced. This allows less time to elapse between exercise bouts.

Cardiac output is the product of heart rate and stroke volume. With exercise, the heart rate increases, and as the heart rate increases the time for ventricular filling decreases. Therefore, a training effect of lower heart rate at a given load will allow more time for ventricular filling, which benefits cardiac output. Because stroke volume increases with endurance training, the result is enhanced cardiac output.

Endurance training induces changes to augment *blood flow* to the muscles. These changes allow more efficient transport of oxygen and tissue nutrients to the muscle and more efficient removal of metabolic waste products and metabolic heat from the tissues. Training increases the number of capillaries in any given area of muscle and induces larger diameters in the existing capillaries. Parallel to the rise in capillary numbers is an increase in the cross-sectional area of the muscle fibers. Active muscle also preferentially increases the portion of the blood volume supply to ensure adequate substrate for muscle work. As a result, the blood flow to inactive muscle beds and less essential organs is decreased, making the blood volume available to meet the demands of active muscle.

Although *blood pressure* is relatively stable during activity in endurance-trained athletes, resting blood pressure drops. This is particularly significant for both athletes and the general population with mild hypertension; regular aerobic exercise is a safe, inexpensive, nonpharmacologic method of reducing systolic and diastolic blood pressure by about 10 mm Hg.

The blood cell mass and intravascular plasma volume both increase because of training to increase the total blood volume. Again, the changes are geared toward increasing the oxygen and nutrient capacity of the blood, and also to provide more fluid for metabolism and thermal homeostasis. The plasma volume increases by about 1 L and the blood cell volume increases by about 0.5 L in an average-sized man. High-altitude training and the illegal use of both erythropoietin (EPO) and blood doping are methods used by athletes to force greater increases in the blood cell mass. Too great an increase in the blood cell mass increases the risk of capillary sludging of the red cells in small capillaries and can result in unexpected sudden death as was seen in several Dutch bicycle racers when EPO first became available commercially.

Intermittent hypoxic training is used to induce EPO by challenging the body at rest to hypoxic conditions and pushing the training stimulus in less hypoxic environments. The concept utilized by many athletes is to live high and train low, as is done by the US Nordic Team living in Park City, Utah, and training at lower elevations in the Salt Lake Valley. Another variation of this technique is to live in houses designed to control the oxygen levels at rest in the house and push the training nearer sea level outside the house. This process improves endurance performance at sea level. The opposite strategy of training at high altitude does not allow the well-trained athlete to overload the systems and improve power or speed.

Respiratory Changes Associated with Endurance Training

The respiratory system is seldom the limiting factor in a healthy endurance-trained athlete. Lung volume changes very little if at all with endurance training. Tidal volume increases with maximal effort as training progresses, in part due to the decrease in residual volume of air that is usually not removed from the lungs with each breath. Respiratory rates may decrease slightly at rest and increase considerably at maximum exercise with training. The combination of increased tidal volume and respiratory rate at maximum exercise results in the marked increase in pulmonary ventilation rate that comes with endurance training. Highly trained athletes can double the ventilation rates of untrained individuals. A typical respiratory ventilation rate is 180 L/min in a healthy trained athlete. Pulmonary diffusion will increase as a result of endurance training following the increases in blood flow through the lung and the increases in pulmonary ventilation rates that when combined force more of the lung diffusion surface into an active role. The arterial-venous oxygen difference increases with training level because the blood volume is more widely distributed throughout the body and the venous blood returning to the heart has less oxygen because the tissues extract more oxygen in a trained athlete. Recent studies suggest that specific respiratory muscle training can improve the endurance and strength of the respiratory muscles in healthy athletes and possibly improve performance. The effects have been small and not widely reproduced.

Neuromuscular Changes

Type 1 muscle fibers are the main aerobic fibers. As activity increases, more type 1 fibers are recruited into action, and as training progresses the number of type 1 fibers increases by up to 25%. When increased power is required, type 2 fibers are recruited. Early training responses increase the recruitment of muscle fibers and more advanced training induces increased muscle size and in some cases increased fiber number. The increased number of fibers is supported by a concomitant increase in the number of capillaries that feed the muscle units.

Metabolic Changes

Muscle work requires the conversion of stored chemical energy to mechanical energy. The ability of the muscle to clear lactate increases and the amount of lactate produced at any workload decreases with high-level training. The result is an increase in lactate threshold; the *lactate threshold* is the point at which lactate begins to rise in the blood. A rise in the lactate threshold allows greater speeds for the same level of fatigue. The *respiratory exchange ratio*, which is the ratio of carbon dioxide produced to oxygen consumed, decreases with training at moderate workloads. The decrease is due to greater utilization of free fatty acids for muscle fuel. The respiratory exchange ratio increases at maximum workloads with the large pulmonary ventilation rates generated by highly trained endurance athletes.

As muscle size and number increase, so does the ability to utilize oxygen and hence the oxygen consumption rises with training. With the rise in VO_{2max} comes an increase in aerobic power and the desired improvement in performance. Repeated muscle contraction early in training induces altered regulation of Na^+-K^+-ATPase membrane protein in the sarcolemma and t-tubule to maintain high Na^+ and K^+ transmembrane gradients. Na^+-K^+-ATPase controls muscle excitation and contraction processes, metabolic flux rates, and contractility.

Endurance exercise increases the mitochondrial volume by 50% in some athletes with training for few weeks. Substrate metabolism moves toward lipids as a source of energy with an intracellular doubling of lipid. Endurance training induces the transcription of protein enzymes required in the energy utilization systems in the mitochondria, including enzymes of the mitochondrial electron transport chain and mitochondrial protein concentration. These protein changes, along with increased capillary blood supply, result in a shift in endurance-trained muscle to burn more fat as a fuel with less dependence on glycolytic flux and more precise control of acid-base status contributing to enhanced performance capacity. The literature suggests that aerobic fitness improves recovery from high-intensity exercise by increasing aerobic response, improving lactate removal from the muscle, and enhanced phosphocreatine regeneration within the mitochondria. Sprint training, in contrast to endurance training, has a greater effect on muscle glycolytic capacity than on muscle mitochondrial content. In highly fit athletes, intense interval training improves performance and seems to support the notion that athletes should train at exercise intensities specific to their event to improve competition performance.

For highly trained athletes, additional increases in the volume of less than maximal training intensity do not appear to improve performance in endurance activity or change the physiologic markers associated with improved endurance capacity. Athletes who are highly fit require greater intensity workloads to show improvement and these loads are achieved through intense interval training. There does not appear to be any change in oxidative or glycolytic enzyme activity in highly fit endurance athletes using intense interval training, even though there are significant improvements in performance. The mechanisms responsible for the improvements in performance have not been determined, but may involve increases in skeletal muscle buffering capacity, changes in plasma volume, or changes in the muscle cation pumps, myoglobin, capillary density, and fiber types.

OVERTRAINING

Highly trained athletes may experience *overtraining* as a consequence of pushing the limits of endurance, especially with high-intensity training. If the metabolic adaptations of the athlete will not support the level of activity, *overtraining syndrome* may occur. In endurance sports, the metabolic aspects of training fatigue appear to be the most relevant parameters that may characterize overtraining when recovery is not sufficient, or when dietary habits do not allow an optimal replenishment of substrate stores. Studies of selected biochemical markers have not been able to demonstrate a specific chemical marker that consistently identifies overtraining in an athlete who clinically demonstrates the syndrome. Studies suggest that energy balance plays a role in overtraining. Well-balanced nutrition with adequate calories to support the level of training activity is critical to avoiding the syndrome of overtraining. Adequate rest and recovery time are also essential. Although it is not proven, tracking first morning pulses can help to determine if adequate recovery time is available for an individual athlete and a first morning pulse of 10 or more above baseline is an indication of inadequate recovery or impending illness.

ENDURANCE EXERCISE AND IMMUNE FUNCTION

Immune function in humans is altered by endurance training. The general perception of physically active people that regular moderate activity increases and vigorous, high-intensity training decreases resistance to minor illnesses is supported by epidemiologic data. The higher incidence of upper respiratory tract infection during intense training may result in impairment of neutrophil function, serum and mucosal immunoglobulin levels, plasma glutamine concentration, and possibly natural killer cell cytotoxic activity. Endurance athletes should avoid overtraining, get adequate rest and recovery, eat well, and avoid exposure to infection. It may be advisable for winter athletes to get an annual influenza immunization.

ENDURANCE TRAINING SCHEDULES

Like strength training, training for endurance in a given sport revolves around the concept of periodization and is broken into macrocycles, mesocycles, and microcycles. The annual plan utilizing the principles of *periodization* should allow an athlete to reach peak performance without the overtraining risk that is prevalent in endurance-trained athletes. The mesocycles should be designed in 3–6 week blocks that concentrate the intense workouts and allow for periods of rest and recovery.

A typical weekly microcycle of workouts integrated into a competitive season might include a hard day, a moderate day, a hard day, a moderate or easy day, a competition day, a moderate or easy day, and a rest day. Within the mesocycles, the volume and intensity of the hard and moderate workouts progressively increase to force an overload and training response. As the peak of competition approaches, the number of easy workouts increases to allow a rested and ready system for the important competitions. The most common training error is to skip the rest and easy days that are in the schedule for recovery.

The *training response* occurs with consistent work that overloads the skeletal and cardiac muscles to the level that allows the energy systems to improve function during exercise. In general, workouts have to increase in intensity and duration at an optimum frequency to provide an overload stimulus and still allow for recovery. Prior to the end of season competitions, it is common for athletes to taper or decrease either the volume or intensity of training. The ideal taper schedule prior the competitions is not well understood. Most studies suggest it is more important to maintain training intensity than training volume. Progressive reductions in training volume in the 2–4 weeks prior to competition can decrease swim times by 2–3% and 5-km running times by up to 6%. The most favorable taper is probably an individual athlete response and may depend on the training intensity and the need for recovery time prior to competition.

Detraining is the loss of training effects that occurs with voluntary or injury-related decreases in training stimulus. Detraining differs based on the length of time away from physical overloads with *short-term detraining* defined as less than 4 weeks duration and *long-term detraining* as more than 4 weeks of insufficient training stimulus. Short-term cardiorespiratory detraining involves rapid decline in Vo_{2max} and loss of the extra blood volume associated with endurance training. Increases in heart rate during exercise are not sufficient to offset the decreased stroke volume, and results in reduced maximal cardiac output. Ventilation volume is also impaired, but is less noticeable in recently trained athletes. Short-term detraining shifts toward carbohydrate metabolism during exercise, increasing the exercise respiratory exchange ratio, and decreasing lipase activity, GLUT-4 content, glycogen level, and lactate threshold. At the level of the muscle, capillary density and oxidative enzyme activities are reduced. For the short term of inactivity, the Vo_{2max} is greatly reduced and recent Vo_{2max} gains are completely lost.

Cross-training may be effective in maintaining and protecting training-induced endurance capacity. The more sport specific the activity, the more carry over to the field of play when the athlete returns to competition. Cross-transfer effect from the uninjured to the injured limb can be utilized to train the injured limb.

HEALTH BENEFITS OF ENDURANCE ACTIVITY

Endurance activity can ease some of the physiologic changes associated with aging and sedentary lifestyle, including decline in fitness level and bone density, onset and severity of chronic disease, and loss of functional independence. Women who participate in lifetime activity are physiologically 20–30 years younger than their sedentary counterparts. An exercise program for life should be functional, enjoyable, and combine endurance and strengthening activities.

Endurance training even at light to moderate levels helps to control weight and counters the recent trend of increasing obesity that is so prevalent in North America. Regular aerobic exercise decreases triglycerides (but not LDL cholesterol) and insulin resistance.

Hypertension is very common in sedentary populations and exercise plays an important role in nonpharmacologic treatment. Regular exercise training decreases blood pressure in the vast majority of patients with hypertension about 10 mm Hg in both systolic and diastolic measures. The effects of training on blood pressure reduction are greatest in women and middle-aged populations, and low to moderate training seems to be as effective as high-intensity training. Exercise in hypertensive patients also improves plasma lipids and insulin sensitivity.

Chronic heart failure guidelines provide little information regarding the value of exercise for patients. A literature review suggests that physical performance and quality of life can be improved, but morbidity and mortality are not affected by regular endurance activity. Exercise training may augment the regression of pathologic left ventricular hypertrophy in hypertensive patients.

The aging and elderly benefit from regular endurance activity. The moderately exercising elderly oxidize more glucose and less fat probably due to age-related changes in skeletal muscle. An active lifestyle into old age reduces the risk of chronic disease, provided the activity is sufficient to maintain or improve maximal oxygen consumption. The response to training in individuals older than 60 years is the same as in younger athletes. However, maximal cardiac output does decline with age and is the main reason that maximal oxygen consumption drops with age.

GLOSSARY OF TERMS USED IN TRAINING

- *Hill training:* uphill and downhill running to produce overload challenge uphill and induce eccentric load downhill; downhill work is also used for leg speed.
- *Intervals:* repeated short to long bouts of an exercise intensity equal or superior to maximal lactate steady-state velocity with recovery periods with a given distance at a set time interval such as twenty 400-m runs starting every 3 minutes.
- *Long slow distance:* running slowly for a set time or distance, used mainly on light days and in the early season.
- *Negative splits:* running the second half of a run faster than the first.
- *Repeats:* same as intervals, with restart of a given distance tied to some marker of recovery like ten 600-m runs starting when the heart rate recovers to 100 bpm.
- *Speed work:* runs at or faster than race pace.
- *Taper:* reduction in training volume prior to competition.
- *Tempo runs:* Changing the pace at given intervals during a long run.

REFERENCES

Billat LV. Interval training for performance: A scientific and empirical practice. Special recommendations for middle- and long-distance running. Part I: aerobic interval training. *Sports Med.* 2001;31:13–31.

Burrows M, Bird S. The physiology of the highly trained female endurance runner. *Sports Med.* 2000;30:281–300.

Carter JB, Banister EW, Blaber AP. Effect of endurance exercise on autonomic control of heart rate. *Sports Med.* 2003;33:33–46.

Coudert J, Van Praagh E. Endurance exercise training in the elderly: Effects on cardiovascular function. *Curr Opin Clin Nutr Metab Care.* 2000;3:479–483.

Durstine JL, Grandjean PW, Cox CA, Thompson PD. Lipids, lipoproteins, and exercise. *J Cardiopulm Rehabil.* 2002;22:385–398.

Echegaray M, Rivera MA. Role of creatine kinase isoenzymes on muscular and cardiorespiratory endurance: Genetic and molecular evidence. *Sports Med.* 2001;31:919–934.

Fitts RH. Effects of regular exercise training on skeletal muscle contractile function. *Am J Phys Med Rehab.* 2003;82:320–331.

Green HJ. Adaptations in the muscle cell to training: Role of the Na^+-K^+-Atpase. *Can J Appl Physiol.* 2000;25:204–216.

Hagberg JM, Park JJ, Brown MD. The role of exercise training in the treatment of hypertension: An update. *Sports Med.* 2000;30:193–206.

Hawley JA. Adaptations of skeletal muscle to prolonged, intense endurance training. *Clin Exp Pharmacol Physiol.* 2002;29:218–222.

Hawley JA, Stepto NK. Adaptations to training in endurance cyclists: Implications for performance. *Sports Med.* 2001;31:511–520.

Hoppeler H, Fluck M. Plasticity of skeletal muscle mitochondria: Structure and function. *Med Sci Sports Exerc.* 2003;35:95–104.

Kubukeli ZN, Noakes TD, Dennis SC. Training techniques to improve endurance exercise performances. *Sports Med.* 2002;32:489–509.

Laursen PB, Jenkins DG. The scientific basis for high-intensity interval training: Optimising training programmes and maximising performance in highly trained endurance athletes. *Sports Med.* 2002;32:53–73.

Levine BD. Intermittent hypoxic training: Fact and fancy. *High Alt Med Biol.* 2002;3:177–193.

Lloyd-Williams F, Mair FS, Leitner M. Exercise training and heart failure: A systematic review of current evidence. *Br J Gen Pract.* 2002;52:47–55.

Mackinnon LT. Chronic exercise training effects on immune function. *Med Sci Sports Exerc.* 2000;32(7 Suppl):S369–S376.

Miszko TA, Cress ME. A lifetime of fitness. Exercise in the perimenopausal and postmenopausal woman. *Clin Sports Med.* 2000;19:215–232.

Mittendorfer B, Klein S. Effect of aging on glucose and lipid metabolism during endurance exercise. *Int J Sport Nutr Exerc Metab.* 2001;11(Suppl):S86–S91.

Mujika I, Padilla S. Detraining: Loss of training-induced physiological and performance adaptations. Part I: Short term insufficient training stimulus. *Sports Med.* 2000;30:79–87.

Mujika I, Padilla S. Detraining: Loss of training-induced physiological and performance adaptations. Part II: Long term insufficient training stimulus. *Sports Med.* 2000;30:145–154.

Naughton G, Farpour-Lambert NJ, Carlson J, Bradney M, Van Praagh E. Physiological issues surrounding the performance of adolescent athletes. *Sports Med.* 2000;30:309–325.

Petibois C, Cazorla G, Poortmans JR, Deleris G. Biochemical aspects of overtraining in endurance sports: A review. *Sports Med.* 2002;32:867–878.

Tomlin DL, Wenger HA. The relationship between aerobic fitness and recovery from high intensity intermittent exercise. *Sports Med.* 2001;31:1–11.

Sheel AW. Respiratory muscle training in healthy individuals: Physiological rationale and implications for exercise performance. *Sports Med.* 2002;32:567–581.

II | INJURY AND ILLNESS

11 | Head Injuries and Concussions

Michael L. Schwartz and Charles H. Tator

Athletic injuries are determined by culture and location and vary widely in incidence and cause from one part of the world to another. In the province of Ontario, Canada, head injuries make up approximately 30% of all major injuries in sports and recreation (Tator, 1996). Motor sports, such as snowmobiling, and bicycling are the most dangerous in this regard and each account for about 25% of the head injuries. The rest of the injuries occur with participation in a variety of other sports including ice hockey, alpine skiing, water sports, baseball, football, and soccer. Because even apparently minor head injuries are irrevocable and severe head injuries can be so devastating, people who are responsible for the safety of athletes must advocate safe practices and take measures that enhance the prevention and the mitigation of brain injuries. Medical providers must be familiar with the mechanisms of brain injury and understand the pathophysiologic principles on which treatment is based.

PATHOPHYSIOLOGY

Most head injuries in sports and recreational activities are caused by falls or collisions and, as a result, are blunt injuries. If the head is buttressed and acceleration of the brain is prevented, there is no significant injury to the brain unless a skull fracture occurs and a bone fragment is driven inward. In depressed skull fractures, there may be a focal injury to the underlying brain.

In most head injuries occurring during athletic activity, there is significant acceleration or deceleration imparted to the head. Although the brain floats in the cerebrospinal fluid, which tends to cushion impact, diffuse damage may occur even if the skull and the coverings of the brain are not broached. The brain is made up of delicate interconnected fibers called axons that may suffer damage with internal shear strains and distortions of cerebral tissue. Indeed, recent research points to diffuse damage to the axons as being a major factor in this type of brain injury, referred to as diffuse axonal injury (Povlishock, 2000). There is also a fine network of blood vessels that has developed to satisfy the high metabolic requirement of neurons. Like the axons, these fine blood vessels may be torn easily because there is no tough internal framework to support the brain. As a result, a blow to the head or the impact when the head strikes the ground or other playing surface literally may tear the brain to pieces by the internal shearing forces that are generated on contact. This shearing injury is usually both diffuse and focal. The cranial cavity, because of its irregular shape, tends to limit rotation forces. Greater internal shearing stress in the region of the sphenoid ridge characteristically causes damage to the adjacent frontal and temporal lobes. Other irregularities of the inner surface of the skull may also cause the bruising (cerebral contusions) that commonly occurs on the undersurface of the frontal lobes and temporal poles. Acceleration/deceleration injuries can cause the brain to move in the opposite direction of the skull or at a different rate, and this differential movement of the brain in relation to the skull can cause contre-coup injuries. For example, a fall backwards striking the occiput can cause coup damage to the occipital lobes and contrecoup damage to the frontal lobes.

121

Rotational forces on the brain that move it relative to the inner table of the skull can shear veins that conduct blood from the surface of the brain to the major venous sinuses. Under these circumstances, blood is released into the subdural space over the surface of the brain, resulting in a subdural hematoma. Severe shear stress in the interior of the brain can cause tearing of blood vessels and the subsequent development of an intracerebral hematoma. Intracranial blood clots also may be produced when a fracture in the temporal or parietal region crosses the middle meningeal artery and blood is released outside the dura to produce an extradural or epidural hematoma. With a hematoma in any of these locations, the patient's level of consciousness declines as the hematoma enlarges, intracranial pressure rises, and the brain is increasingly distorted. There are a myriad of other secondary injury processes in traumatized brain that evolve over hours to days after trauma, including excitotoxicity, electrolyte imbalance, calcium overload, and cytokine and prostaglandin release, that can cause further damage to the brain (Tator, 2002).

RELATIONSHIP BETWEEN THE LOCATION AND AMOUNT OF BRAIN INJURY AND THE SYMPTOMS AND SIGNS

In examining patients who have suffered head injuries, the physician must consider two aspects. First, there is the focal injury that is manifest by the loss of function of the injured part of the brain and the volume of brain diffusely damaged by the effects of deceleration. Injury to the motor strip that is located at the posterior edge of the frontal lobe produces contralateral weakness or paralysis of the arm, leg, or both. For virtually all right-handers and most left-handers, a left posterior frontal injury will interfere with the production of speech. Parietal injuries may cause contralateral impairment of sensation, and occipital injuries can cause hemianopia or loss of vision in one-half the visual field in both eyes. If the focal injury is caused by an in-driven bone fragment or another penetrating object and there is no acceleration of the whole brain, there may be no loss of consciousness. On the other hand, there is a large range of severity of possible injury caused by acceleration of the whole brain that is brief and apparently completely reversible at the mild end of the spectrum and which is prolonged or even permanent when severe. Prolonged unconsciousness is invariably followed by measured changes in cognitive function or in overt neurologic signs.

Recent experience suggests that the least severe concussion can occur without any loss of consciousness, although such concussions usually cause a period of amnesia. However, even these concussions are accompanied by some tissue damage, such as tearing of axons. Widespread axonal injuries have been documented after even mild brain injury, and there is strong evidence that diffuse axonal injury, as noted previously, is one of the major pathologic effects of severe brain injury (Povlishock, 2000). Because concussion is accompanied by subclinical tissue damage, its effect is cumulative and may result in progressive decline of cognitive and motor function when the blows are repeated, as they would be over a long career in boxing, football, soccer, or hockey. There is also experimental evidence for the cumulative effect of repeated brain injury (Laurer, 2001). It appears that there is a genetic factor accounting for the susceptibility to head trauma, the occurrence of repeated trauma, and the risk of the subsequent development of consequences, including the possible development of neurodegenerative disorders such as Alzheimer disease (Graham, 1999, Teasdale, 1997). Individuals with the epsilon 4 allele of apolipoprotein E carry an increased risk.

ADDED EFFECT OF LOSS OF OXYGEN OR LOW BLOOD PRESSURE

Inadequate resuscitation that leads to hypoxia or arterial hypotension can cause inadequate cerebral perfusion and result in a "second injury" (Chesnut, 1993). Thus, the priorities in resuscitation of the fallen athlete are the same as in resuscitation of patients with multiple injuries, known as the ABCs of trauma management. The first three priorities are maintenance or establishment of an adequate airway; maintenance or provision of adequate breathing, even by mechanical ventilation if necessary; and maintenance or provision of adequate circulation. Simultaneously, the cervical spine should be protected if there is any risk that the neck has been injured.

EVALUATION

The person who cares for a fallen athlete must determine rapidly whether there is a condition requiring transfer to a neurosurgical unit, such as a traumatic intracranial hematoma. The probability of significant intracranial bleeding is determined by the mechanism of injury. An equestrian who falls from a horse and strikes his or her head is more likely to harbor an intracranial clot than a hockey player who was stopped by a hard body check and whose head never hit the ice. If the athlete is initially conscious and then his or her level of consciousness declines, or if initially he or she moved all limbs equally but is becoming weak on one side of the body, an expanding intracranial hematoma progressively distorting the brain and raising intracranial pressure should be suspected regardless of the mechanism of injury.

The Glasgow Coma Scale (Teasdale, 1974) is an essential adjunct in the management of patients with suspected brain injuries. The person evaluating the injured athlete is required to repeat, at intervals, a series of stereotyped observations, as described by Teasdale and Jennett. The examiner must determine whether the athlete opens his or her eyes to pain, to voice, or spontaneously; adopts an extensor posture or flexor posture in response to pain, localizes a painful stimulus, or follows simple instructions; or makes no sound, grunts, or answers questions inappropriately or appropriately. Therapeutic decisions may be based on improvement or decline in a 15-point scale. Lesser degrees of brain injury that may not cause a reduction in the Glasgow Coma Scale score are evaluated by methods outlined in the "Concussion" section. Most importantly, any player with a head injury should not be left alone, and should be regularly monitored for deterioration.

RESUSCITATION

ABCs of Trauma Management

As stated earlier, the first priorities in resuscitation are airway, breathing, and circulation (Committee on Trauma, American College of Surgeons, 1994). In the provision of medical services for an organized athletic competition, there should be a prearranged emergency plan to provide personnel and specific procedures and equipment commensurate with the environmental conditions and the level of competition. A system of communication with local emergency services that can supply support personnel and additional equipment also should be established ahead of time. A physician in attendance at an athletic event should be equipped with a blood pressure cuff and a face mask that can be applied so as to provide positive-pressure ventilation should it be required. The remote possibility of having to intubate a patient or establish a surgical airway has to be considered. It should be decided in advance whether the responsible person will acquire the skills to perform endotracheal intubation or to place an intravenous line. Will a large-bore needle and cannula for emergency cricothyrotomy or a small tracheotomy kit be available? Since there is no blood loss in the majority of head injuries in sports, first aid will require maintenance of the airway and ventilation only. With airway and ventilation maintained, athletes who remain unconscious after an injury must be transferred immediately, with cervical spine precautions, to the emergency department of a hospital with a neurosurgical service.

Spine

Any person rendered unconscious has been hit hard enough to have also suffered a broken neck and should be treated accordingly. It is prudent to assume that every unconscious athlete has also sustained a spinal injury, and that the spinal injury is unstable. During resuscitation and transport of the unconscious athlete, precautions should be taken to stabilize the cervical spine in an anatomic position. In general, helmets and other protective equipment should only be removed in the hospital setting with gentle in-line manual traction applied. Personnel in attendance at North American football or hockey games should be familiar with the disassembly of face masks and helmets and be equipped with screwdrivers, wire cutters, and shears to cut the plastic face mask mounting brackets. The proper technique requires the participation of several people to maintain gentle in-line traction on the neck, support of the occiput, and removal and/or disassembly of the chin strap, mouthpiece, face mask, and cheek pads. The reason for these precautions with respect to helmet removal is that extension of the neck occurs when the helmet is removed, especially if the player is wearing shoulder pads, and this may worsen an unstable spinal injury. The design of newer helmets facilitates their removal without manipulation of the neck.

CONCUSSION

When there is significant acceleration or deceleration of the whole brain, a period of cerebral dysfunction follows the impact. There is a continuum of severity of injury, with increasingly severe acceleration causing more severe signs and symptoms with slower and less complete recovery. Recent experience suggests that even the mildest injuries are significant, even those that cause only brief confusion without loss of consciousness and no other symptoms. With more violent acceleration, in addition to confusion, there is a period of amnesia. When the most recent events prior to the impact are lost to memory, the phenomenon is called retrograde amnesia (RGA). The retrograde amnesia initially may be extensive but tends to shorten as time goes by. It is generally considered to be a less reliable measure of injury severity than the duration of posttraumatic amnesia (PTA), the period of memory loss that follows the injury. Some patients may appear normal following a blow to the head, but if questioned later about events surrounding their injury, they may have no recall, even though there was never any loss of consciousness. It has been suggested that this period of PTA should be more correctly termed posttraumatic confusional state (Stuss, 1999). The mildest form of concussion, where there is confusion only, is termed grade 1 in the recently described American Academy of Neurology classification (Kelly, 1999) if it lasts less than 15 minutes, and grade 2 if it lasts longer. In this classification, grade 3 is a head injury with loss of consciousness. The original formulation that we derived (Schwartz, 1994) from the 1986 Cantu classification (Cantu, 1986) of sports-related concussion relied on the presence or absence of PTA to assess the severity of concussion. At that time, PTA could only be assessed in retrospect. As a result, we did not allow the athlete to return to the contest in which he or she was injured. Another modification of the original Cantu classification, adopted by the Colorado Medical Society (Colorado Medical Society, 1990), considers milder injuries causing confusion only and permits return to the game. Amnesia is taken as a criterion of grade 2 severity in the Colorado system.

The American Academy of Neurology system permits a real-time evaluation of concussion severity. In this system, concussion should be diagnosed when there is any of the following symptoms or signs: vacant stare, delayed verbal or motor responses, slurred speech, incoordination, distractibility, disorientation, inappropriate behavior, emotional instability, or memory deficit. A short, structured sideline examination of any athlete suspected of having suffered a concussion should be undertaken as follows.

1. Assessment of mental status: Is the athlete oriented to person, place, and time?
2. Assessment of mental control: Ask the athlete to repeat short digit strings forward and backward, count forward and backward, and to recite the months forward and backward.
3. Memory: Ask the athlete to recall three words after a few minutes interval; test recall of details of the game or prominent, current news events.
4. A very brief neurologic examination to detect asymmetry of sensory and motor function and balance should then be done. Visual fields are tested by finger or hand movements with the subject facing the examiner are compared with the examiner's visual fields. Having the athlete extend the arms forward with eyes closed assesses position sense and arm strength. Balance and lower limb strength and sensation may be evaluated by having the athlete hop a few times on either foot.

Exertional, Provocative Tests

Another feature of the American Academy of Neurology system is the application of exertional provocative tests. They recommend five push-ups, five sit-ups, five knee bends, and when appropriate, a 40-m sprint. The sprint may be adapted to match the athletic activity, for example, having a hockey player skate up and down the rink. Some athletes, who at rest have become asymptomatic after a concussion, will get headache, unsteadiness, or even a return of cognitive dysfunction after physical exertion. These new or recurrent symptoms probably are evoked by changes in cerebral blood flow induced by changes in cardiac output and systemic blood pressure.

Neuropsychological Testing

Neuropsychological testing has been shown to be of value in evaluation of concussed athletes (Aubry, 2002, Collie, 2003, Grindel, 2001). It is especially valuable in cases in which baseline assessments have been performed prior to a concussion to serve as a comparison for post-concussion tests. However, even in the absence of baseline tests, abnormal findings, such as performance variabilty on neuropsychological testing, serve as useful information with respect to determining the advisability of return to play, as discussed as follows. Computerized neuropsychologic testing programs are available at www.cogsport.com and www.impacttest.com. Both systems can be set up on multiple computers to allow easy access to preseason baseline testing.

Neuroimaging

Computed tomography (CT) scans are excellent for detecting structural lesions in acute head injuries in athletes, especially for detecting space occupying lesions, such as hematomas, that require emergent neurosurgical treatment. For the evaluation of post-concussion symptoms and signs, neuroimaging is of less value because there are no identifiable lesions in the majority of cases. Neuroimaging with CT or MRI is indicated for any persistent symptoms, especially in those with focal neurological deficits, seizures, or persistent clinical or cognitive symptoms (Aubry, 2002). Some of the newer MR imaging sequences, such as gradient echo, are sensitive for detecting hemosiderin deposits from small hemorrhages. Also, neuroimaging would detect the presence of rare effects of trauma, such as a chronic subdural hematoma or cerebral atrophy.

Second Impact Syndrome

In a very small number of reported cases, an athlete who had not completely recovered from an earlier concussion suffered a catastrophic outcome after what appeared to be a trivial second blow to the head. These individuals succumbed to a syndrome characterized by immediate, fulminating cerebral edema. The syndrome was given the name *second impact syndrome* by Saunders and Harbaugh (Saunders, 1984). Under normal circumstances, regional cerebral blood flow depends on the metabolic requirements of that particular region and is independent of systemic arterial pressure through a wide range of pressure. This phenomenon is called autoregulation (Lewelt, 1980) We surmise that the cerebral edema develops as a result of increased cerebral blood flow (CBF) in an injured portion of the brain where autoregulation has been lost. When the arterial pressure is very high and exceeds the limits of autoregulation, for example, in hypertensive encephalopathy, or when the brain is injured and CBF varies with systemic arterial pressure, a sufficient rise in arterial pressure may induce cerebral edema. Physical exercise that sufficiently raises arterial pressure in a subject who has lost autoregulation may produce the headache, unsteadiness, and cognitive dysfunction described earlier that preclude a return to athletic activity or, when coupled with a blow to the head, the second impact syndrome. There is experimental evidence that autoregulation of CBF is restored in a matter of weeks. Thus, it is essential for the brain to completely recover from a concussion before another blow is sustained to prevent this syndrome. Currently, it is believed that the incidence of this syndrome is extremely rare, and that most fulminant cases of neurologic deterioration after head injury in sports are really examples of diffuse cerebral swelling (McCrory, 2001). The latter is much more common in children and adolescents than in adults, and does not require a second impact. For clinicians and others involved in sport, there is a need to carefully evaluate postconcussive symptoms, the presence of which should be seen as a significant risk factor for the acute deterioration due to diffuse cerebral swelling (Collie, 2003, Wesner, 2003).

RETURN-TO-PLAY GUIDELINES

It should be emphasized that there is no base of prospectively acquired evidence to validate any of the systems of classification of head injuries or the return to play guidelines. In our view, the most important criterion for determining when it is safe for a player to return to play is the complete return of normal brain function as assessed by examination. A player should not return to training or competition until cognitive function is normal and all symptoms, such as headache, unsteadiness, and cognitive dysfunction, have subsided at rest and after exertion, such as produced by the provocative maneuvers outlined previously. Since there is evidence that subclinical, permanent damage accumulates as repeated concussions occur, the required period of withdrawal from competition for a second concussion of a particular severity is increased as compared with that after the first. After a first grade 1 concussion, a player can return to the contest if after 15 minutes he or she is completely symptom free according to the American Academy of Neurology Classification (Quality Standards Subcommittee, 1997). After a grade 2 concussion, the player is withdrawn from the contest and may play if well for 1 week, after passing an exertional provocative test. A player with a brief (seconds) loss of consciousness (grade 3 concussion) is suspended from play for 1 week, but may then play if completely well at rest and after exertion. For a loss of consciousness lasting minutes, the athlete must be out for 2 weeks and pass the exertion test. As noted previously, there is insufficient research on this topic to satisfy the scientific requirements of evidence-based medicine for definite guidelines about return to play. Indeed, the Canadian Academy of Sport Medicine has issued a statement indicating that there is no evidence to support the use of any one system of classification of head injuries and return to play guidelines over another, and that all athletes with any degree of concussion should be examined by a physician for advice about returning to play, and that athletes must never return to play if symptoms are still present (Canadian Academy of Sport Medicine, 2002). An International Concussion in Sport Group recently echoed the Canadian view that the lack of scientific evidence precludes endorsement of any of the currntly published guidelines (Aubry, 2002). Any athlete who remains drowsy or unconscious must be transported with appropriate airway protection and breathing and circulatory support to the emergency department of a hospital with a neurosurgical service. Neurosurgical consultation and, when indicated, brain imaging must be obtained. The consultant may wish to obtain a complete neuropsychological assessment of the athlete prior to return to competition. Any bruise (contusion) or blood clot (hematoma) or any other sign of recent trauma on CT or MRI precludes return to play for the season. For second concussions, we recommend longer absences or stiffer "penalties" and more

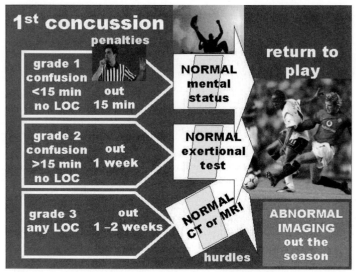

FIG 11-1 The definitions of the grades of severity of concussion are indicated in the left-hand column. Confusion only, without loss of consciousness (LOC), lasting less than 15 minutes is the least severe grade. Confusion lasting longer than 15 minutes is intermediate, and any loss of consciousness is considered the most severe grade. Column 2 indicates the "penalties" for a first concussion of the grades in column 1. Column 3 shows the "hurdle" that the athlete must get over to return to play. An athlete is sidelined for a minimum of 15 minutes but may return to play after a grade 1 concussion if his or her mental status returns completely to normal. If confusion persists for more than 15 minutes (grade 2), then the athlete is withdrawn from the contest but may return to competition on another day if the mental status is normal and the provocative exertional test evokes no symptoms. For grade 3 concussion lasting seconds, the athlete must be out 1 week and may return if completely normal. Neuroimaging and neurosurgical consultation are at the discretion of the treating physician. For more prolonged loss of consciousness, the athlete is sidelined for a minimum of 2 weeks, and neurosurgical consultation and possibly neuroimaging are advisable. Regardless of concussion grade, a contusion, hematoma, or any other sign of recent trauma on CT scan or MRI precludes return to play for the season.

stringent "hurdles" to get over, as indicated in Figures 11-1 and 11-2, before return to play.

After more than one or a series of concussions, an athlete would be allowed to return to play in the following circumstances: the neurologic examination is normal; the player has sustained a small number of concussions, dispersed in time, of low severity (grades 1 and 2), each with complete recovery; the length of time to complete recovery is short, such as only a few days; the neurolopsychological evaluation shows no cognitive deficits; and the MR or CT shows no abnormalities (Tator, 2001). Conversely, after more than one or a series of concussions, an athlete would be advised to never return to play in the presence of the following: neurologic deficits, or

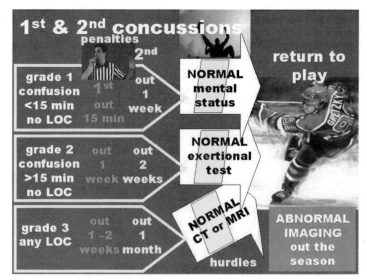

FIG 11-2   The definitions of the grades of severity of concussion are indicated in the left-hand column. The "penalties," that is, the required time out of competition after a first concussion, are indicated in column 2. In recognition of the cumulative effect of repeated concussions, the increased time of withdrawal from play for a second concussion is indicated in column 3. For example, after two grade 1 concussions suffered in the same contest, an athlete is withdrawn from competition and must not return for at least 1 week. The "hurdle" to get over prior to return to play is a symptom-free week, a normal mental status, and a normal provocative exertional test. Similarly, the "penalty" for two grade 2 concussions is a minimum of 2 weeks. The return-to-play "hurdle" is 2 symptom-free weeks, a normal mental status, and a normal provocative exertional test. Neurosurgical consultation and neuroimaging are advisable for any persistent symptoms. More than one grade 3 concussion requires withdrawal from play for at least 1 month. The return-to-play "hurdle" is 1 symptom-free month, a normal mental status, and a normal provocative exertional test. Neurosurgical consultation and neuroimaging are advised. Any persistent symptom at rest or after exertion precludes return to play. Regardless of concussion grade, a contusion, hematoma, or any other sign of recent trauma on CT scan or MRI precludes return to play for the season.

significant persisting symptoms; a history of multiple concussions over a short period of time, and of high severity (grades 2 and 3); recovery was prolonged, for example, several weeks to months; neuropsychological evaluation revealed cognitive deficits; and MR or CT showed the presence of brain lesions (Tator, 2001).

REHABILITATION

A structured, graduated, and supervised rehabilitation protocol is conducive to optimal recovery and safe and successful return to play (Aubry, 2002). The rehabilitation and return to play process should have the following stages.

1. No activity, complete rest: once asymptomatic, proceed to step 2
2. Light aerobic exercise, for example, walking or stationary cycle
3. Sport-specific training, for example, skating in hockey, running in soccer
4. Non-contact training drills
5. Full-contact training after medical clearance
6. Game play

Each step takes a minimum of 1 day. The athlete moves to the next stage only if asymptomatic, and if symptoms recur, the athlete should drop back to the former stage for 1 day.

PREVENTION

Education of all participants, coaches, league officials, and the general public about prevention of head injuries in sports and recreation is essential. Since treatment and rehabilitation of major head injuries or concussions is poor, the emphasis must be on prevention. For example, there must be improved education about the detection of concussion, its clinical features, assessment techniques, and the principles of safe return to play.

Helmets have been of major importance in preventing brain injury in athletes. In certain sports, such as hockey and North American football, helmet use is mandatory. In these sports, major brain injury has been reduced but certainly not eliminated. Major brain injuries still occur in helmeted athletes, and repeated minor brain injuries, with their cumulative and potentially irreversible effects, can occur in helmeted players. In other sports, such as competitive skiing, helmets may not be mandatory but are strongly recommended for all age groups. Bicyclists and equestrians of all ages should wear helmets. Helmets should also be required in many other recreational activities such as all motorsports, snowboarding, and in-line skating. In rugby and soccer, helmets have been considered, but there is no proof that head injuries would be reduced (McIntosh, 2000). Helmets should be fitted properly, maintained in good condition, and certified by one of the recognized testing associations, such as the Canadian Standards Association, and the helmet strap must be secured. Helmets should be replaced after any major impact, and at regular intervals after repeated minor impact.

In many sports, there is a need for additional sport-specific research on prevention of head injuries. For example, in soccer there is considerable uncertainty about the role of repeated heading of the ball in causing long-term cognitive deficits, especially dementia (Kirkendall, 2001, Matser, 1998).

Prevention should be a concern of all those involved in sports, including individual players and participants, parents, league officials, referees, coaches, and trainers. Respect for the opponent and the opponent's long-term health must be part of the psychology of competitive sports. In some sports, concussions could be reduced by eliminating fighting. Athletes should be ambassadors and supporters of brain injury prevention programs, such as Think First (Wesner, 2003).

RECOMMENDED READINGS

Aubry M, Cantu R, Dvorak J. Summary and Agreement Statement of the 1st
    International Symposium on Concussion in Sport, Vienna 2001. *Clin J Sport
    Med.* 2002;12:6–11.
Canadian Academy of Sport Medicine Concussion Committee. Guidelines for
    assessment and management of sport-related concussion, 2000. *Clin J Sport Med.*
    2002;10:209–211.

Cantu RC. Guidelines for return to contact sports after a cerebral concussion. *Phys Sports Med.* 1986;14:75–83.

Chesnut RM, Marshall LF, Klauber MR, et al. The role of secondary brain injury in determining outcome from severe head injury. *J Trauma.* 1993;34:216–222.

Collie A, Maruff P, Makdissi M, McCrory P, McStephen M, Darby D. CogSport: Reliability and correlation with conventional cognitive tests used in postconcussion medical evaluations. *Clin J Sport Med.* 2003;13:28–32.

Committee on Trauma, American College of Surgeons. *Advanced Trauma Life Support. Instructor Manual.* Chicago: American college of Surgeons; 1994.

Graham DI, Horsburgh K, Nicoll JA, Teasdale GM. Apolipoprotein E and the response of the brain to injury. *Acta Neurochir Suppl.* (Wien) 1999;73:89–92.

Grindel SH, Lovell MR, Collins MW. The assessment of sport-related concussion: the evidence behind neuropsychological testing and management. *Clin J Sport Med.* 2001;11:134–143.

Kelly JP, Rosenberg JH. Diagnosis and management of concussion in sports. *Neurology.* 1997;48:575–580.

Kirkendall DT, Jordan SE, Garret WE. Heading and head injuries in soccer. *Sports Med.* 2001;31:369–386.

Laurer HL, Bareyre FM, Lee VM, et al. Mild head injury increasing the brain's vulnerability to a second concussive impact. *J Neurosurg.* 2001;95:859–870.

Lewelt W, Jenkins L, Miller J. Autoregulation of cerebral blood flow after experimental fluid percussion injury of the brain. *J Neurosurg.* 1980;53:500–511.

Matser JT, Kessels AG, Jordan BD, Lezak MD, Troost J. Chronic traumatic brain injury in professional soccer players. *Neurology.* 1998;51:791–796.

McCrory P. Does second impact syndrome exist? *Clin J Sport Med.* 2001;11:144–149.

McIntosh AS, McCrory P. Impact energy attenuation performance of football headgear. *Br J Sports Med.* 2000;34:337–341.

Povlishock JT. Pathophysiology of neural injury: therapeutic opportunities and challenges. *Clin Neurosurg.* 2000;46:113–126.

Report of the Quality Standards Subcommittee: Practice parameter: The management of concussion in sports (summary statement). *Neurology.* 1997;48:581–585.

Report of the Sports Medicine Committee. *Guidelines for the Management of Concussion in Sports, 1990 (revised 1991).* Colorado Medical Society: Denver; 1990.

Saunders RL, Harbaugh RE. The second impact in catastrophic contact-sports head trauma. *JAMA.* 1984;252:538–539.

Schwartz ML, Tator CH. Head injuries in athletics. In: *Oxford Textbook of Sports Medicine,* New York: Oxford University Press; 1994:698–705.

Stuss DT, Binns MA, Carruth FG, et al. The acute period of recovery from traumatic brain injury: Posttraumatic amnesia or posttraumatic confusional state? *J Neurosurg.* 1999;90:635–643.

Tator CH. Spinal cord and brain injuries in ice hockey. In: Bailes JE, Day AL, eds. *Neurological Sports Medicine: A Guide for Physicians and Athletic Trainers.* Rolling Meadows, Ill: American Association of Neurological Surgeons; 2001:261–271.

Tator CH. Strategies for recovery and regeneration after brain and spinal cord injury. *Injury Prevention.* 2002;(suppl iv):33–36.

Tator CH, Edmonds V, Lapczak L. Analysis of 1594 cases of catastrophic injuries in sports and recreation with a view to prevention. *Can J Neurol Sci.* 1996;23(suppl 1):31.

Teasdale G, Jennett B. Assessment of coma and impaired consciousness. A practical scale. *Lancet.* 1974;2:81–84.

Teasdale GM, Nicoll JA, Murray G, Fiddes M. Association of apolipoprotein E polymorphism with outcome after head injury. *Lancet.* 1997;350:1069–1071.

Wesner ML. An evaluation of Think First Saskatchewan. *Can J Public Health.* 2003;94:115–120.

12 | Eye Injuries and Eye Protection

Robert C. Pashby and Thomas J. Pashby

Although the eyes only account for 0.1% of the erect frontal silhouette, they account for 1% of sports injuries. An eye injury can end the career of a professional athlete and destroy the lifestyle and earning power of others. More than 90% of sports eye injuries are preventable, as proven in hockey, racquet sports, and paintball games.

Prevention is the key to reducing eye injuries in sports. Injured participants must be advised of the availability and need for protective eyewear. Tabulation of sports eye injuries is necessary to identify activities causing injury so that protective measures can be introduced with a strong evidence base. Standards for protective equipment are essential. In Canada over the past 25 years, 4449 sports eye injuries have been reported by members of the Canadian Ophthalmological Society (COS), including 512 legally blind eyes. Doctor Paul Vinger, from Boston, in *Duane's Clinical Ophthalmology*, writes: "In 1980 U.S. dollars, the hockey face protector saves society $10,000,000 a year by preventing approximately 70,000 eye and face injuries in 1.2 million protected players" (Tassman and Jaeger, 1994). Table 12-1 lists the sports causing the most eye injuries in various countries.

ASSESSING AN EYE INJURY

When an athlete presents with an eye injury, a minimum amount of equipment should be in the hands of team physicians and trainers. This equipment should include a vision card, a penlight, sterile fluorescein strips, sterile eye pads, eye shields, tape, sterile cotton-tipped swabs, and sterile irrigation solution. Injuries can be segregated into three groups.

1. Injuries that can be treated and the participant returned to action
2. Injuries that must be referred to an ophthalmologist but not on an emergency basis
3. Players that must be treated immediately in a hospital with ophthalmologic care.

A routine eye examination must be made to determine the seriousness of the injury. The penlight is used to obtain an oblique illumination of the eye, which will indicate damage to the conjunctiva, the cornea, the anterior chamber, the pupil, and the lens (Fig. 12-1). The procedure to follow in eye examination is as follows.

1. Inspect the lids and brow for lacerations, bruising, and hematoma.
2. Look in the conjunctival sac for hemorrhage, lacerations, and foreign bodies. Evert the upper eyelid by using a cotton-tipped swab as a fulcrum at the superior tarsal border (8 mm from the lashes) and gently pulling the lashes out and up to expose a foreign body that can easily be brushed away. Such foreign bodies often lodge just inside the upper inner lid margin.
3. Examine the cornea for any foreign body, abrasion, or laceration. Abrasions are well outlined with fluorescein dye, which can be applied by pulling the lower lid downward and dipping a sterile fluorescein strip into the pool of tears in the lower fornix.

TABLE 12-1 The Sport Causing the Most Eye Injuries in
Various Countries

Country	Sport causing most eye injuries
Australia	Cricket
Canada	Hockey
England	Squash
Holland	Soccer
Ireland	Hurling
Japan	Baseball
New Zealand	Squash
Portugal	Soccer
Switzerland	Hockey
Sweden	Hockey
United States	Basketball
The Far East	Badminton

4. Assess the clarity and depth of the anterior chamber, and compare with the other eye.
5. Compare the size, shape, and light reaction of the pupil in the injured eye with the contralateral eye.
6. Compare the iris colors of each eye.
7. Test the visual acuity using a reading card or a newspaper, and compare it with that of the uninjured eye. The examiner should know the patient's vision in each eye with glasses or contact lenses before injury. If the vision after injury is less than 20/40, refer the patient to an ophthalmologist.
8. Test peripheral vision by the confrontation method. Have the patient fix on the examiner's nose, and after occluding the other eye, have the patient identify the number of fingers held up in all fields of gaze. A normal minimal visual field extends 85° temporally, 65° downward, 60° nasally, and 45° upward. Any loss of peripheral field must be referred for specialist's care immediately.
9. Assess the movements of the eye by asking the patient to look to the right, then up, then down. Similarly, look to the left, up, and down.

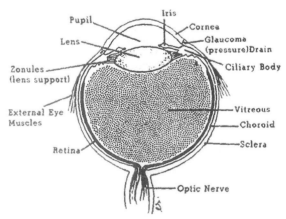

FIG 12-1   Cross-section of an eye.

These are the cardinal positions of gaze. Both eyes moving together should create no double vision when a light is held in the primary position and the six cardinal positions of gaze. Any double vision must be referred for ophthalmologic care.

10. Looking at the eyes, determine whether the injured eye is sunken (enophthalmos), making the palpebral aperture narrower, or proptosed (exophthalmos), in which case the aperture will be enlarged. A fracture of the orbital floor results in a sunken eye, whereas a retrobulbar hemorrhage causes a pushing forward of the eye. Of note in children, orbital floor fractures usually present with no ecchymosis, proptosis, or conjunctival hemorrhage, that is, a quiet white eye, whereas adults are just the opposite.

The examiner should be very careful not to force open an injured eye. If in doubt, it is better to apply a sterile pad and have the patient seen by an ophthalmologist. An exception to this is the case of a chemical burn, which demands immediate treatment by forcibly opening the eye, removing any particles, irrigating the eye with at least a liter of water, soda pop, or Gatorade, and then transporting the patient to the hospital with the eye uncovered.

In summary, injuries that can be treated immediately and the participant allowed to return to play include hematomas around the eye, provided that the eye functions normally, soft tissue injuries that can be sutured, provided that there is no loss of visual function and no lid margin involvement, and foreign bodies on the conjunctiva and cornea easily brushed off with no resulting visual complaints. Injuries that must be referred for ophthalmologic care are those causing loss of vision, whether centrally or peripherally, discoloration of the iris, cloudiness of the anterior chamber, sluggish pupillary reaction to light, inequality of the pupils, diplopia in any field of gaze, a sunken or proptosed eye, or a painful eye. If in doubt, refer to an ophthalmologist!

TYPES OF EYE INJURIES AND THEIR MANAGEMENT

The percentages and types of 4400 serious injuries reported by Canadian Ophthalmological Society (COS) members are listed in Table 12-2. Of the total reported, 11.5% resulted in a legally blind eye. This seems a rather high percentage, but these injuries were those reported only by ophthalmologists and hence needed ophthalmologic care.

Soft Tissue Injuries

Orbital Hemorrhage

Orbital hemorrhages, or black eyes, usually occur after blunt trauma to the orbital region. Proptosis of the eye may occur, and if severe, the eye is pushed forward out of the socket by hemorrhage into the orbit (the area

TABLE 12-2 Serious Eye Injuries

Type of injuries	Percentage
Soft tissue	34
Hyphemas	27
Other intraocular injuries	23
Corneal injuries	9
Orbital fractures	4
Ruptured globes	3

behind the eye), restricting ocular movements. If this retrobulbar hemorrhage is severe, the vascular supply to the optic nerve and retina may be interfered with, and this rarely can result in visual loss. It is therefore urgent that ophthalmologic care be sought immediately. During transport, an ice pack should be applied and the head kept elevated.

Any soft tissue lid injury is not easily assessed before extreme swelling ensues, which can preclude a proper examination of the globe. Such an examination includes visual acuity and fields; pupillary size, shape, and reaction; iris color; and tests for double vision. Any foreign body in the eye must be identified and removed.

Lid Lacerations

Lid lacerations can be caused by sharp objects, blunt trauma, or objects that catch the lid and actually tear it. Bleeding is controlled by direct pressure, allowing the extent of the laceration to be assessed. Lacerations through the lid margin require meticulous surgical repair for proper cosmetic and functional results. Lacerations or punctures of the upper or lower lids should be repaired by an ophthalmologist, who will make anatomic closure of muscle and skin layers. A sterile eye pad should be applied prior to transport to control bleeding and prevent infection.

Lacerations of the Lacrimal Apparatus

Medial lacerations of the upper or lower lid usually involve the lacrimal drainage system. The canalicular laceration is best repaired by an ophthalmologist using a microscope. Rather than simply repairing the lid laceration, refer the patient for canalicular and lid laceration repair immediately.

In the case of severe eyelid trauma, the eyelids may become disinserted from their attachment to the medial or lateral orbital margins, causing a rounded appearance at the lateral canthus or a widened appearance medially. Reattachment of the ligaments to bone is necessary for good functional and cosmetic results. With lid lacerations, as with any wound, control of bleeding (usually not severe) with sterile gauze is essential, and assessment of the globe damage and visual function should be carried out before the application of a sterile eye pad and transport for ophthalmologic care. Tetanus prophylaxis is recommended as in any laceration. Moreover, a record should be kept of visual acuity, peripheral fields, presence or absence of diplopia, and other objective examination findings.

Conjunctival Injuries

In minor lacerations, suturing is not necessary. A search for foreign bodies (as described previously), with removal, must be carried out, antibiotic drops applied, and follow-up examination made in 24 hours. Foreign bodies often lodge just under the margin of the upper eyelid. Eversion of the eyelid (see above) will reveal their presence; removal is achieved by wiping with a moist cotton-tipped swab. The first aid attendant should be familiar with the procedure of everting the upper eyelid. After removal of the foreign body, the player usually can return to play.

Hyphema (Bleeding into the Anterior Chamber)

More than 1200 hyphemas have been reported associated with sports injuries over the past 25 years. Hyphema is a common yet potentially severe injury because it entails hemorrhaging into the anterior chamber of the eye. The person rendering first aid must be familiar with the appearance of a hyphema. A hyphema first appears as a haze in the anterior chamber (the area between the cornea and the iris-lens diaphragm) (see Fig. 12-1). The iris appears somewhat muddy in color compared with the fellow eye, and the pupil is usually irregular in shape and sluggish in reaction to light. Vision is somewhat or extremely blurred. With rest, the blood usually settles down to form a level in the anterior chamber unless bleeding continues, in which case, blood fills the anterior chamber to create a black eight-ball eye. Most hyphemas clear in a few days, but in about 15% of patients, a secondary hemorrhage, may occur usually between the second and fifth days after the initial injury. For this reason, all hyphemas demand ophthalmologic care and advice.

At this time, treatment continues to be controversial; bed rest and even hospitalization for children may be required. Aspirin, NSAIDs, and any other drug that might cause further bleeding must be avoided. The blood usually settles down to form a level in the anterior chamber and absorbs in a matter of 5 or 6 days, depending on the amount. The use of clot-lysing agents still remains controversial, and if the patient has increased risk factors, such as sickle cell disease, extra caution is needed in their use.

Secondary glaucoma and blood staining of the cornea are worrisome complications of hyphema and may result in prolonged or permanent disability. Antiglaucoma medical therapy and even surgical intervention may be necessary by the ophthalmologist to remove the blood and reduce the intraocular pressure.

Other Intraocular Injuries

Injuries to the posterior segment of the eye (see Fig. 12-1) are also common, occurring in 23% of reported patients in our study.

Choroidal Injuries

Choroidal injuries may result when a contrecoup force from a blow by a blunt object in the front of the eye produces a wave of pressure that forces the choroid against the sclera. A split may occur, and if this split involves the macular area, visual acuity is markedly reduced in the injured eye (see Fig. 12-1).

Choroidal hemorrhages may occur without rupture. Such hemorrhages may result in necrosis of the choroid and retina in that area. There is no specific treatment for those injuries, but they should be followed by an ophthalmologist.

Macular Injuries

Macular swelling often follows severe concussion of the globe with contrecoup force. Central vision is seriously affected. The macular swelling may result in the formation of a macular cyst, which can rupture, causing a macular hole and potentially permanent visual impairment. At the present time, macular hole surgery may allow some hope for restored vision.

Retinal Injuries

Hemorrhages in the retina frequently follow blunt injuries to the eye. They are not incapacitating or noted unless they occur in the macular area.

Retinal tears are not uncommon and may lead to retinal detachment. Detachment also may occur at the far periphery of the retina, the ora (the retina's most anterior attachment), and result in a dialysis of the ora. Early recognition and treatment of the tears and holes often will prevent retinal detachment. For this reason, eye injuries of even moderate degree deserve ophthalmoscopic examination. Testing of peripheral field may reveal the presence of a retinal detachment by the confrontation method described previously.

Detachments of the retina require immediate assessment and treatment. If the detachment is allowed to progress, as most do, to involve the macular area, normal central vision cannot be restored even though the retina is reattached successfully. Any loss of visual acuity accompanied by loss of field suggests retinal detachment. Follow-up examination is necessary, and the patient must be warned to report any loss of visual field. Over one-third of retinal detachments due to contusion are sports related. Successful recovery depends on early discovery and treatment by the ophthalmologist.

Rupture and Avulsion of the Optic Nerve

A severe, direct blunt injury to the eye can rupture the optic nerve at its connection to the eye. One injury, seen by us, resulted in immediate blindness to an eye kicked by a boot. This is an unusual but very sickening injury for which there is no chance of visual recovery. The vision is totally absent in the injured eye (i.e., no light perception).

Corneal Injuries

Corneal injuries may cause lacrimation, photophobia, and blepharospasm. In all, there is sudden onset of sharp pain. Foreign bodies, if superficial, can be brushed off using a moist sterile cotton-tipped swab if they cannot be irrigated off using sterile irrigating solution. If not easily removed, a sterile eye pad should be applied and the athlete sent to the primary care physician or referred to an ophthalmologist for removal using the slit lamp and a sterile needle or spud. After removal of the foreign body, a topical antibiotic is applied for 24 hours, at which time, a follow-up examination is carried out. An eye patch may be applied for comfort, but in comparison studies, it was found that this does not alter the healing times.

Corneal abrasions produce similar symptoms and can be outlined with fluorescein, which stains the denuded epithelial area green, as seen with a cobalt blue filter. After determining that no other eye problem exists, medication can be given for pain control and a follow-up examination is done in 24 hours.

Corneal penetrating injuries are accompanied by severe pain with tearing, photophobia, and blepharospasm. If the eye can be opened easily, the pupil will be seen to be irregular, pointing to the area of laceration as the iris plugs the wound; the anterior chamber will seem shallow; and the iris will be adherent to or prolapsed outside the wound. If history suggests a potential penetrating injury, do not open the lids forcibly because this may cause further damage. Immediate ophthalmologic treatment is necessary. A sterile eye pad and shield should be gently taped in place; if these are not available, the bottom third of a disposable coffee or soda pop cup can be used as a shield and the patient transported to hospital for ophthalmologic assessment and repair.

In case of corneal injury or any other intraocular injury, if possible, a record must be kept of visual acuity, fields of vision, and diplopia (if present).

Injuries to the Lens

The lens can be injured by blunt trauma causing a concussion that results in cataract formation. This may occur immediately or after a few days, weeks, or even months. In mild cases, the iris is driven forcibly against the anterior lens capsule, leaving a circular mark like that of a rubber stamp on the anterior lens capsule. This is readily seen as the pupil dilates. As a rule, this type of blow does not lead to cataract formation.

Rarely, more severe blows can cause a rupture of the lens capsule, allowing aqueous humor (the clear fluid in the anterior chamber of the eye) to enter and causing the lens to become opaque (see Fig. 12-1). Localized cataracts may develop after a blow without capsular rupture. Such opacities often take the form of a rosette in the subcapsular area of the lens. Blunt injury may cause the lens zonules, the fibers that support the lens in the eye, to rupture so that the lens loses its moorings. If all the zonules rupture, the lens becomes dislocated and may disappear back into the vitreous or even migrate forward to appear in the anterior chamber. If only some of the zonules rupture, subluxation occurs, and the lens may shift away from its central location.

Treatment of cataracts entails removal of the cataractous portion of the lens and restoration of visual function with an intraocular or contact lens. Some professional athletes have continued their careers under these circumstances. Direct injuries to the lens by penetrating wounds of the cornea are not uncommon. The cataractous lens material is removed at the time of corneal repair. Injuries to the lens must be recognized by the person rendering first aid and referred for ophthalmologic care. Decreased vision and pupillary and anterior chamber changes must be recognized (see Fig. 12-1).

Traumatic Glaucoma

Following blunt injury to the eye, the intraocular pressure may rise and fall, swinging between hypertension and hypotension for a few days before settling back to normal. In such cases, there is usually no permanent structural damage within the eye. However, blunt injury may damage the anterior chamber angle, resulting in a split of the ciliary body with deepening of the angle and interference with aqueous outflow (see Fig. 12-1). Glaucoma develops in 10% of patients with split angle; it may occur soon after injury or even many years later. Problems of this type should be followed by an ophthalmologist, who can monitor intraocular tensions, because the development of glaucoma is usually insidious, causing damage to the optic nerve without the patient being aware of anything happening. Any loss of peripheral vision (field loss) resulting from glaucoma cannot be restored. A dislocated lens is another cause of secondary glaucoma. In this case, it is necessary to remove the lens for control of intraocular pressure.

Secondary glaucoma is not uncommon with hyphema, especially with secondary hemorrhages. Irrigation of the anterior chamber and removal of the blood clot may be indicated if the intraocular pressure cannot be adequately controlled medically (i.e., with drugs). Should the intraocular pressure remain high with blood in the anterior chamber, not only is the optic nerve in danger, but blood staining of the cornea may occur. Even when the intraocular pressure is controlled, the blood staining rarely may remain, often taking years to absorb.

Orbital Fractures

There are two theories of orbital floor fracture. The first suggests that with blunt trauma the pressure within the orbit increases sufficiently to cause the weak point, the orbital floor, to fracture and decompress into the maxillary sinus. The second theory, probably more likely, especially in children, is that the inferior orbital rim is pushed posteriorly, causing a buckling of the orbital floor bones and a trapdoor fracture with or without entrapment of tissues, including the inferior rectus muscle. Subsequently, limitation of ocular movement, especially on elevation, will ensue. Diplopia is commonly present and more marked on upward or downward gaze.

Ophthalmologic examination of the globe and investigation of the fracture with x-rays and computed tomography (CT), notably coronal views, are necessary, but not on an emergency basis. In addition, it may be necessary to free the entrapped muscle and insert a support along the orbital floor to cover the fracture.

Additional orbital fractures may occur in the maxilla or other portions of the orbital rim. They often can be recognized by direct palpation, an appropriate x-ray, and clinical evaluation. Fractures of the roof with potential cerebrospinal fluid leak necessitate neurosurgical assessment, with the ophthalmologist in the secondary position.

Fracture into any of the sinuses may leak air into the orbital cavity, producing crepitus (a crackling sound) when finger pressure is applied on the swollen area. The air and fracture are usually readily demonstrated on x-ray. Resolution without surgical intervention is usual unless a muscle is trapped. Systemic antibiotics are used often because a sinus cavity has direct connection with the orbit.

Ruptured Globe

Ruptured globes usually result from contact with an object such as a hockey stick or puck, a golf ball or club, a ski tip, a squash ball or racquet, a tennis ball, or a baseball. They are usually caused by high-velocity, low-mass missiles. Rupture also can occur when a slower-moving, high-mass object, such as a fist or large ball, strikes the eye with a glancing blow. This type of rupture usually occurs near the limbus, where the sclera is thinnest. Unfortunately, most of these injuries result in enucleation. A direct blow on the front of the cornea by an object larger than the orbital opening is more likely to produce a blowout fracture.

When ruptured, the globe often will appear soft or collapsed or sunken in the orbit. Such an eye must be gently covered with a sterile eye pad and shield, and the patient must be transported directly to hospital for ophthalmologic assessment and repair.

CONTACT LENSES

Because spectacles may present a problem when playing contact sports, many athletes in hockey, football, baseball, and other sports have found that contact lenses, when correction of refracting errors is necessary, are the answer to their problem. Historically, in the 1940s, large scleral contact lenses were custom made for proper fit and rested on the sclera. The central dome cleared the cornea and contained the refraction correction.

In the late 1940s, a young hockey player, future Hall of Famer, National Hockey League, Toronto Maple Leaf Tim Horton, turning professional, needed corrective glasses. Scleral contact lenses were fitted that were filled with normal saline solution and inserted underneath the lids to cover the front of the eyes. In the first preseason hockey game, Horton engaged in a fight with another player, and this caused concern. However, no damage occurred, and Horton continued to wear his contacts. The balanced salt solution in the contacts clouded over during play and had to be replaced with fresh normal saline between periods.

In the 1950s, hard corneal lenses became available. They were easier to fit and to insert but also more easily displaced after a blow. They might migrate off the cornea into the lower fornix or more commonly up under the upper lid. The displaced lens could be removed by irrigating the eye with sterile eye solution or could be lifted off by applying a small suction cup. We have seen a hard contact split in two halves from a blow in a hockey game with resulting corneal abrasion but, fortunately, no permanent visual defect. Both halves were found in the fornix and preserved as a trophy. At times, small foreign bodies could becomes trapped under these hard contacts, scratching the cornea, causing much pain, and preventing continuation of play.

In the 1960s, soft contact lenses became available. They were more comfortable but more fragile and required nightly disinfection and cleaning to prevent possible bacterial or fungal growth. They did not dislocate easily from the cornea and sealed out foreign bodies because of their larger size and snug-fitting edge. There was no spectacle blur on switching to regular glasses, as had commonly been the case with hard contacts. Soft contacts usually were replaced every 6 to 12 months because of the buildup of tear deposits.

Subsequently, a wide range of soft hydrophilic lens materials became available with higher water content and greater oxygen permeability. The very thin, high-water contact lenses were approved for extended wear, but ophthalmic experience showed that this regime could lead to a substantial increase in ocular infections.

Recently, disposable soft contact lenses have become available. They are available in powers up to 9 diopters of myopia and will compensate for up to 2 diopters of astigmatism. Because of their high water content, they are generally comfortable, and because they are discarded after 1 week of wear, there is less chance of a problem with protein deposits on the lens.

The advantage of contact lenses over regular glasses is an improved peripheral field of vision, less tendency to be displaced, and no fogging. It must be stressed, however, that they provide no protection against injury. Safety glasses or other types of eye protection must be worn where indicated.

PREVENTION

The old saying "prevention is better than a cure" sums up what has been proven in the effort toward the prevention of sports eye injuries, particularly in hockey, racquet sports, and war games. Paul Vinger, in *Duane's Clinical Ophthalmology*, writes: "Injury is probably the most unrecognized major health problem facing the nations today" (Tassman and Jager, 1994). He

TABLE 12-3 Sports Eye injuries in Canada, 1972–1997

Sport	Years	Injuries	Blind eyes
Hockey	23	1860	298
Racquet sports	21	1099	47
Baseball	21	490	31
Ball hockey	21	371	33
Football	21	189	9
War games	13	75	32
Golf	21	61	19
Basketball	21	48	1
Skiing (water and snow)	21	39	11
Volleyball	21	28	4
Lacrosse	21	19	0
Guns (BB)	21	19	4
Snowmobiling	21	11	5
Other sports	21	115	16
TOTAL		4424	510

further states the impossibility of injury reduction without knowledge of injury incidence and severity.

In Canada since 1972, sports eye injuries have been reported by members of the Canadian Ophthalmological Society (COS). The data to date are listed in Table 12-3.

Hockey

Hockey is the sport causing most eye injuries in Canada, Sweden, and Switzerland. In Canada, 1860 hockey eye injuries were reported, including 298 legally blind eyes. Of the 298 blind eyes reported, none were suffered by players wearing Canadian Standards Association (CSA)–certified full-face protectors, but seven were suffered by players wearing CSA-certified half-shields (visors).

In the preprotector season (1974–1975), 258 eye injuries were recorded, including 43 blind eyes. In the 1996–1997 season, 12 hockey eye injuries were recorded, including three blind eyes.

Because the face protectors available in 1972 were unsafe (the hockey stick blade could penetrate the wire mesh mask immediately over the eye areas), a standard was needed to eliminate unsafe products. A CSA standard was published, manufacturers produced safe products, the Canadian Hockey Association (CHA) demanded that all minor league players to wear CSA-certified protectors, and the Canadian government ruled that only certified protectors could be imported into or sold in Canada (see Fig. 12-2).

The percentage of hockey eye injuries treated at the Hospital for Sick Children in Toronto decreased from 11% in 1973 to 3% in 1978—a gratifying decrease. Several recent studies have shown the superior protection of the full shield eye facial protection in ice hockey. If all hockey players wear full face CSA-certified protectors, and wear them properly, hockey eye injuries will cease to be a concern.

Racquet Sports

Between 1987 and 1997, the number of injuries reported in racquetball players was greater than reported in hockey players; in fact, 322 racquet sports eye injuries were recorded compared with 282 hockey eye injuries.

TABLE 12-4 Racquet Sports Eye Injuries in Canada, 1976–1997 (1106 Injuries, 47 Blind Eyes)

Year	No. of injuries	Racquetball and squash (%)	Badminton (%)	Tennis (%)
1982[a]	90	73	13	14
1983	87	59	22	19
1984	115	58	16	26
1985	82	50	33	17
1986	83	39	33	28
1987	68	36	38	26
1988	46	39	46	15
1989	62	35	47	18
1990	40	35	55	10
1991	35	23	40	37
1992	33	24	52	24
1993	31	23	55	22
1994	27	26	56	18
1995	14	28	58	14
1996	19	21	68	11
1997	18	17	66	17

[a]CSA standard published.

Racquet sports are presently the leading cause of sports eye injuries worldwide. Squash, racquetball, tennis, and badminton are included in our study.

Doctor Michael Easterbrook, of Toronto, discovered in the late 1970s that 17% of eye injuries reported in racquet sports were suffered by players wearing an open-type eye protector, one they had purchased believing that they were protected when, in fact, they were not. Subsequently, in 1982, a CSA standard for racquet sports eye protectors was published, and most racquetball and squash players began to wear CSA-certified protectors. Now badminton players, not wearing protectors, account for more racquet sports eye injuries than squash, racquetball, and tennis players combined (Table 12-4).

Of interest, the CSA-certified face protectors with polycarbonate lenses in a sturdy frame give protection from ball contact with the eye of the headform at speeds of 90 miles per hour.

Baseball

While baseball is the third leading eye injury sport in Canada, it is the leader in Japan and was the leader in the United States until recently overtaken by basketball-related injuries. Of the 490 reported eye injuries in Canada, 31 were blinding injuries, and 90% of the injured players were injured by the baseball.

An American Standard for Testing and Materials (ASTM) standard for baseball face protectors has been established in the United States and gives protection with contact of the ball at speeds of 70 miles per hour. These protectors, made of polycarbonate or wire, are firmly attached to the batting helmet and are commonly worn in Little League baseball programs throughout the United States.

Ball Hockey

Ball hockey is a common sport in Canada, played on the streets and in school yards throughout the country. A ball, often an old tennis ball, is slapped at great speed with a hockey stick toward the net. To date (1997), Canadian records total 371 ball hockey eye injuries, including 33 blind eyes. Most blinding injuries are suffered by goaltenders not wearing eye or face protectors. They wear leg pads, belly pads, and goaltender gloves and hold a stick, but unfortunately, they usually have no protection above the neck. Ball hockey goalie masks are readily available and must be worn.

Soccer

Soccer is noted as causing the most sports eye injuries both in Holland and in Portugal. Fingers, elbows, and the ball are the usual injuring weapons. An underinflated ball can cause severe eye injury on contact.

Football

Many American football linemen are now attaching polycarbonate shields to the bars of their face protectors to prevent injury, mostly by opponents' fingers. In Canada, soccer and American football together have accounted for 189 reported eye injuries, including nine blind eyes.

War Games (Paintball Games)

These games originated in New Hampshire in 1981 and by 1984 became popular in Canada, where 26 eye injuries were reported, including 14 blind eyes. By 1997, 75 reported injuries were recorded in Canada, including 32 blind eyes. None of the blind eyes were suffered by a player wearing appropriate eye protection.

Paintball games are usually comprised of two teams of 25 to 50 players in a playing field, and players are equipped with repeater guns with a carbon dioxide–powered muzzle capacity of 250 feet per second. The gun fires 14-mm colored gelatin bullets. When struck by a bullet, the opponent is dead and out of play.

Eye injuries occur when the eye protectors provided are not worn, either taken off because they are dirty or brushed off by trees or bushes. Doctor Paul Vinger, of Boston, has impacted paintballs on pigs' eyes. The eyes ruptured when fired on from a distance of 4 m. Doctor Vinger has been instrumental in establishment of the ASTM standard for paintball game eye protectors. Protectors must be worn by everyone in the environment of the games at all times, whether a participant or not. Eye injuries can be prevented.

Golf

Golf balls travel at speeds of up to 200 miles per hour with a club head speed up to 150 miles per hour. In 20 years (1960–1980), Dr. Vinger, at the Massachusetts Eye and Ear Infirmary in Boston, reports eight eyes enucleated because of golf ball injuries and three eyes enucleated because of club head contact.

As a precaution, one-eyed golfers always should wear polycarbonate-lensed spectacles whether prescription or not. Golf eye injuries continue to occur even though it is a sport not highly associated with eye injury.

In Canada from 1976 to 1997, 61 eye injuries, including 19 blind eyes, have been reported. Some injuries have been club induced, but the majority are caused by a ball, often a ricochet from trees. Certainly one should never look to see who has called fore.

Basketball

Basketball is presently the number one sport causing sport eye injuries in the United States, whereas in Canada it accounts for only 1%, likely due to the number of participants. One in 10 college basketball players in the United States (10%) sustains an eye injury each year, mostly corneal abrasions caused by fingers and elbows. Many players are now, wisely, wearing certified racquet sports eye protectors.

Skiing

Both snow and water skiers can suffer eye injuries. In fact, 39 such injuries have been recorded in Canada, including 11 blind eyes, caused by skis, ski poles, and even the ski lift. The types of eye injuries include corneal abrasions to cross-country skiers and ski pole injuries to both cross-country and downhill skiers. *Snow blindness* is also a concern; ultraviolet light–absorbing polycarbonate goggles should be worn. Water skiers must be aware of the ski tip when falling and a fellow skier's rope handle when he or she drops off. The boat driver and observer also must be alert to the skier's rope handle as it ricochets from the water.

Snowmobiling

Five blinding injuries among the 11 injuries reported by COS members resulted from contact with wire fences, tree branches, and the breaking or fracturing of nonpolycarbonate lensed goggles that shattered. Care must be taken on starting a dead machine battery. The proper way to connect battery cables when trying to recharge a discharged battery is available in the information book accompanying each machine.

Boxing

In Canada, boxing eye injuries have not been a serious problem; very few have been reported. Doctor Albert Cheskes, of Toronto, however, examined boxers for the local boxing commission and found several eye problems neither reported nor treated. Boxers may come from other areas seeking money for bouts, under assumed names, even if suspended in other areas.

In the United States, serious recorded boxing eye injuries also are few. The boxers tend not to seek care because such injuries are considered part of the game. Even loss of vision in one eye may not be reported for fear of disqualification and loss of income.

Doctor Paul Vinger reports the following:

1. Of 13 US Olympic boxers examined, three had eyes with retinal holes and one was amblyopic with reduced vision to 20/400.
2. Another study of 23 eye injuries over a 10-year period included one retinal detachment and one eye that had been ruptured in a fight in a soldier at West Point. This eye had to be enucleated.
3. Among 70 boxers examined at the Manhattan Eye, Ear and Throat Hospital over a 2-year period (1984–1986), 43 had significant eye injuries; 2 of the boxers had 20/200 in the injured eye, and 24% had retinal tears.

4. In New Jersey, of 284 boxers examined, 19% had retinal tears and 15% had cataracts.
5. Another study of 505 boxers, all professionals, revealed that 18% had retinal tears, 39% had damaged anterior chamber angles, and 6% had cataracts.

The recommendation has been made that boxers wear thumbless gloves so that the glove thumb cannot be poked in the eye of the opponent. These gloves are also suggested for all nonchampionship bouts. In the 1930s, a Toronto boxer, Sammy Luftspring, fighting in New York for the world championship, was struck in the eye with his opponent's thumb. He subsequently lost the eye, ending his boxing career. An annual ophthalmologic examination is recommended, and perhaps one should be done before each scheduled fight. One-eyed boxers should not be allowed to perform owing to the obvious risk to the remaining eye.

ONE-EYED ATHLETES

A person is functionally one-eyed when the loss of the better eye would result in a significant change in lifestyle owing to the poor vision in the remaining eye. Realistically, a person is considered one-eyed if vision in one

TABLE 12-5 COS Survey: Eye Injuries in Canadian Sports, 1972–2002

Years	Hockey	Racquet sports	Baseball	Ball hockey	Football
1972–5	545(63)				
1976–7	90(12)	43(3)	19(2)	24(3)	13(1)
1977–8	52(8)	12(1)	2	8	2
1978–9	43(13)	28(1)	2	9(2)	3
1979–80	85(21)	58(1)	10	27(2)	1
1980–1	68(20)	103(4)	15	22(4)	8
1981–2	119(18)	100(3)	41(5)	10(2)	4
1982–3	115(13)	88(5)	68(3)	19(3)	27(1)
1983–4	124(12)	115(6)	56(3)	25(2)	22(1)
1984–5	121(18)	81(6)	43(2)	29(1)	15(1)
1985–6	123(22)	83(1)	32(3)	28	10
1986–7	93(18)	66(3)	34	18(1)	20(1)
1987–8	62(11)	45(4)	16	31	12(1)
1988–9	37(8)	62(3)	24(2)	24(1)	10(1)
1989–90	33(6)	40(2)	15(1)	14(1)	8
1990–1	21(3)	35(1)	14(1)	20(2)	6
1991–2	28(7)	33	18(1)	12(2)	6
1992–3	32(5)	31(1)	17(1)	16(2)	3(1)
1993–4	16(7)	27	23(2)	11(3)	5(1)
1994–5	19(5)	14(1)	17(2)	7	4
1995–6	22(7)	17	11(2)	4	2
1996–7	12(3)	18(1)	13(1)	13(1)	8
1997–8	23(4)	12	10	7	2
1998–9	8(5)	5	5(1)	8(2)	5
1999–2000	13(1)	11	4	5	1
2001–2	4(2)	1			4(1)
TOTAL	1914(311)	1135(47)	513(33)	397(35)	202(10)

eye is less than 20/40, because loss of the better eye would render him or her unable to drive an automobile in most areas.

Years ago, a young man named Bailey lost an eye in an accident. He was an outstanding hockey and football player at school. He was upset when he was told to not play hockey or football because of danger to his remaining eye. Subsequently, he became a track and field star, successfully representing Canada at the Olympic Games.

Presently, in the United States (because of better protection), one-eyed players are allowed to participate, providing racquet sports–certified eye protectors are worn under the other protection required in hockey, football, lacrosse, and baseball.

Finally, all one-eyed people (people who have useful vision in only one eye) must wear polycarbonate lenses, even in street wear glasses, whether they require prescription correction or not. The remaining functional eye must be protected. Table 12-5 presents the COS survey results.

REFERENCE

Tassman, Jaeger, eds. *Duane's Clinical Ophthalmology*. Philadelphia: Lippincott; 1994.

TABLE 12-5 (*Continued*)

War games	Golf	Basketball	Skiing	Volleyball	Broomball
	5(1)		1(1)	3(3)	2(2)
		1	1		
	1		3(2)		
	1			6	2
		2		3	2
	5(4)	4	3(2)	2	3
	7(2)	3		3	3
	3(2)	5	2(1)	4(1)	2
26(14)	4(1)	1	4		
8(2)	5(2)	2	2(1)	2	1
9(1)	4(1)	7	6(1)		4
2	1		1		3
6(4)	3	2		3	1
4(2)	5(1)	2	4		2
4	4	2	3(1)	1	
3(2)	4(1)	2	1		
1(1)	1(1)	4(1)	2		
3(3)	2	5			
2(1)	1	1	3(1)		
3(1)	1	2	1		
4(1)	4(3)	3	2(1)	1	
1	3(1)	3(1)	1		
1(1)	1			1	
1					
2		1			
80(33)	65(20)	52(2)	40(11)	29(4)	25(2)

(*Continued*)

TABLE 12-5 (*Continued*)

Years	Lacrosse	Hunting and BB guns	Snowmobiling	Other	TOTAL
1972–5					545(63)
1976–7	3		2(1)	6	211(29)
1977–8	1				79(9)
1978–9	1		1	1	92(18)
1979–80				7	197(24)
1980–1		4(1)		3	230(29)
1981–2			1(1)	6(1)	298(36)
1982–3	3			6(1)	342(28)
1983–4	4	1	1	9(2)	373(30)
1984–5	1	5(2)	1	19(2)	350(47)
1985–6	1	1	2(1)	7(1)	307(33)
1986–7			1(1)	5(1)	267(28)
1987–8			1(1)	9(3)	183(20)
1988–9		3(1)		7(1)	182(19)
1989–90	1		1	6(2)	135(16)
1990–1	2	1		5	118(8)
1991–2		1		8(1)	116(14)
1992–3	1			2	110(13)
1993–4				3	95(16)
1994–5					68(10)
1995–6	1			2(1)	66(11)
1996–7		3		4	85(11)
1997–8			4(1)	9	75(7)
1998–9	1			1	36(9)
1999–2000		1(1)	2	2(1)	40(3)
2001–2					12(3)
TOTAL	20	20(5)	17(6)	128(17)	4638(535)

Note: Numbers in parentheses indicate numbers of blind eyes. Send injury reports to Dr. Tom Pashby, 20 Wynford Drive (215), Don Mills, ON (Canada) M3C 1J4; Tel.: (416)441-1313; Fax: (416)441-6138.

13 | Ear, Nose, and Throat Injuries

Mark Snowise and William W. Dexter

QUICK REFERENCE

- Acute airway management: use jaw thrust, oral airway, nasoendotracheal tube, or cricothyroidotomy; can all be used with unstable cervical spine.
- Human bites need antibiotic treatment for at least 5 days.
- Lacerations through the cartilage in the ear and nose require stabilizing sutures through the cartilage.
- Lacerations involving the lip can pose a significant cosmetic deformity.
- Lacerations of the nasolacrimal apparatus (laceration over the medial third of the lower lid), the parotid duct, and facial nerve require referral.
- Auricular hematomas need to be drained with pressure dressing for 2–3 days.
- Tympanic membrane perforation may return to play immediately, but swimming should be avoided until the perforation is completely healed.
- Nasal fractures: it is essential to rule out a septal hematoma.
- Septal hematoma is treated with needle aspiration and nasal packing for 7 days.
- Endotracheal intubation is usually contraindicated with a laryngeal fracture.
- Stridor, hoarseness and hemoptysis are signs of serious laryngeal injury.
- Orbital fractures are associated with diplopia with or without enophthalmos, and an inability to look upward.
- Nasal discharge in a midface fracture should be considered cerebrospinal rhinorrhea.
- Mandible dislocations should be reduced before the onset of significant muscle spasm and edema.

INTRODUCTION

Head and neck injuries in the athlete are fairly common and are mostly seen in contact collision sports. The contact can be with an opponent's head, elbow, fist, or other body part, equipment (bats, sticks, balls, pucks, or goal posts), and the ground. Injuries involving the face and neck can affect the soft tissue or underlying bone. Most injuries in this region can be managed safely on the sidelines, but occasionally severe injuries will need immediate stabilization and transport to a medical facility.

EPIDEMIOLOGY

Most maxillofacial injuries involve contusions, abrasions, and lacerations to the scalp, forehead, nose, lips, and mouth. Fractures involving the nose and mandible are the two most common head and neck fractures seen in athletes, but more severe injuries to the maxilla, zygoma, and larynx can occur, and the physician needs to be aware of these injuries and how to stabilize them initially. The incidence of maxillofacial injuries, including dentoalveolar trauma, varies depending on the sport, and has been reported in 6–20% of soccer injuries, 4% of skiing injuries, approximately 17% of collegiate hockey players, and 28–52% of professional hockey players. Whiteside and associates reported on the fracture rate over an 11-year

149

period at Pennsylvania State University, and documented 23 nasal fractures and 5 facial fractures out of a total of 18 teams and 7784 athletes (Whiteside et al., 1981). Most of the nasal fractures were seen in football and female lacrosse players. Perkins and colleagues reviewed the incidence of facial fractures in children and found that sports injuries accounted for 42% of all facial fractures, and involved the nose 63% of the time (Perkins et al., 2000). In addition, this study found that 21% of the facial fractures and 29% of the nasal fractures occurred in athletes under the age of 17. In a review of injuries to youth soccer players, head and face injuries accounted for 5–22% of injuries, of which 20% were concussions.

ACUTE MANAGEMENT

With the rare severe maxillofacial injury, the immediate focus should be on stabilizing the airway, controlling bleeding, treating shock, and identifying associated injuries such as cervical spine trauma and closed head injuries. Airway management in a conscious patient without cervical spine injury can be accomplished by sitting the patient upright and slightly forward. In an unconscious patient or when there is concern for a potential underlying cervical spine injury, the airway needs to be managed while maintaining cervical stabilization. Use of the jaw thrust technique, oral airway, nasoendotracheal tube, or in extreme cases tracheotomy or cricothyroidotomy can all be utilized to maintain an open airway in such patients. Most hemorrhages in the head and neck area, despite being profuse due to the copious blood supply, can be controlled with direct pressure. Shock, although rare in maxillofacial injuries can be managed in the usual manner by laying the patient flat, elevating the legs, and administering a colloid solution such as lactated Ringer's.

GENERAL PRINCIPLES

Contusions

Most contusions are simple and require no specific treatment except for local ice application. Ice can be applied to the injured area for 10–15 minutes at a time, with care being taken not to cause frostbite to the skin. Application of a thin protective cloth layer or massage with a block of ice can ease the discomfort from icing. Very rarely contusions may result in the formation of a large hematoma. In most instances these will resolve spontaneously over a few weeks, but occasionally when the hematoma is extremely large, drainage via needle or incision is warranted. Early drainage within a few weeks will decrease the incidence of scar tissue and capsular formation. Hematomas of the external ear are a separate entity and are addressed below.

Abrasions

Commonly seen in bicyclists, skateboarders, and in-line skaters, abrasions vary in severity depending on the depth of the injury. With isolated epidermal involvement, simple cleaning followed by the application of topical antibiotic ointment for a few days is all that is required. Deeper abrasions require more careful attention and vigorous cleaning. Once foreign material becomes embedded in the dermis, removal is necessary to avoid traumatic tattooing and infection. Foreign material becomes attached to the tissues in

10–12 hours, so good careful cleaning within this time helps avoid subsequent complications. Topical anesthetics can be used in smaller abraded areas. Occasionally, with very deep abrasions that require significant cleaning, analgesics should be administered to ease the pain of the procedure.

Puncture Wounds

Any puncture wound should be examined with a sterile probe to gauge its depth and to evaluate for associated injuries to nerves and vessels. X-rays are occasionally helpful to identify foreign material embedded in the skin. Wounds should be copiously irrigated with saline solution and most can be left to heal by secondary intention. Antibiotics are usually not needed with the exception of human bites.

The puncture wound associated with the most risk is that caused by a human bite, either intentional or unintentional. Intentional bites are not an uncommon injury in rugby, and have even been seen in championship boxing. Human bite wounds are invariably associated with infection and should be treated as a serious entity. Wounds should be thoroughly cleaned and left to heal via secondary intention. If the bite involves the lip and the vermilion border, the skin can be closed loosely with care taken to properly align the vermilion border. All human bites should be treated immediately for 5 days with broad-spectrum antibiotics, including a beta-lactam penicillin or a second- or third-generation cephalosporin. For individuals with a penicillin allergy, clindamycin along with a fluoroquinolone or trimethoprim-sulfamethoxazole is adequate. Close follow-up is essential for these wounds.

Lacerations

Lacerations are common in contact sports and can occur anywhere on the face or neck. They need to be cleansed thoroughly with an antiseptic solution and then closed. Most small lacerations may be temporarily closed with steri-strips to achieve hemostasis and allow for rapid return to play as long as the wound is covered. Most if not all lacerations of the face should eventually be closed with cyanoacrylates ("skin glue") or with sutures. If the wound is gaping, a few absorbable deep sutures are helpful to better approximate the edges. Skin closure should be done with 5.0 or smaller nonabsorbable suture and optimally achieved within 8–12 hours. This can be extended to 24 hours for clean facial lacerations if necessary. Sutures about the face should be removed within 5–7 days.

Lacerations about the nose, eye, lip, tongue, and mouth require special attention. Lacerations through the cartilage in the ear and nose require stabilizing sutures through the cartilage with 4-0 chromic or monofilament nylon. Lacerations involving the lip can pose a significant cosmetic deformity and require meticulous care when closing. The vermilion border (mucocutaneous line) should be aligned first with a temporary stitch, and deep closure should then be performed followed by superficial closure. For through-and-through lacerations around the mouth, prophylactic antibiotics are generally recommended. Intra-oral lacerations can be loosely sutured to help reduce healing time. Lacerations of the tongue can be loosely closed with 3-0 or 4-0 absorbable deep sutures, and it is important to note that tongue lacerations can occasionally cause enough swelling to obstruct the airway. Other complications that can arise from lacerations to the face may involve the nasolacrimal apparatus (laceration over the medial third of the lower lid), the parotid duct, and the facial nerve. These injuries need to be evaluated by a specialist as they will require complex treatment.

Return to play after most lacerations can occur once hemostasis is achieved via temporary or permanent closure and the wound is covered. As with any laceration, ensure that the patient's tetanus booster is up to date.

EAR INJURIES

General

The most common injuries involving the ear occur to the external ear and are seen most often in wrestling, boxing, and rugby. Athletes may also suffer infections of the outer ear canal as seen with swimmers and surfers. Perforations of the tympanic membrane can occur from scuba diving, water skiing, high diving, and occasionally boxing. Finally, injuries to the inner ear due to barotrauma are seen in scuba diving.

Otitis Media

Though not a specific sports-related injury, but seen in many athletes, otitis media involves an infection of the middle ear. Up to 85% of middle ear infections may be viral in nature, and thus require only supportive treatment. The most common bacterial pathogens include *Streptococcus pneumoniae*, *Haemophilus influenzae* and *Moraxella catarrhalis*. Most patients will have a history of a recent upper respiratory infection and fever, and may complain of ear pain and fullness with or without hearing impairment. The diagnosis is made by otoscopy and visualization of an erythematous, bulging, non-mobile tympanic membrane. If antibiotic treatment is entertained, first-line treatment is amoxicillin with repeat examination in 2 weeks to ensure resolution of symptoms. Complications are rare, but may include perforation of the tympanic membrane, mastoiditis, labyrinthitis, and rarely meningitis. Return to play is allowable when the athlete is afebrile. It is important to remember that certain over-the-counter and prescription cold remedies are banned by the IOC and NCAA, so care should be taken not to provide these medicines to athletes competing at these levels.

Otitis Externa

Infections of the outer ear canal are mostly seen in swimming, waterskiing, scuba diving, surfing, or other sports that involve prolonged water exposure. Most commonly, these infections are due to *Pseudomonas*, *Proteus*, or fungal infections, and respond well to antibiotic drops. Athletes will complain of ear pain and drainage with occasional hearing loss. On otoscopy, the external canal is edematous and erythematous with occasional discharge. Pain on manipulation of the auricle is pathognomonic of otitis externa. The mainstay of treatment initially involves cleaning the external canal with the subsequent application of antibiotic drops with or without steroids. In cases of severe canal edema, a small cotton wick is inserted to assist with penetration of the antibiotic drops. When tympanic membrane perforation is suspected, only suspension drops should be used as opposed to solutions. The ear should be kept as dry as possible while antibiotic treatment is continued for a total of 7 days. Return to swimming can occur after 3–4 days of treatment, but most would recommend the avoidance of water sports for 7–10 days. Malignant otitis externa can occur as a complication, usually involves a *Pseudomonas* infection, and is seen most commonly in diabetics. Prevention includes the application of a few drops of baby oil prior to swimming, and the use of acidifying and drying ear drops afterwards. An easy home remedy to use after swimming consists of the application of a few drops of a 50/50 mixture of white vinegar and 70% isopropyl alcohol.

Auricular Hematoma

Auricular hematomas are commonly seen in wrestling, boxing, rugby, and judo, when trauma and friction cause hematoma formation at the junction of the perichondrium and elastic cartilage of the ear. Left untreated, the underlying cartilage is resorbed, resulting in the well-known cauliflower ear. These lesions are most commonly seen in the anterior aspect of the ear when athletes present with gross edema and pain on palpation (Figs. 13-1 and 13-2). Once an auricular hematoma is identified it needs to be drained to prevent cauliflower ear.

After anesthetization, drainage can usually be performed under sterile conditions via needle aspiration, but occasionally an incision is needed. After drainage, if the hematoma does not recur within 1 hour, no compression dressing is needed. However, if the hematoma recurs, a pressure dressing will

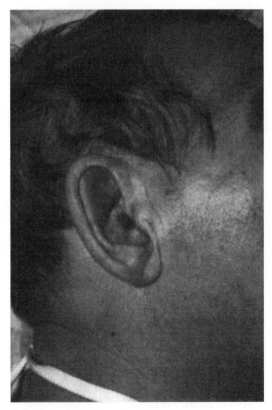

FIG 13-1   Acute hematoma of the ear.

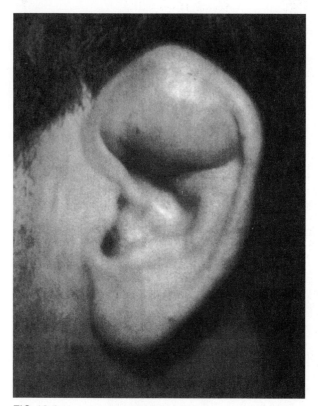

FIG 13-2 Loculated hematoma of the ear.

be needed for 2–3 days. Options for pressure dressings include compression suture dressings, colloid-cotton casts, plaster of Paris casts, silicone molds (dental molding pastes), or mastoid dressings. Antibiotic use after drainage is not necessary unless a compression suture dressing is applied, but it may help prevent perichondritis after any incision and drainage procedure. These patients should be instructed to avoid NSAIDs and aspirin, and daily follow-up is necessary to ensure that the hematoma completely resolves.

Ear protection can decrease the incidence of auricular hematomas by 50%, but does not eliminate the injury completely. Athletes with apparent irritation in this region may benefit from icing immediately after practice and games. Return to play is controversial. Some authors advocate return to play immediately, but most recommend return to full competition only when the hematoma is completely healed. Given the choice of delayed return or cauliflower ear, many wrestlers choose to leave the hematoma untreated. Complications include pressure necrosis, infection, or allergic reaction to the dressing.

Barotrauma

Barotrauma is mostly seen in divers, but can also result from air travel and activities at high altitude. These injuries are caused by the inability to equilibrate pressure across the tympanic membrane, resulting in injuries from the external auditory canal to the inner ear, and can range from varying degrees of hearing loss to severe nausea and vertigo as a result of a perilymphatic fistula. The most common injuries include vessel rupture within the tympanic membrane and tympanic membrane rupture. Athletes usually present with otalgia, blood-tinged sputum, tinnitus, decreased hearing, ear fullness, and in extreme cases vertigo, nausea, and vomiting. On examination, the tympanic membrane is usually erythematous and depressed (ear squeeze) or bulging (reverse ear squeeze). Mild cases of barotrauma are treated with rest and decongestants and restriction from diving or pressure changes until symptoms are resolved and the ear is healed. In severe cases of barotrauma, when the symptoms do not clear within 48 hours, a perilymphatic fistula should be suspected and ENT referral is indicated. These fistulas can be plugged with fat or muscle, which may improve the vertigo and nausea, but the hearing loss is permanent.

Preventative measures include correcting underlying ear problems (ie, cerumen impaction, sinus polyp, osteoma, or exostosis), avoiding diving with a sinus infection, allergic rhinitis, or severe upper respiratory tract infection, and properly equilibrating ear pressure while descending. When diving with a significant cold or congestion, decongestants should be used to minimize the risk of injury. It is important to note that even with mild barotrauma, there is evidence that deterioration can occur despite abstaining from diving. Athletes should be counseled to avoid diving until their symptoms are completely resolved and the exam is normal.

Tympanic Membrane Perforation

Perforations are most commonly seen in scuba diving but can occur from a direct blow to the ear during water skiing, boxing, water polo, diving, or even football. Athletes present with otalgia, otorrhea, vertigo, tinnitus, and a conduction hearing loss. Once visualized it is essential that nothing enter the ear. Most perforations will heal spontaneously within 8 weeks and require follow-up until completely healed. ENT referral is appropriate as a small flap can occasionally be seen and replaced which may assist in healing. Athletes may return to play immediately if the injury is mild, but swimming should be avoided until the perforation is completely healed.

NASAL INJURIES

General

Because of its prominent position the nose is very easily injured and is said to be the most commonly fractured bone in the body. Usually injury occurs from a direct blow and is seen most commonly in rugby, football, boxing, hockey, basketball, and wrestling. In addition to fractures, nose bleeds and septal hematomas can be seen when treating athletes.

Nasal Fractures

Most fractures are compound and associated with mucosal lacerations and epistaxis. Players will often hear a crack and present with significant epistaxis and occasional difficulty breathing through one or both sides of the nose. A clinical deformity is usually evident (Fig. 13-3) and in most cases x-rays do not change management. When evaluating a nasal fracture it is essential

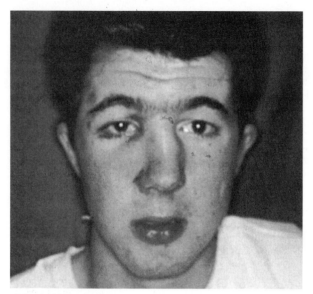

FIG 13-3 Fractured nose.

to rule out a septal hematoma (see below). Initial sideline treatment involves stopping the bleeding (see below) and attempting a reduction. Occasionally, displaced nasal fractures can be reduced gently without anesthesia if they are seen immediately before the onset of significant swelling. Once swelling has occurred, reduction is usually delayed until edema has resolved. Ice should be applied frequently over the next 24–48 hours and antibiotics are only required if a septal hematoma has been drained. Return to play after a nasal fracture depends on the sport and whether protective gear can be worn without impeding performance. Nasal protection should be used for 4–5 weeks following injury and boxers should not fight for at least 1 month after a fracture. Complications from nasal fractures can include septal hematomas, permanent saddle-nose deformities, and in severe fractures, injuries to the cribriform plate.

Epistaxis

Nose-bleeds can be a result of trauma or may occur spontaneously in dry climates or high altitudes, and are especially prevalent in wrestlers. Anterior epistaxis accounts for 90% of nose-bleeds while nasal fractures can result in anterior and posterior bleeding. With persistent epistaxis the physician needs to look for an occult nasal fracture, and if the bleeding becomes more dilute, a basal skull fracture should be suspected. On examination, the site of bleeding should be identified whenever possible. The athlete should be instructed to sit upright with the head elevated and slightly forward. Direct pressure is applied to the nose for approximately 20 minutes. Additional pressure can be applied at the midline of the upper lip, as this is where the septal branch of the superior labial artery supplies the anterior portion of the nasal septum. In addition, gently blowing one nostril at a time will help remove clots, allowing the vessels to contract and retract thus decreasing bleeding. If the bleeding stops with pressure, no further treatment is needed and follow-up should be in 48 hours. If the bleeding persists, the source should be identified. Placement of a cotton pledget soaked in epinephrine 1:1000 or a vasoconstrictor such as phenylephrine or oxymetolazone in the anterior nose can assist in vasoconstriction and allow better visualization. If an anterior source is found it should be cauterized with silver nitrate and topical antibiotic ointment used for a few days. If the bleeding site cannot be identified or controlled with cautery, anterior nasal packing can be applied for 72 hours using a nasal tampon, conformable sponge, or gauze. A hemostatic agent, if available, should be used. Patients should be instructed to avoid hot liquids and hot showers while the packing is in place. Posterior bleeding often cannot be controlled with pressure and requires packing with a commercially available kit, or a 16 or 18 French Foley catheter inserted and then inflated with 10–15 mL of saline. These patients should usually be referred to an ENT for treatment and follow-up. Return to play can be immediate if the bleeding is controlled with pressure and does not recur with exertion, but once nasal packing is used, return to play should be delayed until the packing has been out for 2 weeks.

Septal Hematomas

By far the most serious injury that affects the nose involves the nasal septum. Any-time the nose is fractured the nasal septum needs to be evaluated carefully. The chance of a septal hematoma forming is high in nasal fractures, and if overlooked, absorption of the septal cartilage, with or without abscess formation, can occur. In children, this is critical for the development of the nose, and if a septal hematoma, with or without an abscess, is neglected, a saddle-nose deformity will result in a significant cosmetic and therapeutic problem. On inspection of the injured nose an enlarged, bluish, discolored septum that can obstruct the nasal passage is evident (Fig. 13-4). On palpation, septal hematomas are boggy and

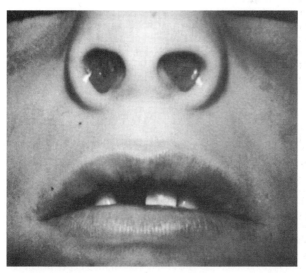

FIG 13-4 Septal hematoma.

fluctuant. Once identified, these hematomas need to be treated via needle aspiration or small incision in the dependent portion of the hematoma, and after evacuation of the hematoma with nasal packing applied for 7 days. Prophylactic antibiotic treatment is warranted in the case of septal hematomas.

THROAT INJURIES

Fortunately, serious throat injuries are not common in sports, but can occur in ice hockey, baseball, and other stick/projectile sports, as well as high-velocity snowmobile and motorcycle accidents. The larynx is susceptible to blunt trauma such as a blow from a hockey stick or puck, a karate chop, or a forearm check in football or hockey. In laryngeal injuries, the head is usually extended, which brings the larynx closer to the surface, rendering it more vulnerable to the assault. The severity of the injury can vary from a simple contusion to fracture. The major consideration when dealing with throat injuries is the adequacy of the airway. Initial treatment involves assessment of the airway, and any signs or symptoms of airway compromise necessitates evaluation in an acute care setting. If the athlete is able to inflate and expand his or her chest wall despite stridor, there is time to get the patient to the hospital for definitive care. With complete airway obstruction an airway needs to be established immediately, usually via cricothyroidotomy. Endotracheal intubation is usually contraindicated with a laryngeal fracture.

With significant injuries, athletes will note varying degrees of respiratory distress, pain and discomfort in the neck, dysphagia, swelling, and crepitus over the anterior neck. Stridor, hoarseness, and hemoptysis are signs of serious laryngeal injury. The obliteration of the normal cartilage landmarks about the neck is suggestive of a fracture. Fortunately, most injuries to the trachea are hematomas or small cracks. These are usually treated with close observation, preferably in a hospital setting, until the symptoms are resolved. Athletes with no signs or symptoms of laryngeal fracture and normal exam after neck trauma can return to play immediately with close monitoring. Athletes with a laryngeal injury need to be held from practice and competition until symptoms are completely resolved.

FACIAL BONE FRACTURES

General

As with throat injuries, the evaluation of maxillofacial fractures starts with the assessment of the airway. Severe injuries are uncommon and usually seen in augmented speed sports, but approximately 50% of severe injuries will require tracheostomy when significant nasal and cheek swelling is present. Also, it is essential to evaluate for associated injury to the head or neck with any significant facial bone fracture. CT scans are the preferred way to image facial fractures.

Zygoma Fractures

Fractures of the zygoma result from a direct blow to the face and usually result in a tripod fracture, with the zygoma being displaced medially and inferiorly. The zygoma forms the lateral and most of the inferior rim of the orbit. The athlete usually complains of localized pain and varying degrees of trismus (difficulty opening the mouth) due to the zygoma impinging on the coronoid process of the mandible. If there is displacement of the lateral canthal ligament of the eye, which is attached to the zygoma, then diplopia may also be a complaint. On examination there can be obvious flattening of the cheek with significant tenderness over the fracture site. Patients may also have numbness of the cheek, nose, and upper lip, and many patients have unilateral epistaxis on the injured side due to blood from the maxillary sinus. Ocular and periorbital changes are also common and include periorbital ecchymosis, subconjunctival hemorrhage, and diplopia. X-rays will reveal the location of the fracture and opacification of the maxillary sinus due to blood. Most zygomatic fractures require surgical reduction. Return to play is usually delayed until the fracture is completely healed, but may be facilitated with proper protection.

Orbital Fractures

Blowout fractures of the orbit usually result from a blow to the orbital rim that compresses the contents of the orbit, causing a fracture at the weakest site (usually the floor of the orbit). Racquet balls, tennis balls, and baseballs are the usual offending projectiles, but these fractures can occur due to elbow or foot blows in contact collision activities. Athletes present with diplopia, with or without enophthalmos, and the inability to look up is a pathognomonic finding on examination. The diagnosis is confirmed with x-rays and most surgeons utilize CT scanning to obtain a detailed evaluation of the orbital floor. Most of these injuries need to be repaired surgically to free the entrapped orbital contents and repair the fracture defect. If a fracture occurs through the ethmoid sinuses, the patient often will report that the eyelid swells up when blowing the nose. This is due to air being forced into the orbital area and requires no specific treatment except the avoidance of blowing the nose. Return to play is delayed until the fracture is completely healed or adequate protection can be provided.

Maxilla Fractures

Fractures of the maxilla are rare in sports, and usually are a result of high-velocity injuries seen in augmented speed sports as with a hockey puck hitting the face. These fractures are divided into three categories based on the degree of structural involvement and maxillary mobility. LeForte type 1 fractures extend horizontally across the maxilla at the level of the floor of the nose and result in a mobile upper gingival area, together with varying amounts of mobility of the hard palate. LeForte type 2 fractures are characterized by a fracture to the central third of the face with the nasal, middle, and lower portions of the maxilla separated from the zygomatic and frontal bones. In LeForte type 3 fractures, there is complete separation of the zygomatic, maxillary, and ethmoid regions from the frontal and cranial regions. This is usually caused by an anterior injury forcing the facial bones backward and downward, causing the classic "dish face" deformity.

Combinations of all three may occur, and the important areas to assess immediately, after ensuring a stable airway, are the state of the eyes and the teeth. If the eyes are moving well together without diplopia, and if the dental occlusion has not changed, then the fracture can be treated conservatively. However, if it is clear that there are problems with the eyes, teeth, or central face, then these patients must be treated in a hospital setting. On examination, these fractures are usually made evident by the loss of facial symmetry, gagged or open bite occlusion, and the ability to move the midface. Gentle manual manipulation can be used to assess the degree of fracture. The thumb and index finger are used as reference points and are initially placed on either side of the nose. The opposite hand is used to grip the maxilla on the anterior alveolar ridge. Movement of one hand relative to the other indicates a LeForte type 1 fracture. The reference hand is then placed over the zygomatic arch area and then the forehead, and movement relative to each of these positions indicates a LeForte type 2 or 3 injury, respectively. In addition to evaluating these athletes for cervical spine and skull fractures, the treating physician needs to look for signs of cerebrospinal rhinorrhea, which is common in type 2 and 3 fractures. Nasal discharge associated with a midface fracture should be considered cerebrospinal rhinorrhea until proven otherwise. Treatment of these fractures involves surgery, and when cerebrospinal rhinorrhea is present, antibiotics are administered. Great care must be taken with these injuries, and it may be weeks to months before it is advisable for the patient to return to full competition.

Mandible Fractures

Due to its vulnerable position the mandible is the second most commonly fractured facial bone, and like the nose, most fractures to the mandible occur from a direct blow. More than 50% of these fractures are multiple owing to the fact that this U-shaped bone transmits the forces around the curved mandible resulting in a contrecoup injury. Usually the athlete will report hearing a crack and complain of severe pain and some degree of malocclusion. In addition to malalignment of the teeth, ecchymosis in the floor of the mouth is almost pathognomonic of a mandible fracture. A simple clinical method to test if the mandible is fractured is to place the thumbs on the chin and the fingers on the angle of the mandible and press between the two. This maneuver will usually cause pain over the area of the fracture. If a blow has been sustained directly to the chin, the forces may be transmitted up the mandible, causing either unilateral or bilateral subcondylar fractures. These fractures may be associated with hemotympanum and even bleeding from the ear. A condylar fracture should be suspected when the examiner cannot palpate condylar movement by placing a little finger in the patient's external ear canal while opening the jaw.

Mandibular fractures are classified by the location of the fracture. The most common sites of mandibular fractures are the gonial angle, condyle, mental foramen, and symphysis. The numerous muscle attachments to the mandible make displacement of the fracture quite common. Mandibular fractures can further be classified by the nature of the break. A *simple mandibular fracture* is one in which the bone is completely broken but the overlying oral mucosa is intact. A *greenstick mandibular fracture* is an incomplete fracture of the bone. This type of fracture is often seen in children when the bone bends rather than breaks. Missed diagnosis of a greenstick mandibular fracture may result in nonunion during healing due to displacement by muscle pull. A *compound mandibular fracture* is a complete fracture of the bone with an external wound, usually though the oral mucosa. These fractures must be considered contaminated and appropriate antibiotic therapy used in conjunction with reduction and stabilization. A *comminuted mandibular fracture* is one in which the bone is splintered or crushed. These fractures may be simple or compound.

Initial evaluation of mandibular fractures should include assessment of the airway and inspection and removal of any fractured or foreign materials including teeth, which may occlude the airway during stabilization. These fractures can be stabilized with a circumferential compression bandage, or Barton bandage, that is wrapped under the chin and over the top of the head. With the exception of condylar fractures in adults and some subcondylar fractures, which can be treated with a soft diet and protection, most mandible fractures require immobilization via attachment of the mandible to the maxilla or direct plating of the fracture. Immobilization is usually required for 6–8 weeks, during which time the athlete should avoid contact sports. Due to the location of a growth plate in the condyles, condylar fractures in children pose several problems. Most of these fractures are treated conservatively with fixation for 10–14 days with subsequent close follow-up. If malocclusion occurs, then fixation is continued for a longer period of time. As with all mandible fractures, return to play is delayed until the fracture is completely healed.

Mandible Dislocations

In some instances the mandible can become dislocated and not fractured due to a lateral blow with the mouth open. Dislocations are mostly seen in hockey and basketball where there is a high incidence of elbow trauma to the face. The mandible is most commonly displaced anterior to the eminence of the glenoid fossa. These athletes will present with an obvious deformity in the temporomandibular region and the inability to open the jaw. It is best to try and reduce these dislocations before the onset of significant muscle spasm and edema prevent an easy reduction. To reduce the mandible, the physician should be facing the patient, and place his or her hands bilaterally on the mandible with the thumbs on the anterior region of the mandible and the index and middle fingers around the mandibular eminence. Reduction is accomplished by depressing the mandible and applying posterior pressure. Ice should be applied immediately after the reduction. It is recommended that athletes use a mouth guard continuously for 2–4 weeks after a dislocation to enhance soft tissue healing and to stabilize the joint, and some authorities recommend the continued use of a mouth guard during all athletic activity to prevent chronic, recurrent luxations. These injuries can also be prevented by the use of mouth guards in all players. Return to play after mandible dislocations should be delayed for 2–3 weeks.

PREVENTION

Preventative strategies for specific injuries have been discussed in each section. In general, most maxillofacial injuries occur in contact collision sports, and the incidence can be reduced with proper headgear and face protection. In a nonrandomized prospective cohort study of youth baseball players, injuries to the face were reported 28% less in the group wearing face guards when compared to the group not using face guards. This study relied on self-reported data from players, coaches, and parents, which makes the results less valid, but there clearly is an indication that this is a reasonable intervention that needs further study. Several studies in ice hockey have shown the effectiveness of full face shields in reducing facial injury. Mouth guards have been shown to reduce dentoalveolar trauma and may also protect players from dislocations of the mandible and reduce the incidence of concussion. More data are clearly needed to assess the extent of facial injuries in sports and the effectiveness of various protective measures.

REFERENCES

Bertz JE. Maxillofacial injuries. *Clin Symp*. 1981;33:1–32.

Committee on Sports Medicine and Fitness 1999–2000. Injuries in youth soccer: A subjective review. *Pediatrics*. 2000;105:659–661.

Dannis RP, Hu K, Bell M. Acceptability of baseball face guards and reduction of oculofacial injury in the receptive youth league players. *Inj Prev*. 2000;6:232–234.

Felix AC. Ear, nose and throat problems. In: Sallis RE, Massimino F, eds *ACSM's Essentials of Sports Medicine*. St Louis: Mosby; 1997;118.

Hussain K, Wijetunge DB, Grubnic S, et al. A comprehensive analysis of craniofacial trauma. *J Trauma*. 1994;36:34–47.

Lephart SM, Fu F. Emergency treatment of athletic injuries. *Dent Clin North Am*. 1991;35:707–717.

McGrail JS. Ear, nose, and throat injuries. In: *Bull's Handbook of Sports Injuries*, 1st ed. New York: McGraw-Hill; 1998;33–46.

Perkins SW, Dayan SH, Sklarew EC, et al. The incidence of sports-related facial trauma in children. *Ear Nose Throat J*. 2000;79:632–638.

Tu HK, Davis LF, Nique TA. Maxillofacial injuries. In: Mellion MB, Walsh WM, Shelton GL, eds. *The Team Physician's Handbook*, 2nd ed. Philadelphia: Hanley and Belfus; 1997;26.

Whiteside JA, Fleagle SB, Kalenak A. Fractures and refractures in intercollegiate athletes. *Am J Sports Med*. 1981;9:369–377.

14 | Dental Injuries

Mark Roettger

QUICK LOOK

- A simple tooth fracture does not involve the dental pulp and a complex fracture does involve the dental pulp.
- Transport the patient and any tooth fragments to a dentist as soon as possible.
- A tooth luxation is at least partially in the bony socket, but out of position.
- An extruded tooth appears longer than adjacent teeth and should be repositioned in the socket with finger pressure.
- A lateral luxation is pushed back or forward in relation to adjacent teeth and should be repositioned with finger pressure.
- An avulsed tooth is completely removed from its bony socket.
- Do not handle the tooth by the root.
- If there is debris on the tooth, gently rinse it with water or saline.
- Reimplant the tooth using the adjacent teeth as a guide to the final position.
- Stabilize by biting on sterile gauze and transport the patient to a dentist.
- If unable to reimplant the tooth, transport the tooth with the patient to the dentist.
- Proper transport media for avulsed teeth include:
    Hank's balanced salt solution
    Cold milk
    Normal saline or sterile saline for contact lenses
    Plastic bag
- Teeth reimplanted within 30 minutes of injury have the best chance for normal healing.

INTRODUCTION

Participation in athletics has greatly increased in recent years, and with this comes an increased risk of orofacial soft and hard tissue injuries (Fig. 14-1). Dental injuries are often complex, involving numerous specialized tissues such as enamel, dentin, periodontal ligaments, dental pulp, bone, oral mucosa, and temporomandibular joint structures. These injuries are in many cases permanent, and dental injury prevention strategies will reduce these potentially disfiguring injuries. Complicated injuries require proper evaluation and initial management to ensure proper healing. Dental injuries are often overlooked in sports medicine because in many cases dental injuries do not limit athlete participation in competition, and many times athletes do not even report these injuries to athletic trainers (Kvittem et al., 1998). These injuries can be significant, can be expensive to manage, and deserve the full attention of the sports medicine community. A dentist should be an integral part of the sports medicine team.

EPIDEMIOLOGY

Review of the literature regarding epidemiology of athletic dental trauma reveals a large variation in incidence of these injuries. These variations may be attributed to differing study designs and the lack of a national dental

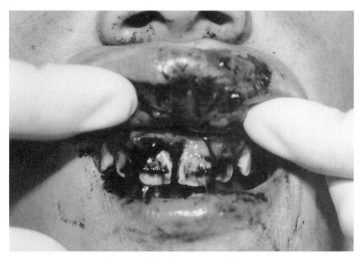

A

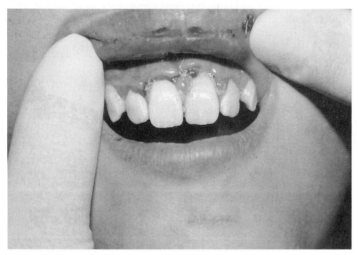

B

FIG 14-1 Soccer injury. A. Shows complex injury involving teeth, oral soft tissue and alveolar bone. B. Five days postinjury; proper management has allowed proper healing to occur. Photo courtesy of Mark Roettger, DDS.

injury surveillance system (Tesini et al., 2000). Published studies indicate that dental injuries occur at a significant rate in sports in which mouthguards are not required. In a 1995 Flanders and Bhat study of high school basketball players, orofacial injuries accounted for more than 30% of all injuries suffered. In 1998 Kvittem and Roettger studied the incidence of dental trauma in Minnesota high school basketball, soccer, and wrestling. They found that approximately 25% of soccer players, 50% of basketball players and 75% of wrestlers sustained a dental injury during the season studied.

The literature suggests that there are a few factors that predispose an athlete to dental injury. The National Youth Safety Foundation found that the number of dental injuries increases with age (National Youth Sports Safety Foundation, 1992). Athletes with excessive overbite or maxillary anterior tooth protrusion are more susceptible to injury. Finally, fixed orthodontic appliances were shown to increase the risk of athletic dental injury (Kvittem et al., 1998).

PATHOPHYSIOLOGY

Enamel, dentin, and dental pulp are each unique and different from other tissues. Tooth enamel has no reparative capability, while dentin and dental pulp have limited reparative capability. Once a tooth is fractured it is damaged forever. Modern dental materials and techniques allow aesthetic restoration of damaged teeth, but not without a significant investment of time and money.

Dental injuries can be the result of either direct or indirect trauma. *Direct trauma* usually results from a blow delivered straight to the teeth, resulting in fracture or luxation of the anterior teeth, along with soft tissue injuries to the lips or gingiva. *Indirect trauma* results from a blow to the face or jaws, causing the mandibular teeth to suddenly strike the maxillary teeth. This mechanism can produce laceration of the tongue, fracture of the posterior teeth, temporomandibular joint injury or mandibular fracture.

The energy of impact is also a factor in the type of damage generated by dental trauma. The energy of impact relates to mass and velocity. High-velocity and low-mass impacts to the mouth tend to cause more tooth fractures. Low-velocity and high-mass collisions tend to cause more injuries to the supporting structures of the teeth, causing tooth luxation or avulsion.

INJURIES

Soft Tissue Injuries

Oral soft tissue injuries are commonly seen in athletes. These injuries can vary widely in severity and complexity. Oral abrasions, hematomas, lacerations, and tissue avulsions are encountered in sports medicine. It is important to remember that any oral soft tissue injury may indicate the presence of an underlying dentoalveolar injury. A full dental evaluation is indicated for orofacial soft tissue injuries. When multiple injuries exist, many times it is prudent to treat the tooth injuries prior to repairing the soft tissues. Dental consultation before suturing can be helpful in making this decision.

Oral lacerations should undergo careful debridement and be closed in anatomic layers. Aesthetics must be considered in repairing a laceration that crosses the vermilion border of the lip to ensure proper alignment of the tissue (Fig. 14-2). Lacerations of the lip or tongue that occur in conjunction with tooth fractures must be carefully evaluated for the presence of tooth fragments in the wound (Fig. 14-3). This can be verified only by taking a radiograph of the injured soft tissue to search for radiopaque tooth fragments

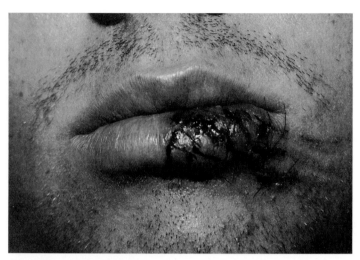

A

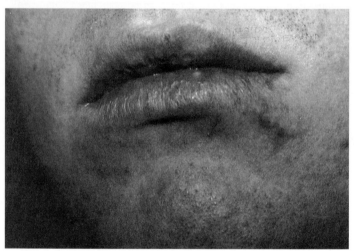

B

FIG 14-2 Lip laceration. A. Laceration crossing the vermilion border of the lip is sutured with careful tissue alignment. B. Five months postinjury, and the integrity of the vermilion border has been preserved. Photo courtesy of Mark Roettger, DDS.

in the radiolucent soft tissue. Through-and-through lip lacerations require careful evaluation and treatment. First, radiographic evaluation for foreign bodies is done. Then, both the mucosal side and the skin side of the wound must be repaired. Repair of only the skin side of such wounds without repair of the mucosal side allows oral bacteria to percolate through the wound resulting in scarring of the skin.

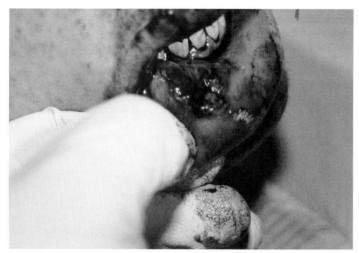

A

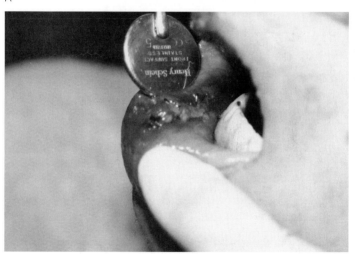

B

FIG 14-3 Baseball injury. A. Large laceration of the lower lip caused by baseball impact. B. Laceration is sutured after radiographic verification that the lip was free of tooth fragments. Photo courtesy of Mark Roettger, DDS.

Tooth Fractures

Tooth fractures can occur in the crown of the tooth or in the root. Crown fractures are much more common than root fractures (Fig. 14-4). Tooth fractures occur most frequently in the upper anterior teeth as a result of high-velocity direct trauma, and are most easily classified by the dental tissues that are injured.

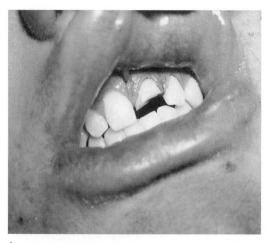

A

B

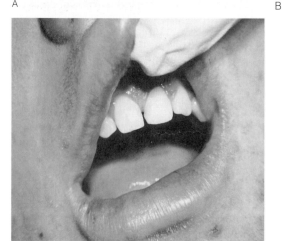

C

FIG 14-4 Basketball injury. A. The left central incisor was fractured by contact with the floor. B. The tooth fragment was retrieved by the player and brought to the dentist. C. The tooth fragment has been rebonded to the tooth. Photo courtesy of Mark Roettger, DDS.

Crown Fractures of Enamel Only

Enamel-only crown fractures are usually not emergencies by themselves. These injuries seldom cause problems for the athlete other than feeling rough on the tongue. Nonemergency dental consultation is recommended.

Crown Fractures of Enamel and Dentin

Fractures of enamel and dentin may be sensitive to changes in temperature. These fractures are not always true dental emergencies; however, the exposed dentin should be covered in order to protect the underlying dental pulp from bacterial invasion. Dental consultation and treatment is recommended as soon as possible.

Crown Fractures Involving the Dental Pulp

These injuries are often termed *complex crown fractures* because their management is more difficult than fractures that do not involve the dental pulp. A fracture that involves only the crown can still affect the pulp of the tooth and expose the nerve and blood vessels. Involvement of the pulp is a more important indicator of severity than the actual amount of the tooth involved. The exposed nerve also causes pain that is not seen in minor fractures of the tooth. The fractured tooth that involves the pulp can be identified by a bleeding site or by a pink or red dot in the middle of the dentin. Diagnosis is normally made by observation of hemorrhage from the exposed pulp chamber. A fracture that exposes the pulp can be very painful, and limiting nerve exposure to air, saliva, temperature changes, and the tongue will decrease the pain. Covering the nerve with a drop of cyanoacrylate glue will seal the root canal for immediate sideline management. Medical grade cyanoacrylate is recommended to minimize palpal histotoxicity. Complex crown fractures are true dental emergencies and the athlete should be referred for dental treatment immediately. If left untreated, complex crown fractures can lead to necrosis of the dental pulp, along with severe pain and possible temporary disability. Treatment for this type of injury may range from pulpotomy to endodontic therapy.

Root Fracture

Root fractures are difficult to distinguish from luxation injuries without radiographic evaluation (Fig. 14-5). Teeth with root fractures are usually mobile and appear to be displaced. These are true dental emergencies and should be referred immediately for dental evaluation and treatment.

Tooth Luxation, Displacements, and Avulsion

Luxation injuries to the teeth are caused mainly by low-velocity direct trauma. These displacement injuries can occur in different directions. The teeth can be displaced forward or backward, usually termed lateral luxation, and can also be intruded or extruded from their normal position in the bone. These are potentially very damaging injuries to the periodontal ligament and the dental pulp. All luxation injuries should be treated as dental emergencies and be referred immediately for dental evaluation and treatment. Luxation injuries can be reduced using finger pressure prior to transport to the dentist. If the displaced tooth is not easily repositioned by finger pressure, transport the athlete directly to the dentist. Many times these injuries are too painful to reposition and require the use of local anesthetic. Luxation injuries may have concomitant alveolar bone fracture that may complicate reduction of the injury.

Avulsion is the most extreme luxation injury. In this injury the tooth is completely exarticulated from its bony socket (Fig. 14-6). Avulsions are also true dental emergencies.

Avulsed teeth must be re-implanted within 30 minutes of injury to maximize treatment success. The goal of tooth re-implantation is complete redevelopment of the periodontal ligament. The redevelopment of the periodontal

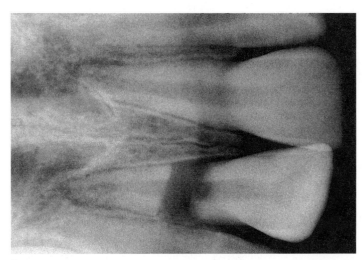

A

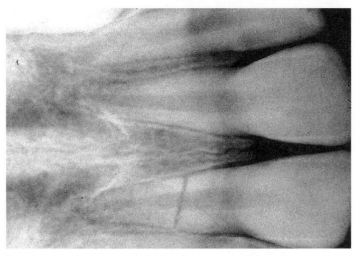

B

FIG 14-5 Baseball injury. A. Radiograph confirms the horizontal root fracture with coronal displacement of the right central incisor. B. Radiograph of the tooth after reduction and prior to placement of splint. (Photo courtesy of Mark Roettger, DDS).

ligament depends on the viability and vitality of the periodontal ligament cells that remain on the root surface of the avulsed tooth. The avulsed tooth should never be handled by the root nor should there be any attempt to scrub debris from the root surface. If there is debris on the tooth it should be gently rinsed with water prior to re-implantation. Holding the tooth by the crown, firmly place the tooth back into the bony socket using adjacent

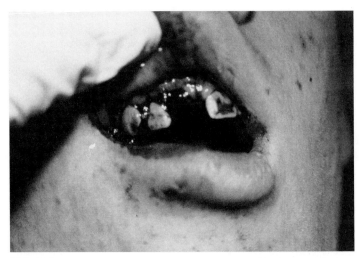

FIG 14-6 Baseball injury. Avulsion of the right central incisor caused by baseball impact. The tooth was lost in the grass of right field. Photo courtesy of Mark Roettger, DDS.

teeth as a guide to proper position. There is often a "click" as the tooth seats into the socket. After the tooth has been re-implanted, stabilize it by having the athlete bite on sterile gauze during transport to the dental office or hospital.

When the tooth can not be re-implanted on the sideline, the athlete and the tooth must be transported immediately to the dentist. In order to protect the vitality of the periodontal ligament cells on the root surface, an appropriate transport medium must be used. The osmolality of the transport medium should match the osmolality of the periodontal ligament cells. Hank's balanced salt solution is thought to be the best transport medium, but it is not always available. Milk is the next best medium available, followed by normal saline and saliva. If these are not available, place teeth in a plastic bag and transport to the dentist immediately.

Once the patient is seen by the dentist, final positioning and splinting of the re-implanted tooth will be accomplished. Most of these teeth will need root canal treatment as a part of total treatment, depending on the degree of root development at the time of injury. If the periodontal ligament cells do not survive the accident, the periodontal ligament will not redevelop and the tooth will become ankylosed. Ankylosis of the tooth and bone will cause the root of the tooth to be resorbed and replaced with bone. When this happens the tooth will ultimately be lost.

Facial Fractures

Every athlete who has suffered a head or facial injury should be examined for the possibility of a jaw fracture. Many times jaw fractures are overlooked at the time of injury, only to be discovered days or weeks later. Late diagnosis may complicate treatment and compromise the final outcome of treatment. The most common sports-related facial fractures include nasal, mandibular, maxillary, and orbital. If a fracture of the jaws is suspected the patient should be stabilized, paying special attention to the airway, and transported to the hospital. The patient can be made more comfortable by placing temporary fixation in the form of a head bandage or Barton's bandage. This bandage is looped under the chin and tied at the top of the head with the teeth gently in contact. Facial fractures are covered in detail in Chapter 13.

On-field evaluation of athletes suspected of having a mandibular fracture should include a careful examination of the dental occlusion. A step or disruption of the normal plane of occlusion of the mandibular teeth could indicate a fracture. Ecchymosis or hematoma in the floor of the mouth could also indicate the presence of a fracture.

Temporomandibular Joint Injuries

The mandibular condyle and the glenoid fossa of the temporal bone form the temporomandibular joint (TMJ). The articular disc separates these bones. The TMJ is one of the most complex joints in the body. The TMJ is capable of hinge or rotational movements in one plane as well as gliding or translational movement. This complexity makes the TMJ susceptible to injury. Direct blows to the chin result in superior posterior transmission of forces through the articular disc and retrodiscal tissues, which are compressed between the condyle and the temporal bone. This results in local soft tissue injury and swelling. Oblique forces may result in injury to the ligaments of the TMJ. The mandible receives important support when the teeth are clenched. Trauma to the mandible with the mouth closed produces less severe TMJ injury than open mouth trauma. Traumatic joint effusion and hemarthrosis are often seen after impact trauma to the mandible. These injuries may lead to more serious long-term problems such as joint derangement, chronic pain, facial skeletal remodeling, and growth disturbances.

TMJ injuries can mimic jaw fractures and appropriate dental referral should be made to complete a radiographic evaluation and examination to make a proper diagnosis.

The most common complaint at the time of TMJ injury is pre-auricular pain and limited range of motion. The patient may also report that the bite is uneven, being unable to occlude the teeth on the injured side. This is usually due to joint effusion or hemarthrosis. TMJ injuries require supportive care and careful management to minimize the risk of long-term sequelae.

The TMJ can be dislocated as a result of a lateral or oblique blow to the mandible while the athlete has an open mouth. In this case the athlete cannot close the mouth properly and the mandible seems locked out of place. Immediate reduction of the dislocation should be attempted because over time the muscles will go into spasm, increasing the pain and difficulty in reduction. Reduction can be accomplished by placing the hands on either side of the mandible and gripping the chin. Exert downward pressure first, then posterior pressure to place the mandible in its proper position. Another method of reduction is to stand behind the athlete and place the thumbs bilaterally over the occlusal surfaces of the posterior teeth, pushing the mandible gently downward, then pulling it gently back into position. Once the mandible has been reduced, ice should be applied, and the athlete referred to the dentist for evaluation and management.

EMERGENCY EVALUATION OF DENTAL INJURIES

Dental and orofacial injuries range from minor to life threatening. Complete evaluation of the athlete with dental injuries is imperative. It is necessary to have access to the patient's medical history and consider the physical status of the patient prior to injury treatment.

The principles of basic life support must be followed before dental evaluation can begin. Evaluation of the airway, breathing, and circulation are completed prior to dental injury assessment. Some orofacial injuries may compromise the patient's airway. Dislodged dental appliances, fractured or avulsed teeth, or severe jaw fracture may contribute to airway obstruction.

When evaluating the patient with dental injuries, consideration must be given to the fact that there may be a concomitant head injury. Neurologic assessment to determine the patient's awareness and orientation should be completed. If the patient is unconscious it must be assumed that the athlete has suffered a head or neck injury and further radiographic and neurologic attention is needed prior to treatment of the dental injuries.

It is important in emergency evaluation of dental injuries to consider trauma beyond the obvious problem. An underlying dental fracture or luxation may accompany an obvious lip laceration. All aspects of the craniofacial complex must be assessed prior to clearing an athlete to return to the field. The dental occlusion should be evaluated for any steps or disruption. The teeth should be examined for proper positioning within the dental arch and for fracture. The gingiva should be inspected for any tears or laceration. The temporomandibular joint should be palpated and the mandibular range of motion tested. Normal interincisal opening for the mandible is 40–60 mm. Pain or deviation of the mandible to the right or left during opening should be noted and referred to the athlete's dentist for follow-up and treatment.

The team dentist or the patient's private dentist should follow all dental injuries noted on a trauma evaluation.

MANAGEMENT OF DENTAL INJURIES

Management of dental injuries is highly specialized, requiring dental training and specialized equipment. All dental injuries should be referred to the team dentist or the athlete's private dentist for management. Treatment of dental injuries may consist of bonding restorative materials to the tooth to replace fractured enamel or dentin (Fig. 14-7). Pulp tissue irreversibly damaged by trauma must be treated by endodontic therapy. Severely fractured teeth may require full crown restoration. Teeth too badly injured to restore need to be extracted, and restoration of the dental arch may include removable prosthetics, fixed bridgework, or dental implants. The patient's age or athletic situation may influence treatment planning. Some athletes choose to restore the dental arch with removable prosthetics until their competitive days are over and then pursue more definitive restoration such as bridgework or dental implants. All athletes should be advised never to wear removable dental prosthetics during athletic competition.

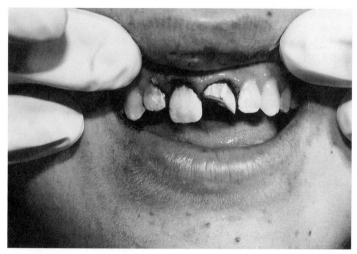

A

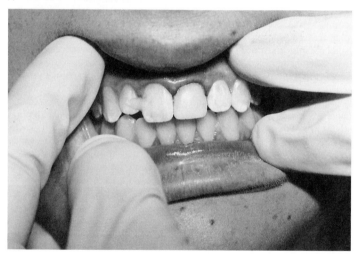

B

FIG 14-7 Soccer injury. A. Head-to-head contact has caused displacement of the right central incisor and complex fracture of the left central incisor. B. The right central incisor has been repositioned and splinted. The left central incisor was restored with composite resin after completion of a partial pulpotomy. Photo courtesy of Mark Roettger, DDS.

CONFOUNDING CONDITIONS

The single most common confounding condition of dental injuries is that many of these injuries have hidden future sequelae. What may seem to be a minor dental injury on the field, if unmanaged or mismanaged, could lead to pain, infection, and tooth loss, resulting in facial deformity, expensive restoration, and disability. Having sports medicine personnel refer all dental injuries to a dentist, no matter how trivial they may seem, can minimize these sequelae.

PREVENTION OF ATHLETIC DENTAL INJURIES

Many athletic dental injuries are easily preventable. The use of protective equipment has been successful in preventing numerous dental injuries in sports. Helmets, facemasks, and mouthguards have been particularly helpful in preventing dental injuries in football and ice hockey. Many sports do not require the use of helmets or facemasks, so the properly fitted mouthguard becomes the single most important piece of equipment used in the prevention of dental injuries.

The function of the properly fitted mouthguard is multifactorial. First, the mouthguard provides cushioning from direct trauma to the teeth, preventing tooth fracture and luxation. Second, the mouthguard provides a barrier between the teeth and the oral soft tissues, preventing laceration and other soft tissue injuries. Third, the mouthguard prevents violent contact of the upper and lower teeth caused by mandibular trauma, preventing tooth fracture, luxation, and tongue laceration. Finally, the mouthguard acts as a shock absorber to prevent traumatic posterior superior displacement of the mandible. This can minimize the risk of temporomandibular joint injury and mandibular fracture caused by a blow to the chin. The shock absorber function of the mouthguard has also been credited with preventing or decreasing the severity of concussions caused by trauma to the mandible. This phenomenon has to date been supported mainly by empiric and anecdotal evidence. Careful scientific studies are underway to more accurately define the role of the mouthguard in concussion prevention.

The American Society for Testing and Materials (ASTM) has established a classification system for mouthguards (American Society for Testing and Materials, 1999). This system was introduced in 1980 and is still useful today. Mouthguards are classified based on the level of sophistication involved in the customizing process used to provide fit, comfort, and protection for the athlete. This classification includes type I (stock mouthguards), type II (mouth-formed mouthguards), and type III (custom-fabricated mouthguards).

Stock mouthguards are ready-made and require no customizing. The fit is poor and athlete satisfaction is low with this type of mouthguard. These mouthguards are held in place by clenching the teeth, making breathing difficult and speech impossible. Because of poor fit, stock mouthguards are considered the least desirable of all mouthguards.

Mouth-formed mouthguards are customized intraorally using a thermoplastic process. The mouthguard is placed in boiling water to soften it, and inserted into the mouth to attempt to form the internal aspect of the guard to fit the teeth and other oral structures. The forming procedure is almost always carried out entirely by the athlete at home or at school with no supervision. This type of mouthguard is by far the most common one in use by athletes today. The fit of mouth-formed mouthguards is usually unacceptable and athlete satisfaction is low due to poor fit and large variation in thickness.

Custom-fabricated mouthguards are the most sophisticated mouthguards available. A dentist fabricates it over a model of the athlete's mouth (Fig. 14-8). Custom-fabricated mouthguards offer the best fit, protection, and comfort available. These mouthguards do not interfere with speech or

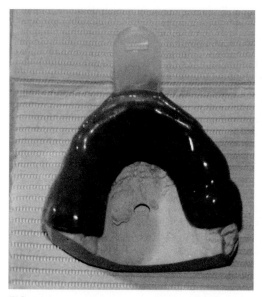

FIG 14-8 Custom-fabricated mouthguard. Formed over a cast of the athlete's teeth, this type of mouthguard is the best available for fit, comfort, and protection. Photo courtesy of Mark Roettger, DDS.

breathing and are more dimensionally stable than other types of mouthguards. Athlete satisfaction is high with custom-fabricated mouthguards compared to stock or mouth-formed types.

It is clear that custom mouthguards are the best choice to prevent dental injuries. The main objections to this type of mouthguard are availability and cost. Despite these objections, it is still desirable to prevent a dental injury rather than endure the expense, discomfort, and time involved in repairing the injury. Sports medicine personnel should have significant influence over athletes and coaches, and can use this influence to promote the use of custom-fabricated mouthguards.

SIDELINE TIPS

Preparation is the key to providing proper treatment to athletes with dental injuries. Many dental injuries require treatment within the first 30 minutes postinjury to ensure a favorable outcome. Whether during practice or games, on-field medical staff must be prepared with some basic knowledge regarding dental injuries. These medical personnel should also be prepared with some basic dental emergency equipment and supplies (Table 14-1). Ideally all athletic teams should include a dentist as a part of the sports medicine team to be available on the sideline or on call for practice and games.

SUMMARY

Dental injuries occur at a significant rate in sports participants. These injuries seldom limit athlete playing time, but they should not be considered insignificant. They can cause pain, infection, growth disturbances, and facial

TABLE 14-1 Suggested Contents for Dental Emergency Kit
Anesthetic (local and topical)
Aspirating syringe (local anesthetic)
Bandage (stabilization of jaw fracture)
Biohazard bags
Butane torch (mouthguard repairs)
Calcium hydroxide paste
Cotton rolls
Curing light (composite resins)
Dental needles (anesthetic)
Emergency dental treatment card[a]
Flashlight
Flowable composite resin (tooth splint)
Gauze
Gloves
Hank's balanced salt solution (tooth preservation)
Cold milk (tooth preservation)
Contact lens saline (tooth preservation)
Mouth mirror
Mouthguards (extra)
Suture kit
Cyanoacrylate glue (e.g., Colgate Orabase Sooth-n-Seal)
Tongue depressors
Ruler

[a] Available from The International Academy for Sports Dentistry.

deformity. These injuries also fall outside the scope of traditional sports medicine, requiring management and treatment by a dentist. This makes the dentist a valuable member of the sports medicine team. Dental injuries are also preventable in many cases by the use of a properly fitted mouthguard. All dentists, sports medicine personnel, and coaches should encourage the use of mouthguards for athletes in collision and contact sports.

REFERENCES

American Society for Testing and Materials. *Standard Practice for Care and Use of Mouthguards.* Designation: F 697-80 (reapproved 1992). Vol. 15. American Society of Testing and Materials; 1999.
Flanders RA, Bhat M. The incidence of orofacial injuries in sports: A pilot study in Illinois. *J Am Dent Assoc.* 1996;126:491–496.
Kvittem B, Roettger M. Incidence of orofacial injuries in high school sports. *J Public Health Dent.* 1998;58:288–293.
National Youth Sports Safety Foundation. Dental Injuries Fact Sheet. Needham, MA, 1992.
Tesini D, Soporowski N. Epidemiology of orofacial sports-related injuries. *Dent Clin North Am.* 2000;44:1–19.

RECOMMENDED READING

Andreasen JO, Andreasen FM. *Textbook And Color Atlas of Traumatic Injuries To The Teeth*, 3rd ed. Copenhagen: Munksgaard; 1994.
Information on sports dentistry and team dentists can be obtained by contacting The International Academy for Sports Dentistry at (800) 273-1788.

15 | Dermatology Issues in Athletes

Wilma F. Bergfeld and Joshua M. Berlin

INTRODUCTION

Athletes are prone to a variety of skin problems that can hinder performance. In some instances a dermatologic disorder can disqualify an athlete from participation. The various dermatoses that bring the athlete to the attention of a physician are categorized by the underlying cause: mechanical problems, physical factors, and infections.

MECHANICAL PROBLEMS OF THE SKIN

Corns

Corns are thickening of the stratum corneum in areas of increased pressure that are due to mechanical forces and protect underlying structures. Corns are frequently found in skiers, ice skaters, and snow boarders. A hydrocolloid dressing such as Duoderm will pad and protect the area during treatment. Prior to application of the hydrocolloid dressing, pare down the corn with a scalpel, pumice stone, or keratolytic emollient such as Lac-Hydrin. The dressing can be left on for several days and often will stay in place with training and showering. Cotton socks are worn over the dressing. Padding can be added to footwear for comfort and to prevent sliding of the feet.

Blisters

Blisters commonly occur in novice athletes or athletes with new footwear while running or competing for a long period of time. They primarily occur on weight-bearing or equipment contact surfaces of the feet and hands. Frictional forces cause dissolution of keratinocytes in the epidermis and the loss of adhesion of keratinocytes. The effect of friction is exacerbated by heat, humidity, and sweat-soaked clothing. Unless symptomatic or impeding with further activity, there is no treatment necessary for blisters. When treatment is required, the blister should be prepped with alcohol or povidone iodine, and then incised with a sterile #11 blade or needle. The blister fluid is evacuated by gentle pressure and the surrounding necrotic epidermis can be left in place. The re-epithelialization process is enhanced by the application of an antibiotic ointment such as bacitracin. An occlusive hydrocolloid dressing like Duoderm can then be applied to serve as a physical barrier to infection and further trauma. Blisters on the feet can be reduced by applying an antiperspirant with aluminum chlorhydrate on a regular basis to decrease sweating.

Subcorneal Hemorrhage

With vigorous exercise, capillaries in the superficial papillary dermis may rupture, leading to hemorrhagic bullae. At times, small hemorrhagic blisters may not be noticed, and as they resorb, they may leave pigmentation within the stratum corneum that is often mistaken for melanoma. The black discoloration due to blood in the stratum corneum is known as a calcaneal puncture or talon noir. Talon noir commonly occurs at the upper edge of the heel due to shearing forces from sudden stops and starts, and is commonly seen in tennis players and gymnasts. No treatment is necessary as the lesions will spontaneously resolve with discontinuation of the activity. If the diagnosis is in question, a talon noir can be confirmed by paring the skin to the stratum corneum that houses the hemoglobin pigment. If paring does not remove the pigment, a biopsy should be considered to exclude the possibility of melanoma.

Splinter Hemorrhage

Splinter or subungal hemorrhages, like subcorneal hemorrhages, occur in sports that involve rapid starts and stops such as squash, tennis, racquetball, and basketball, and is often confused with an underlying pigmented neoplasm. Subungal melanoma is often preceded by an erroneous history of prior trauma; therefore clinicians must be wary of this pitfall. A pigmented lesion in the nail bed should be evaluated closely (Fig. 15-1). A punch biopsy can be obtained through the nail plate. If hemorrhage is suspected, the area of hemorrhage underneath the nail will grow out in an orderly fashion at approximately 2 mm per month, and the outgrowth should be monitored. If the pigmented area does not grow out or if it spreads out laterally, a biopsy is indicated.

A variant of splinter hemorrhage is called golfer's nails. This disorder is due to gripping the club too tightly and loosening the grip will lead to spontaneous resolution. "Tennis toe" refers to subungal hemorrhage from repetitive slippage of the foot anteriorly against the shoe toe box. Advise athletes to trim their

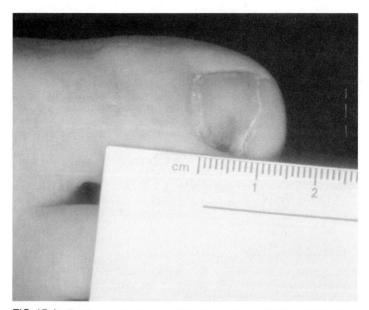

FIG 15-1   Black discoloration involving the great toenail due to blood in the stratum corneum. This discoloration is commonly seen in tennis players, gymnasts, and ballerinas. It is important to rule out subungal melanoma if the pigment does not resolve.

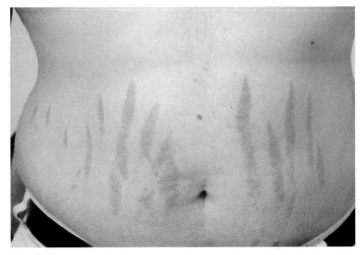

FIG 15-2   Multiple striae on the abdomen due to extensive stretching of the skin with fragmentation of elastic supporting fibers.

toenails as short as possible and to wear shoes with a toe box that has a thumb-width sized space between the great toe and the end of the shoe.

Striae Distensae

Striae distensae or stretch lines are a result of extensive stretching of the skin with fragmentation of elastic supporting fibers (Fig. 15-2). Weight gain or increased muscle mass lead to rupture of elastic fibers into the reticular dermis. The most common sites for striae are the shoulders, back, and thighs. Weightlifters and wrestlers are particularly prone to striae. Treatment options are limited with laser therapy offering only modest results and top-ical retinoids and alpha-hydroxy acids producing limited improvement in studies done to date.

Abrasions

Abrasions are superficial erosions or ulcerations that occur due to shearing forces directed to the skin, and they are prevalent throughout all sports participants. The underlying etiology is direct epidermal trauma, so the best intervention is wearing protective clothing, especially on artificial turf. Once abrasions occur, gentle cleansing and application of a topical antibiotic ointment will prevent secondary infection, and an occlusive dressing may speed healing. If the abrasion becomes secondarily infected, systemic antibiotics such as dicloxacillin or cephaloxin 500 mg three times a day for 10 days may be indicated. Debridement of crusts will help improve the final cosmetic appearance.

PHYSICAL FACTORS

Sunburn

Sunburn is a phototoxic reaction due to excessive skin exposure to ultraviolet light. Clinically, it presents as an intense erythema with or without blistering

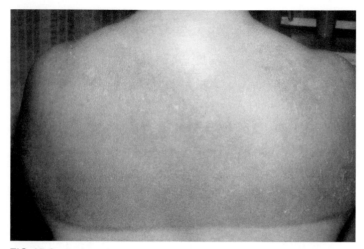

FIG 15-3 Sunburn is most likely occur between 10 AM and 2 PM because of the intensity of ultraviolet B rays at that time of day. It is important to advise athletes on the importance of using broad-spectrum sunscreens.

at the sites of sun exposure (Fig. 15-3). It is common in athletes with fair complexion and blond or red hair. Athletes who train between the hours of 10 AM and 2 PM, when ultraviolet light is at its greatest intensity, are at greatest risk for developing sunburn. Skiers, paddlers, and sailors are exposed secondary to reflection of the sun on snow and water, and often develop sunburn on normally shaded areas of the face and body. Athletes should use broad-spectrum sunscreens applied 30 minutes prior to activity to allow the active ingredients to combine with the stratum corneum, and sunscreens should be reapplied every 2 hours. Many athletes do not receive optimal benefit from traditional sunscreens because they are removed by sweating. A sunscreen with a sun protective factor (SPF) of at least 30 should be used. The SPF is calculated by dividing the amount of time required to produce erythema in skin covered with a sunscreen by the time required to produce erythema in skin without sunscreen. For example, an SPF of 10 would allow a person who normally burns in 10 minutes to be exposed as long as 100 minutes before burning occurs. Acute sunburn can trigger many skin disorders including herpes simplex, solar urticaria, and lupus erythematous. In addition, athletes taking medications like tetracycline and sulfa products can have phototoxic reactions following sun exposure. Sunburn interferes with the sweating mechanism, decreasing evaporative heat exchange and increasing the risk of heat stroke.

The treatment of sunburn is directed towards decreasing inflammation and temperature of the skin. Cool compresses are effective in reducing skin heat and local discomfort. A low-potency topical corticosteroid applied twice daily can hasten resolution of the local inflammatory response. Nonsteroidal anti-inflammatory agents such as aspirin or indomethacin interfere with the prostaglandin mediators that initiate cutaneous damage, and help relieve pain. Emollients are important to reduce dehydration of the epidermis that results from extensive ultraviolet exposure.

INFECTIONS

Herpes

Infections with herpes simplex virus types I and II can affect any part of the body, and recurrent infection commonly occurs around the lips and vermilion border. Although it will classically present as grouped vesicles on an erythematous base, early cases may exhibit no lesions and late lesions may show only erosions (Fig.15-4). Herpes virus is known to shed before skin manifestations are visible, and the moist lesions of herpes simplex are highly contagious through contact. Athletes with prodromal symptoms of burning or tingling and with active lesions should be closely monitored and kept from participating in contact sports. Treatment with a systemic antiviral agent for at least 5 days will suppress the infection and decrease the risk of athlete-to-athlete transmission, and allow athletes to return to contact sports. Once the lesions are crusted and dry, participation in sports is also considered safe. Treatment is directed to alleviate pain and promote early healing. Oral antiviral agents such as acyclovir (400 mg five times a day for 10 days), famciclovir (250 mg three times a day for 10 days), or valacyclovir (1000 mg twice a day for 10 days) are effective if started early in the course of the infection or during the prodrome, when patients will often note tingling prior to the onset of a skin eruption.

Genital herpes is characterized by the development of vesicles and pustules on an erythematous base. Lesions tend to be clustered and the patient may experience flu-like symptoms such as myalgia and headache. Treatment with oral antiviral agents given in daily doses is indicated. Unless the athlete feels ill, and assuming there will be no contact with the affected area, genital herpes does not require disqualification from sports.

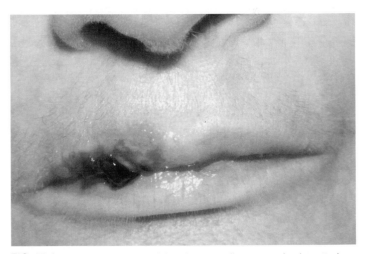

FIG 15-4 Crusted plaque involving the upper lip commonly characterizes herpes simplex infections. When the lesions are moist, the virus is highly contagious and athletes should be held back from competition.

Herpes Gladiatorum

Herpes gladiatorum or scrum pox is the spread of herpes simplex via direct skin-to-skin contact. It is common among wrestlers and other athletes with direct skin-to-skin contact, and some studies found that up to one-third of wrestlers have experienced the disease. The lesions commonly affect the head and neck, upper extremities, and trunk, and are commonly masked by the hairline. If spread to the eye occurs, the athlete can be blinded for life. When the diagnosis is suspected, the wrestler should be quarantined from contact, the lesion cultured, and systemic antiviral medications started. A Tzanck smear or immunofluorescence study can also provide confirmation of herpes simplex infection, but require a trained reader for accurate results. Widespread blisters can develop in individuals with pre-existing dermatoses such as atopic dermatitis and Darier's disease. Therapy with an antiviral agent is warranted to stop the transmission within and between teams. In addition, transmission to other wrestlers can be reduced by showering immediately after practice, cleaning workout clothing daily, not sharing equipment, and cleaning the mats daily. Covering isolated lesions during practice sessions and competitions does not assure safety for uninfected wrestlers. Outbreaks and recurrences can be reduced by suppressive therapy with valacyclovir 500 mg a day for affected athletes.

Molluscum Contagiosum

Molluscum contagiosum is caused by a poxvirus that commonly affects athletes. It presents as discrete, flesh-colored 2- to 5-mm papules with central umbilication (Fig. 15-5). The disease is easily spread by autoinoculation and from one individual to another. Widespread outbreaks have been reported in swimming, rugby, and wrestling teams. The lesions of molluscum contagiosum occur on exposed surfaces such as the face, trunk, and extremities.

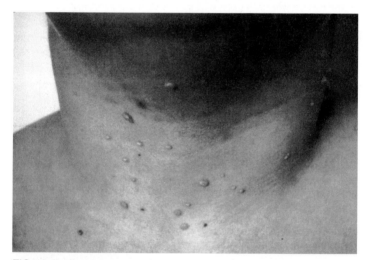

FIG 15-5 Multiple umbilicated papules are characteristic of molluscum contagiosum. Widespread outbreaks can occur among swimming, rugby, and wrestling teams.

Contact sports should be avoided until lesions have been resolved for 24 hours, and wrestlers should have the treated lesions covered with a bio-occlusive dressing. Treatment is aimed at destruction of the poxvirus lesion with liquid nitrogen cryotherapy, electrocautery, chemical lysis, or curettage. Athletes with dark complexions are at risk for hypopigmentation and liquid nitrogen cryotherapy should be used with caution. The use of a topical anesthetic such as lidocaine (ELA-Max) applied 30 minutes prior to the procedure may be helpful in young children. Less invasive treatment options include the application of tretinoin (Retin-A), topical salicylic acid preparations (eg, Duofilm), or an immunomodulator such as imiquimod (Aldara) cream.

Warts

Warts are common benign growths caused by infection with the human papilloma virus. Common warts are typically skin-colored or tan in appearance with a rough surface. If the diagnosis is in question, paring the warts will reveal stippled blood vessels and loss of normal dermatoglyphics. Warts are often located on the hands and feet and may interfere with sports participation. Treatment of warts varies and no one treatment is uniformly effective. Destructive techniques include the use of chemical agents, liquid nitrogen for cryocautery, and electrodesiccation. During the competitive season, these destructive techniques may result in an erosion or ulcer that may interfere with an athlete's performance. Topical salicylic acid preparations can also be effective, with greater concentrations of salicylic acid producing results more quickly. We favor the use of 40% salicylic acid plasters (Mediplast) cut to the size of the wart and applied each night at bedtime. Covering a topical salicylic acid preparation with duct tape overnight can also speed the wart's destruction. A novel therapy involves the topical immunomodulator Aldara cream applied to the wart on a scheduled basis to stimulate the body's immune response and destroy the papilloma-virus.

Human Immunodeficiency Virus Infection

HIV infection in high-profile athletes has helped raise the awareness of this disease. Athletes with recalcitrant herpes zoster, candidiasis, or extensive molluscum contagiosum may be exhibiting the cutaneous manifestations of AIDS. Current information suggests that there is no risk of acquiring HIV through sports activity or intact skin-to-skin contact, but athletes are not immune from the disease. It is important for sports physicians and athletic trainers to practice universal precautions with all treated individuals.

Folliculitis

Folliculitis is infection of the upper portion of the hair follicle. Sweating during practice and competition are risk factors for developing folliculitis. On examination there are discrete pustules with hair follicles in the center (Fig. 15-6). Once the pustule ruptures, a superficial crust or erosion can be noted. Treatment involves daily use of a benzoyl peroxide wash followed by application of a topical antibiotic such as clindamycin (Cleocin) solution or erythromycin gel. For widespread or refractory folliculitis, oral erythromycin or minocycline are usually effective.

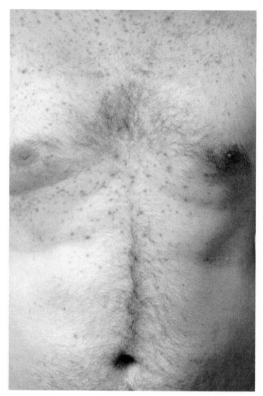

FIG 15-6 Folliculitis. Discrete pustules centered around a hair follicle on the chest.

Impetigo

Impetigo is a highly contagious, superficial skin infection that commonly occurs in wrestlers, rugby, and football players. *Staphylococcus* and *Streptococcus* species are the most common culprits. It often occurs around the mouth as pustules that rupture, resulting in erosions which form honey-colored crusts on healing (Fig. 15-7). The disease is easily spread through minor skin trauma. Athletes should be withheld from contact sports until the lesions of impetigo have fully healed, which generally occurs in 7–10 days. Topical treatment should include the use of a benzoyl peroxide wash and application of an antibacterial ointment such as mupirocin. For more widespread eruptions, the use of oral antibiotics such as dicloxacillin (500 mg three times a day for 10 days) or erythromycin (250 mg three times a day for 2 weeks) is indicated. Treatment is enhanced by using moist, warm packing to debride the crusts. Wrestlers with impetigo and other bacterial skin infections should be on antibiotics for at least 72 hours with no draining, oozing, or moist lesions before returning to contact practice or competition.

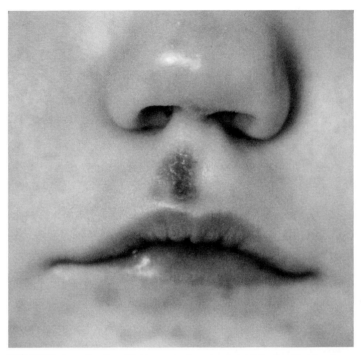

FIG 15-7   Impetigo is a highly contagious bacterial infection that begins as pustules that rupture, leaving a honey-colored crust. Athletes should be withheld from contact sports until the lesions have fully healed.

Erythrasma

Erythrasma is an infection caused by *Corynebacterium minutissimum* that presents as well demarcated red to reddish-brown plaques in the axillae and inguinal folds. The diagnosis can be confirmed by the presence of coral-red fluorescence while exposing the rash to a Wood's ultraviolet lamp. These patients do very well with a benzoyl peroxide wash and application of a topical erythromycin cream twice a day for 7 days. The alcohol-based erythromycin products should be avoided because of the irritation they create in the body folds.

Tinea Infections

Fungal infections are common in athletes, and can be spread by direct contact. Skin fungal infections thrive in dark, damp places, but can occur anywhere on the body.

Tinea cruris is an infection of the inguinal folds that presents as scaly annular plaques with central clearing (Fig. 15-8). The scrotum is spared and this condition is commonly seen in the summer months. Topical antifungals such as econazole (Spectazole) or terbinafine (Lamisil) applied twice daily for 6 weeks usually resolve the infection.

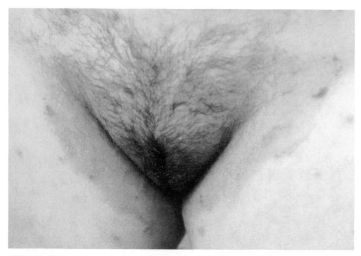

FIG 15-8 Tinea cruris, a fungal infection, presents as scaly, erythematous patches with discrete borders. It responds well to topical antifungals.

Tinea capitis is a fungal infection of the scalp that is characterized by scaling, erythema, patchy hair loss, and pustule formation. In severe cases, kerion formation occurs, consisting of a boggy, indurated mass with purulent discharge. Treatment with an antifungal shampoo such as keto-conazole (Nizoral) coupled with oral antifungals such as griseofulvin 500 mg a day for 4–6 weeks, terbinafine 250 mg a day for 6 weeks, or itraconazole (Sporanox) 200 mg twice a day for the first week of each month for 2–3 months is effective.

Tinea pedis or athlete's foot usually involves interdigital web spaces of the toes, but can present in several different ways. Some individuals have widespread scaly plaques involving the soles of their feet in a moccasin like distribution, while others present with inflammatory vesicles along the instep. Topical treatment with antifungals is usually effective. Nail infection or onychomycosis can commonly occur with tinea pedis.

Tinea infections are especially prevalent in wrestlers and have been termed *tinea corporis gladiatorum. Trichophyton tonsurans* is the most common fungus leading to this condition, and it is easily transmitted through direct skin contact. Wrestlers are prone to develop infections due close skin-to-skin contact during training and competition. The head, neck, and upper extrem-ities are commonly affected. The wrestler should not be allowed to compete if active lesions are present on the neck or head, and lesions on other body parts must be covered with an occlusive dressing. A bio-occlusive dressing like Tegaderm covered with prewrap and secured with elastic tape makes an effective and adherent dressing. Oral antifungals are the most effective agents for treating and controlling the spread of tinea in wrestlers, and a wrestler should be treated for 24 hours for skin lesions and 14 days for scalp lesions before returning to contact practice and competition. Potential therapeutic regimens include Lamisil 250 mg a day for 2–4 weeks, griseofulvin 500 mg twice a day for 4 weeks, or itraconazole (Sporanox) 100 mg a day for 15 days. These agents can be combined with a topical antifungal.

INFESTATIONS

Scabies

Scabies infestation is common in young athletes and easily spread with close contact to other individuals. It is characterized by an intensely pruritic eruption that may involve the flexural surfaces of the wrists and extremities, the lower abdomen and genitalia, and the interdigital web spaces. Although burrows may be seen, often the only clinical finding will be excoriations. A skin scraping viewed under oil immersion microscopy can sometimes demonstrate the mite. Treatment involves the use of permethrin (Elimite) cream applied to the entire body at night and subsequently washed off the next morning. All clothing and bedding should be laundered and everyone living in the same household as the index case should be treated. The treatment should be repeated 1 week later.

Lice

Lice infection (*Pthirus corporis* and *P. pubis*) may be spread through close contact between individuals. Lice can remain in clothing, equipment, or bedding, so infection is often acquired while traveling if the accommodations are not properly sanitized. For scalp involvement, shampoos such as Nix or Pronto provide improvement. A nit brush can then be used following shampoo treatment to remove eggs from the hair. This treatment can be repeated after 10 days if the infection persists. All individuals on a team warrant examination if one member is infected. Athletes may return to practice the day after treatment.

Miscellaneous Dermatoses

Green Hair

Swimmers with blond or light hair can develop a greenish tint to their hair. This occurs due to long-term exposure to copper ions found in the water. Treatment with penicillamine-containing shampoos or application of 2-3% hydrogen peroxide will clear the color.

Jogger's Nipples

This condition refers to redness and irritation of the nipples from chronic friction between the nipples and clothing. If the runner does not seek medical attention, erosions will develop. These athletes should apply petroleum jelly and adhesive tape over the nipples before running. Some athletes may need to have cotton patches sewn into jerseys if the problem persists.

Cold Panniculitis

Some athletes, especially young women, may develop panniculitis on the lateral thighs. This has been noted most often in equestrian sports. The cold may lead to solidification of the panniculus, which in turn leads to formation of painful erythematous nodules. Wearing protective clothing will help prevent recurrence.

Foot Contact Dermatitis or Sweat Sock Dermatitis

Foot contact dermatitis is a red, scaly rash, sometimes associated with deep splitting of the skin, located on the dorsal and plantar surfaces of the feet, sparing the interdigital web spaces. Foot dermatitis is often confused with tinea pedis and the sparing of the interdigital spaces is the key physical finding. It is due to sensitivity or allergic reaction to the glues and dyes used in shoe manufacturing that leach onto the skin with heavy sweating or wet footwear. The foot dermatitis is controlled with topical steroid creams and antiperspirants to decrease the inflammatory reaction and stop the chemical leaching onto the skin. Frequent sock changes and wearing sandals will decrease the intensity and duration of the rash.

CONCLUSION

Proper diagnosis for common skin conditions that affect athletes will improve comfort, decrease risk of spread, and return athletes to peak performance. Skin ailments that do not resolve with the usual interventions should be evaluated by a dermatologist familiar with the demands sports puts on athletes to ensure the athlete will be able to return to practice and competition without undo delay.

REFERENCES

Adams BB. Tinea corporis gladiatorum. A cross-sectional study. *J Am Acad Dermatol*. 2000;43:1039–1041.

Bergfeld WF, Elston D. Skin problems of athletes. In: Fu F, Stone D, eds. *Sports Injuries*. Baltimore: Williams & Wilkins; 1994;781–795.

Bergfeld WF, Helm TN. The skin. In: Strauss RH, ed. *Sports Medicine*, 2nd ed. Philadelphia: Saunders; 1991;117–131.

Bergfeld WF, Taylor JS. Trauma, sports, and the skin. *Am J Ind Med*. 1985;8: 403–413.

Pharis DB, Teller C, Wolf JE. Cutaneous manifestations of sports participation. *J Am Acad Dermatol*. 1997;36:448–459.

Powell FC. Sports dermatology. *J Eur Acad Dermatol Venereol*. 1994;3:1–15.

Adams BB. Sports dermatology. *Adolesc Med*. 2001;2:305–322.

16 | Neck, Spinal Cord, and Back

Michael H. Ford and Ken Fern

QUICK LOOK

- Assume all injured athletes have a potentially unstable spinal injury until proven otherwise.
- Treat injuries with an organized team approach using ATLS (advanced trauma life support) protocols.
- Stabilize the head and shoulders while assessing and managing the ABCs (airway, breathing, and circulation).
- Four people should log-roll the injured athlete onto his or her back with the head and shoulders supported as a unit.
- Removal of helmet and shoulder pads should be carried out in a monitored hospital setting as an "all or none" procedure.
- Do a quick assessment of gross active motor function and of sensory levels without delaying transport to hospital for imaging studies and definitive management.
- Numerous benign spinal pathologies (spondylolysis, spondylolisthesis, disk herniations, mechanical neck and back pain) may limit activities but do not cause harm; full recovery to preinjury level of function can usually be expected.
- Awareness of proper techniques, equipment, and training are critical to reduce the incidence of catastrophic injury.
- Rehabilitation should focus on functional restoration using an active exercise program aimed at preventing stiffness and weakness while avoiding programs that emphasize passive modalities of treatment.

INTRODUCTION

Recreational and elite-level sports are statistically safe endeavors when compared with everyday activities such as driving a car. Nevertheless, injuries to the spine do occur. These injuries range from the benign and brief discomfort of a paraspinal muscle strain to catastrophic quadriplegia. The relatively low incidence of spinal injuries during athletic activities can leave on-site medical personnel with less experience and a lower comfort level in dealing with these types of injuries.

Registries in Canada and the United States have been established to track the more catastrophic injuries (Tator et al., 1997). These registries have allowed for the early recognition of trends and for an assessment of the effectiveness of specific interventions. Primary goals in the approach to spinal injury in sports are prevention, recognition and management of the acute injury, and rehabilitation.

EPIDEMIOLOGY

A number of series clearly demonstrate that football contributes the greatest number of catastrophic injuries, followed by ice hockey, gymnastics, and wrestling (Mueller et al., 1990; Bruce et al., 1984; Keene et al., 1989). While the majority of spine injuries in football are minor, cervical spine injuries account for a significant number of permanently disabling injuries. A large series of college athletes demonstrated a back injury rate of 7 per 100 participants (Keene et al., 1989). Eighty percent of the injuries occurred in practice, 6% occurred in competition, and 14% occurred during preseason conditioning. Muscle strains were the most common (59%), whereas 29% were associated with preexisting conditions.

In a study funded by the National Collegiate Athletic Association (NCAA) from 1977 through 1998, there were 200 cases of permanent cervical cord injuries due to participation in football (Cantu et al., 2000). This study also documented that 118 athletes died due to playing football. Defensive players were more at risk than offensive players for sustaining a cervical cord injury. The act of tackling with an axial loading mechanism was identified in 27% of injuries.

An international registry established through Sport Smart Canada reported an average of 16.8 cases per year of major spinal injury as a result of hockey between 1982 and 1993 (Tator et al., 1997). Children younger than age 11 more often had ligamentous injuries of the upper cervical spine, whereas older children typically had adult patterns of injury involving the middle and more caudal cervical spine (McGrory et al., 1993).

Significant costs to society result from spinal cord injuries. A recent study estimated the costs of spinal cord injuries caused by sports to be $295,643 (U.S.) in first-year charges, and $27,488 annually, with an average lifetime cost of $950,973 per person (DeVivo et al., 1997). The annual direct total cost of spinal cord injuries secondary to sports was estimated at 694 million in the United States (DeVivo et al., 1997).

PATHOPHYSIOLOGY

The spine is a segmental structure comprised of 7 cervical, 12 thoracic, and 5 lumbar vertebrae. The caudal end of the spine consists of the sacrum and coccyx. The primary function of the spine is to house and protect the neural elements. It is capable of withstanding considerable forces before yielding.

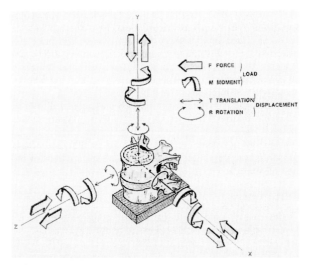

FIG 16-1   A functional spinal unit or FSU, demonstrating degrees of freedom and forces transmitted. (Reprinted with permission from White AA, Panjabi M: *Clinical Biomechanics of the Spine*, 2d ed.)

Injury occurs when the yield point of the tissues involved is exceeded. The forces required to reach this threshold are rate-dependent. Faster rates of application require less force to produce a pathologic change.

Besides being a shock absorber, the intervertebral disk is also the primary stabilizer of the spine. The facet joints and interspinous ligaments further contribute to stability. The disk is relatively stiff in flexion and extension, as well as in lateral flexion. It is weakest when exposed to torsional forces. The outer annular fibers of the disk are firmly attached to the vertebral end plates. Suprathreshold forces result in yield at the level of the bone before disruption of the disk–bone interface occurs.

Two contiguous vertebrae and the intervening disk and ligamentous and muscular attachments constitute the functional spinal unit (FSU) (Fig. 16-1). Studying the biomechanics of one small section of the spine allows for the validation of complex finite-element modeling studies.

The biomechanical properties of the FSU change with age. Postmortem studies have demonstrated degenerative changes in the intervertebral disk as

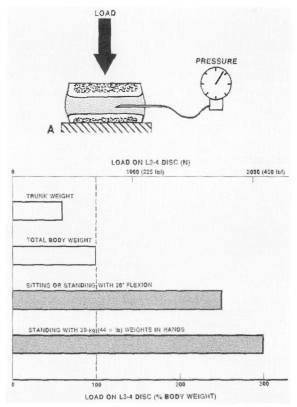

FIG 16-2   Variation in intradisk pressure depending on position. (Reprinted with permission from White AA, Panjabi M: *Clinical Biomechanics of the Spine*, 2d ed. Philadelphia: Lippincott William & Wilkins; 1990)

we approach our late teens. By age 50, all of us have degenerative disks that typically are most advanced at the L3–4, L4–5, and L5–S1 levels (Miller et al., 1988). Degeneration is a process of desiccation, with the water content of the disk dropping from 90–63% with aging. The disk becomes stiffer and stronger with age. This is the reason why disk herniations are relatively rare over age 50. The intradiscal pressures can vary greatly depending on the position of the body (Fig. 16-2).

A disk herniation occurs when the outer annular fibers fail, allowing for migration of disk nucleus material (which has the texture and appearance of crab meat), typically posterolaterally. This can cause secondary nerve compression and radicular pain. With greater forces applied to the FSU, components will be disrupted and fail, potentially leading to instability. Instability is defined as the lack of the ability to withstand normal physiologic forces, resulting in the potential for injury to the neural elements.

The first priority in the assessment of a spinal injury is the determination of stability. This can be difficult to do. Criteria have been established that define instability in the cervical and lumbar spine. These criteria are listed in Tables 16-1 and 16-2.

The presence of instability requires immobilization and bracing and/or surgery. A stable injury, however, can be treated with early mobilization. Missing an unstable injury can lead to permanent and catastrophic neurologic damage.

The spinal cord is the caudal extension of the brainstem, beginning at the level of the foramen magnum of the skull and extending down to approximately L1 or L2. Distal to this are peripheral nerve roots that make up the cauda equina. Therefore, injuries below L1 or L2 typically result in peripheral nerve or lower motor neuron injuries, whereas higher injuries result in

TABLE 16-1 Checklist for the Diagnosis of Clinical Instability in the Middle and Lower Cervical Spine

Element	Point value
Anterior elements destroyed or unable to function	2
Posterior elements destroyed or unable to function	2
Positive stretch test	2
Radiographic criteria	4
A. Flexion/extension x-rays	
1. Sagittal plane translation >3.5 mm or 20% (2 pts)	
2. Sagittal plane rotation >20° (2 pts)	
OR	
B. Resting x-rays	
1. Sagittal plane displacement >3.5 mm or 20% (2 pts)	
2. Relative sagittal plane angulation >11° (2 pts)	
Abnormal disk narrowing	1
Developmentally narrow spinal canal	1
1. Sagittal diameter <13 mm	
OR	
2. Pavlov's ratio <0.8	
Spinal cord damage	2
Nerve root damage	1
Dangerous loading anticipated	1
Total of 5 or more = unstable	

SOURCE: Reprinted with permission from White AA, Panjabi M: *Clinical Biomechanics of the Spine*, 2d ed.

TABLE 16-2 Checklist for the Diagnosis of Clinical Instability
in the Lumbar Spine

Element	Point value
Anterior elements destroyed or unable to function	2
Posterior elements destroyed or unable to function	2
Radiographic criteria	4
A. Flexion/extension x-rays	
1. Sagittal plane translation >4.5 mm or 15% (2 pts)	
2. Sagittal plane rotation	
>15° at L1–L2, L2–L3 & L3–L4 (2 pts)	
>20° at L4–L5 (2 pts)	
>25° at L5–S1 (2 pts)	
OR	
B. Resting x-rays	
1. Sagittal plane displacement >4.5 mm or 15% (2 pts)	
2. Relative sagittal plane angulation >22° (2 pts)	
Cauda equina damage	3
Dangerous loading anticipated	1
Total of 5 or more = unstable	

SOURCE: Reprinted with permission from White AA, Panjabi M: *Clinical Biomechanics of the Spine*, 2d ed.

spinal cord or upper motor neuron damage. The spinal cord itself has no inherent resistance to injury. It has a very low yield point. The surrounding cerebrospinal fluid (CSF) and bony canal are instrumental in maintaining the integrity and function of the cord. Failure of the surrounding protective elements can result in a spectrum of injury to the cord ranging from transient edema, which results in temporary partial dysfunction, to cord transection, which is a permanent and complete injury.

SCREENING OF ATHLETES TO PREVENT SPINAL INJURIES

Routine x-ray screening of all sport participants is not a cost-effective approach to prevention. The very low yield does not justify this approach. There are, however, high-risk populations that do warrant screening.

The growth of the Special Olympics has resulted in many individuals with Down's syndrome participating in sports. Spinal hypermobility at C1–C2 has a prevalence rate of 25%, and 33% will demonstrate instability below C1–C2 as they become adults. Only 3%, however, have neurologic deficits (Pizzutillo, 1993).

Surgical stabilization and refraining from sporting activities are recommended in these individuals if the atlanto-dens interval (ADI) is greater than 9 mm on a standard lateral flexion view of the cervical spine. An ADI of 5–8 mm requires repeat x-rays every 3–5 years, with yearly neurologic assessments consisting of an accurate history and detailed physical examination.

Pseudosubluxation in non–Down's syndrome children is common. Typically, the child is less than 8 years old, and translations of less than 4.0 mm are seen at C2–3 and C3–4. An ADI of less than 4.5 mm is normal (Cattell et al., 1965).

Congenital fusion of segments of the cervical spine is known as Klippel-Feil syndrome. Stresses applied to the spine are concentrated above and below the fused segment. When congenital fusion of C2–C3 is combined with occipitalization of the atlas, 75% will develop instability at C1–C2. These individuals require careful assessment prior to playing contact sports.

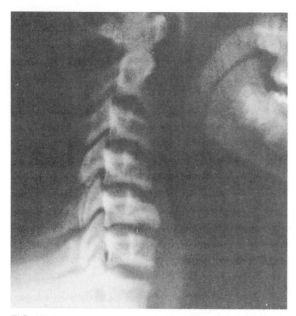

FIG 16-3 Spear tackler's spine. Note the flattened cervical lordosis with secondary degenerative changes and narrowed cervical canal indicative of congenital stenosis with secondary acquired changes. (Reprinted with permission from Joseph S. Torg.)

A significant percentage also will have unilateral absence of the renal system, which has obvious significance in the event of a renal injury.

Routine lateral x-rays of the cervical spine should be carried out in all adults playing football. Radiologic features consistent with "spear tackler's spine" are a contraindication to continued play (Torg et al., 1993; Fig. 16-3). The Torg ratio is the ratio of the diameter of the spinal canal to that of the vertebral body. A ratio of 0.8 or less has been found to have a high sensitivity for transient neurapraxia, but does not predispose to permanent catastrophic injury (Torg et al., 1996). Spinal canal stenosis with a Torg ratio of less than 0.8 is a predictor of probable frequent "burners" or "stingers" but is not a contraindication to play (Meyer et al., 1994). The incidence of initial "stinger" experience in some series ranges up to about 8% with average Torg ratios of 0.9, while multiple "stingers" occur with significantly smaller Torg ratios (0.75 vs. 0.87) (Castro et al., 1997). Recurrence rates of cervical cord neurapraxia of up to 56% have been associated with significantly smaller Torg ratios (Torg et al., 1997). In the older athlete, degenerative changes may be present. In the absence of spear tackler's spine changes, there is no contraindication to play. However, these changes may be a predictor of an increased probability of mechanical neck pain.

Spondylolysis, or a defect in the pars interarticularis, is common in the athlete (Fig. 16-4) and typically involves the L5 vertebra. Prevalence rates of 6–47% have been demonstrated. This lesion is not a contraindication to play. A grade I or grade II spondylolisthesis (Fig. 16-5) is not a contraindication to play. Higher-grade slips, however, typically are symptomatic and

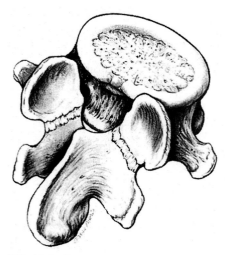

FIG 16-4   Spondylolysis.

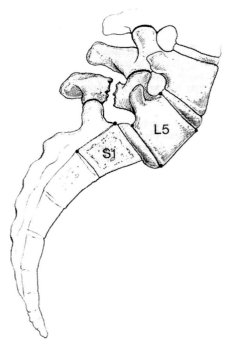

FIG 16-5   Spondylolisthesis.

may prevent participation in sports on the basis of the functional limitations this condition typically imparts.

EVALUATION AND MANAGEMENT

The evaluation and management of the acutely injured athlete is no different from that of the multiple-trauma patient. It is strongly recommended that the team leader be advanced trauma life support (ATLS) qualified. Worst-case scenarios should be practiced (eg, the motionless, unconscious athlete lying face down and not breathing, wearing a tight-fitting helmet and full-face mask, with full equipment).

The team leader takes charge. The team members should know what their defined roles are. A maximum of four individuals is recommended. Those not on the team should stay clear. The athlete is log-rolled as a unit onto his or her back. The team leader supports the head and shoulders as a unit (Fig. 16-6).

The helmet and shoulder pads of a football player should not be removed on the field unless absolutely necessary. The emergency medical service providers should assume that all unconscious football players have a significant spinal injury until proven otherwise. The face mask can be removed to allow access and monitoring of the airway. Only trained personnel (minimum of 3 or 4) should remove the helmet and shoulder pads, preferably in a hospital setting. Studies support leaving the helmet and shoulder pads on in the prehospital setting; moreover, there are no studies or case reports of increased morbidity resulting from leaving equipment on prior to arrival to hospital (Waninger et al., 1998).

Removal of equipment is an "all or none" procedure. Shoulder pads must be removed at the same time the helmet is removed. Cadaveric studies and radiographic studies in humans have shown that significant movement of the

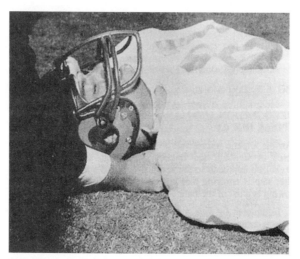

FIG 16-6 Note that the head and shoulders are supported as a unit. (Reprinted with permission from Hochschuler SH (ed): *Spinal Injuries in Sports.* Philadelphia: Hanley & Belfus; 1990).

cervical spine occurs when only the helmet or only the shoulder pads are removed (Gastel et al., 1998; Donaldson et al., 1998; Palumbo et al., 1996; Swenson et al., 1997). Removal of equipment should also take place prior to obtaining cervical radiographs to allow for adequate visualization (Davidson et al., 1991).

The team leader then proceeds through the ABCs of trauma management. With the head and shoulders stabilized, an airway is established and maintained by whatever means required:

1. Jaw thrust
2. Oropharyngeal airway
3. Orotracheal mask
4. Nasotracheal tube
5. Endotracheal tube
6. Cricothyroidotomy
7. Tracheostomy

Medical personnel should always ensure that the neck is adequately stabilized during any of these procedures. Ventilation is required if the athlete is not breathing. Cardiopulmonary resuscitation (CPR) is initiated if there is no palpable carotid pulse. The athlete is then rolled to one side, the back board is placed behind, and the athlete is rolled back. The head is taped to the board. Transport by ambulance to the nearest appropriate facility should be done expediently. A cell phone is required to call for ambulance services and to notify the receiving hospital. The appropriate phone numbers should be taped to the phone along with directions to the site.

Causing further neurologic injury to the athlete because of an ill-conceived and ill-equipped approach to the problem is completely preventable. In the conscious patient complaining of spinal pain and altered sensation or loss of movement, the emphasis on stability and preventing further harm is paramount. A brief description of the mechanism of injury should be obtained. Tender sites should be determined and documented. A quick neurologic examination assessing gross active motor power and a rough assessment of sensory level should be sought. Quick transport to an appropriate facility should be carried out. Checking reflexes and posterior column function on the field is not necessary and only delays transport.

The athlete complaining of neck pain with no neurologic symptoms can provoke a difficult on-field judgment process. The presence of marked tenderness along the posterior spine should be treated as a serious injury until proven otherwise. Erring on the side of caution is the appropriate approach.

At the hospital, appropriate imaging (plain x-ray, CT, MRI) will be carried out. Treatment will be established, dictated by the presence or absence of stability.

MANAGEMENT OF BENIGN AND CONFOUNDING SPINAL PATHOLOGIES

Statistically, the athlete is far more likely to experience pain and functional limitations from benign spinal pathology than from a serious fracture/dislocation. The serious injuries are associated with a uniform and widely accepted approach to the problem. Ironically, it is the larger and more benign group of spinal problems that is associated with a controversial and heterogeneous approach.

Spondylolysis and Spondylolisthesis

The bridge of bone between the superior and inferior articular facets is the pars interarticularis. In the general population, approximately 6% of individuals have a genetically weakened pars that can fracture with everyday normal use. It is typically a slow-onset, fatigue-type fracture and is usually evident by age 5 or 6. Most such fractures are asymptomatic in children. The pars defect typically involves L5, but other levels can be affected.

During the growth spurt, a spondylolysis can result in the development of a spondylolisthesis, or a forward slip of one vertebra on another, typically L5 on S1. The grading of spondylolisthesis reflects the percentage of the anteroposterior (AP) dimension of the vertebral body of L5 that has slipped in relation to the sacrum. A slip of up to 25% of L5 on S1 is a grade I spondylolisthesis. A slip of 25–50% is grade II, 50–75% is grade III, and 75–100% is a grade IV.

Many of the lower-grade slips are asymptomatic. However, they may be responsible for an acceleration of degenerative change and the onset of back pain in adulthood. Higher-grade slips are more likely to be symptomatic at a younger age and often undergo stabilization surgery with reliable outcomes.

Spondylolysis without a slip can be occult, acute, or chronic. The adolescent athlete who experiences sudden-onset low back pain should be investigated for the presence of a spondylolysis. Oblique plain films usually demonstrate the lesion, although in 14% it is seen only on the lateral x-ray. In many cases, plain x-rays are normal. The lesion is reliably demonstrated in single photon emission computed tomographic (SPECT) scans. Planar technetium-99m bone scans are not as sensitive (Read, 1994). Acute lesions may heal with bracing in a lumbosacral orthosis for 6 to 12 weeks. However, many will not heal.

Chronic, well-defined pars defects are unlikely to heal with bracing. In the adolescent with persistent pain secondary to a pars defect, elective repair may relieve many of the symptoms. In the symptomatic adult, elective fusion surgery is usually the surgical treatment of choice.

It should be made clear, however, that spondylolysis with or without a slip is a benign condition. Slip progression is rare in the adolescent and does not occur in the adult. Intermittent radicular symptoms are common, but neurologic injury does not occur. Therefore, the medical imposition of activity restriction is not justified. The acute spondylolytic lesion is the only exception.

Adolescent Idiopathic Scoliosis

This is a female-predominant genetic condition. Significant curves should be followed by a spine specialist to monitor progression and for management. The presence of scoliosis, however, should not preclude full participation in sports.

Thoracic and Lumbar Scheuermann's Kyphosis

Abnormalities in the vertebral end plates in adolescence can result in contiguous wedging of vertebrae and herniation of disk material into the vertebral bodies. This can result in an accentuated thoracic kyphosis or flattened lumbar lordosis. This can be associated with the development of large, misshapen lumbar vertebrae, with disk height reduction. Again, despite dramatic x-ray changes, these are totally benign conditions. Scheuermann's kyphosis may cause some deformity as well as low back pain. Nevertheless, surgery is rarely indicated. Correction of severe thoracic deformities is primarily a cosmetic procedure. Once again, there is no need to impose activity restriction.

Mechanical or Degenerative Causes of Neck and Back Pain

This is the most common cause of neck and back pain and has been demonstrated to be very prevalent, even among adolescent athletes (Kujala, et al., 1996). The incidence increases with age, with a peak between the ages of 29 and 39 years.

The natural history is extremely variable, and the pain can last days to years, but 70–80% of patients experience resolution within 2–3 months. In the acute phase, this problem can be virtually indistinguishable from a muscle strain clinically. The diagnosis is clinical, with a typical pattern of aggravation of symptomatology with activity and some relief with rest. The physical examination may be relatively noncontributory. The adolescent should have a SPECT scan if symptoms persist to rule out a potentially treatable spondylolysis.

Imaging studies of any kind (x-ray, CT, MRI) in the adult rarely yield information that dramatically changes management. Treatment is typically conservative. Rest beyond 2–3 days is detrimental and does not improve the natural history. Muscle loss and bone density reduction occur at an alarming rate with protracted bed rest. Early mobilization is the key to preventing secondary changes of disuse. Treatment should be an active program that is exercise based, with functional restoration as the intended goal of treatment. Accompanying this is an education program to reassure the athlete that ongoing symptomatology does not mean further structural damage (hurt versus harm concept). Various therapeutic modalities [ie, transcutaneous electrical stimulation (TENS), interferential current (IF or IFC), laser, ultrasound, massage, traction, and VAX-D] are widely used, but their efficacy has never been demonstrated in peer-reviewed literature (Griffin, 1993; Basford, 1995; van der Heijden et al., 1997; Deyo et al., 1990; Sawyer et al., 1986).

More invasive therapeutic modalities, such as epidural steroids, facet blocks, and rhizolysis, are also of limited benefit when compared with placebo or natural history. In the small minority of individuals with chronic, persistent, disabling mechanical neck or low back pain, surgery may be indicated. Management is typically an elective stabilization or fusion procedure. This is somewhat controversial with variable outcomes. Return to sports is rarely a reasonable expectation.

Disk Herniation

A herniated nucleus pulposus (HNP) in the cervical or lumbar spine typically results in arm- and leg-dominant pain, respectively. This may be associated with a conduction deficit (altered or decreased sensation, reduced or lost motor power). In the absence of severe cord compromise causing myelopathic symptoms or a central lumbar HNP causing a cauda equina syndrome, treatment is always conservative initially.

In the individual who has continued severe pain 6–12 weeks after onset, appropriate imaging studies are indicated, with an aim toward elective surgical decompression. The individual who experiences urinary retention with or without overflow or bowel incontinence should be managed surgically on an emergent basis. The prognosis postoperatively is dictated by the speed of onset. Rapid-onset cauda equina syndrome is associated with a poor prognosis regardless of the timing of surgery.

Conservative treatment of a HNP is again an active exercise-oriented approach to avoid the secondary changes of disuse. The McKenzie approach is used commonly and may help centralize the pain. Between 60 and 70% of disk herniations resolve within 6–12 weeks. Those which are still painful and functionally limiting are appropriately imaged.

In the cervical spine, the imaging modality of choice is the MRI. In the lumbar spine, however, plain CT and MRI are close to being equivalent with respect to sensitivity and specificity. If there is a history of previous surgery of the spinal canal, a gadolinium-enhanced MRI is the imaging tool of choice to help differentiate scar tissue from disk material.

The surgical management of a cervical HNP is typically an anterior decompression and fusion, whereas a simple discectomy is all that is required in the lumbar spine. Thoracic disk herniations are very rare. Those which cause an intercostal radiculopathy only are managed conservatively. However, thoracic cord compression causing myelopathy is dealt with surgically.

Burners and Stingers

A "burner" or "stinger" is very common in football. It is typically initiated by a tackle. It has also been reported in other sports such as wrestling, basketball, hockey, and weight lifting. Clinically, the individual experiences a transient radiating pain, numbness, and tingling down an arm. It is felt to be due to a C6 root traction injury secondary to flexion and lateral deviation of the neck (Rockett, 1982). These injuries are typically transient and self-limiting. The existence of congenital and/or secondary acquired cervical canal stenosis increases the probability of experiencing these symptoms.

PREVENTION

Education

Education programs such as the Spinal Awareness and Prevention Program in Australia demonstrated a 20% reduction in spinal cord injuries (Yeo, 1993). Spearing in football (head-first tackling) is illegal and enforcing this rule has been the single most important intervention to reduce spinal cord injuries in football.

Likewise illegal body checking such as hitting from behind in ice hockey should not be tolerated, since this has been recognized as a common mechanism for spine injuries and causes significantly more catastrophic injuries than legal checking maneuvers (Juhn et al., 2002). Helmets and face masks have virtually eliminated facial and ocular injuries, but unfortunately, have been linked to an increase in spinal injuries. This has occurred not because of biomechanical reasons, but because of a false sense of security among players that leads to excessive and unwarranted risks (Murray et al., 1995).

Equipment and Training

Over the years, recognition of hazardous field conditions has resulted in simple modifications to on-field equipment that are directly responsible for reductions in serious injuries. In football, a switch to a single padded-pole goal post reduced the frequency and injury severity of collisions. The break-away hockey net has also done the same.

However, there is no evidence at present that the modern-day equipment worn by players has reduced spinal injury frequency and severity. Given that a large percentage of injuries occur during practice, the advisability of high-intensity, full-contact practices is brought into question.

The frequency of injuries associated with the use of the trampoline and minitrampoline has prompted Torg to state that these devices have no place in gymnastics (Torg, 1985). The use of harness suspension devices in gymnastics and the development of aerated water landings in free-style aerial skiing are certainly training steps in the right direction. Moreover, there has been a call to eliminate some of the more dangerous head holds in wrestling, but to our knowledge, this has not been done (Wu et al., 1985).

Factors have been identified that predispose the athlete to accelerated degenerative changes. A too-early start at ages younger than 10 years and high-intensity training in gymnastics are associated with an increased incidence of juvenile osteochondroses and subsequent magnetic resonance imaging (MRI) changes associated with degeneration (Pollähne et al., 1995). Given the permanence of many spinal injuries, prevention is the most important first step in the care of the athlete.

REHABILITATION

After stability has been established rehabilitation can begin. The benign conditions typically are stable, so there is no reason for delay of therapy. Treatment is a program of functional restoration. Stiffness is addressed with an exercise program aimed at regaining range of motion, and weakness is treated with a resistive strengthening program. This should always be combined with an education program. Any program that emphasizes the use of passive modalities should be discouraged.

PROGNOSIS AND RETURN TO SPORT

Spinal cord concussion secondary to transient edema of the cord typically results in very early and often complete return of neurologic function. The incomplete lesion will have varying degrees of recovery, but in many instances the return is not functional. The individual who still has complete or profound loss of function beyond the period of spinal shock (return of the bulbocavernosus reflex) typically does not experience any return of useful function.

The benign spinal pathologies statistically are associated with a good prognosis and ultimate return to sport without restriction. Athletes with spondylolysis or spondylolisthesis treated surgically can in some cases return to sport, but this is not a reasonable expectation. The individual with a surgically treated HNP of the lumbar spine has a high probability of returning to sport without significant functional limitation.

However, a patient with a cervical HNP treated with an anterior decompression and fusion is at risk for injury of adjacent levels. There are no well-established guidelines, but we would be somewhat reluctant to allow someone who has had a surgical fusion to return to contact sports such as football.

Prior to clearing an athlete to return to sport, two important questions must be answered: (1) Is there a significant potential for further structural harm? and (2) Is performance going to be significantly hampered by residual symptoms? These questions must be answered by careful clinical assessment that includes a history, physical examination, and possibly imaging studies. The first question usually can be answered objectively by establishing the presence of clinical and radiologic stability. The second question is a decision made jointly by the medical personnel and the athlete based on functional capacity assessments performed during practice sessions. These are best done in a stepwise fashion.

SIDELINE TIPS

For the athletic trainer and physician involved in the care of athletes in football, ice hockey, wrestling, and gymnastics, an organized approach to the seriously injured athlete is a must. The first step is ensuring that proper equipment is available. The following is a list of the bare essentials:

- Equipment for face mask removal (ie, screwdriver and shears to cut the plastic mask clips)
- Oropharyngeal airway
- Intubation equipment
- Tracheostomy and crichothyrotomy equipment
- Semirigid cervical orthosis (Aspen or Philadelphia collar)
- Back board
- Heavy scissors
- Cellular phone

An organized team approach is mandatory, and there must be a team leader coordinating efforts. The leader should be designated well in advance. Serious consideration should be given to practice drills, as this will go a long way toward eliminating the panic that invariably permeates the air around the motionless, unconscious athlete who is not breathing.

It is always prudent to err on the side of caution and approach any injured athlete as if he or she has sustained an unstable spine injury. Making assumptions can lead to errors in diagnosis with potentially catastrophic consequences. A high index of suspicion coupled with a systematic and thorough approach will help prevent this.

SUMMARY

The medical team's responsibility is to the athlete and the athlete only. Prevention is the primary goal, with the teaching of proper techniques and safety protocols playing an important role. The goals of management are the same as those for acute spinal trauma from a motor vehicle accident, namely to preserve life and function, prevent further harm, provide for a stable spine to maintain neurologic integrity, and to prevent the stiffness and weakness associated with prolonged immobility. Recognition of significant injury is extremely important, and a tendency to err on the side of caution should be adopted. Subsequent rehabilitation should be evidence based, avoiding the adoption of useless treatments.

REFERENCES

Basford JR. Low-intensity laser therapy: Still not an established clinical tool. *Lasers Surg Med.* 1995;16:331–342.

Bruce DA, Schut L, Sutton LN. Brain and cervical spine injuries occurring during organized sports activities in children and adolescents. *Prim Care.* 1984;11:175–194.

Cantu RC, Mueller FO. Catastrophic football injuries: 1977–1998. *Neurosurgery*. 2000;47:673–675.

Castro FP Jr, Ricciardi J, Brunet ME, et al. Stingers, the Torg ratio, and the cervical spine. *Am J Sports Med*. 1997;25:603–608.

Cattell HS, Filtzer DL: Pseudosubluxation and other normal variations in the cervical spine in children. *J Bone Joint Surg*. 1965;47A:1295–1309.

Davidson RM, Burton JH, Snowise M, et al. Football protective gear and cervical spine imaging. *Ann Emerg Med*. 2001;38:26–30.

DeVivo MJ. Causes and costs of spinal cord injury in the United States. *Spinal Cord*. 1997;35:809–813.

Deyo RA, Walsh NE, Martin DC, et al. A controlled trial of transcutaneous electrical nerve stimulation (TENS) and exercise for chronic low back pain. *N Engl J Med*. 1990;322:1627–1634.

Donaldson WF 3rd, Lauerman WC, Heil B, et al. Helmet and shoulder pad removal from a player with suspected cervical spine injury. A cadaveric model. *Spine*. 1998;23:1729–1732.

Gastel JA, Palumbo MA, Hulstyn MJ, et al. Emergency removal of football equipment: a cadaveric cervical spine injury model. *Ann Emerg Med*. 1998;32:411–417.

Griffin LY. Introduction: Applications of rehabilitation modalities in the treatment of acute injuries, in Instructional Course Lectures, Vol. 41. Park Ridge, IL, American Academy of Orthopaedic Surgeons, 1993, p. 437.

Juhn MS, Brolinson PG, Duffey T, et al. Position statement. Violence and injury in ice hockey. *Clin J Sport Med*. 2002;12:46–51.

Keene JS, Albert MJ, Springer SL, et al. Back injuries in college athletes. *J Spinal Disord*. 1989;2:190–195.

Kujala UM, Taimela S, Erkintalo M, et al. Low-back pain in adolescent athletes. *Med Sci Sports Exerc*. 1996;28:165–170.

McGrory BJ, Klassen RA, Chao EY, et al. Acute fractures and dislocations of the cervical spine in children and adolescents. *J Bone Joint Surg*. 1993;75A:988–995.

Meyer SA, Schulte KR, Callaghan JJ, et al. Cervical spine stenosis and stingers in collegiate football players. *Am J Sports Med*. 1994;22:158–166.

Miller JAA, Schmatz C, Schultz AB. Lumbar disc degeneration: Correlation with age, sex, and spine level in 600 autopsy specimens. *Spine*. 1988;13:173.

Mueller FO, Cantu RC. Catastrophic injuries and fatalities in high school and college sports, fall 1982–spring 1988. *Med Sci Sports Exerc*. 1990;22:737–741.

Murray TM, Livingston LA. Hockey helmets, face masks, and injurious behavior. *Pediatrics*. 1995;95:419–421.

Palumbo MA, Hulstyn MJ, Fadale PD, et al. The effect of protective football equipment on alignment of the injured cervical spine. Radiographic analysis in a cadaveric model. *Am J Sports Med*. 1996;24:446–453.

Pizzutillo P. Spinal considerations in the young athlete, in Instructional Course Lectures, Vol. 41. Park Ridge, IL, American Academy of Orthopaedic Surgeons, 1993, p. 463.

Pollähne W, Teichmüller HJ, Ahrendt E. Spinal injuries from the radiologic point of view in children in intensive training for competitive sports. *Radiol Diagn (Berl)*. 1990;31:479–487.

Read MT. Single photon emission computed tomography (SPECT) scanning for adolescent back pain: A sine qua non? *Br J Sports Med*. 1994;28:56–57.

Rockett FX. Observations on the "burner": Traumatic cervical radiculopathy. *Clin Orthop*. 1982;164:18–19.

Sawyer M, Zbieranek CK. The treatment of soft tissue after spinal injury. *Clin Sports Med*. 1986;5:387–405.

Swenson TM, Lauerman WC, Blanc RO, et al. Cervical spine alignment in the immobilized football player. Radiographic analysis before and after helmet removal. *Am J Sports Med*. 1997;25:226–230.

Tator CH, Carson JD, Edmonds VE. New spinal injuries in hockey. *Clin J Sports Med*. 1997;7:17–21.

Torg JS, Corcoran TA, Thibault LE, et al. Cervical cord neurapraxia: Classification, pathomechanics, morbidity, and management guidelines. *J Neurosurg.* 1997;87:843–850.

Torg JS. Epidemiology, pathomechanics, and prevention of athletic injuries to the cervical spine. *Med Sci Sports Exerc.* 1985;17:295–303.

Torg JS, Naranja RJ Jr, Pavlov H, et al. The relationship of developmental narrowing of the cervical spinal canal to reversible and irreversible injury of the cervical spinal cord in football players. *J Bone Joint Surg Am.* 1996;78:1308–1314.

Torg JS, Sennett B, Pavlov H, et al. Spear tackler's spine: An entity precluding participation in tackle football and collision activities that expose the cervical spine to axial energy inputs. *Am J Sports Med.* 1993;21:640–649.

van der Heijden GJ, van der Windt DA, de Winter AF. Physiotherapy for patients with soft tissue shoulder disorders: A systematic review of randomised clinical trials. *Br Med J.* 1997;315:25–30.

Waninger KN. On-field management of potential cervical spine injury in helmeted football players: Leave the helmet on! *Clin J Sport Med.* 1998;8:124–129.

Wu WQ, Lewis RC. Injuries of the cervical spine in high school wrestling. *Surg Neurol.* 1985;23:143–147.

Yeo JD. Prevention of spinal cord injuries in an Australian study (New South Wales). *Paraplegia.* 1993;31:759–763.

17 | Evaluation and Treatment of Shoulder Injuries

Edward G. McFarland, Hyung Bin Park,
Tae Kyun Kim, and Atsushi Yokota

INTRODUCTION

The shoulder complex presents unique challenges to those who evaluate and treat injuries to athletes. First, the shoulder includes three joints (the sternoclavicular, the acromioclavicular, and the glenohumeral) and one articulation (scapulothoracic), which should work integrally to create normal shoulder function for sports and activities of daily living. When examining an athlete, all four areas potentially have influence upon the final function of the shoulder and all should be carefully evaluated. Secondly, the physical examination of the shoulder is thought by many to be difficult, with good cause. Shoulder pain is often nonspecific and nonlocalized, and patients have difficulty isolating the exact place that they hurt. Thirdly, some symptoms which are considered to be due to one disease entity may be secondary to another, such as rotator cuff tendinitis pain, which is presumably due to an entirely different entity such as instability.

Fourth, the physical examination of the shoulder reflects this complexity such that many physical findings may be present or elicited by more than one condition. For example, an apprehension maneuver for shoulder instability can cause pain in a patient with shoulder instability, but it can also produce pain in a patient only with rotator cuff tendinitis. Fifth, the patient may have more than one condition that confounds the examination, such as a superior labrum lesion associated with shoulder instability. Lastly, the treatment of shoulder injuries can produce more predictable results in some conditions than others, which reflects the inexact knowledge of the pathophysiology of many of the conditions that affect the shoulder. Consequently, patients with shoulder conditions require the clinician to be something of a detective, assimilating the mechanism of injury, the pattern of symptoms, the physical examination, and the results of tests and radiographs.

Because of these factors it is important to obtain a good history, particularly of the mechanism of injury, since this often provides information that can assist in making a diagnosis. Some patients with instability are not aware of the direction their shoulder subluxates or dislocates, and a careful history of the arm position at the time of injury is important. Patients who have symptoms with the arm in an abducted and externally rotated position are probably experiencing anterior instability, while the patient with the arm in front of the body with an axial load along the arm in a posterior direction typically is experiencing posterior instability. Hyperabduction and hyperextension injuries can cause tears of the subscapularis tendons, with or without associated anterior instability. Patients with pain over shoulder level without trauma typically have rotator cuff tendinitis, but if they have it with throwing or volleyball spiking maneuvers it may indicate excessive laxity in the shoulder as a contributing factor to the symptoms of tendinitis. Patients with symptoms of a heavy or "dead" arm after throwing may have occult instability contributing to their symptoms. A history of an axial load on an outstretched arm can be a factor in rotator cuff tears or superior labrum anterior and posterior lesions (SLAP lesions). A fall on the top or lateral side

207

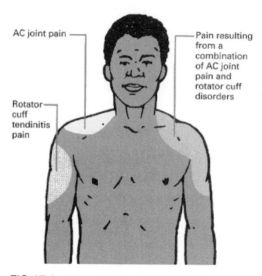

FIG 17-1   Diagram of the distribution of acromioclavicular joint pain versus impingement pain. (Reproduced with permission from McFarland EG, Hobbs WR. The active shoulder: AC joint pain and injury. *Your Patient & Fitness* 1998;12:23–27.)

of the top of the shoulder can be the cause of a wide variety of lesions, including acromioclavicular (AC) contusions, AC separations, rotator cuff tears, greater tuberosity fractures, proximal humerus fractures, and superior labrum lesions.

Clicks and pops in the shoulder are non-specific and tend not to be diagnostic of any one clinical entity. In patients who feel grinding or a click with motion, it is important to have them demonstrate how it happens. Patients with snapping scapula syndrome typically can demonstrate the arc of crepitus and pain. Patients with voluntary shoulder subluxations can often demonstrate the maneuvers that are causing their symptoms, and it is important to establish if these are anterior or posterior subluxations.

The distribution of pain is an important historical factor to ask patients about. Pain from the AC joint tends to be local to the AC joint, but typically radiates into the trapezius proximally (Fig. 17-1). This pattern of pain was substantiated in a study by Gerber and associates, in which they injected saline into the AC joint and the subacromial space of the shoulders of volunteers with no previous problems in their shoulders (Gerber et al., 1998).

PHYSICAL EXAMINATION

There are four important axioms to follow when examining an athlete with shoulder complaints (Table 17-1). The first is to undress the patient. This allows the detection of subtle conditions, such as infraspinatus wasting or ecchymosis (Fig. 17-2). The second is to compare sides, which allows comparison of the scapular positions, muscle atrophy, swellings, and color and temperature of both extremities (Fig. 17-3). The third is a standard orthopedic exhortation to always consider a joint above and below the site of

TABLE 17-1 Orthopaedic Axioms for
Examination of Shoulder Injury
- Undress the patient
- Compare sides
- Consider joints above and below
- Do a neurovascular exam
- Obtain radiographs in two planes

injury when evaluating complaints of pain, and in the shoulder examination that would include the cervical spine proximally and the elbow distally. Cervical injuries in athletes are common, and they should particularly be considered in patients with pain that radiates down the arm. Pain along the medial scapula and the medial half of the trapezius typically have origins in the cervical spine. Elbow and forearm conditions, such as posterior interosseous nerve entrapment or carpal tunnel syndrome, can cause arm and shoulder pain.

The fourth axiom is to consider a neurovascular examination an important part of every shoulder evaluation (Tables 17-2 and 17-3). Testing of shoulder range of motion, muscle strength, and sensation are not only crucial components of a complete shoulder examination, they also provide an excellent opportunity to rule in or out neurological causes of a patient's pain. While they may be seen due to musculoskeletal conditions, paresthesias and weakness are important signs of neurologic conditions or nerve injury. More and more people are athletically active as they get older, and it is especially important to be cognizant of neurologic symptoms in this population.

A comprehensive review of the physical examination of the shoulder is beyond the scope of this chapter, but Table 17-4 lists the most common

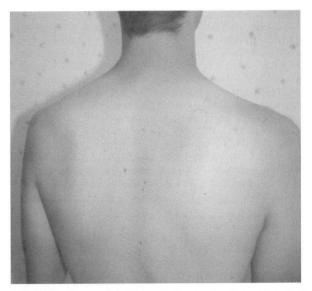

FIG 17-2 Photograph of infraspinatus wasting in female volleyball player which would go unnoticed if the patient was not undressed.

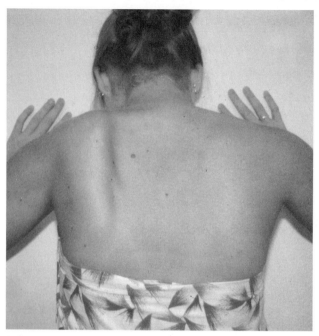

FIG 17-3 Photograph of unilateral scapular winging which demonstrates the need to compare sides.

physical examination maneuvers for examining the shoulder (McFarland et al., 1996a). We recommend that the examination begin with observation, followed by range-of-motion and strength testing. Palpation and provocative maneuvers are typically saved for last since they may cause the patient pain.

There is increasing appreciation that when examining the shoulder a distinction should be made between laxity and instability. A certain degree of laxity is normal and necessary for shoulder movement and function. Two maneuvers designed to describe anterior and posterior shoulder laxity include the load and shift test and the drawer signs (McFarland et al., 1996b; Gerber et al., 1984). The load and shift test is performed with the patient sitting (Fig. 17-4), while the posterior drawer test is performed with the patient supine (Fig. 17-5). The goal of these maneuvers is to try to translate or move the humeral head over the rim of the glenoid, and this translation over the

TABLE 17-2 Dermatomes and Areas to Test Sensation

Level	Sensory
C5	Lateral deltoid
C6	Thumb
C7	Middle finger
C8	Ulnar border, little finger
T1	Medial side, proximal arm

TABLE 17-3 Which Muscles to Test for Peripheral Nerves and Dermatomes

Peripheral nerves	Dermatomes	Muscles
Suprascapular nerve	C5–C6	Supraspinatus
		Infraspinatus
Axillary nerve	C5–C6	Deltoid
		Teres minor
Radial nerve	C5–C8, T1	Triceps
		Wrist extensors
		Finger extensors
Long thoracic nerve	C5–C6	Serratus anterior
Musculocutaneous nerve	C5–C7	Coracobrachialis
		Biceps
Spinal accessory nerve	Cranial nerve XI, C3–C4	Trapezius
Subscapular nerve	C5–C6	Subscapularis
		Teres major
Dorsal scapular nerve	C5	Levator scapulae
		Rhomboid major
		Rhomboid minor
Lateral pectoral nerve	C5–C6	Pectoralis major
		Pectoralis minor
Thoracodorsal nerve	C6–C8	Latissimus dorsi

TABLE 17-4 Examinations of the Shoulder

Observation
1. Range of motion elevation—normal range (170–180°)
2. External rotation at 90 degrees—normal range (90–100°)
3. Internal rotation at 90 degrees—normal range (80–90°)
4. External rotation arm at side—normal range (80–90°)
5. Internal rotation up back—normal range (T5–T10)

Strength testing
Tenderness
Reflexes
Provocative maneuvers:
1. AC joint
   Crossed arm adduction
   Arm extension test
   Active compression test
   Local tenderness
2. Impingement/tendinitis
   Neer impingement sign
   Hawkins impingement sign
   Speed's test
   Coracoid impingement sign
3. Instability signs
   Anterior apprehension sign
   Posterior apprehension sign
   Increased external rotation sign
   Sulcus sign
   Relocation test
4. Laxity signs
   Anterior and posterior drawer
   Load and shift test
   Sulcus sign
5. SLAP lesion signs
   Speed's test
   Compression rotation
   Active compression
   Anterior slide test
   Biceps load test II

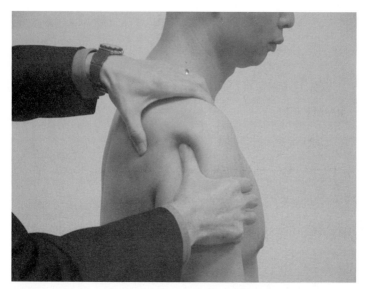

A

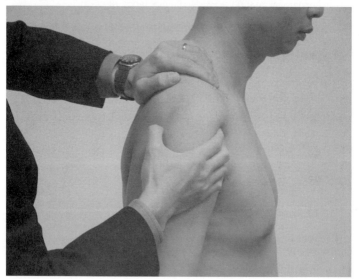

B

FIG 17-4 Load and shift test is done with the patient sitting and an anterior force (A) or posterior force (B) is directed to the shoulder.

rim is called a subluxation of the shoulder. There are three ways to measure the translation of the humeral head using these maneuvers. One is to estimate the translation in millimeters and the second is to guess the percentage of the humeral head diameter that translates out of the socket. Neither of these measures is practical and their accuracy has not been established.

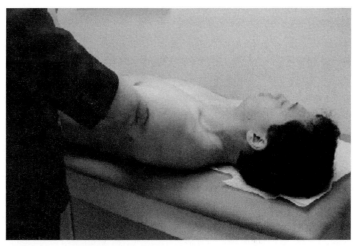

A

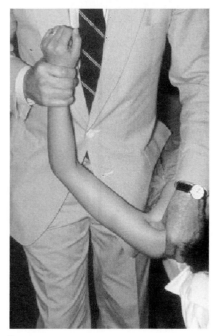

B

FIG 17-5   Anterior (A) and posterior drawer (B) test.

The most commonly utilized measure of translation is a modified Hawkins scale, which describes what the examiner feels when performing these tests. A grade I laxity indicates that the humeral head cannot be subluxated over the rim, a grade II indicates that the humeral head can be

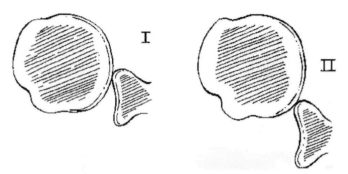

FIG 17-6 Modified Hawkins classification for shoulder laxity. Type I shows the translation of the head is to the rim, and type II demonstrates the head translating over the rim. In type III, the head locks out over the rim. (Reproduced with permission from McFarland EG, Campbell G, McDowell J. Posterior shoulder laxity in asymptomatic athletes. *Am J Sports Med.* 1996;329:240–243.)

subluxated over the rim, and a grade III indicates that the head dislocates and stays out of the socket without the examiner holding the shoulder (Fig. 17-6). Studies have shown that grade III is uncommon even under anesthesia, and it is not recommended that it be provoked in the office (McFarland et al., 1996c). However, the ability to subluxate the shoulder anteriorly or posteriorly is common in symptomatic and asymptomatic athletes. As a result, the ability to subluxate the shoulder over the rim (a Hawkins II) is essentially a normal variant and should not be interpreted as demonstrating instability unless it reproduces the patient's symptoms. If the shoulder can be subluxated over the rim, we recommend asking the patient if their symptoms are reproduced by this maneuver. Pain alone with translations is not adequate for making the diagnosis of instability, and the patient with shoulder instability should report that they feel their shoulder sliding in a fashion similar to the movement produced by these maneuvers.

A sulcus sign is also a measure of shoulder laxity, and is typically graded I–III (Fig. 17-7). This gradation is somewhat subjective, with a grade I being 0.5–1.5 cm, a grade II as 1.5–2.0 cm and a grade III as over 2.0 cm. This sign can be performed with the patient standing, sitting, or supine, but we recommend that it be performed with the patient sitting with their arms resting in their lap (Fig. 17-7). This allows the patient to relax and allows a more accurate test. The sign should be performed with the arm in neutral rotation and then again with the arm externally rotated. If the sulcus sign remains the same, then it has been postulated that the patient does not have laxity of the superior ligaments of the shoulder and does not have an open rotator cuff interval. This is important when considering surgery on patients who may have an inferior component to their instability. The patient should be asked if the sulcus sign causes pain or reproduces their symptoms of instability. In our experience it is rare for a patient to have symptoms of instability with a sulcus sign. While a positive sulcus sign has been interpreted in the past as indicative of multi-directional instability, it is now known that it measures only inferior laxity of the shoulder. True inferior instability in which the shoulder dislocates inferiorly (luxatio

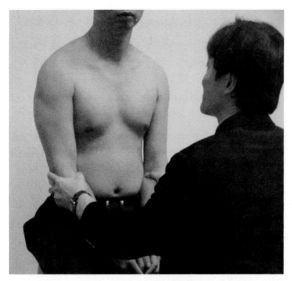

A

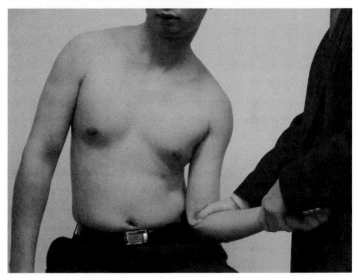

B

FIG 17-7 The sulcus sign should be performed with the arm at the side (A) and again with the arm externally rotated (B).

erecta) is rare, and symptomatic inferior subluxation of the shoulder is also an rare finding in patients with shoulder instability. The exact role of the sulcus sign and inferior laxity in producing symptoms in the shoulders of athletes is controversial. However, no specific treatment needs to be

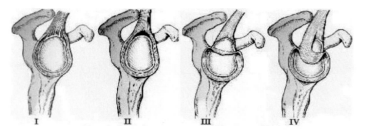

I   II   III   IV

FIG 17-8 Four different types of SLAP lesions. (According to Snyder SJ, Karzel RP, Del Pizzo W, et al. SLAP lesions of the shoulder. *Arthroscopy.* 1990;6:274–279.)

directed to a positive sulcus sign unless the patient is symptomatic in that direction.

Another area of controversy is the physical examination for superior labrum lesions of the shoulder, also known as SLAP (superior labrum anterior and posterior) lesions (Fig. 17-8). This detachment of the biceps tendon to the superior glenoid tubercle and of the attachments of the superior labrum to the glenoid can be seen in athletes, but they can also be seen due to dislocations, the stress of overhead throwing, and to falls on an outstretched arm. They often coexist with other shoulder pathologies, so it is difficult to ascribe symptoms specifically to SLAP lesions. There is no one pain pattern unique to these lesions, and sometimes they produce impingement pain or sometimes pain in the posterior-superior shoulder.

There have been numerous physical examination tests for making the diagnosis of SLAP lesions. While many have been touted as having high accuracy and sensitivity, many of these tests are nonspecific (Table 17-5) (McFarland et al., 2002; Kim et al., 2003). A click in the shoulder is usually nonspecific and cannot be used reliably as a sign of a labral tear. The diagnosis of this entity by physical examination will continue to evolve and requires further study.

IMAGING

When evaluating shoulder injuries it is important to begin with plain radiographs first. When evaluating the glenohumeral joint, the radiographs should include an anteroposterior radiograph in internal and external rotation. A third view can be either the scapular Y view or an axillary lateral view. Both are equally effective in an emergency room setting, where the goal is to determine if the humeral head is located or not. However, there are many advantages of an axillary lateral view over a scapular Y view. Axillary view radiography gives more information about the glenoid, the acromion, and the coracoid. There are specialized views of the acromio-clavicular joint which also provide more information about that joint. The Zanca view is angled upward 15° and coned down to give more detail (Zanca et al., 1971). Comparison views can also be helpful (Phillips et al., 1998). Weighted views of the AC joint are no longer recommended since they typically do not influence treatment (McFarland et al., 1997).

Once plain radiographs are obtained, the choice of imaging modality depends on what information is being sought. For detailed bony anatomy

TABLE 17-5 Review of Diagnostic Accuracy for SLAP Lesions as Reported in the Literature

Test	Study (year)	Disease	Sensitivity (%)	Specificity (%)	PPV (%)	NPV (%)	DV (%)
Compression rotation test	Snyder et al. (1990)	SLAP	22				86
	Holovacs et al. (2000)	Glenoid labral tear	80	19	9	90	
	McFarland et al. (2002)	SLAP	24	76	84	87	71
Anterior slide test	Kibler (1995)	Superior labral tear	78	92	5	90	77
	McFarland et al. (2002)	SLAP	8	84	95	100	99
Active compression test	O'Brien et al. (1998)	Superior labral tear	100	99	42	88	57
	Morgan et al. (1998)	Anterior type-II SLAP	88	42	17	27	20
		Posterior type-II SLAP	32	13	42	85	56
		Combined type-II SLAP	85	41	60		
	Stetson et al. (2002)	SLAP	67	41			
	Guanche et al. (2000)	SLAP	50	50			
	Holovacs et al. (2000)	Glenoid labral tear	69	50			
	Parentis et al. (2002)	SLAP (type II)	65				
	McFarland et al. (2002)	SLAP	47	55	10	91	54

Abbreviations: PPV, positive predictive value; NPV, negative predictive value; DV, diagnostic value.

217

and evaluation of fractures, computed tomography (CT) scanning is the recommended examination. When evaluating soft tissue injuries, the magnetic resonance imaging (MRI) provides the best information. For evaluation of the labrum, MRI with an arthrogram with gadolinium or saline offers increased resolution. Ultrasonography (US) can be utilized for evaluating the rotator cuff, specifically the supraspinatus. US depends on an experienced operator to perform and interpret the test, and it will not yield information about the bones, labrum, or occult mass lesions. Three-phase bone scanning can also be utilized for patients with suspected stress fractures or when looking for occult lesions.

ACUTE INJURIES

Acute traumatic lesions of the shoulder complex are common in athletes, particularly those participating in contact sports. The severity of the lesion can often be ascertained by a thorough history and physical examination, but it is important to follow the evaluation axioms mentioned above. This chapter will discuss many of these injuries, but some will be discussed in more detail elsewhere in this book. This discussion is meant to be an overview of these injuries and more detailed information can be obtained from other sources.

Sternoclavicular Joint

Sternoclavicular joint injuries are less common than injuries to other parts of the shoulder complex. Acute injuries include fractures and instability. Since the growth plate of the medial clavicle is one of the last to close (up to the age of 22), deformity of the SC joint typically is either a fracture of the growth plate or a subluxation or dislocation of the joint (Fig. 17-9). Anterior subluxations or dislocations of the clavicle relative to the sternum are

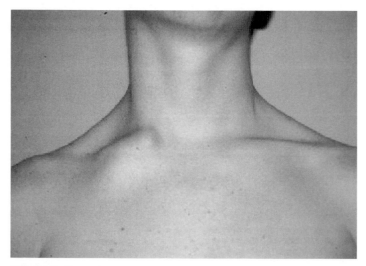

FIG 17-9 Deformity of proximal sternoclavicular fracture in an adolescent.

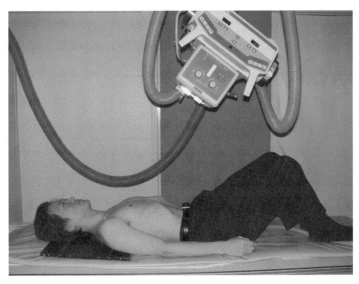

FIG 17-10 Serendipity view. The x-ray tube is tilted 40° from the vertical position and is aimed directly at the manubrium. In children, the tube's distance from patient's shoulder be 45 inches. In thicker-chested adults the distance shoulder be 60 inches.

the most common injuries seen. These do not need reduction or surgery since most patients recover with no long-term sequelae. While the deformity may be less than desirable, the risks and the poor results with surgery warrant a nonoperative treatment course with ice, pain pills or nonsteroidal anti-inflammatory drugs, and physical therapy as needed until full recovery.

Posterior dislocations of the sternoclavicular joint are serious injuries that require immediate medical attention. If the displacement of the clavicle posteriorly is severe, it can compress the great vessels, the trachea, or the esophagus. Symptoms can be due to any of these, and the patient may have difficulty swallowing, speaking, or breathing. These should be evaluated and treated in the emergency room setting. The physical examination should give some hint of the diagnosis, and plain films should be done including a serendipity view (Fig. 17-10). A CT scan is the best imaging modality to use in these cases. If a closed reduction of the deformity is undertaken, it should be done where surgeons are available to deal with any complication due to vessel disruption or other complications. Reduction is performed by placing a bolster behind the thorax and hyperabducting the shoulder (Kirkley et al., 1999; Geiger et al., 1997). The shoulder is then splinted for 4–6 weeks with a figure-of-8 bandage to allow ligament healing.

Clavicle Fractures

Clavicular fractures are among the most common fractures encountered in sports. They are divided into fractures of the proximal clavicle, fractures of the shaft of the clavicle, and distal clavicle fractures. Shaft fractures are the most common and typically heal with no sequelae. Treatment is supportive

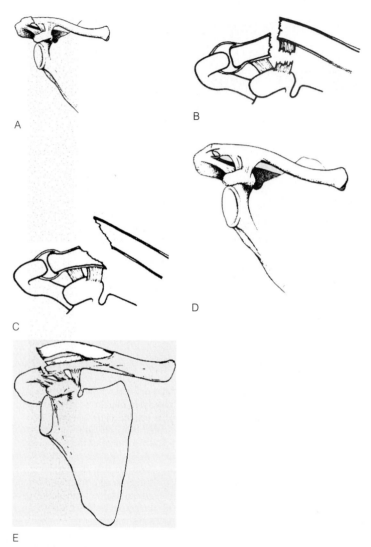

FIG 17-11 Distal clavicular fracture.

with pain medication, cryotherapy, and an arm sling. Figure-of-8 bandages have no advantage except for the rare patient who thinks they give more support. Range of motion of the fingers, wrist, and elbow can begin right away, and pendulum exercises can begin as the pain allows. Range of motion of the shoulder typically can begin within 7–10 days and can progress as tolerated.

There is increasing debate over indications for surgical intervention for clavicle fractures. Some studies suggest shortening of over 2 cm is an indication for surgery (Wick et al., 2001). Some surgeons have designed special plates or screws for immediate fixation. Since these fractures heal

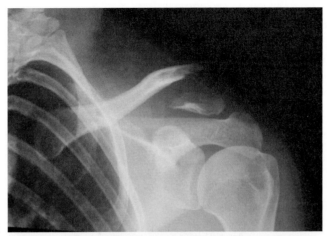

A

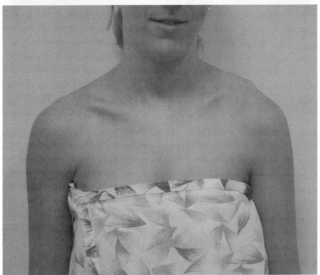

B

FIG 17-12 Type II distal clavicle fractures in which the ligaments are partially or totally torn, resulting in displacement of the clavicle upward, giving the shoulder the appearance of an acromioclavicular separation.

without surgery in a majority of cases, there is little rationale for operative intervention in most cases. Surgical intervention should be reserved for those fractures that do not heal; most heal within 3 months.

Distal clavicle fractures are controversial; operative intervention has been recommended for some subtypes. Nondisplaced fractures do not require surgery and can be treated like clavicular shaft fractures. In some variants of these fractures, ligaments are partially or totally torn, resulting in displacement of the clavicle upward (Fig. 17-11), giving the shoulder the appearance of an AC separation (Fig. 17-12). Surgical repair of these has been advocated, but some surgeons do not feel immediate surgery is necessary. These cases should be discussed with surgeons familiar with this injury.

Acromioclavicular Joint Injuries

Acromioclavicular joint injuries are very common in athletes, especially in those involved in contact sports, such as hockey, and high velocity sports, like mountain biking. The most commonly accepted classification is a modified Allman scale, which describes six types of injury (Fig. 17-13). Type I injuries are sprains of the AC ligaments and typically take 1–3 weeks to recover. They can be treated with cryotherapy, NSAIDs, and early range of motion. Athletes can return to sport once they have full motion and strength, and they can keep the AC area padded if needed. These injuries rarely

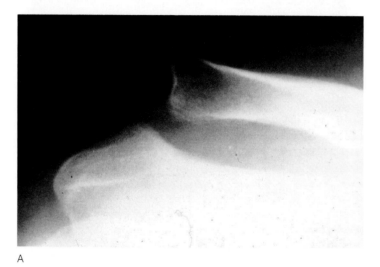

A

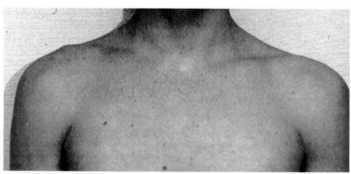

B

FIG 17-13 Modified Allman classification of acromioclavicular joint injuries. (Reproduced with permission from Rockwood CA, Matsen FA III [eds]: *The Shoulder* [2 Vols], 2nd ed. Philadelphia: WB Saunders, 1998.)

require surgery acutely, although a small percentage continues to have pain. In type II AC joint injuries the AC ligaments and the coracoclavicular (CC) ligaments are torn enough that the clavicle subluxes superiorly but does not dislocate. These injuries are typically treated like type I, and full recovery may take 4–6 weeks. Surgery is rarely indicated in this injury acutely.

Type III injuries produce a deformity at the AC joint since all the ligaments (AC and CC) are disrupted, allowing the clavicle to dislocate superiorly (Fig. 17-14). These injuries are very painful and early treatment as described above may need to be supplemented with narcotics for a couple of weeks. Often the patient has difficulty sleeping and may have to sleep sitting up for a short period of time. Most of these injuries can be treated nonoperatively and the athlete can expect nearly full recovery within 8–12 weeks.

Surgical correction of these lesions remains controversial, but there is no evidence that operative intervention produces a result superior to no surgery in a majority of cases (Phillips et al., 1998). Some physicians suggest that

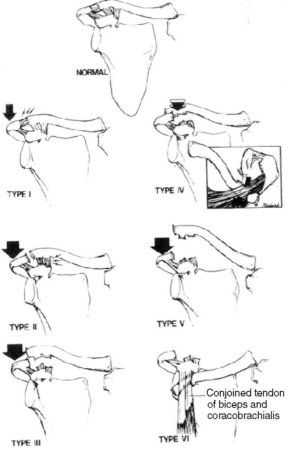

FIG 17-14   Injury of AC joint.

a grade III AC separation alters the shoulder biomechanics such that overhead athletes will be particularly affected, but these cases are so rare that consensus about treatment is lacking. A survey of major league baseball physicians revealed that two-thirds would initially treat this injury non-operatively (McFarland et al., 1997). A reasonable approach is to let the athlete return to sports and see if the injury affects their function. Surgery can always be done later if the athlete becomes symptomatic, and there is no indication that delaying surgery causes any technical difficulties with the repair or any changes in the results of the procedure.

More severe AC separations in which the clavicle is dislocated posteriorly into the trapezius fascia (type IV) or dislocated significantly superiorly (type V) may be candidates for early surgical intervention. These injuries should be treated nonoperatively at first and decisions to operate made based on each individual case. The recovery time from surgery is typically 4–6 months and this should be considered when deciding upon surgery.

Glenohumeral Joint Fractures

Injuries to the glenohumeral joint in athletes include fractures, instability, rotator cuff tears, and labrum lesions. Fractures to the scapula and proximal humerus are beyond the scope of this text and the reader is referred to other sources (Rockwood et al., 2001; Browner et al., 1998). However, in the older athlete over the age of 40, fractures of these bones should be seriously considered in the differential diagnosis in patients with shoulder trauma. For example, a fall on the shoulder may produce symptoms similar to those of a rotator cuff tear, with pain into the deltoid muscle, but frequently the older athlete will have sustained a fracture of the greater tuberosity or the proximal humerus. Fractures of the proximal humerus can occur with falls off of a bicycle, falls skiing, or with other moderate- to high-impact injuries.

Shoulder Instability

Shoulder instability is one of the most common injuries to athletes. Instability may be classified by direction (anterior, posterior, or inferior) or by etiology (traumatic or atraumatic). Instability can also be classified by degree, such as subluxation where the head does not totally leave the confines of the glenoid, and a dislocation where the humeral head does leave the confines of the joint. This discussion will focus on traumatic instability patterns. Occult instability which produces impingement pain found in overhead athletes will be discussed later.

Traumatic anterior instability is the most common type of instability seen in athletes, and occurs with the arm in an abducted, externally rotated position. Less common mechanisms causing anterior instability include a blow from the back of the shoulder or having the arm pulled away from the body, such as by a ski rope or when being pulled to the ground. If the shoulder does not relocate spontaneously it will need to be reduced. Usually a closed reduction can be accomplished without surgery. A thorough neurovascular exam is recommended before reduction is undertaken, with particular attention paid to the axillary nerve.

There are several techniques for reducing a dislocation, but the four most popular include axial distraction, a Stimson maneuver which is done with the patient supine, a Kocher maneuver, or a scapular stabilizing maneuver. All of these maneuvers are best accomplished with some form of sedation, either intravenously or by direct injection into the joint of local anesthetic. Axial traction is performed by pulling on the arm with the chest stabilized. The Stimson maneuver is performed the same way only with the patient prone, and the arm can be pulled manually (our preference) or weights can be hung from the wrist. In the Kocher maneuver, the humeral head is levered on the anterior glenoid and the shaft is levered against the anterior thoracic wall until reduction is complete. Various forms of scapular stabilizing maneuvers have been described, all of which involve manipulating the scapula while elevating and rotating the arm (Anderson et al., 1982).

After the reduction, the neurovascular exam should be repeated and radiographs should be repeated to make sure no fractures have occurred or been missed by the premanipulation radiographs. The patient can then be treated with an arm sling, or cryotherapy and an arm sling. Range of motion can begin immediately but the patient should avoid a position of abduction and external rotation. Typically full motion and strength return after 6 weeks.

The decision to return to sports depends on many factors, and the decision for surgery or non-operative treatment is individualized for every athlete. Many studies have documented that patients under the age of 25 have over a 90% chance of another instability episode, but this may be related more to their activity level and their level of risk-taking in sports (Hovelius et al., 1983). The position played in the sport is a factor, along with the type of sport that is being considered. A dominant arm dislocation may be at higher risk than a nondominant arm dislocation in some sports. The time of year in the sport is a factor, and some players may need only to finish the season before giving up the sport. The patient's future in the sport may be a factor, along with the monetary or scholarship implications of further instability. There may be an increased risk of arthritis of the shoulder with multiple dislocations, but this has not been convincingly proven (Marx et al., 2002). While it has been demonstrated that early surgical stabilization for traumatic anterior instability is better at preventing subsequent instability than nonoperative treatment (Kirkley et al., 1999), the decision for surgery is not that clear cut and immediate stabilization is typically not necessary. Some players can participate in their sport with braces that restrict elevation and external rotation, but a vast majority of athletes cannot function well with these devices.

If a decision is made to operate on the shoulder, this can be performed with open techniques or with arthroscopic techniques. Using either technique the repaired tissues take approximately 6 weeks to heal to bone and another 6 weeks to gain strength. With either technique contact sports are not typically recommended before 4–6 months. Open techniques are the time-proven method with redislocation rates of 3–5% at 2 years after surgery. While some studies show that arthroscopic stabilizations can produce stability rates similar to those of open procedures, this has not uniformly been the case. Arthroscopic operations have approximately twice the redislocation rate at 2 years compared to open operations (Geiger et al., 1997; Guanche et al., 1996).

Posterior dislocations are much less common (5%) than anterior dislocations. They typically occur with a fall with the arm flexed in front of the body with a posteriorly directed force, or there may be a push posteriorly on the arm standing, such as is seen in offensive linemen in American football. Upon examination the arm will be held in an adducted, internally rotated position. There may or may not be a prominence on the posterior shoulder, but the patient will be unable to externally rotate the shoulder.

Many of these posterior instability episodes reduce spontaneously. However, if the patient presents with a posterior dislocation, reduction is best performed with some form of anesthesia. The reduction is performed by axial traction on the arm with gradual external rotation and abduction. Once relocated, a neurovascular examination and repeat radiographs should be performed. Postreduction treatment is the same as for anterior dislocations, except the patient is urged to avoid elevation with internal rotation. The decision for surgery is individualized in every patient, and since posterior instability does not seem to have the same recurrence rate, a program of physical therapy to strengthen the shoulder is recommended for most patients. If they fail this program, the surgery is recommended. However, the failure rate after surgery for posterior instability has been reported to be between 15 and 20% at 2 years follow-up, so this should be factored into the discussion of risks and benefits of surgery (Antoniou et al., 2001). Recovery time after surgery is typically 4–6 months.

Inferior dislocations are quite rare and typically do not occur in athletics. The arm is typically stuck abducted 90° and these types of dislocations are associated with greater tuberosity fractures and neurovascular injury (Matsen et al., 1998). Few athletes describe a true sense of unidirectional inferior instability with sports or with laxity testing. This has important implications for making the diagnosis of multidirectional instability, which historically has been based on symptomatic inferior instability.

Rotator Cuff Tears

Rotator cuff tears in athletes can occur as the result of trauma, but the most common association of rotator cuff tears is with the performance of overhead sports. While full-thickness rotator cuff tears are uncommon in athletes due to trauma, they do occur and should be considered in the differential diagnosis (Blevins et al., 1996). Physical examination may not provide convincing signs initially in athletes, but continued pain or weakness with resisted abduction or external rotation may warrant study of the rotator cuff. Ultrasound, arthrography, or MRI can be utilized to make the diagnosis. Repair of the tendons typically eliminates the pain and returns the athlete to competition in most instances. In the more mature patient over the age of 40, cuff tearing is common as a result of trauma and the initial treatment should be cryotherapy, early range of motion, and NSAIDs. A decision to image the shoulder in these patients depends on the severity of the injury and the subsequent symptoms.

CHRONIC INJURIES

Sternoclavicular Injuries

Chronic sternoclavicular problems in athletes are uncommon. Degenerative problems of the SC joint typically do not appear until the fourth decade. The optimum treatment of arthritis of the SC joint is nonoperative, including activity modification, ice, and NSAIDs. Surgical intervention for intractable pain and loss of function due to arthritis of this joint involves excision of 5 mm of the proximal clavicle. While pain may be resolved, the ability to return to sports after this surgery is limited.

Another condition of the SC joint seen primarily in the second decade is voluntary subluxation of the SC joint. This typically occurs spontaneously without trauma, and patients can demonstrate the subluxation usually by moving the arm around with a specific maneuver. This condition rarely leads to arthritis and the athlete can typically live with any symptoms. One study suggested that the results of surgical excision for this situation is contraindicated due to the poor results (Rockwood et al., 1997).

Acromioclavicular Injuries

Two common chronic conditions of the AC joint include degenerative arthritis and osteolysis. Degenerative arthritis can be due to a number of etiologies, but the most common is an injury that initiates the degenerative process. Osteolyis is a disease of bone turnover due to abnormal stress at the AC joint (Cahill, 1992). However, its presentation and symptoms mimic that of degenerative arthritis. However, osteolysis usually has no history of trauma and is more frequently bilateral than osteoarthritis. The pain is typically exacerbated by exercise, and the most common exercises that stress the AC joint include bench press, push-ups, and dips. Some patients with these conditions complain of pain in the AC joint with the follow-through of golf. Upon physical examination there may be swelling of the AC joint compared to the opposite side. Local tenderness of the AC joint is frequent and other positive physical findings include the crossed-arm adduction stress test (Clarke et al., 2000; Shaffer, 1999), the active compression test (O'Brien et al., 1998), and the forced arm extension test. Diagnostic injections into the AC joint are uniformly positive in AC arthritis but may not be positive in osteolysis. Plain radiographs are the diagnostic modality of choice and bone scans may demonstrate the degree of inflammation. However, MRI and CT scanning are usually not of benefit in evaluating these lesions.

Treatment of these lesions initially includes relative rest and activity modification, cryotherapy, and NSAIDs. If this is not effective, cortisone shots into the AC joint can sometimes resolve the inflammation. After the shot the patient should see resolution of the symptoms due to the local anesthetic. If they do not get any relief, then consider the possibility of another source of the pain. The AC joint is a small joint with a small meniscus, so when injecting the joint it is helpful to inject the periosteum around the joint as well. If cortisone shots do not provide permanent relief, then operative excision of the distal 0.5–1.0 cm of the clavicle is indicated. This excision can be done arthroscopically or through a small incision. The recovery time is approximately 6 weeks for full motion and 3 months to return to sports. A majority of patients can return to full sports activity with few restrictions, although there may be some local tenderness for a longer period of time (Shaffer, 1999).

Glenohumeral Joint

The most common chronic conditions affecting the athlete include shoulder instability and rotator cuff disorders. In the younger athlete it has been postulated that instability may lead to cuff disorders, but either condition can exist as an isolated condition. There are several theories of how shoulder instability is related to rotator cuff disease. Frank Jobe first postulated that due to the repetitive motions of overhead activities such as baseball, tennis, and swimming, the ligaments of the shoulder begin to stretch (Jobe et al., 1991). This stretching leads to a subtle form of instability that is characterized by pain typical of cuff tendinitis. This pain can radiate into the deltoid and down the arm like primary rotator cuff problems.

As the condition of subtle instability progresses, other pathologies can develop in the shoulder. These include partial rotator cuff tears, anterior labrum tears typical of instability, and superior labrum tears (SLAP lesions). The superior labrum tears typically produce posterior and superior shoulder pain, particularly with the arm in abduction and externally rotated position. Upon physical examination the athlete should have a positive relocation maneuver as described by Kvitne and Jobe (Kvitne et al., 1993). In this sign, with the patient supine and the arm in a cocking position, the patient should have pain posteriorly and superiorly. The humeral head is then stabilized by placing posterior pressure on the head, and the pain should be eliminated. The patient may have increased external rotation and decreased internal rotation compared to the other extremity when the arm is abducted 90°. This GIRD (glenohumeral internal rotation deficit) has been postulated by some physicians to be a contributing factor to the development of pain, but it is not entirely clear if the motion lost is a cause of the problem or just an adaptation due to the forces seen by the athletic shoulder (Ellenbeker et al., 2002). Weakness in external rotation is frequently seen in overhead athletes, but its exact relationship to pain or instability is not entirely clear. Plain radiographs should be obtained as the first imaging modality in these patients.

Treatment of this condition in its early stages includes relative rest, cryotherapy, and NSAIDs. Cortisone shots are typically not recommended in the younger athlete, but in some instances they may allow function enough to prevent surgical intervention. Physical therapy to eliminate any rotator cuff weakness or weakness of any of the scapular stabilizing muscles is typically utilized to improve the mechanics of the shoulder. Nonoperative treatment should be utilized as long as possible to avert surgical intervention. If these treatments are not curative or the athlete's performance is significantly impeded, then a decision must be made about whether the athlete should proceed with surgical intervention or to have further imaging studies. The best imaging study in this situation is an arthrogram-MRI since it gives the best detail of the labrum and rotator cuff. However, it should be mentioned that interpretation of the labrum is fraught with difficulties, particularly with distinguishing normal variants from pathological lesions (McFarland et al., 2003). As a result, in the athlete with shoulder pain with no history of trauma, an MRI is not absolutely necessary before surgery can be considered. An MRI does provide information about other structures and can rule out masses such as synovial cysts, so there are other reasons to consider MRI imaging prior to surgery.

Other theories of why athletes get rotator cuff tears include (1) normal senescence of the tendon, (2) a vascular etiology due to inadequate blood supply of the distal tendon, (3) tension overload of the tendon due to traction when throwing, and (4) internal impingement or contact of the rotator cuff tendon on the superior glenoid. Normal senescence of the tendon probably is the cause of tears in patients over the age of 30, unless there is a distinct history of trauma. In these cases with no history of trauma, nonoperative treatment is considered first, and cortisone shots can be beneficial. While it is controversial how or why cortisone shots into the subacromial space work, most physicians do not recommend more than a couple shots before imaging of the shoulder is indicated. MRI, arthrograms, or ultrasound can be utilized after plain radiographs are obtained.

The surgical treatment of rotator cuff tears is beyond the scope of this chapter but the main factor influencing the result of surgical repair is the size of the tear (Cofield et al., 2001). Partial tears of the tendons upon MRI are common and do not need surgical treatment unless the patient remains symptomatic after nonoperative treatment. When treatment is necessary, arthroscopic or open partial acromioplasty is effective in relieving the pain in a majority of patients. However, the results of these procedures in throwing athletes are less predictable, and in these patients the possibility of underlying occult shoulder instability should be considered. Conversion of a partial tear to a full-thickness tear during the surgical procedure is controversial, and some recommend this if the tear is more than 50% of the thickness of the tendon, while other surgeons suggest the tear should be 90% of the thickness of the tendon. Repair of full-thickness rotator cuff tears with either arthroscopic or open techniques provides pain relief in a majority of patients, and a majority will be satisfied with their surgery. However, recovery of full strength and function may take 9–12 months depending on the size of the tear (Cofield et al., 2001; Grana et al., 1994). In these older, more mature athletes who wish to return to tennis, only 80% will achieve their previous level of function (Sonnery-Cottet et al., 2002).

Another theory of cuff tears in overhead athletes suggests that the partial rotator cuff tears are due to a form of "superior" instability and impingement. The theory is that with the arm in abduction and external rotation, the rotator cuff and greater tuberosity make contact with the superior glenoid where the labrum and biceps tendon attach. This repetitive wear causes the labrum to "peel back" from the glenoid rim and eventually the labrum tears. The theory suggests that the resulting SLAP lesion creates pathological laxity in the shoulder which is a form of "superior instability." SLAP lesions have been classified by Snyder as type I (fraying only), type II (detachment of the biceps attachment to the superior glenoid and detachment of the labrum to the superior glenoid), type III (flap tear of the superior labrum) and type IV (flap tear with tear into the biceps tendon) (Snyder et al., 1990). Type II SLAP lesions have been subdivided by Morgan and associates into three types: anterior lesions alone with detachment of the labrum anterior to the biceps attachment, posterior lesions alone with detachment of the labrum posterior to the biceps attachment, or combined lesions in which the whole biceps anchor is detached (Fig. 17-15; Morgan et al., 1998). Each type has characteristic physical examination findings and location of partial cuff tearing, reflecting their different pathophysiologies. A review of the literature suggests the treatment for each type, and is outlined in Table 17-6.

The surgical options for the athlete with pain and presumed instability include an open capsular shift, an arthroscopic capsular shift, or a thermal capsular shift (Levine et al., 2001; Treacy et al., 1999). Other procedures that may be performed depending on the pathology found include repair of a SLAP lesion, repair of the rotator cuff interval, and release of posterior shoulder capsular tightness. After surgery most soft tissue repairs require at least 3 months of protected activity to allow healing of the tissue to bone. Progression of activity to include throwing typically begins around 4–6 months, and average time to return to throwing with no limitations occurs between 10–14 months. In a patient returning to contact sports, the recommendation is to wait at least 4 months or until full motion and strength have returned. As a result, surgery for instability of the shoulder should be undertaken with an understanding that it is not a quick fix and

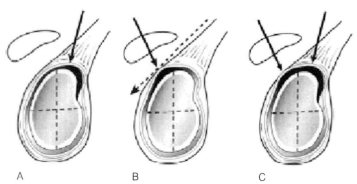

A   B   C

FIG 17-15 Type II SLAP lesions have been subdivided into three types: (A) anterior lesions alone with detachment of the labrum anterior to the biceps attachment, (B) posterior lesions alone with detachment of the labrum posterior to the biceps attachment, or (C) combined lesions in which the whole biceps anchor is detached. (Reproduced with permission from Morgan CD, Burkhart SS, Palmeri M, Gillespie M. Type II SLAP lesion: three subtypes and their relationships to superior instability and rotator cuff tears. *Arthroscopy.* 1998;14:553–565.)

that rehabilitation is lengthy. After surgery, most studies indicate that 70–80% of athletes will get back to their previous level of throwing (Snyder et al., 1990; Morgan et al., 1998; Burkhart et al., 2001). A majority of patients who have surgery for traumatic instability of the shoulder should be able to return to sports as well. Thermal procedures do not seem to be as effective for traumatic multidirectional instability or for patients with congenital multidirectional instability (Samani et al., 2001). Surgical repairs in athletes continue to evolve and many aspects remain controversial. Each patient's needs and goals should be considered in any decision to proceed with surgical intervention.

MISCELLANEOUS CONDITIONS

Little League Shoulder

There are a variety of lesions that occur in the athlete that are not common, but which should be considered in the differential diagnosis in the painful

TABLE 17-6 Subclassification of Type II SLAP Lesion

	Anterior Lesion	Posterior Lesion	Combined
Etiology	Trauma	Overhead/throwing athletes	Overhead/throwing athletes
Physical examination	O'Brien test/ speed test	Jobe relocation test	Nonspecific
Location of partial cuff tear	Anterior	Posterior	Nonspecific
Drive through sign	Negative	Positive	Positive
Treatment	Repair with anterior anchor	Repair with posterior anchor	Repair with anterior and posterior anchors

Adapted from Morgan et al, 1998.

shoulder. In adolescent athletes with open growth plates, pain in the shoulder with throwing typically indicates a stress injury to the proximal humeral physeal growth plate, and is known as "little league shoulder." Radiographs will typically demonstrate a widened growth plate of the proximal humerus. Pain in an adolescent who is not a throwing athlete should be carefully evaluated for other causes. Treatment is rest from throwing only for 4–6 weeks and then return to throwing as the athlete is capable.

Synovial Cysts

Synovial or ganglion cysts can occur in the shoulder of athletes and cause shoulder pain and weakness. In some instances they can compress the suprascapular nerve or they may affect only the infraspinatus branch of the suprascapular nerve. Atrophy of the infraspinatus or of the infraspinatus and supraspinatus may or may not be present. Electromyography can isolate the location of the nerve entrapment, and MRI imaging is the best imaging modality to delineate the location and extent of the cyst. Nonoperative treatment is indicated typically and surgery is indicated in those patients who continue to have pain and dysfunction. Aspiration of the cyst has been shown to be effective in only 64% (Joseph et al., 2003). Surgical intervention can be performed via an incision to excise the cyst and in some instances decompression of the cyst can be done arthroscopically.

Nerve entrapments around the shoulder can occur as a result of athletic participation. The most common nerve palsies are the long thoracic nerve and the infraspinatus branch of the supraspinatus nerve. Long thoracic nerve palsies do not have a predictable etiology, and can occur after weight lifting or simply doing push-ups. Typically patients describe an ache in the shoulder which generally goes away, but they sense that their shoulder "just isn't right." Usually they notice or someone else notices their scapula winging, and occasionally the winging is severe enough that it affects their performance. It is important to do a complete neurologic evaluation to rule out other causes of the winging, such as a cervical disc problem. Electromyography can localize the injury to the nerve and can help determine if the lesion is partial or complete. A vast majority of these lesions are incomplete and will recover over 6–9 months. Until that time the athlete is allowed to participate as much as symptoms allow. If the nerve does not recover and the symptoms are limiting, surgery can be performed but it rarely restores normal function.

Entrapment of the infraspinatus branch of the suprascapular nerve results in weakness and atrophy of the infraspinatus muscle. This injury is seen frequently in volleyball players and is believed to be due to the overhead motion of hitting the volleyball, which produces traction on the nerve as it courses around the spine of the scapula. This injury is also common in baseball players due to throwing but not batting. On physical examination the patient will have weakness with resisted external rotation but few other signs. There may be signs of anterior impingement due to the loss of infraspinatus function in the rotator cuff. Electromyography can verify an isolated lesion to the infraspinatus branch of the suprascapular nerve and that there is no other etiology for the injury. MRI scanning is helpful to rule out synovial cysts, which can frequently cause similar symptoms. The initial treatment is nonoperative with symptomatic treatment of any pain or weakness. If the player is incapable of performing physical activity, then surgery to decompress the nerve can be helpful in relieving symptoms. However, recovery of the atrophied muscle is less predictable and depends upon chronicity of the lesion and other variables (Romeo et al., 1999).

Vascular lesions of the shoulder are also quite rare but can produce symptoms that mimic rotator cuff disease or nonspecific shoulder pain. Vascular lesions can be divided into venous or arterial lesions. Venous lesions have been reported after a variety of sports and most frequently occur either at the thoracic outlet beneath the clavicle or just distal to that in the axillary vein. Symptoms of swelling and discoloration of the extremity are common, but pulmonary embolus is rare. The diagnosis can be made by plethysmography or with venogram. Athletes who develop upper extremity clots should be considered for evaluation of hypercoagulable states. These lesions are treated with urokinase or streptokinase if necessary, followed by longer-term anticoagulation. Surgery is indicated only for clear obstructive lesions such as at the thoracic outlet or clavicle-first rib complex.

Arterial lesions of the shoulder area present with pain, paresthesias, weakness, and intermittent discoloration or coolness of the hand. Rarely punctate lesions in the fingers due to emboli may occur. These lesions require a high index of suspicion but should be considered anytime an athlete complains of a cold extremity after sports activity. The lesions producing arterial compromise include aneurysms of the artery or compression of the arteries due to aberrant anatomy. The tests of choice for the diagnosis include plethysmography and MRI angiography. If a lesion is discovered or suspected, then arteriography remains the gold standard for evaluating these lesions. Surgical intervention can be beneficial in symptomatic lesions and patients can usually return to their previous level of participation.

TENDON RUPTURE

Biceps Long Head Tendon Rupture

The long head of the biceps tendon is one of the most commonly torn tendons in the body in individuals over 50 years of age, but it is uncommon in young, athletic individuals. The most common cause of the long head of biceps tendon rupture is degenerative change within the tendon, and it frequently is accompanied by subacromial pathology, such as subacromial impingement or rotator cuff tears (Piatt et al., 2002). Rupture of the biceps may be preceded by a history of anterior shoulder pain that quickly resolved after a painful audible pop (Neer, 1983). But in most cases the patient will not have had any prodromal symptoms at all. Bruising down the front of the arm and the characteristic "Popeye arm" due to the tendon and muscle balling up in the anterior arm may follow the acute rupture. The initial treatment of a biceps tendon rupture is symptomatic with ice, range of motion, and acetaminophen or NSAIDs. Most people recover within 3 weeks and can resume their normal activities.

There are almost no long-term sequelae of this injury and there is rarely any noticeable loss of strength at the shoulder (Yamaguchi et al., 1999). One study compared operative treatment versus nonoperative treatment of biceps tendon ruptures (Carroll et al., 1968). This study reported an earlier return to work in the conservatively treated patients, but they had had an 8% loss of elbow flexion strength and a 21% loss of forearm supination strength compared with the surgically treated patients. In patients with chronic rupture of the biceps tendon, Habermeyer and Walch recommended arthroscopic evaluation of the proximal stump to assess for potential entrapment in the joint and to evaluate the labrum (Habermeyer et al., 1996). They suggested arthroscopic resection of the stump should it become entrapped in the joint. While some surgeons have suggested that tenodesis be performed in younger (<30 years old) athletes, there is no objective evidence to suggest this is better than nonoperative treatment. However, surgery is almost never indicated for isolated biceps tendon ruptures. Rarely patients will consider surgery because of the cosmetic appearance, but they trade a bump in the arm for a scar.

Pectoralis Major Rupture

Pectoralis major rupture is an uncommon injury which typically occurs in active individuals while they are participating in sports or manual labor. Sports-related injuries usually occur during weight training, particularly the bench press. Most reported sports-related ruptures are complete and are located at the insertion to the humerus (Bak et al., 2000). Diagnosis of pectoralis major injuries can usually be made based on the patient history and physical examination. Most patients will demonstrate ecchymosis down the arm and chest, and a defect in the tendon is usually palpable. MRI can be helpful if the diagnosis is unclear, but it is usually not necessary. Specific treatment options should be based on the severity of the injury and on the patient's individual needs. Nonoperative management consisting of immobilization and physical therapy can offer a functional result with return of shoulder motion and activities of daily living. However, according to some studies, surgical repair of rupture of the pectoralis major results in greater recovery of peak torque and work performance than conservative management of patients, particularly in competitive athletes (Bak et al., 2000). Although complications such as re-rupture, infection, and heterotopic ossification do occasionally occur, surgical treatment, preferably within the first 8 weeks after the injury, has a significantly better outcome than conservative treatment or delayed repair (Hanna et al., 2001).

Subscapularis Tendon Rupture

Isolated complete rupture of the subscapularis tendon is a rare injury which is often missed initially. The injury occurs in either forceful hyperextension or external rotation of the adducted arm. Most reported subscapularis tears have been associated with traumatic anterior dislocation and have been followed by symptoms of recurrent instability (Hauser, 1954; Neviaser et al., 1988). Gerber and colleagues reported on another group of patients with rupture of the subscapularis tendon caused by a traumatic event without combined instability. The symptoms were anterior shoulder pain and weakness of the arm when used above and below shoulder level. Upon physical examination, the injured shoulders exhibited increased external rotation and decreased strength of internal rotation. The lift-off test and the belly press test are reliable diagnostic clinical tests. Confirmation of clinical diagnosis was best achieved by MRI. Repair of the ruptured tendon is recommended when possible. Partial tears of the subscapularis tendon are common and their exact clinical significance is not known (Kim et al., submitted).

SCAPULAR DYSKINESIS

Another area of recent interest has been the relationship of scapulothoracic mechanics and shoulder function. Efficient transfer of torque from the legs to the upper extremities is recognized as important in the biomechanics of sports, and in the development of and recovery from shoulder problems. It has been recognized that strength in the lower extremities can affect upper extremity mechanics, and some physicians emphasize a need to evaluate upper and lower extremity function when evaluating athletes involved in overhead sports.

Abnormal biomechanics or shoulder pathology can result in "scapular dyskinesis." This abnormal relationship of the scapula to the shoulder blade may contribute to shoulder pathologies, but the exact relationship has not been fully elucidated. Four patterns of scapular dyskinesis have been described by Kibler and associates, and they require special expertise to discern accurately (Kibler et al., 2002). Once the abnormality has been recognized, therapy can be directed at the scapulothoracic articulation, the rotator cuff, and the scapular stabilizing muscles. If physical therapy fails, then surgical intervention is directed at the occult instability, SLAP lesions, or cuff problems, which are contributing to the problem (Kibler, 1998).

REFERENCES

Anderson D, Zvirbulis R, Ciullo J. Scapular manipulation for reduction of anterior shoulder dislocations. *Clin Orthop*. 1982;164:181–183.

Antoniou J, Harryman DT 2nd. Posterior instability. *Orthop Clin North Am*. 2001;32:463–473.

Bak K, Cameron EA, Henderson IJ. Rupture of the pectoralis major: A meta-analysis of 112 cases. *Knee Surg Sports Traumatol Arthrosc*. 2000;8:113–119.

Blevins FT, Hayes WM, Warren RF. Rotator cuff injury in contact athletes. *Am J Sports Med*. 1996;24:263–267.

Browner BD, Jupiter JB, Levine AM, Trafton PG, eds. *Skeletal Trauma*, 2nd ed. Philadelphia: W-B Saunders, 1998.

Burkhart SS, Morgan C. SLAP lesions in the overhead athlete. *Orthop Clin North Am*. 2001;32:431–441, viii.

Cahill BR. Atraumatic osteolysis of the distal clavicle. A review. *Sports Med*. 1992;13: 214–222.

Carroll RE, Hamilton LR. Rupture of biceps brachii—a conservative method of treatment. *J Bone Joint Surg Am*. 1968;49:1016.

Clarke HD, McCann PD. Acromioclavicular joint injuries. *Orthop Clin North Am*. 2000;31:177–187.

Cofield RH, et al. Surgical repair of chronic rotator cuff tears. A prospective long-term study. *J Bone Joint Surg Am*. 2001;83:71–77.

Ellenbeker TS, Roetert EP, Bailie DS, Davies GJ, Brown SW. Glenohumeral joint total rotation range of motion in elite tennis players and baseball pitchers. *Med Sci Sports Exerc*. 2002;34:205–206.

Geiger DF, et al. Results of arthroscopic versus open Bankart suture repair. *Clin Orthop*. 1997;April:111–117.

Gerber C, Galantay RV, Hersche O. The pattern of pain produced by irritation of the acromioclavicular joint and the subacromial space. *J Shoulder Elbow Surg*. 1998;7:352–355.

Gerber C, Ganz R. Clinical assessment of instability of the shoulder. With special reference to anterior and posterior drawer tests. *J Bone Joint Surg Br*. 1984;66:551–556.

Gerber C, Krushell RJ. Isolated rupture of the tendon of the subscapularis muscle. *J Bone Joint Surg Br*. 1991;73:389–394.

Grana WA, et al. An analysis of rotator cuff repair. *Am J Sports Med*. 1994;22:585–588.

Guanche CA, et al. Arthroscopic versus open reconstruction of the shoulder in patients with isolated Bankart lesions. *Am J Sports Med*. 1996;24:144–148.

Guanche CA, Quick DC. Prospective correlation of clinical examination with arthroscopy in the diagnosis of glenoid labral tears [abstract]. *Arthroscopy*. 2000;16:432–433.

Habermeyer P, Walch G. The biceps tendon and rotator cuff disease. In: Burkhead WZ Jr, ed. *Rotator Cuff Disorders*. Philadelphia: Lippincott Williams & Wilkins; 1996;142.

Hanna CM, Glenny AB, Stanley SN, Caughey MA. Pectoralis major tears: Comparison of surgical and conservative treatment. *Br J Sports Med*. 2001;35:202–206.

Hauser EDW. Avulsion of the tendon of the subscapularis muscle. *Am J Bone Joint Surg*. 1954;36:139–141.

Holovacs TF, Osbahr D, Singh H, et al: The sensitivity and specificity of the physical examination to detect glenoid labrum tears. Presented at the specialty day meeting of the American Shoulder and Elbow Society, Orlando, Florida, March 2000.

Hovelius L, Eriksson K, Fredin H, et al. Recurrences after initial dislocation of the shoulder. Results of a prospective study of treatment. *J Bone Joint Surg Am*. 1983;65:343–349.

Jobe FW, et al. Anterior capsulolabral reconstruction of the shoulder in athletes in overhand sports. *Am J Sports Med*. 1991;19:428–434.

Joseph TA, Williams JS Jr, Brems JJ. Laser capsulorrhaphy for multidirectional instability of the shoulder: an outcomes study and proposed classification system. *Am J Sports Med*. 2003;31:26–35.

Kibler WB. Specificity and sensitivity of the anterior slide test in throwing athletes with superior glenoid labral tears. *Arthroscopy*. 1995;11:296–300.

Kibler WB. The role of the scapula in athletic shoulder function. *Am J Sports Med*. 1998;26:325–337.

Kibler WB, Uhl TL, Maddux JW, Brooks PV, Zeller B, McMullen J. Qualitative clinical evaluation of scapular dysfunction: a reliability study. *J Shoulder Elbow Surg*. 2002;11:550–556.

Kim TK, Queale WS, Cosgarea AJ, McFarland EG. Clinical features of the different types of SLAP lesions: An analysis of one hundred and thirty-nine cases. *J Bone Joint Surg Am*. 2003;85:66–71.

Kim TK, Rauh PB, McFarland EG. Partial tears of the subscapularis tendon during shoulder arthroscopy: A statistical analysis of sixty cases. *Am J Sports Med*. (submitted).

Kirkley A, et al. Prospective randomized clinical trial comparing the effectiveness of immediate arthroscopic stabilization versus immobilization and rehabilitation in first traumatic anterior dislocations of the shoulder. *Arthroscopy*. 1999;15:507–514.

Kvitne RS, Jobe FW. The diagnosis and treatment of anterior instability in the throwing athlete. *Clin Orthop*. 1993;291:107–123.

Levine WN, Prickett WD, Prymka M, Yamaguchi K. Treatment of the athlete with multidirectional shoulder instability. *Orthop Clin North Am*. 2001;32:475–484.

Mariania EM, Cofield RH, Askew LJ, et al. Rupture of the tendon of the long head of the biceps brachii: Surgical versus nonsurgical treatment. *Clin Orthop*. 1988;228:223–229.

Marx RG, McCarty EC, Montemurno TD, Altchek DW, Craig EV, Warren RF. Development of arthrosis following dislocation of the shoulder: A case-control study. *J Shoulder Elbow Surg*. 2002;11:1–5.

Matsen FA III, Thomas SC, Rockwood CA Jr, Wirth MA. Glenohumeral instability. In: Rockwood CA Jr, Matsen FA, eds. *The Shoulder*, 2nd ed. Philadelphia: WB Saunders; 1998.

McFarland EG, et al. Treatment of grade III acromioclavicular separations in professional throwing athletes: Results of a survey. *Am J Orthop*. 1997;26:771–774.

McFarland EG, Campbell G, McDowell J. Posterior shoulder laxity in asymptomatic athletes. *Am J Sports Med*. 1996c;24:468–471.

McFarland EG, Kim TK. Clinical features of SLAP lesions. *J Bone Joint Surg Am*. 2003;85:12–15.

McFarland EG, Kim TK, Savino RM. Clinical assessment of three common tests for superior labral anterior-posterior lesions. *Am J Sports Med.* 2002;30:810–815.

McFarland EG, Kim TK, Savino RM. Clinical assessment of three common tests for superior labral anterior-posterior lesions. *Am J Sports Med.* 2002;30:810–815.

McFarland EG, Shaffer B, Glousman RE, Conway, Jobe FW. Clinical and diagnostic evaluation: Anterior shoulder instability, impingement, and rotator cuff tear. In: Jobe FW, ed. *Operative Techniques in Upper Extremity Sports Injuries.* St. Louis, Missouri: Mosby-Year Book; 1996a.

McFarland EG, Shaffer B, Glosman RE, Conway JE, Jobe FW. Clinical and diagnostic evaluation. In: Jobe FW, ed. *Operative Techniques in Upper Extremity Sports Injuries.* St. Louis, Missouri: Mosby-Year Book; 1996b.

Morgan CD, Burkhart SS, Palmeri M, Gillespie M. Type II SLAP lesions: Three subtypes and their relationships to superior instability and rotator cuff tears. *Arthroscopy.* 1998;14:553–565.

Neer CS 2nd. Impingement lesions. *Clin Orthop.* 1983;173:70–177.

Neviaser RJ, Neviaser TJ, Neviaser JS. Concurrent rupture of the rotator cuff and anterior dislocation of the shoulder in the older patient. *Am J Bone Joint Surg.* 1988;70:1308–1311.

O'Brien SJ, Pagnani MJ, Fealy S, et al. The active compression test: A new and effective test for diagnosing labral tears and acromioclavicular joint abnormality. *Am J Sports Med.* 1998;26:610–613.

Parentis MA, Mohr KJ, El Attrache NS. Disorders of the superior labrum: Review and treatment guidelines. *Clin Orthop.* 2002;400:77–787.

Phillips AM, Smart C, Groom AF. Acromioclavicular dislocation. Conservative or surgical therapy. *Clin Orthop.* 1998;353:10–17.

Piatt BE, et al. Clinical evaluation and treatment of spinoglenoid notch ganglion cysts. *J Shoulder Elbow Surg.* 2002;11:600–604.

Rockwood CA, Jr., et al. Resection arthroplasty of the sternoclavicular joint. *J Bone Joint Surg Am.* 1997;79:387–393.

Rockwood CA Jr, Green DP, eds. *Fractures in Adults*, 5th ed. Philadelphia?: Lippincott Williams & Wilkins; 2001.

Romeo AA, Rotenberg DD, Bach BR Jr. Suprascapular neuropathy. *J Am Acad Orthop Surg.* 1999;7:358–367.

Samani JE, Marston SB, Buss DD. Arthroscopic stabilization of type II SLAP lesions using an absorbable tack. *Arthroscopy.* 2001;17:19–24.

Shaffer BS. Painful conditions of the acromioclavicular joint. *J Am Acad Orthop Surg.* 1999;7:176–188.

Snyder SJ, et al. SLAP lesions of the shoulder. *Arthroscopy.* 1990;6:274–279.

Sonnery-Cottet B, Edwards TB, Noel E, Walch G. Rotator cuff tears in middle-aged tennis players: Results of surgical treatment. *Am J Sports Med.* 2002;30:558–564.

Stetson WB, Templin K. The crank test, the O'Brien test, and routine magnetic resonance imaging scans in the diagnosis of labral tears. *Am J Sports Med.* 2002;30:806–809.

Treacy SH, Savoie FH 3rd, Field LD. Arthroscopic treatment of multidirectional instability. *J Shoulder Elbow Surg.* 1999;8:345–350.

Wick M, et al. Midshaft fractures of the clavicle with a shortening of more than 2 cm predispose to nonunion. *Arch Orthop Trauma Surg.* 2001;121:207–211.

Yamaguchi K, Bendra R. Disorders of the biceps tendon. In: Iannotti JP, Williams GR Jr, eds. *Disorders of Shoulder: Diagnosis and Management.* Philadelphia: Lippincott, Williams & Wilkins; 1999;159–190.

Zanca P. Shoulder pain: Involvement of the acromioclavicular joint. (Analysis of 1,000 cases). *Am J Roentgenol Radium Ther Nucl Med.* 1971;112:493–506.

18 | The Chest and Abdomen

William W. Dexter

INTRODUCTION

Thoracoabdominal injuries are unusual in sports. Requiring significant force, they are most commonly seen in augmented speed sports such as bicycling and skiing, but can also be seen in high-energy contact sports. While representing less than 2% of sporting injuries, chest and abdominal trauma can have dire consequences with the potential for significant morbidity and possible mortality. The presentation of these injuries may be subtle and thus are often missed or under-diagnosed and require the sideline practitioner to have a high index of suspicion.

THORACIC INJURIES

Chest wall injuries can range from soft tissue injuries of the muscles, ligaments, and fascia, to bony injuries. Intrathoracic injuries can occur to the lung, pleura, heart, and great vessels, as well as the trachea, esophagus, and diaphragm. While blunt trauma from a direct blow is the most common etiology, indirect injury can be seen in augmented speed sports from sudden deceleration. Many chest injuries are self-limited and resolve with conservative treatment. Some can be life threatening, thus a high level of suspicion is necessary along with a plan for rapid assessment and triage. The on-field evaluation includes identification of the location of the pain/injury and a rapid determination of hemodynamic stability. Obviously, any hemodynamically unstable athlete should be immediately transported to the emergency room. Assessment includes a quick review of mental status and execution of the trauma "ABCs," focusing on the quality and character of respirations and determination of pulsations in the neck and upper and lower extremities. Inspection of the neck is done to assess the neck veins and position of the trachea and to evaluate any welts or cuts on the neck, chest, upper back, shoulders, and abdomen. Following this the bony structures are first palpated, followed by soft tissues, and concluding with evaluation of all organs. Auscultation is then done to determine decreased, increased, or adventitial breath sounds and evaluation of heart sounds—particularly looking for added or muffled sounds. Finally, percussion of the lungs and abdomen searching for dullness or hyperresonance in the thorax and for rebound tenderness and boarding or guarding in the abdomen is performed.

Musculoskeletal Injuries about the Chest

Contusions

Contusions are a frequent chest wall injury and simple bruising is commonly seen in contact collision sports. Deep hematomas are unusual but can present problems, particularly when in the pectoralis muscles anteriorly or the paraspinals and trapezius posteriorly. Diagnosis is often straightforward; however, one should be aware that swelling in these large muscle groups may obscure a tear. Treatment is conservative and return to play is as tolerated by the athlete, allowing for protection of the injured area. As with any hematoma there is the potential risk for myositis ossificans.

Muscle Strains

Pectoralis. Common muscle strains about the chest include the pectoralis muscles and are not uncommon, such as those seen in weightlifting with the bench press and power cleans. Diagnosis is facilitated by checking active range of motion and strength and discomfort on resisted range of motion (push-ups). Palpation at the insertions of the pectorals at the muscle tendon junctions of the coracoid and humerus will often reveal tenderness. Mild to moderate strains of the pectoralis usually respond to conservative measures including physical therapy with gradual return to play as tolerated. Complete ruptures should be surgically repaired.

Serratus Anterior. A strain of the serratus anterior is an unusual injury caused by a sudden pull and can be seen in rowers or with dead lifting in weightlifters. There often will be a bony avulsion of the serratus at its insertion, so radiographs should be obtained if this injury is suspected. Diagnosis is suggested by the athlete's inability to abduct their arm and palpation of a mass on their lateral chest wall. Treatment is typically conservative.

Fractures

Clavicle. Clavicle fractures are one of the more common fractures encountered in sports medicine. Typically occurring from a direct blow to the shoulder, the clavicle pivots over the first rib, thus fracturing (80% of the time) in the middle third of the clavicle. Diagnosis is straightforward from the history and physical exam, which will reveal an obvious deformity, swelling, crepitus, tenderness, and ecchymosis. The shoulder should always be checked for concomitant injury and a careful neurovascular evaluation performed. Treatment of midclavicular fractures is conservative and comfort measures are usually all that is needed. Use of a sling for several days will provide reasonable pain relief; a swathe or figure-of-8 brace is not necessary. Return to play is dictated by the athlete's symptoms combined with evidence of clinical and radiographic healing.

Thoracic Spine. Acute fractures of the thoracic spine are uncommon but can occur from direct blows. Clinically the athlete will exhibit pain and tenderness, particularly with resisted motion at the thoracic spine. There usually will be modest soft tissue swelling over the area of the fracture, and x-rays of the thoracic spine, including a PA and lateral chest, are diagnostic. These injuries typically require a significant amount of force, so one must have a high index of suspicion for potential injury to underlying structures such as the great vessels and lung (pneumothorax). Assuming no associated injuries, treatment is with relative rest, and return to play is usually feasible after healing occurs in about 6–8 weeks.

Older athletes may sustain compression fractures of the thoracic spine. Typically these occur in the older athlete who has osteopenia or osteoporosis and an overuse etiology such as the golf swing. Diagnosis is based on the history, clinical findings, and radiographs. Treatment is functional with bracing, modification of technique, and pain control.

Ribs. Rib fractures, particularly to the lower ribs (4th–9th), are one of the most common thoracic injuries. Any time a lower rib is fractured, an abdominal or diaphragmatic injury must be considered. If the upper ribs (1st–3rd) are fractured, injury to the neck and the potential for great vessel trauma should be suspected. As upper rib fractures typically require a great deal of force, it is probably prudent to manage them in a controlled setting. Most rib fractures, if not displaced, are not serious injuries and can be managed symptomatically. The most common location for rib fractures is at the posterior angle and often a step-off and crepitus may be palpated at the fracture site. The patient will be tender and may splint this area. Acute symptoms include hypoventilation with mild tachypnea. Diagnosis is made from a history of blunt trauma, though ribs can fracture from a violent twist or sudden action such as a hard cough, and is confirmed with radiographs. Either a rib series or standard PA and lateral chest films will suffice, but if the diagnosis remains unclear, CT scanning is the recommended imaging modality. Differential diagnosis includes rib contusion, costochondral separation or strain, and thorough soft tissue and abdominal examination should be undertaken to rule out underlying organ injury. Treatment is typically conservative, aimed at achieving pain relief. If respirations are moderately impaired, a local anesthetic block may be utilized, but taping and bracing may be counterproductive and thus are not recommended. Return to play occurs as the ribs heal, usually in 6–8 weeks, but may be hastened through appropriate protection with "flak jackets." Athletes resume training as symptoms permit, usually in 3–4 weeks.

There are several situations involving rib fractures that deserve mention. First, any rib fracture in a child must be considered a serious injury. In children the ribs are very elastic and rib fractures represent injury from significant force, so the pediatric athlete must be closely monitored for potential underlying injuries. Another injury that requires significant force is a flail chest. This occurs when three or more ribs are fractured or with costochondral separation in association with a lateral rib fracture. Fortunately these are rare in sports, but rapidly progress to significant respiratory compromise, so these patients should be stabilized and transported immediately. Finally, rib stress fractures are not uncommon. Typically seen in golfers in the posterior lateral ribs (4th–6th) on the leading side, these fractures are caused by repetitive motion coupled with an imbalance between weak serratus and rhomboid musculature. Diagnosis is made clinically and with bone scan for confirmation. Treatment is conservative with relative rest, technique modification, and appropriate conditioning.

Sternum. Sternal injuries are uncommon and result from a direct blow. Sternal fractures require significant force and usually occur in a transverse fashion at the junction of the manubrium. Diagnosis can be difficult to make either clinically or with typical radiographs (lateral sternal view) so CT scanning is recommended. If this injury is detected or suspected, consider possible injury to the heart, aorta, and underlying bronchus. Treatment for nondisplaced sternal fractures is nonsurgical, while displaced fractures should be treated with surgical reduction and fixation. Return to play with protection is as pain allows and with clinical and radiographic healing.

Sternoclavicular joint dislocations can occur either from a direct blow or indirectly with injury to the shoulder. Anterior dislocation is far more common than posterior dislocation, and though painful, is not a dangerous injury and can be treated conservatively. A posterior dislocation has significant potential for complications (disruption of the major vessels) and should be treated surgically. Diagnosis is usually straightforward; the area is quite painful, tender, and swollen, with an obvious deformity, abnormal motion, and crepitus at the joint.

Effort Thrombosis

Effort thrombosis can occur in either the subclavian or axillary veins from a repetitive overhead motion (eg, a baseball pitcher), or from a single trauma to the shoulder or clavicle. The athlete presents with diffuse aching pain and significant circumferential swelling in the arm with prominent veins and diffuse complaints of numbness and tingling in the limb. Imaging should include a chest x-ray to rule out a cervical rib and ultrasound/doppler. The gold standard is venography. Treatment of this injury includes rest, elevation of the arm, and anticoagulation with either standard or low molecular weight heparin therapy followed by long-term warfarin. Return to play can be problematic as there are frequent recurrences off anticoagulation. The exception may be when the condition is caused by compression of the vessels by a cervical rib or fibrous band that can be treated via surgical resection.

Pulmonary Injuries

Pneumothorax

Simple pneumothorax occurs when air enters the pleural space. This is a common injury and can result from blunt trauma, spontaneous rupture of a bleb, direct lung tissue injury secondary to rib fracture/puncture, and any injury to the trachea or esophagus. While a simple pneumothorax is usually not a life-threatening situation and will not progress, it can cause significant morbidity. Symptoms include tachypnea, dyspnea, and respirophasic chest pain. Diagnosis is made clinically by noting diminished breath sounds and hyperresonance to percussion on the side with the pneumothorax. While diagnosis is confirmed via a standard PA and lateral chest x-ray, further evaluation may be warranted with CT scanning. Treatment of a small pneumothorax (less than 20%) with minimal symptoms consists of careful observation and repeated chest films. For a larger (greater than 20%) pneumothorax, or those with significant symptoms, a tube thoracostomy with negative suction at 20 cm H_2O is the treatment of choice and can be discontinued once the air leak is resolved. The athlete can resume most activities once the pneumothorax is completely resolved. A return to contact/collision activities may warrant a delay of 2–4 weeks. Concerns have been expressed regarding returning to scuba diving and other activities that result in significant changes in barometric pressure. Typically these activities should be constrained only in those who have an underlying pulmonary etiology for their pneumothorax. The military allows a soldier to fly and return to full duty 2 weeks after a normal chest x-ray.

Tension Pneumothorax

Tension pneumothorax is rarely seen in athletics and represents a progressive accumulation of air in the pleural space, creating an increase in intrapleural pressure. This causes decreased venous return, which results in a clinical picture of neck vein distention and hypotension. The significant intrapleural pressure increase typically causes deviation of the trachea and a mediastinal shift that compresses the contralateral lung. Tension pneumothorax can be life threatening and treatment should be immediate decompression. This can be achieved on the sideline with needle aspiration via insertion of a large-bore needle in the second intercostal space in the midclavicular line. Definitive treatment is with a chest tube.

Hemothorax

Hemorrhaging from damage to arteries, aorta, or lung tissue into the pleural space is an uncommon injury in athletics and can prove to be a fatal injury. A large amount of blood can accumulate and there may be little external evidence that this injury has occurred, so there must be a high index of suspicion for this entity. Clinically, the athlete will present with tachypnea and dyspnea, and on the involved side decreased breath sounds and dullness to percussion. The injured athlete may quickly become hypotensive and will require immediate stabilization and transport to an emergency center. Imaging includes chest x-rays, or even better, CT scanning. Treatment includes replacing volume, supportive care, draining of the hemorrhage, and surgical repair of the torn vessels.

Pulmonary Contusion

Pulmonary contusions or "bruised lungs" represent hemorrhage and/or edema in the lung parenchyma and can occur through direct trauma, a deceleration type injury, or rib fracture. Children tend to be at higher risk for this as the elastic ribs may not fracture, thus imparting the force of the blow to the underlying tissue. Symptoms include cough, dyspnea, tachypnea, and often hemoptysis. Diagnosis is made both clinically and radiographically. On auscultation crackles and decreased breath sounds are appreciated over the injured area and the chest x-ray varies from a fluffy, patchy infiltrate to complete consolidation. Lung contusions are self-limited so treatment is conservative. Fluid intake should be limited to maintenance needs to avoid overload. If severe, the injury may warrant ventilatory support. Return to play is advanced as tolerated by the athlete. There are few complications from this injury.

Cardiac Injuries

Commotio Cordis

Commotio cordis is an almost always fatal arrhythmia that occurs from a low-energy direct blow to the anterior chest, and is typically a result of being stuck by a moving projectile such as a baseball, hockey puck, or lacrosse ball, or it can be seen with player contact. While the mechanism is unknown, it is probably a form of ventricular fibrillation that occurs secondary to disruption of the cardiac cycle by impulses from the blow. In pigs, a baseball striking the chest at 40 mph over the left ventricle during depolarization of the T wave will uniformly induce fatal arrhythmias. Diagnosis of commotio cordis is based on observation of the mechanism of the injury, followed by sudden collapse and a subsequently unresponsive and pulseless athlete. Treatment may not be effective, but one should immediately and aggressively pursue CPR and ACLS protocols. A primal thump to the sternum may be effective.

Myocardial Contusion

Myocardial contusion, while still an unusual injury, is being seen with increasing frequency. The mechanism of injury is similar to that of commotio cordis, typically from a direct blow or perhaps from a rapid deceleration. A wide spectrum of injury can be observed and while significant cardiac events are rare, they do occur. Histologically the injury pattern is similar to that observed in myocardial infarction. Various forms of arrhythmias often occur within the first 24–48 hours after injury. Diminished cardiac output and pericardial effusion are natural consequences of myocardial contusion and may lead to cardiac tamponade. Clinically the athlete complains of chest pain and presents with dyspnea and tachycardia and possibly an overlying sternal injury. Management includes obtaining an electrocardiogram (which usually will demonstrate an ST injury pattern, particularly with severe injuries), a CPK-MB (not particularly sensitive for contusion), and echocardiographic and nuclear scans, which while useful to define the extent of the injury, will not necessarily predict the outcome. Fortunately the vast majority of cardiac contusions seen in athletes will be self-limited, though these individuals should be monitored closely for several days on telemetry. Return to play is gradual when there are no abnormal ECG, echocardiographic, or laboratory findings, and the athlete is asymptomatic, usually in about 4–6 weeks. Left ventricular aneurysms can be a late sequela of this injury.

UNUSUAL COMPLICATIONS OF THORACIC TRAUMA

The sideline physician must always be aware of a number of somewhat uncommon though potentially devastating thoracic injuries. Great vessel injury can occur either from blunt or penetrating trauma, and can lead to significant morbidity with a high degree of mortality. Thus one must have a high clinical suspicion for disruption of the great vessels, particularly when fracture to the first three ribs, sternum, or thoracic spine are encountered. Chylothorax may occur as a rare complication from blunt trauma and may be associated with thoracic vertebral fractures. Diaphragmatic injury should be suspected in a high force blunt injury or penetrating injury below the 6th rib. Finally, tracheobronchial injuries (also rare) can be life threatening and require urgent treatment. In all of these injuries, while the urgency is somewhat greater than the injuries previously discussed, the same basic approach to evaluation and triage should be employed. The sideline physician must be well versed in the trauma ABCs and have a plan for rapid assessment and transport of these injured athletes.

ABDOMINAL INJURIES

The first step in assessing an abdominal injury is, as always, to note the mechanism of injury, proceed with the standard ABCs of trauma, and then through a step-wise examination that includes inspection, palpation, percussion, and auscultation. Particularly with abdominal trauma, close observation and repeat examinations can be invaluable in determining the progression of intra-abdominal injury. The most common reason for missed diagnosis in abdominal trauma is the failure to follow the athlete with serial exams, depending solely on the initial findings and clinical impression.

The first distinction to make is whether an injury is to the abdominal wall only or whether there is intra-abdominal damage. Abdominal wall contusions and strains are common, often painful, and present little risk to the athlete. A distinguishing characteristic of abdominal wall injuries is focal pain that increases with tensing of the muscles. Occasionally there may be a significant hematoma in the rectus or the deep posterior muscles such as the psoas or iliacus. In these cases, a CT scan may be useful to distinguish these from an intra-abdominal process. Intra-abdominal processes result in a variety of additional findings. For instance, intra-peritoneal bleeding from solid organ damage to the spleen, kidney, and liver (more common than hollow organ damage) result in irritative peritoneal findings. A ruptured viscus causes severe pain which is almost always referred and results in "surgical abdomen" with boarding, guarding, and rebound tenderness. Retroperitoneal bleeding can be substantial but may not result in peritoneal findings. Finally, in female athletes, one must always consider the possibility of pelvic organ damage and/or pregnancy.

Spleen

The spleen is the most commonly injured solid organ. The risk of injury is increased with splenomegaly, for instance secondary to mononucleosis. Injuries occur from a blow to the left upper quadrant, particularly those resulting in a lower rib (10th–12th) fracture, or from a sudden deceleration. Splenic injury ranges from bruising or hematoma through mild to severe lacerations to disruption of the vascular pedicle. Clinical findings are somewhat nonspecific. The abdomen will be painful and tender, Kerr's sign (shoulder pain secondary to diaphragmatic irritation from blood) may be present, and the athlete will be tachycardic and tachypneic, and may progress to hypotension and shock. The best radiographic imaging test to assess the potentially injured spleen is a CT scan. Most of these athletes can be managed nonoperatively if clinically stable and the CT scan does not worsen. This requires bed rest and careful monitoring over 5–10 days in the hospital with serial CT scans. Up to 90% of children and 70% of adults can be conservatively managed. Operative management is recommended if the athlete is unstable, there is a pedicle injury, or with failure of nonoperative management. There is some debate over whether to repair the injury or perform splenectomy. This determination can usually be made within the first several days. Return to play is likewise controversial. When to exercise, and how hard, depends on the severity of the injury, and the clinical course will dictate an individual athlete's status. Most would recommend a minimum of 3–4 months out of sports for conservatively managed athletes. If splenectomy is the route taken, typically 6–8 weeks will suffice.

Hepatobiliary Injury

The gallbladder is well protected and rarely injured. When injured, this organ will usually present with peritoneal signs and require cholecystectomy. The liver is more commonly injured, ranging from minor contusions to life threatening exsanguination from lacerations. The liver is well protected, but a direct blow to the side or back and fractured ribs (10th–12th) or a rapid deceleration mechanism should raise suspicion for liver trauma. The signs, symptoms, and examination findings are not specific or reliable. The athlete will complain of pain and tenderness in the right upper quadrant and often have referred right shoulder pain. Nausea and vomiting may be associated symptoms, along with intraperitoneal signs, and eventually, hemodynamic instability.

Evaluation should include serial exams with any suspicion of liver damage leading to immediate transport to an emergency facility. While CT scanning can help quantify the injury, it may not be useful in clinical decision making, and determining operative versus nonoperative treatment is based on clinical status. Nonoperative management is recommended if the athlete is hemodynamically stable and without evidence of peritoneal signs, other abdominal injury, or associated head injury. This consists of bed rest, serial CT scanning, and monitoring laboratory values, and is as with splenic injury, often more successful in children. Operative treatment is undertaken if there is severe injury. An unstable patient with peritoneal signs or concomitant closed head injury makes assessment difficult. Return to play is controversial with no evidence-based data to guide decisions. For minor injuries such as contusions or subcapsular hematomas, the athlete may be able to return to play about 1 month after resolution of CT findings. With a severe injury there is no consensus, and many would advocate no return to contact or high-risk sports.

Pancreatic Injuries

These are uncommon injuries which can be quite severe and are typically caused by a direct blow, such as from a bicycle handlebar or a kick in martial arts. Signs and symptoms include mid abdominal pain that radiates through to the back with peritoneal findings. Conservative management is often successful and the need to undertake surgery depends on the integrity of the pancreatic duct. As with all intra-abdominal injuries, CT scanning is the imaging modality of choice. Return to play can be entertained when the athlete is asymptomatic with a normal examination and laboratory results.

Hollow Viscus Injury

Injury to the hollow organs in the abdomen is fortunately extremely rare. Typically these are seen from rapid deceleration in augmented speed sports or from a crush injury. The range of injuries to the hollow organs includes contusions, hematomas, and (rarely) ruptures. The milder injuries can be difficult to diagnose, but management is conservative and return to play is acceptable when the athlete is asymptomatic.

When there is a rupture of a hollow viscus peritoneal signs will ensue, although they may be somewhat focal on examination. Immediate and early referral to the hospital for management is mandatory. Return to play after repair can usually be accomplished in 6–8 weeks time.

Kidney

The kidney can be injured from either single or repeated blows (eg, in boxing) to the flank. Children seem to be more susceptible to this injury due to the plastic deformation of the young rib. There is a wide range of kidney injury with contusions and hematomas representing the vast majority. Lacerations, with or without renal pelvic involvement, are the next most common injuries, and fortunately, vascular injuries are quite rare. The clinical presentation may be somewhat subtle with minimal presenting symptoms. While hematuria is common, it is not seen 100% of the time and is not reliable for diagnosis. The athlete may present with a flank mass, pain, tenderness, and ecchymosis. The more severe injuries present with tachycardia, hypotension, and gross hematuria. These unstable patients require immediate transport and hospital evaluation. The best imaging test for assessing these injuries is a CT scan, which allows one to distinguish between contusions, hematomas, lacerations, hilar injury, and to assess retroperitoneal bleeding. While many kidney injuries can be treated nonoperatively and will resolve within 6–8 weeks, operative management is required for the unstable athlete and most vascular injuries.

Nonoperative treatment is acceptable if the hematocrit and the athlete are clinically stable. Monitor with repeat CT scans and expect resolution for mild to moderate injuries within 6–8 weeks. Microscopic hematuria may persist for many weeks to months. Return to play with minor injuries can take place when the athlete is asymptomatic, usually in about 3 weeks. For more significant injuries the CT scan should normalize and there should be no sequelae.

Other Urologic Injury

Bladder

The most common type of bladder injury is a contusion which occurs from repetitive trauma such as the "kissing bladder" lesion common in runners. This presents as asymptomatic hematuria and resolves uneventfully within 24–48 hours; no evaluation is usually necessary. "Kissing bladder" is prevented by evacuating the bladder 15–20 minutes before running rather than immediately before a race or workout. Bladder contusion or laceration (very rare) can occur from blunt trauma in contact and augmented speed sports. These present with gross hematuria and significant pain. The diagnosis is best made with an intravenous pyelogram. Treatment is surgical.

Ureter

The ureter can be injured from a straddle-type injury seen in gymnastics and bicycling. Urethral trauma presents with gross blood at the meatus and penile or peritoneal hematoma. Diagnosis is made via retrograde urethrogram and treatment often requires stent placement, and on occasion, surgery.

BIBLIOGRAPHY

Amaral JF. Thoracoabdominal injuries in the athlete. *Clin Sports Med.* 1997;16:739–753.

Diamond DL. Sports related abdominal trauma. *Clin Sports Med.* 1989;8:91–99.

Ikonomidis JS, Boulanger BR, Brenneman FD. Chylothorax after blunt chest trauma: A report of 2 cases. *Can J Surg.* 1997;40:135–138.

Kshettry VR, Bolman RM. Chest trauma: Assessment, diagnosis, and management. *Clin Chest Med.* 1994;15:137–146.

Link MS, Wang PJ, Pandian NG, et al. An experimental model of sudden death due to low energy chest wall impact (commotio cordis). *N Engl J Med.* 1998;338:1805–1811.

Powell M, Courcoulas A, Garner M, et al. Management of blunt splenic trauma: Significant differences between adults and children. *Surgery.* 1997;122:654–660.

Ray R, Lemire JE. Liver laceration in an intercollegiate football player. *J Athletic Train.* 1995;30:324–326.

Ryan JM. Abdominal injuries and sport. *Br J Sports Med.* 1999;33:155–160.

Stricker PR, Hardin BH, Puffer JC. An unusual presentation of liver laceration in a 13 year old football player. *Med Sci Sports Exerc.* 1993;25:667–672.

van-Amerongen R, Rosen M, Winnik J, et al. Ventricular fibrillation following blunt chest trauma from a baseball. *Pediatr Emerg Care.* 1997;13:107–110.

19 | Wrist and Hand Injuries

C. Stewart Wright

QUICK LOOK

- Injuries to the wrist and hand are very common in sports
- They may be bony and/or soft tissue injuries
- Look for bony tenderness or deformity
- Splint and ice suspected injuries on the sidelines
- Reduce dislocations of digits as soon as possible after injury
- Watch out for scaphoid fractures; x-ray if at all suspicious
- Early unloaded range of motion is suitable for most digital fractures

Wrist and hand injuries are very common sports injuries and may be bony or soft tissue in nature. Bone and joint injuries include fractures, dislocations, and epiphyseal injuries. Ligaments and tendons may be partially or fully torn. While there are numerous mechanisms of injury, falling on the outstretched hand (FOOSH) is especially common and is often made worse if the player is holding something like a stick, racquet, or ski pole on impact with the ground. Injuries also occur when the hand is on the receiving end of a blocked shot, a kick, or a mishandled ball. Hand and wrist injuries may prove frustrating for players, trainers, and physicians due to difficulties in making a diagnosis and obtaining a successful outcome.

WRIST INJURIES

Bony injuries of the distal radius and ulna are usually secondary to considerable force such as that from a fall, flying off a speeding vehicle, or being struck with a stick. These may be extra-articular, the so-called Colles' fracture, or enter the joint. A high index of clinical suspicion is necessary and point tenderness over the distal radius is a fracture until proven otherwise. Impacted or undisplaced fractures may be amenable to functional bracing for 2–3 weeks. Whether intra- or extra-articular, the displaced injuries require accurate reduction. If a reduction cannot be maintained by closed means, then percutaneous pins or an open reduction may be necessary. Occasionally, external fixation may be needed and can be used alone or in conjunction with open procedures. These injuries will usually require up to 6 weeks in a cast. Although the fracture may heal in 6 weeks, full recovery may be protracted and often require considerable rehabilitation. It is not uncommon to see patients continue to gain range of motion, strength, and function for up to 18 months.

Fracture dislocations of the wrist may occur with a volar lip (Barton's fracture), dorsal lip (reverse Barton's), or radial styloid fracture (chauffeur's fracture). Closed reduction is usually possible, but maintenance of reduction often requires pins and/or plate fixation.

Distal radioulnar joint (DRUJ) injuries usually occur with rotational forces through the forearm. One should always examine the elbow to look for injuries to the radial head or proximal radioulnar joint. DRUJ injuries may result in subluxation or dislocation in either a dorsal or volar direction. This may be associated with a number of fractures including Colles', radial shaft, radial head, ulnar, and radial epiphyseal injuries. The joint itself may be involved with a variety of injuries, including fractures of the sigmoid notch of the radius, ulnar head fractures, cartilage injuries of the ulnar head, and ulnar styloid fractures. DRUJ instability will usually require a long arm cast for 4–6 weeks. Dorsal displacement is managed in full supination and volar instability is held in neutral rotation. Pin fixation across the DRUJ may occasionally be necessary.

Also at risk of injury is the triangular fibrocartilage complex (TFCC), including the articular disk or meniscus, dorsal and volar ligaments, and the ulnar collateral ligament. TFCC injury may occur in conjunction with other wrist injuries. Once the obvious acute injury has been diagnosed, there may be concern about damage to the TFCC. The pain is localized to the fossa just distal to the end of the ulna. Symptoms are usually provoked by fore-arm rotation as well as radial and ulnar deviation. A wrist arthrogram or MRI is helpful in diagnosing a full-thickness tear. If symptoms persist after a reasonable period of time (8–12 weeks), wrist arthroscopy may be considered. As in the knee, the meniscus may be arthroscopically debrided and occasionally repaired. Players usually return to sport in 2–3 weeks after arthroscopy, using a wrist support for comfort and protection.

Carpal injuries represent a wide spectrum of sprains, strains, flake fractures, and both undisplaced and displaced carpal bone fractures. The dorsum of the triquetrum is the most common flake fracture. There are reported cases of fractures to each of the carpal bones including the pisiform. Displaced scaphoid fractures and scapholunate dissociation with rotatory subluxation of the scaphoid are more severe injuries (Fig. 19-1). The worst injuries have a perilunate component. This represents an injury to the intrinsic and extrinsic ligaments that hold the scaphoid, lunate, triquetrum, and capitate together. These injuries may be a pure perilunate dislocation or they may be associated with a bony injury. The three most common are trans-scaphoid, transcapitate or transradioulnar. These will usually require open reduction and should be referred to a hand surgeon.

An often missed diagnosis is a fracture of the hook of the hamate. This is usually from a direct blow or load through a bat, golf club, hockey stick, or racquet. There is localized tenderness 2.5 cm distal to the pisiform on a line from the pisiform to the second metacarpophalangeal joint. Like undisplaced scaphoid fractures this injury may not be appreciated on plain x-rays. A specific hamate view may show the fracture (Fig. 19-2 and Fig. 19-3A). It may also be seen on a carpal tunnel view (Fig. 19-3B). If necessary, additional studies are used including bone scan, tomograms, or CT scans.

Hamate hook fractures are slow to settle and are not aided by a cast. They should be treated expectantly as there are reported cases taking up to 2 years to settle. Additional padding in the area may allow the athlete to return to competition once the acute pain has settled. Bicycle gloves are often a useful adjunct. If pain persists the hook fragment may be excised, but there is a risk of damage to the motor branch of the ulnar nerve.

Scaphoid fractures require special mention because they are frequently missed and may result in a nonunion. They are the second most common wrist injury, behind fractures of the distal radius. The typical patient is a young adult male who has fallen on his outstretched hand. The injury may initially be dismissed as a sprain or strain and not fully evaluated. Any athlete with pain in the anatomic snuffbox or over the scaphoid tubercle requires radiologic evaluation and presumptive casting for 2 weeks before assuming that the injury is not a fracture.

Routine wrist x-rays may miss the fracture and scaphoid views must be ordered (Fig. 19-4). If these are normal and clinical suspicion persists then

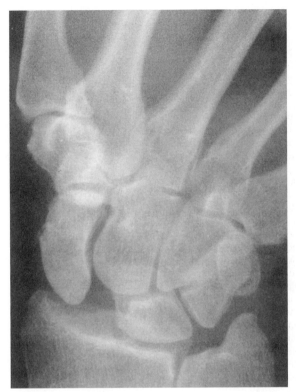

FIG 19-1   Scapholunate dissociation.

other studies are needed. A nuclear bone scan or tomograms may help in the diagnosis. A CT or MRI scan will usually provide a definitive answer. If the initial studies are normal but the athlete is very sore, then a splint is used for 2 weeks and the studies repeated.

The most common site of scaphoid fracture is through the middle third of the bone ("waist fracture"). The navicular blood supply circulates from the distal pole to the proximal pole, so the more proximal the fracture, the

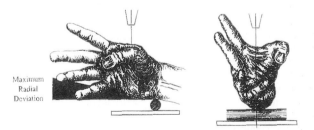

Maximum
Radial
Deviation

FIG 19-2   The forearm is in the neutral position. The wrist is maximally deviated, and the thumb is maximally opposed.

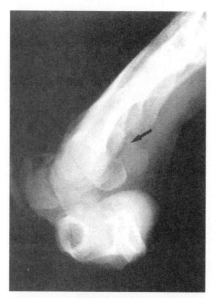

A

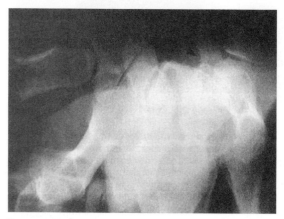

B

FIG 19-3 A. Hook of the hamate fracture. B. Carpal tunnel view with hamate hook fracture.

more likely that the circulation has been disrupted to the proximal pole (Figs. 19-5 and 19-6). A navicular fracture may also be associated with an unrecognized carpal instability.

Undisplaced fractures of the scaphoid can be managed in a scaphoid cast but may take 3–4 months to heal. If there is no sign of union by 3 months or if the fracture is displaced initially by more than 1–2 mm, then open reduction and internal fixation should be employed. As with wrist fractures

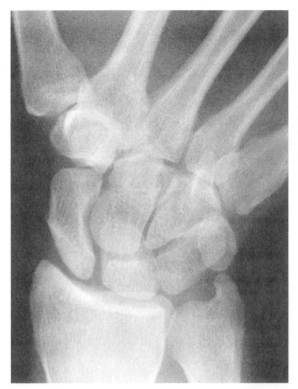

FIG 19-4   Scaphoid view with wrist in ulnar deviation.

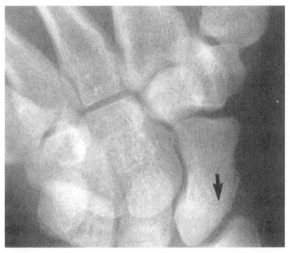

FIG 19-5   Fracture of the proximal pole of the scaphoid.

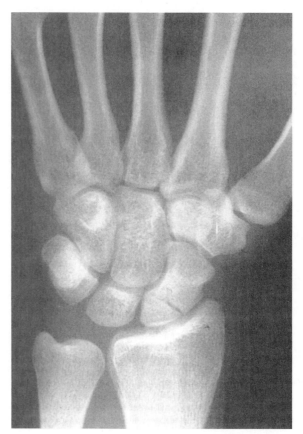

FIG 19-6 Fracture of the proximal scaphoid.

there is a long period of rehabilitation to regain motion and strength. The athlete may need to use a scaphoid splint upon return to sports until good function has been restored.

With longstanding nonunion of the scaphoid there is a high likelihood of osteoarthritis of the wrist. This may take 10–15 years to develop, but occurs in a predictable manner. It begins at the radioscaphoid joint initially and then at the capitolunate joint. This long-term complication can be avoided with increased vigilance in assessing the painful wrist in an athlete.

In the adolescent one needs to be aware of Salter type I epiphyseal injuries to the distal radius and ulna that are normal radiographically. It is a clinical diagnosis with tenderness just proximal to the radial or ulnar styloid. A splint or cast may be necessary as dictated by the severity of symptoms.

When one encounters a bony injury around the wrist, care must be taken to assess for any associated neurologic damage. The radial sensory nerve is at risk with direct trauma on the radial side of the wrist from stick slashing injuries in hockey or lacrosse. Median nerve dysfunction with an acute carpal tunnel syndrome may occur even with a simple undisplaced distal radius fracture. There may be damage to the ulnar nerve with injuries to the elbow or ulnar side of the wrist in hamate fractures. If there is neurologic injury associated with dislocation, the joint should be reduced as expeditiously as possible. Prophylactic median nerve release may be needed with the severe carpal injuries as there can be considerable swelling in the first 24 hours after injury. Either an open or arthroscopically assisted release of the carpal tunnel can be done. The complication rate is slightly higher with the closed techniques (neurologic and vascular), but it is purported to have less down-time for the patient.

Tendon injuries at the level of the wrist are uncommon, although there are occasional skate-related lacerations that involve the wrist tendons. More common is posttraumatic tendonopathies of the flexor carpi radialis, flexor carpi ulnaris, the first extensor compartment (deQuervain's), the radial wrist extensors, or extensor carpi ulnaris. These often prove slow to settle but usually respond to a combination of splinting, oral nonsteroidal anti-inflammatory drugs (NSAIDs), therapeutic modalities, stretches, and corticosteroid injections. Functional braces may allow athletes to continue playing while these conditions settle. Extracorporeal shock wave therapy may prove beneficial for these injuries in the future. A small percentage of patients may require surgical release of a tendinitis at the wrist.

The retinaculum surrounding the extensor carpi ulnaris may be disrupted when rotational force is applied to the wrist. This may happen with a shanked golf shot when the club strikes a root or rock (watch out for hook of the hamate fracture as well). If this results in subluxation of the tendon, reconstruction of the retinaculum may be necessary. Again, a functional brace may be needed to return to sports.

Over the last 10 years wrist arthroscopy has been playing an increasingly larger role in managing athletic injuries. It allows patients to return to sport more quickly than when open procedures are performed. Arthroscopy is used for both diagnosis and in treatment. It can be used as an adjunct to limited open reduction of a wrist fracture, intercarpal ligament reconstruction or percutaneous fixation of a scaphoid fracture. TFCC debridement or repair is also done arthroscopically.

It is not uncommon to see normal wrist x-rays and yet find pathology arthroscopically. Partial ligament tears, chondromalacia of articular surfaces, and synovitis of the joint can be diagnosed and debrided with use of the arthroscope. As in the knee, osteoarthritis of the wrist can also be treated arthroscopically with patients returning to sports in 2–3 weeks. A wrist support or taping may be necessary for the first few weeks and range of motion exercises may begin the day of the surgery.

HAND INJURIES

The vast majority of hand fractures seen in the athlete (up to 90%) can be handled by closed means. The goal is for early unloaded range of motion of the digits within 1 week of the injury. This helps to lessen swelling and prevent joint and tendon adhesions. Extension block splinting, buddy taping (adjacent finger strapping), and the use of Coban and unloaded range of motion exercises are used to achieve these objectives.

Fractures in the hand may be oblique, transverse, or comminuted (Fig. 19-7). Excessive shortening must be avoided (especially with the proximal phalanx), or the extensor mechanism will not function properly.

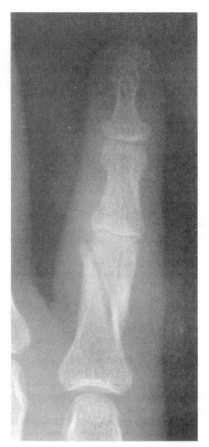

FIG 19-7 Oblique fracture of the proximal phalanx.

Malrotation and excessive angulation must also be corrected (Fig. 19-8). With the metacarpophalangeal (MCP) and proximal interphalangeal (PIP) joints in flexion, rotation is checked by ensuring that the nail plate points toward the scaphoid tubercle. When obvious malalignment of a digit is seen on the playing field it should be gently realigned and taped to the adjacent digit.

With metacarpal neck fractures (boxer's fracture) up to 35–40° of volar angulation may be accepted in the fourth and fifth metacarpal. This relates to mobility of the subjacent carpometacarpal (CMC) joints. Less angulation is acceptable as metacarpal fractures become more proximal. No more than 15–20° is acceptable with the second and third metacarpals. Many metacarpal neck fractures are stable and can be managed with early motion, buddy taping, and a compressive bandage to help with the swelling. Unstable fractures may require pin fixation and a gutter splint.

Many phalangeal fractures are stable in flexion and unstable in extension. If a stable range can be established then extension block splinting using buddy taping allows motion through that range. Position of the fracture should be

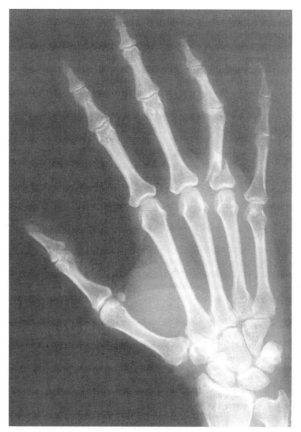

FIG 19-8   Proximal phalanx fracture with malrotation.

checked weekly with an x-ray over the first 3 weeks. A fracture that is unstable through all ranges or has an intra-articular component may require operative fixation. Range of motion is started once stability has been obtained.

Most displaced hand fractures can be reduced under a digital or metacarpal block. Gentle traction will usually allow correction of the deformity. If successful reduction cannot be either obtained or maintained, then open reduction or percutaneous pinning may be necessary.

Crush injuries of the fingertip are often associated with a fracture, and most are amenable to a splint. If the nail is avulsed it can be replaced to act as a splint. A laceration of the nail bed with a bony injury represents a compound fracture. This should be managed with thorough debridement and antibiotic coverage. The nail bed may also require repair with a fine absorbable suture. The nail may be replaced to splint the nail bed while it heals.

Dislocation may occur in any of the joints in the hand. They are usually in a dorsal direction and can often be reduced on the playing field by applying traction to the digit. Occasionally soft tissue becomes interposed in the joint, making reduction difficult. This can occur at the MCP level with the flexor tendons or at the interphalangeal level with a volar plate caught in the joint. Dorsal MCP joint dislocations are often difficult to reduce when the volar plate is caught behind the joint, or the lumbrical muscle and flexor tendon are by the metacarpal head, and such injuries may require general anesthesia with operative intervention. Dislocations are also managed with early unloaded range of motion employing buddy taping and occasionally extension block splinting. CMC joint dislocations may be unstable and require pin fixation.

Ligament injuries are very common at both the MCP and interphalangeal joint level. It is useful to think of these joints as a box with four sides. These sides include the volar plate, radial and ulnar collateral ligaments, and the extensor mechanism. Each structure can be palpated and stressed in turn to assess for injuries. If the injury site is too painful for an adequate examination of the support structures, a digital block may be necessary, but the sensory integrity of the distal finger should be documented prior to anesthesia. At the MCP joint the collateral ligaments are in maximum tension with the joint in flexion, and are tested in this position as well as in extension.

MCP injuries to the collateral ligaments and volar plate are often slow to heal and may require long-term use of buddy taping. Volar plate injuries may need extension block splinting. The thumb MCP ulnar collateral ligament (UCL) injury is referred to as a "ski-pole" or "gamekeeper's" thumb. Ski poles with strap bindings are a common source of injury, although it can occur with any FOOSH injury.

Sprains of the UCL of the thumb are managed with a removable splint and early unloaded range of motion. The splint is discontinued once local discomfort has settled. Much of the hand surgery literature suggests that completed UCL tears require surgery, but general experience supports the use of closed treatment using 3–4 weeks in a short arm- or hand-based thumb spica cast followed by a removable thumb spica splint. The exception is the grossly unstable joint, which was likely a dislocation and represents damage to more than the UCL. A large bony fragment will usually render the joint unstable and require repair. Whether UCL injuries are treated operatively or with casting/splinting, the athlete may need to use prophylactic splinting or taping once they resume their sporting activities.

Boutonniere injuries occur at the PIP finger joint with a disruption of the central slip of the extensor tendon mechanism as a result of longitudinal force to the finger such as that from a basketball that is miscaught. Once the central slip is disrupted, the lateral bands may sublux volarly and result in a PIP flexion deformity. There may also be a secondary hyperextension deformity of the distal interphalangeal joint (DIP). If the injury is appreciated initially, the PIP joint is splinted in extension for 6–8 weeks and the DIP joint left free for motion. Often this injury is overlooked or does not fully develop for 10–14 days. If the athlete presents with a PIP flexion contracture, dynamic splinting is used during the day and static splinting at night. Prophylactic splinting is used at sport until the injury has completely healed, which may be 6 months or longer. A late boutonniere may not respond to splinting alone and may require surgical repair. This involves release of the collateral ligaments and volar plate. The lateral bands are released and moved dorsally, and the central slip of the extensor is reconstructed. Six months of splinting and therapy may be needed for a successful outcome.

At the DIP joint, injury to the extensor mechanism results in a mallet finger. This may be an injury to the tendon alone, involve a bony fragment, or go through the epiphysis in the adolescent athlete. Most of these are managed with splinting unless the bony fragment renders the DIP joint unstable. Full-time splinting of the DIP joint in full extension for 6 weeks results in successful tendon healing for the vast majority of cases. Night splinting is continued for a further 3–4 weeks. A delay in treatment for up to 6 weeks may still result in a favorable result as long as there is an inflammatory reaction over the DIP joint when the splinting is commenced, but may require up to 6 months of splinting. A late mallet finger can be reconstructed by removal of an ellipse of skin and tendon dorsally (tenodermatodesis). The defect is closed to correct the flexion deformity and the DIP joint pinned for 6 weeks. A protective splint is employed for a further 6 weeks for sports.

A more serious tendon injury is the "rugger jersey" or "jersey" finger. This is an avulsion of the profundus tendon from the distal phalanx. The ring finger is most commonly involved, because it is functionally the longest finger when the hand is in a reaching and grasping position. The injury usually occurs when the opponent's jersey is tightly gripped and is forcibly pulled away. This results in forced extension of the digit while the flexor profundus is maximally contracted. The tendon may be avulsed or a fragment pulled off of the distal phalanx. Commonly, the tendon retracts to the PIP level but may end up in the palm. The injury is often not initially appreciated. Ideally it is repaired within 10 days, although success is possible up to 8 weeks post-injury. If seen several months later, the profundus stump may be excised and the DIP joint fused if unstable. Restoration of tendon function at that time often requires a two-stage tendon reconstruction with significant down-time from sport.

The extensor expansion is a retinaculum that stabilizes the extensor tendon over the MCP joint. This structure may be forcibly disrupted (typically the radial side) with subluxation or dislocation of the tendon in an ulnar direction. These occur most commonly in the index and long fingers. Patients present with swelling, pain, and complaints of weakness. They may also be aware of the tendon snapping over the metacarpal head as the joint is flexed. A minor disruption is managed by buddy taping and it may be slow to settle. Most will require surgical reconstruction of the radial sagittal band.

Ring avulsion injuries occur when a ring catches on something while the athlete is pulling away or falling. They run a spectrum from a crush of the soft tissues to amputation. Any suggestion of circulatory compromise should be referred to a hand surgeon. Rings should not be allowed in competition and practice when there is an obvious risk for this injury. An athlete who insists on wearing rings while competing should be encouraged to purchase a breakaway-type of ring to minimize the occurrence of this injury.

Human bites can also occur to the hand and wrist. These can happen when the hand ends up in an opponent's face or mouth. The typical injury is over the dorsum of the MCP joints. These wounds require thorough debridement, should be left open, and require antibiotic treatment as prophylaxis for infection.

INVESTIGATION OF WRIST AND HAND INJURIES

Routine radiographs are usually adequate to evaluate injuries to the distal radius, ulna, carpal bones, metacarpals, and phalanges. When the injury is more complex, a CT scan may be necessary. It is particularly helpful when

TABLE 19-1 Imaging for Hand and Wrist Injuries
Osseous trauma
  Distal radius/ulna
    Routine radiographs
    CT for complex injuries
    MRI for soft tissues
  Carpal bones
    Routine radiographs
    CT for complex injuries
    MRI for AVN
  Metacarpals, phalanges
    Routine radiographs

Soft tissue injuries
  DRUJ subluxation
    CT
  Ligament and wrist capsule
    Arthrography or MRI
  Muscle, tendon, nerve
    MRI

evaluating the DRUJ. MRI is useful in the assessment of soft tissue injuries such as to ligament, capsule, muscle, tendon, and nerve. It is also helpful to examine bone marrow with problems such as avascular necrosis (AVN) or infection. Wrist arthrography is used in the evaluation of capsular and ligamentous injuries such as to the scapholunate ligament or the TFCC. Table 19-1 summarizes when these investigations are employed.

20 | Knee Injuries

Peter G. Gerbino

QUICK LOOK

- Traumatic effusion indicates internal derangement and hemarthrosis.
- Immediate sideline examination is frequently the best examination.
- Consider injuries to be medial, lateral, patellofemoral, or global.

INTRODUCTION

Injuries about the knee are most easily diagnosed by a careful history. If there was a specific traumatic event, it means that all overuse injuries are immediately excluded. Likewise, if there was no acute trauma, the injury is unlikely to be a meniscus tear or ligament rupture, except in older athletes with degenerative menisci that can tear with a seemingly innocuous load and twist maneuver.

EPIDEMIOLOGY

The knee is one of the most commonly injured joints among athletes. It accounts for the majority of injuries that require surgery in a sports medicine practice. Each sport has its own incidence of knee injury that varies with intensity, age, and gender. Sports with high levels of traumatic knee injury are football, soccer, and basketball. Anterior cruciate ligament (ACL) tears occur 4–10 times more often in female soccer and basketball players than in males (Moeller et al., 1997). Sports with high numbers of overuse injuries to the knee include track, soccer, and swimming (breast stroke).

PATHOPHYSIOLOGY

Each specific knee injury has its own mechanism of occurrence and underlying risk factors. These variables are useful for both diagnosis and injury prevention. For example, ACL injuries are known to increase as the coefficient of friction between the athlete's foot and the playing surface increases (Powell et al., 1992). Similarly, patellofemoral pain and other anterior knee pain increase as cyclic loading and extensor mechanism loading increase (Brechter et al., 2002).

TRAUMATIC INJURIES

A direct blow to the knee, or more often, an indirect load to the knee leads to injury. The key aspects of the history when there has been trauma are (1) mechanism of injury, (2) whether or not a "pop" was heard or felt, and (3) the rapidity of swelling (minutes to hours). Valgus stress to the knee causes stress to the medial collateral ligament (MCL), compression to the lateral knee (bone bruises), and if great enough, stress to the ACL. Valgus stress with twisting adds the possibility of a lateral meniscus tear.

Varus stress stretches the lateral collateral ligament (LCL) and compresses medially leading to bone bruises. If there was a rotational component, the medial meniscus may be torn. Hyperextension stresses the posterior capsule and ACL. Posterior translation to the tibia (such as a fall from a horse) can cause posterior cruciate ligament (PCL) injury.

259

Hearing or feeling a "pop" will most often indicate an ACL tear. A tearing sensation is typically associated with MCL, LCL, or meniscal injury. A "pop" followed by a second "pop" is usually patella dislocation followed by relocation. When swelling and pain occur rapidly and prevent return to play, a torn ACL is most often the cause. A patella dislocation or osteochondral fracture can cause similar rapid bleeding. Swelling that is unilateral is usually MCL or LCL. Slow (8–12 hours) of swelling is more common with a meniscus tear.

With the history concluded, the injury will have been isolated to the medial, lateral, or patellofemoral compartment of the knee, and strong suspicion of the specific injury or injuries should be present.

Evaluation

If the patellofemoral joint is suspected, palpation for a defect in the medial retinaculum, a positive patella lateral translation apprehension test, or pain with anteroposterior loading of the patella is found. Examination of the medial compartment of the knee after trauma focuses on the MCL, medial bones, and medial meniscus. MCL tears are more painful at the femoral or tibial attachment, rather than over the joint line. Valgus stress will be painful medially and the knee will gap open variable amounts depending on severity. Comparison to the contralateral side is frequently necessary.

Medial joint line pain can indicate meniscus tear or bone bruise. If meniscal stress tests such as the McMurray test or hyperflexion with tibial rotation test are painful, meniscal tear rather than bone bruise is more likely.

Lateral compartment injuries include LCL, lateral bone bruises, and lateral meniscus injury. LCL injuries are more painful at the attachments rather than midjoint and may gap with varus stress. Meniscus versus bone bruise can be difficult to differentiate, but meniscus stress tests can help. Magnetic resonance imaging (MRI) is definitive.

Whenever there is medial or lateral compartment injury, the cruciates should be tested and consideration given as to whether the posteromedial or posterolateral corners have been injured. The ACL is tested by translating the tibia anteriorly with the knee slightly flexed (Lachman test) (Torg et al, 1976). The PCL is tested by posterior translation with the knee flexed 90° (posterior drawer) or quadriceps activation when the tibia is posteriorly subluxated (Daniel, 1988). A variety of tests exist to assess the posterior corners. All involve techniques that check for increased anteroposterior translation combined with internal rotation (lateral corner should be tight if intact) or external rotation (medial corner should be tight if intact). Careful comparison to the contralateral side is necessary with these tests.

Imaging studies of the acutely injured knee almost always include plain radiography. Anteroposterior, lateral, tunnel, and patellofemoral (sunrise/skyline/Merchant) views are obtained. If necessary, MRI can provide detail about the ligaments, meniscus, and bone bruising or occult fracture not visible with any other study (Fig. 20-1A–E).

MANAGEMENT OF TRAUMATIC INJURIES

Meniscus

Few meniscal tears heal of their own accord. Repair within a few weeks of injury, resecting only portions that are not repairable is recommended.

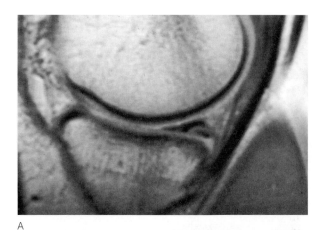

A

B

C

FIG 20-1 MRI images of acute knee pathology. **A.** Posterior horn medial meniscus tear. **B.** Complete ACL tear. **C.** Bone bruise to lateral femoral condyle.

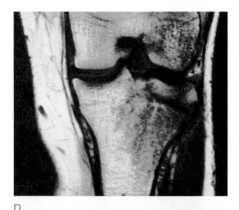

D

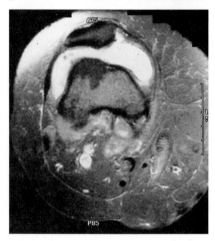

E

FIG 20-1 *(Continued)* **D.** Occult fracture of tibial plateau.
E. Hemarthrosis, medial retinacular defect, and lateral femoral condyle bone bruise following patella dislocation.

A locked knee that will not fully extend usually indicates a large ("bucket-handle") tear incarcerated in the joint centrally. These should be reduced if possible by widening the joint space of the affected side (varus or valgus stress) and gently flexing and extending the knee with internal or extended rotation of the tibia. Failure to unlock the knee is cause for more urgent operative intervention (DeHaven et al., 1994). Following meniscal repair, the athlete is kept out of competition for a minimum of 4 months, during which the repair matures and the muscles are rehabilitated.

Anterior Cruciate Ligament

Initial management includes removal from the field and thorough ligament assessment before swelling becomes severe. Waiting longer than 1 hour may be too long to get an accurate exam. It may then take 2 weeks for the swelling to subside enough to get another accurate exam. In athletes at the professional or Division I level, ACL reconstruction surgery is sometimes performed within 48 hours to minimize atrophy and stiffness. For others, the decision must be made whether or not to reconstruct the ligament and therapy is undertaken to resolve swelling and restore range of motion prior to surgery. Indications for surgery are high demand activity, concomitant meniscal repair, or instability despite adequate rehabilitation.

Ideal graft selection is controversial with evidence that patella tendon and hamstring autografts and various types of allografts can all be effective in appropriately selected patients (Malinin et al., 2002; Marder et al., 1991; Pinczewski et al., 2002). Standard rehabilitation is 6 months; however, some 4-month protocols are being used (Howell et al., 1996). There is no lower age limit for ACL repair. Near maturity, soft tissue grafts through the physes are used and at younger ages, physeal sparing techniques are used successfully (Bisson et al., 1998). No young athlete should be left with an unstable knee in order to delay surgery (Millet et al., 2002).

Posterior Cruciate Ligament

The isolated PCL tear does not necessarily need to be reconstructed (Keller et al., 1993). Instability and pain despite rehabilitation or combined injuries are indications for surgery. An allograft is usually utilized and rehabilitation is similar to that for ACL reconstruction.

Medial and Lateral Collateral Ligaments

Collateral ligament tears range from minimal strain to complete rupture. Complete MCL and LCL tears can be managed nonoperatively, but when combined with other instabilities may require repair (Indelicato, 1983). An isolated MCL or LCL tear is managed by symptomatic treatment of pain and swelling with rest, ice, compression, and elevation. A hinged knee brace to prevent varus or valgus motion in the early weeks of healing is used for all collateral ligament sprains. A hinged knee brace with a 15–30° extension block to check full extension in the early weeks of healing has been used successfully for more severe tears with the intention of healing the ligament "short" to prevent laxity. Both methods work in practice and neither is evidence based. The key to rapid recovery and return to full function is protecting the ligament from a second stretch injury during the healing process. The athlete can return to sports in a hinged brace as soon as comfort allows. Complete healing is usually achieved within 6 weeks for mild to moderate sprains, and full tears may take up to 12 weeks.

Lateral compartment injuries that involve the posterolateral corner of the knee in addition to the LCL require surgical repair to avoid instability after the LCL heals. These structures are frequently injured when the LCL is completely disrupted. A complete tear of the MCL is more forgiving and will usually heal without instability.

Knee Dislocation

A knee dislocation is an emergency because of the high incidence of arterial injury (Welling et al., 1981). The patency of the popliteal artery is assessed and plans made to address all torn ligaments. Timing of the repairs is controversial and no consensus exists as to whether to repair every structure. Direct repair is performed on all injured structures using allograft for structures without sufficient native tissue. Post-operative stiffness can be a problem in these patients and early motion is mandatory (Noyes et al., 1997).

Patella Dislocation

There are two types of lateral patella dislocation. The most common type occurs in adolescent females with generalized ligament laxity. They are more likely to have patella alta and a history of patellofemoral syndrome (PFS) (Atkin et al., 2000). The dislocation typically occurs with a change of running direction and minimal trauma. The patella can spontaneously reduce and swelling is moderate. Treatment is symptomatic using ice, compression, and a lateral buttress brace or knee immobilizer. Physical therapy is begun to decrease swelling and restore quadriceps balance. These patients are cautioned that an already unstable patella is now more unstable and may require operative realignment if subluxation recurs.

The second type of athlete sustaining patella dislocation is more often male and has taken a direct blow, driving the patella laterally. These athletes have a larger hemarthrosis and more pain. A medial retinacular defect is sometimes palpable and radiographs frequently demonstrate the presence of medial avulsion fracture at the patella or an osteochondral fracture at the patella distal pole or lateral femoral ridge. Fragments usually require operative repair or excision and the patella retinaculae should be rebalanced. Quadriceps strength is slow to recover after these injuries and may take 3–6 months to match the contralateral side.

Osteochondral Fracture

A final acute injury to the knee is the osteochondral fracture. This will present with an acute hemarthrosis and possibly a locked knee. Physical examination may be very difficult if the knee is locked and radiographs will show the fragment. Treatment is urgent operative repair of the fragment if possible, excision if not. Depending on the size of the defect, further cartilage restoration procedures might be necessary later on.

The majority of traumatic knee injuries can be sorted out rapidly and accurately. The comfort level of the examiner and availability of subspecialty care will determine whether to treat locally or refer. An algorithm for managing acute hemarthrosis is provided (Fig. 20-2).

OVERUSE INJURIES

A practical way to think about overuse knee problems is to decide whether or not the injury is related to the extensor mechanism. Extensor problems include patellofemoral syndrome (PFS), quadriceps tendinitis, patellar tendinitis, apophysitis of the patella (Sinding-Larsen-Johansson syndrome), or apophysitis of the tibial tubercle (Osgood-Schlatter syndrome). Other overuse problems include iliotibial band (ITB) syndrome, pes anserine bursitis, osteochondritis dissecans (OCD), and osteoarthritis.

Extensor Mechanism Overuse

Extensor mechanism problems are extremely common and differentiating among them is the source of much frustration among practitioners. Perhaps the easiest way to approach extensor mechanism problems is to first establish that the problem is from overuse and then search for focal tenderness.

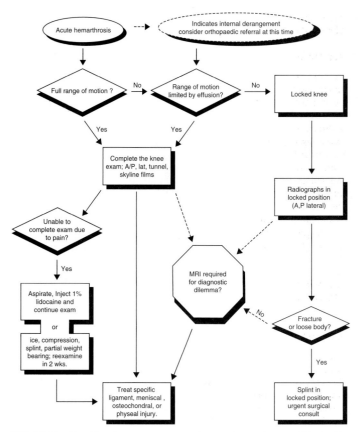

FIG 20-2 Algorithm for management of acute hemarthrosis. (Used with permission from Gerbino et al., 1996.)

Increased anterior knee pain with running, climbing stairs, or after prolonged sitting is the classic history. Focal tenderness is usually found with antero-posterior loading of the patella, at the distal pole of the patella, in the region of the medial plica, and along the nonarticular medial femoral condyle. Less often, the lateral retinaculum, patella tendon, or tibial tubercle will be tender. A lateral apprehension test to try to dislocate the patella can help determine if pathologic lateral tracking is present. A variety of other signs can indicate if the patella is tracking laterally, but lateral tracking per se has never been directly shown to cause PFS; more likely it is one risk factor for PFS. Despite the fact that the essential lesion in patellofemoral syndrome is unknown, certain interventions are known to help. Quadriceps strengthening (Kannus et al., 1994), physical therapy intervention (Crossley et al., 2002), and hamstring stretching are the standard interventions known to help decrease pain. Many other interventions are less well proven. If there is patella maltracking, McConnell taping (Crossley et al., 2002) or bracing can be helpful. Over 1–3 months, flexibility and strengthening are maximized. If pain persists and maltracking is present, lateral retinaculum release has

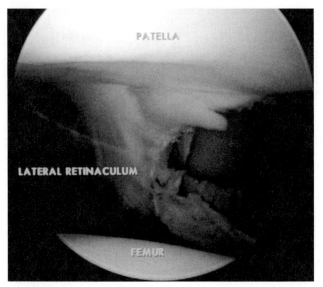

FIG 20-3   Arthroscopic photograph demonstrating lateral retinacular release for patellar lateral tracking.

been shown to help (Micheli et al., 1981; Fig. 20-3). If a painful plica is present, it can be removed at the same time.

Osgood-Schlatter apophysitis occurs when the tibial tubercle apophysis in an immature athlete becomes painful. Most feel that this represents a stress fracture to the physeal cartilage and will heal with rest. Ensuring adequate flexibility and quad strength are felt to be protective. An algorithm for managing anterior knee pain is provided (Fig. 20-4).

Other Overuse Knee Injuries

Osteochondritis dissecans is another condition that occurs in the immature athlete. Its etiology is unknown, but the condition is felt to be subchondral stress fracture from overuse in a predisposed bone (Campbell et al., 1966). The medial femoral condyle is most often involved and is tender to palpation. Both radiographs (Fig. 20-5) and MRI (Fig. 20-6) are needed for full assessment. Treatment depends on stage of injury. Intact, stable lesions are treated with relative rest to the area. This has been accomplished several ways including activity modification, bracing, and casting. For stable lesions that fail to heal or for unstable lesions, surgical evaluation and repair is necessary (Fig. 20-7). Irreparable lesions are treated with microfracture of the base (Steadman et al., 1997) or with cartilage regeneration techniques.

Iliotibial band (ITB) syndrome is a bursitis or tendinitis of the posterior band of the ITB at the lateral knee. Sometimes confused with lateral meniscus or ligament pathology, ITB syndrome will have occurred atraumatically. Sometimes the athlete will have a recent history of downhill running, but more often no specific cause is found. A tight ITB is found with the Ober test (Fig. 20-8). The inferior ITB at the knee is tender to palpation.

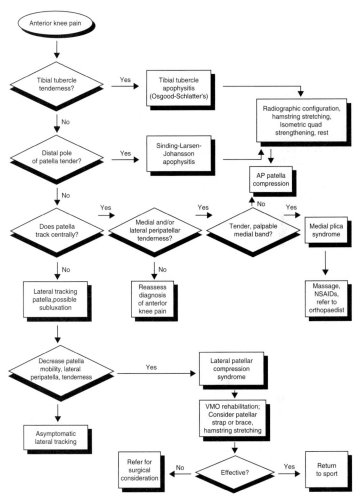

FIG 20-4 Algorithm for evaluation and management of anterior knee pain (Used with permission from Gerbino et al., 1996.)

Treatment includes rest, ITB stretching, and a general pelvic and lower extremity strengthening program. Oral nonsteroidal anti-inflammatory drugs (NSAIDs) can help, as can a local corticosteroid injection to the bursa just deep to the ITB. Severe, persistent ITB syndrome can sometimes require release of the posterior band at the knee.

Pes anserine bursitis is an inflammatory problem that occurs with excessive hamstring use. Pain and swelling can be seen and palpated at the pes anserine attachment medially on the proximal tibia. Like ITB syndrome, NSAIDs and corticosteroid injection can be helpful. Lower extremity stretching and core strengthening are utilized. Surgery is rarely indicated.

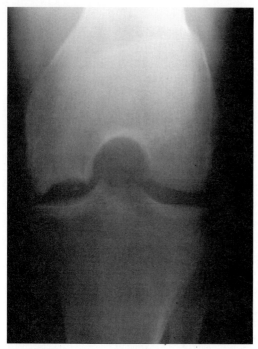

FIG 20-5 Radiograph demonstrating osteochondritis dissecans (OCD) of the medial femoral condyle.

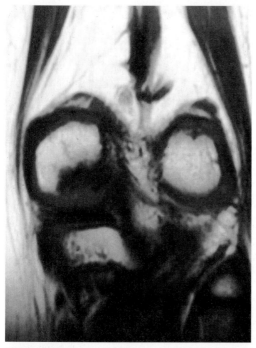

FIG 20-6 MRI of OCD of the medial femoral condyle.

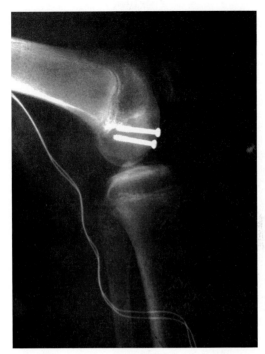

FIG 20-7   Radiograph of OCD repair using cannulated screws (screws are removed before weight-bearing is permitted).

Osteoarthritis can occur in the posttraumatic knee or idiopathically in predisposed individuals. Early on, pain with activity, morning stiffness, and weather-related pain are common. Infection and other types of arthritis are excluded. Radiographs may be normal or show early degenerative changes. Treatment requires stabilizing an unstable knee, consideration of osteotomy for severe varus or valgus, consideration of meniscal transplantation if postmeniscectomy, and use of glucosamine sulfate, activity modification, and hyaluronate injections.

CONFOUNDING CONDITIONS

Occasionally an athlete presents with persistent knee pain and no obvious diagnosis. Rheumatoid arthritis, Lyme disease, infection, and neoplasm should be considered in these cases. Laboratory analysis including CBC, differential, ESR, CRP, rheumatoid factor, anti-nuclear antibody, and Lyme titer will identify some; others are diagnoses of exclusion. Neoplastic processes are rare, but both benign and malignant lesions can present as overuse knee pain (Fig. 20-9).

PREVENTION

Improved strength training, field conditions, equipment, coaching, and adherence to the rules of play can decrease traumatic injuries. Overuse injuries are prevented in the same way, but more important is being aware

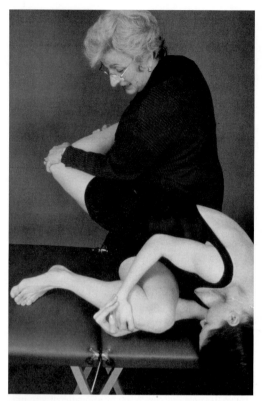

FIG 20-8 The Ober test places the iliotibial band on tension to assess relative tightness. The knee should come to the midline without pelvic motion if the ITB has no excessive tightness.

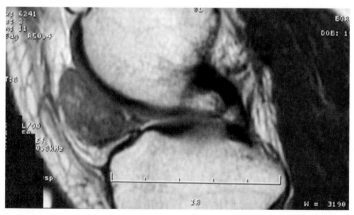

FIG 20-9 Gadolinium-enhanced MRI of the knee demonstrating benign tumor at the anterior fat pad causing patellofemoral pain.

that they can and do occur. Preparticipation screening can identify athletes at risk for both types of injury (Goldberg et al., 1980). The ideal prevention strategy is to identify the specific risk factors for each injury in each sport and devise specific interventions.

SIDELINE TIPS

- A "pop" indicates ACL tear or patella dislocation.
- Examine the knee immediately on the sideline.
- Have crutches available for acutely injured players.
- Have a system in place for rapid diagnosis and treatment.

SUMMARY

Sports injuries to the knee are common. Traumatic injuries frequently require consideration of operative repair. Atraumatic pain usually indicates extensor mechanism overuse. Breaking the knee down into the medial, lateral, and patellofemoral compartments and systematically evaluating the structures in each compartment eases analysis. Treatment and rehabilitation are injury specific and constantly evolving. Prevention requires knowing the specific etiologic factors for a specific injury in a particular individual.

REFERENCES

Atkin D, Fithian D, Marangi K, Stone M, Dobson B, Mendelsohn C. Characteristics of patients with primary lateral patellar dislocation and their recovery within the first 6 months of injury. *Am J Sports Med.* 2000;28:472–479.

Bisson L, Wickiewicz T, Levibson M, et al. ACL reconstruction in children with open physes. *Orthopedics.* 1998;21:659–663.

Brechter J, Powers C. Patellofemoral stress during walking in persons with and without patellofemoral pain. *Med Sci Sports Exerc.* 2002;34:1582–1593.

Campbell C, Ranawat C. Osteochondritis dissecans: The question of etiology. *J Trauma.* 1966;6:201–221.

Crossley K, Bennell K, Green S, Cowan S, McConnell J. Physical therapy for patellofemoral pain. A randomized, double-blind, placebo-controlled trial. *Am J Sports Med.* 2002;30:857–865.

Daniel D. Use of the quadriceps active test to diagnose posterior cruciate-ligament disruption and measure posterior laxity of the knee. *J Bone Joint Surg.* 1988;70A:386–391.

DeHaven K, Aronoczky S. Meniscus repair: Basic science, indications for repair, and open repair. Rosemont, IL: American Academy of Orthopaedic Surgeons; 1994. Schafer M, ed. Instr Course Lect; No. 42.

Gerbino P, Micheli L. The lower extremity. In: Scuderi G, McCann P, eds. *The Pediatric Athlete.* Philadelphia, PA: Elsevier Science; 1996.

Goldberg B, Saraniti A, Whitman P, et al. Pre-participation sports assessment: An objective evaluation. *Pediatrics.* 1980;66:736–745.

Howell S, Taylor M. Brace-free rehabilitation, with early return to activity, for knees reconstructed with a double-looped semitendinosus and gracilis graft. *J Bone Joint Surg.* 1996;78A:814–823.

Indelicato P. Non-operative treatment of complete tears of the medial collateral ligament of the knee. *J Bone Joint Surg.* 1983;65A:323–329.

Kannus P, Niittymaki S. Which factors predict outcome in the nonoperative treatment of PF pain syndrome? A prospective follow-up study. *Med Sci Sports Exerc.* 1994;26:289–296.

Keller P, Shelbourne K, McCarroll J, Rettig A. Nonoperatively treated isolated posterior cruciate ligament injuries. *Am J Sports Med.* 1993;21:132–136.

Malinin T, Levitt R, Bashore C, Temple H, Mnaymneh W. A study of retrieved allografts used to replace anterior cruciate ligaments. *Arthroscopy.* 2002;18:163–170.

Marder R, Raskind J, Carroll M. Prospective evaluation of arthroscopically assisted anterior cruciate ligament reconstruction. Patellar tendon versus semitendinosus and gracilis tendons. *Am J Sports Med.* 1991;19:478–484.

Micheli L, Stanitski C. Lateral patellar retinacular release. *Am J Sports Med.* 1981;9:330–336.

Millet P, Willis A, Warren R. Associated injuries in pediatric and adolescent anterior cruciate ligament tears: Does a delay in treatment increase the risk of meniscal tear? *Arthroscopy.* 2002;18:955–959.

Moeller J, Lamb M. Anterior cruciate ligament injuries in female athletes. Why are women more susceptible? *Physician Sports Med.* 1997;25:31–48.

Noyes F, Barber-Westin S. Reconstruction of the anterior and posterior cruciate ligaments after knee dislocation. Use of early protected postoperative motion to decrease arthrofibrosis. *Am J Sports Med.* 1997;25:769–778.

Pinczewski L, Deehan D, Salmon L, Russell V, Clingeleffer A. A five-year comparison of patellar tendon versus four-strand hamstring tendon autograft for arthroscopic reconstruction of the anterior cruciate ligament. *Am J Sports Med.* 2002;30:523–536.

Powell J, Schootman M. A multivariate risk analysis of selected playing surfaces in the National Football League: 1980–1989. An epidemiologic study of knee injuries. *Am J Sports Med.* 1992;20:686–694.

Steadman J, Rodkey W, Singleton S, et al. Microfracture technique for full thickness chondral defects. Technique and clinical results. *Oper Tech Orthop.* 1997;7:300–307.

Torg J, Conrad W, Kalen V. Clinical diagnosis of anterior cruciate instability in the athlete. *Am J Sports Med.* 1976;4:84–93.

Welling R, Kakkasseril J, Cranley J. Complete dislocations of the knee with popliteal vascular injury. *J Trauma.* 1981;21:450–453.

21 | The Athlete's Arthritic Knee

Glen Richardson and William D. Stanish

Athletics are an integral part of life for many people. It is well known that physical activity confers longevity and a sedentary lifestyle is associated with an increased mortality rate. With increased societal awareness of the benefits of physical activity, a new group of athletes with unique problems is beginning to emerge, the masters athlete (senior runners: over 35 years; masters runners: over 40 years; this varies from sport to sport). One of the medical problems that aging athletes must face is osteoarthrosis of the knee. This condition can be very disabling, thus discouraging a healthy physically active lifestyle. Unfortunately, osteoarthrosis of the knee is a chronic disease affecting the social and psychological well-being of an athlete. Therefore it is imperative that the sports medicine physician be adept at diagnosing and treating osteoarthrosis of the knee.

THE SCIENCE OF OSTEOARTHROSIS

The knee is often thought of as a simple hinge joint, but it is really an unconstrained joint with a number of complex movements. There are many structures that support the knee joint, and any abnormalities of these structures can result in disability. In osteoarthrosis, the soft tissues of the knee joint are involved, but the key pathologic process is loss of articular cartilage. To fully understand the pathologic process occurring in osteoarthrosis, it is necessary to know about normal articular cartilage.

Articular cartilage is connective tissue with unique mechanical properties created by its biologic structure. Articular cartilage consists of two components, cells and extracellular matrix. Chondrocytes are the cell type found in articular cartilage. They are responsible for the formation and maintenance of the extracellular matrix that forms the articular cartilage. Since the articular cartilage is a relatively avascular environment, the chondrocytes receive most of their metabolic requirements from the synovial fluid. The low oxygen tension of the articular cartilage forces the chondrocytes to rely mostly on anaerobic metabolism. Chondrocytes have been shown to replace degraded matrix and remodel the articular surface. Chondrocytes have a number of important functions in growing children, but in the aging athlete, function is restricted to the degradation and synthesis of the extracellular matrix. The interactions between chondrocytes and the articular cartilage are controlled in part by cytokines such as IL-1, TGF-β, and IGF-1. Science has shown that with aging, the ability of chondrocytes to synthesize certain proteoglycans and respond to stimuli such as growth factor decreases. The inability of the chondrocytes to maintain the homeostasis of the articular cartilage leads to degeneration.

The extracellular matrix is composed of fluid and various macromolecules. Approximately 80% of articular cartilage is water. It is the interaction of water with the macromolecules that determines the structure and properties of articular cartilage. The structural macromolecules of articular cartilage include collagen, proteoglycans, and noncollagenous proteins. Collagen is the main structural element of articular cartilage. Type II collagen forms 90–95% of collagen found in articular cartilage. Type IX collagen is felt to form covalent bonds in the extracellular matrix. Type XI collagen also forms covalent bonds to type II collagen. Both of these collagens are thought to

273

provide stabilizing crosslinks within the extracellular matrix. Type VI collagen is found concentrated around chondrocytes and may help their attachment to the matrix.

Proteoglycans are another important component of articular cartilage. It consists of a protein core that is attached to glycosaminoglycan chains. The most common glycosaminoglycan chains include hyaluronic acid, chondroitin sulfate, and dermatan sulfate. The two main classes of proteoglycans are the large aggregating proteoglycan monomers called aggrecans, and the small proteoglycans, such as decorin, biglycan, and fibromodulin. There is little data on noncollagenous proteins. Research suggests that along with glycoproteins they help to stabilize the extracellular matrix.

Articular cartilage is not a homogenous layer of extracellular matrix and chondrocytes, but instead has distinct zones. There are four histologically different layers in articular cartilage. Zone 1 is the superficial layer. This very thin layer is relatively acellular and its composition creates its resistance to shear forces in joints. In addition, it may also filter the influx of fluid from the synovium, thereby shielding the articular cartilage from the immune system. Zone 2 is the transitional zone. The tide mark separates the middle, or zone 3, from the fourth zone of calcified cartilage. Zone 4 is a thin zone of calcified cartilage which separates the uncalcified zones from the subchondral bone.

There is an important interrelationship between chondrocytes and the matrix. The matrix filters nutrients, waste products, cytokines, and synthesized molecules that all have effects on chondrocytes. Thus any stimulus that affects the matrix will have indirect effects on chondrocytes, thereby allowing the chondrocytes to respond to stimuli affecting the matrix.

DEVELOPMENT OF OSTEOARTHROSIS

The primary derangement of osteoarthrosis of the knee is the degradation of articular cartilage. The loss of articular cartilage leads to changes in the subchondral bone, with sclerosis and osteophyte and cyst formation. Furthermore, all tissues of the knee are involved in osteoarthrosis, including the synovium, ligaments, capsule, and muscle. The soft tissue contractures and muscle weakness from inactivity result in the clinical picture of osteoarthrosis, with pain and loss of function.

The earliest histologic change in articular cartilage is the fraying or fibrillation of the superficial zone. With time and further degeneration of the matrix, clefts develop in the articular cartilage. These eventually extend through the transitional zone to the subchondral bone. The formation of clefts and fibrillation causes instability of the articular cartilage. Consequently, fragments of the cartilage are liberated into the joint. Eventually all the articular cartilage is removed, leaving eburnated bone.

This progression of articular cartilage failure occurs at the molecular level, and is divided into three stages. The first stage involves an increase in the water content of the matrix with a decrease in the aggrecan concentration. There is also a decrease in the length of the glucosaminoglycans. At this point there is no change in the collagen composition. It is felt that the increase in water content decreases articular cartilage stiffness and thus makes it more likely to fail. The second stage involves the chondrocyte response to stress on the matrix. The increased anabolic and metabolic activity of the chondrocytes in the second stage allows the matrix to withstand the forces of degradation. Eventually, the chondrocytes fail to respond to the changes in the matrix and the third stage develops. The chondrocytes are unable to maintain homeostasis, and the balance shifts in favor of matrix destruction.

Hyaline cartilage becomes degenerative principally under two conditions. The first is hyaline cartilage overload. In situations of disturbed joint mechanics such as genu varum, hyaline cartilage degeneration can occur depending on the degree of exogenous demand. Following the initial blistering, the joint surface progresses to frank erosion with eburnation if the mechanical disturbance is not rectified. The second condition is hyaline cartilage underloading. Although unusual, the situation of persistent underload can offer an unfavorable situation for hyaline cartilage survival. This situation occurs far less frequently than overload, but does require the same type of mechanical adjustment.

PRIMARY AND SECONDARY OSTEOARTHROSIS

The classification of osteoarthrosis is based on the presumed etiology. Primary osteoarthrosis is the most common, when the condition is idiopathic with no known cause. Inflammation is not an important component of primary osteoarthrosis, and the inflamatory processes associated with osteoarthritis may be due to release of crystals from the affected cartilage. Secondary osteoarthrosis occurs when the etiology can be identified. The secondary causes of osteoarthrosis are varied and should be addressed in the athlete. Intra-articular fracture, high-intensity impact joint loading, ligament injuries, dysplasia of the joint, and aseptic necrosis, to name a few, have been identified as causes of osteoarthrosis. Identification of a secondary cause may initiate treatment before the development of end-stage osteoarthrosis.

EVALUATION OF THE MASTERS ATHLETE

As always, a thorough history is necessary when evaluating the aging athlete. The physician must be aware of the secondary causes of osteoarthrosis, other causes of a painful knee, and any comorbid medical conditions. A careful history helps to discriminate conditions such as rheumatoid arthritis, seronegative arthropathies, or crystalline disease. Typically the patient with osteoarthrosis of the knee will complain of pain with activity and decreased range of motion. Quite often, patients will complain of pain localized to one particular region of the knee, often the medial joint. There may be a history of knee effusions, but not to the extent found in other inflammatory conditions.

The physical examination of the painful knee provides invaluable information for diagnosis and treatment. It is important to determine the alignment of the knee as altered joint mechanics play a significant role in the development of osteoarthrosis. Furthermore, treatment options may depend on the alignment of the knee. For example with genu varum, the medial compartment of the knee must be unloaded. The physical exam should identify any ligamentous instability, which may be found in the masters athlete with a chronic anterior cruciate ligament deficiency. The presence of a significant effusion may suggest inflammatory disease or infection. A sterile aspiration of the effusion should be performed if there is any doubt in a diagnosis.

Plain x-ray films of both knees in the standing position (AP and intra-condylar notch views) provide information regarding the integrity of the joint space. The amount of articular cartilage can be evaluated by measuring the joint space on the standing films. Bony changes of osteoarthrosis are evident, such as sclerosis, cysts, and osteophytes.

NONINVASIVE THERAPY

Nonsteroidal Anti-inflammatory Drugs

Certainly osteoarthritis of the knee in an athlete can be quite painful and relief of this pain is one of the chief reasons for seeking medical attention. For many years the first line of medical analgesia has been nonsteroidal anti-inflammatory drugs (NSAIDs). This family of drugs is very effective in reducing inflammation and pyrexia, but the main role of NSAIDs in OA of the knee is analgesic except for the periodic flares associated with a crystal-induced inflammatory response. The anti-inflammatory effect is accomplished through NSAID interference with cyclooxygenase. This enzyme catalyzes the reaction that synthesizes cyclic endoperoxidases from arachidonic acid. These are the precursors to prostaglandin. There are COX 1 and COX 2 NSAIDs on the market that are useful in treatment of osteoarthritic pain, but the COX 2 medications are expensive and are used only after the COX 1 alternatives have failed.

Prostaglandins

Prostaglandins D_2, E_1, E_2, and F_2 are major components in the acute inflammatory response to trauma. They cause dilation of blood vessels and leakage of fluid into the surrounding tissues. The amount is usually much more than the body needs for healing, and this results in significant pain. NSAIDs have an antiprostaglandin effect.

A number of studies have demonstrated the effectiveness of NSAIDs in the symptomatic treatment of osteoarthrosis of the knee. In a systematic review of randomized controlled trials of NSAIDs for treatment of osteoarthrosis, they were found to be superior to placebo in all short-term studies. Although there are more than 50 different brands of NSAIDs on the market, only 5 of 32 studies demonstrated any clinically significant difference between use of NSAIDs in osteoarthritis.

Despite the obvious effectiveness of NSAIDs for the treatment of the symptoms of osteoarthrosis, there are serious side effects associated with NSAID use. The most common complication is gastrointestinal (GI) problems. These can range from simple dyspepsia to severe bleeding or perforation. The symptoms of GI upset are often masked by other medications, including H_2 blockers, hydrogen ion pump blockers, or misoprostol. Other toxic side effects of NSAIDs include intestinal nephritis, hepatic dysfunction, allergic reactions, and drug interactions. It is important for physicians to remember that NSAIDs may be too costly for less affluent athletes. Ironically, certain NSAIDs may have deleterious effects on articular cartilage. In a randomized controlled study, indomethacin was shown to cause a significant decrease in joint space compared to placebo.

Some investigators have suggested the use of local NSAID gels instead of oral agents to avoid the most common side effects. In a randomized controlled clinical trial with 290 patients with osteoarthritis of the knee, there was no statistical difference between the active treatment groups and placebo. However, in patients with more painful osteoarthritis prior to treatment, both active intervention groups were statistically more effective than the placebo. The authors also found that GI reactions were three times higher with oral NSAIDs. Based on this evidence, certain athletes with painful osteoarthrosis of the knee may benefit from an NSAID gel.

Dimethylsulfoxide (DMSO) is a chemical solvent that is rapidly absorbed through the skin. Thus other chemicals can be transported into tissues adjacent to the knee joint, such as NSAIDs, local anesthetics, or corticosteroids. A 70% solution of DMSO has its own anti-inflammatory action. This is enhanced by the addition of Voltaren (diclofenac) and is available commercially as Dimethaide-D or Pennsaid. A daily or twice-daily application of 6–8 drops on the arthritic joint usually relieves pain and decreases swelling. DMSO is not approved for use in humans in the United States, but it is often used.

Acetaminophen

Acetaminophen is a first-line analgesic for pain control in OA of the knee and an important alternative to NSAIDs. This drug has a safer toxicity profile as compared to the NSAIDs. There have been a number of studies comparing the efficacy of acetaminophen to NSAIDs. Acetaminophen has consistently been shown to be superior to placebo. Furthermore, at a dose of 4 g/d, acetaminophen is equally effective as an analgesic dose of ibuprofen. A prospective randomized, controlled study found that after 6 weeks of treatment, acetaminophen and naproxen both caused a modest improvement in pain. The difference between groups was not significant. There was also a high drop rate in the study, suggesting that the long-term use of either drug for osteoarthrosis is not very successful.

Ultrasound

The high-frequency sound waves of ultrasound are felt to penetrate into the soft tissues surrounding the knee joint and facilitate pain relief and increased mobility. A randomized clinical trial was performed to examine this effect on patients with osteoarthritis of the knee. In this study patients were subjected to an exercise regimen, and a randomly selected group received ultrasound while the other group received a sham treatment. Although the treatment group did experience an improvement in pain, gait velocity, and range of motion, there was no statistical difference between the treatment and sham groups. The effect of the exercise program may have masked any benefits provided by ultrasound. Further research into ultrasound may prove it to be a useful modality.

Exercise

For the masters athlete with osteoarthrosis of the knee, continued participation in exercise may be perceived as worsening the condition. Research has not supported this opinion in all cases. There is evidence that repetitive, high-impact loading of the knee is a risk factor for the development and progression of osteoarthrosis of the knee. However, low-impact exercise may be beneficial. In a randomized controlled study examining the effect of exercise in 102 patients with osteoarthritis, the treatment group reported statistically significant improvements in pain and physical activity based on arthritis impact measurement scale (AIMS) tests. Walking distance improved in the treatment group compared to the control group as well. The benefits of aerobic activity for patients with osteoarthrosis have been reported elsewhere. These data suggest that the aging athlete should not completely stop physical activities, but may have to change to low-impact exercises to maintain physical and mental health.

Another important benefit of exercise is the maintenance of appropriate body weight. There is evidence that an increased body mass index (BMI) above normal can increase the risk for development of osteoarthrosis of the knee. Furthermore, weight loss may help decrease the symptoms of osteoarthrosis. Unfortunately, the once-active aging athlete can be trapped in a vicious circle of osteoarthrosis and decreased activity that leads to weight gain, which worsens arthritic symptoms.

Capsaicin Cream

Capsaicin is an extract from chili peppers that is used in a cream base and rubbed into the affected joint. The effect of capsaicin is felt to be its inhibition of substance P. In a randomized blinded study, 70 patients with osteoarthritis of the knee with moderate to severe pain were given 0.025% capsaicin cream or placebo every 4 hours. After 4 weeks there was significant improvement in visual analog pain scores as well as the physician's global assessment of pain. The most bothersome side effect is the burning sensation that occurs.

Laser Therapy

The use of laser therapy has been investigated for the treatment of osteoarthritis. Researchers found that patients receiving red and infrared radiation applied to the affected knee did better than placebo on visual analog pain scales and the short-form McGill pain questionnaire. How laser therapy exerts its effect is unknown. Beware of the laser, however, as there is concern over the use of the laser related to several cases with massive loss of articular cartilage and avascular necrosis of the femoral condyle following laser debridement.

Acupuncture

Once considered an exotic Asian therapy, acupuncture has recently gained considerable acceptance as a legitimate therapy. In a study of 40 patients with osteoarthritis, researchers compared the effect of acupuncture versus a sham acupuncture. All patients improved after 3 weeks, but none could be attributable to the traditional acupuncture.

Transcutaneous Electrical Nerve Stimulation

Transcutaneous electrical nerve stimulation (TENS) has been used in the treatment of various chronic pain conditions, including osteoarthrosis of the knee. There are some theoretical advantages of using TENS as opposed to medical therapy for pain because of its lack of toxic side effects. Published research has been divided on the benefits of TENS for osteoarthrosis of the knee. In one randomized study of 30 patients with a 12-month history of osteoarthrosis of the knee, both the TENS and sham groups reported pain relief. There was no significant difference between the two groups. Another study did find a clinically significant improvement in pain control; however, most of the pain relief occurred only when using the device. Researchers have compared TENS to naproxen in a clinical trial. There appeared to be no difference in the ability of TENS or naproxen to relieve pain. Nevertheless, a large placebo effect was found to be just as effective. TENS may be effective, but there has been no study with enough statistical power to demonstrate it.

Bracing and Wedged Insoles

Often the disease process in osteoarthrosis in the masters athlete involves only one compartment of the knee. Therefore any physical modalities that facilitate unloading of the involved compartment should improve pain and function. Both bracing and wedged insoles have been used to address the problem of mechanical malalignment in osteoarthrosis of the knee. The use of the Generation II knee brace was evaluated in 20 patients with medial compartment disease. Nineteen of 20 patients experienced pain relief and 17 of 20 had an increase in quadriceps muscle strength. Conclusions drawn from case series should be analyzed critically, but the use of proper bracing could provide enough relief to allow the aging athlete to continue active exercise. Lateral heel wedges have been evaluated as a treatment for medial osteoarthrosis of the knee. Theoretically the lateral heel wedge imparts a valgus stress across the knee joint, thus reducing the pressure through the medial compartment. In a study of 149 patients with medial osteoarthrosis, lateral heel wedges were more effective in patients with mild to moderate osteoarthrosis than in those with advanced changes.

INVASIVE THERAPIES

Intra-articular Corticosteroid Injections

Unlike diseases such as rheumatoid arthritis, osteoarthrosis often is not associated with significant inflammation. It is not surprising that the use of intra-articular steroid injections is associated with some debate. Deciding which patient should receive an injection can be difficult, as many predictors of inflammation are not predictors of a patient's response to the injection. Intra-articular methylprednisolone acetate has demonstrated a significant reduction in visual analogue pain scores at 3 weeks in a randomized study. It is important to note that research into steroid injections is associated with a large placebo effect. In a randomized controlled study of triamcinolone hexacetonide intra-articular injections in patients with osteoarthrosis, a statistically significant improvement was found only at 1 week, and thereafter placebo was just as efficacious. Based on these results, the sports medicine practitioner should use intra-articular steroids carefully as complications such as septic arthritis may be difficult to justify in a healthy athlete.

Intra-articular Hyaluronan Injections

In articular cartilage, aggrecan molecules bind to a chain of hyaluronate-forming macromolecular complexes that are immobilized within the articular cartilage. In osteoarthrosis it is hypothesized that the hyaluronate synthesized is abnormal, preventing aggregation, or there is rapid degradation of hyaluronate. The effect of injecting hyaluronan (hyaluronic acid derivative) into the knee joint is unknown. It is described as viscosupplementation and is thought to improve arthritic knees by increasing the viscosity of synovial fluid. A randomized placebo-controlled study of intra-articular hyaluronan injections found no difference between treatment and placebo groups at 20 weeks as both groups had improvement above baseline. Stratification of their results found a clinically significant improvement in pain in patients over 60 years of age with a number of symptoms. Although no significant side effects were reported in the study, the sports medicine physician should choose patients carefully for this treatment. The cost and multiple injections required may be inappropriate for most aging athletes.

ARTHROSCOPIC SURGERY

Surgical interventions often begin with arthroscopy in the masters athlete with osteoarthritis of the knee. The indications for arthroscopy in the older athlete include failure of conservative treatment or clinical suspicion of a mechanical derangement that is correctable with arthroscopy, such as a meniscal tear. Studies have shown patients with short duration of symptoms or mechanical symptoms of unstable meniscal tears or loose bodies will do better after arthroscopy. It is essential to have a candid discussion with older athletes about what can reasonably be expected from arthroscopy, as patients may have unrealistic goals for surgical results. Doctor Don Johnson says, "Some of my most unhappy patients in the past have been the middle-aged jocks with unrealistic expectations for an arthritic knee." Washout arthroscopy of the knee was recently shown to have no greater effect than a sham procedure. It was felt that lavage removed debris and inflammatory mediators from the joint. Arthroscopic partial meniscectomy in the degenerative joint can produce good results. This effect is especially true with acute tears. Degenerative tears are not as rewarding. A review of arthroscopic debridement studies found an average 68% good results and 32% poor outcomes at a mean follow-up of 35 months. Clearly the results of meniscectomy deteriorate with time.

Finally, arthroscopic debridement of the osteoarthritic knee can provide pain relief for the older athlete with obvious fibrillation of the articular cartilage with unstable edges. It is apparent that patients who have significant varus or valgus malalignment with medial or lateral compartment osteoarthritis have a worse response to arthroscopic debridement. The use of arthroscopy in osteoarthrosis of the knee is a purely palliative procedure, before more definitive surgery is required.

Arthroscopic Debridement of the Osteoarthritic Knee

Robert Jackson presented his results of arthroscopic debridement of the osteoarthritic knee (Jackson, 1995). He considers a debridement to be removal of all loose flaps of articular cartilage, trimming of a degenerative meniscus, and removal of symptomatic spurs. He feels that if in doubt, one should err on the conservative side of surgical excision.

The patients were divided into four categories (Table 21-1).

The patients in stages 1 and 2 had good results and were improved in the short term in 85%. At 3 years 60% of the patients were still enjoying good results. This makes it a reasonable procedure to offer patients. Stage 3 patients had only fair results and took a long time to rehabilitate. The patients in stage 4 had poor results. Thus the message is there is no benefit

TABLE 21-1 Four Categories of Arthroscopic Debridement

	Symptoms	X-Ray findings	Arthroscopic findings
Stage 1	Postexercise pain	Normal	Softening
Stage 2	Activity pain Taking NSAIDs	Decreased joint space	Fibrillation
Stage 3	Rest pain	Angular deformity	Fragmented
Stage 4	Limited function Decreased ROM	Severe changes Osteophytes	Erosion to bone

in arthroscopic debridement in the severe stage 4 patient. He found that abrasion arthroplasty was no better than joint lavage.

OSTEOTOMY

In patients over 30 and under 60 with a varus deformity between 2° and 15°, an osteotomy should be considered. The medial compartment collapse creates a varus (bowlegged) knee with constant medial pain and effusion. A valgus osteotomy is indicated when relief cannot be obtained by NSAIDs and physiotherapy, the patient's job is compromised, or if there is severe limitation in sports participation. The osteotomy is usually high tibial (HTO), but a low femoral procedure can be done when the deformity is in the femur. A small incision is used, and an oscillating saw removes a wedge from the bone. The lower tibia is straightened, closing the wedge against a medial periosteal hinge. Thus the weight-bearing forces are swung into the lateral compartment, unweighting the medial compartment. This can be held in place with staples or a plate and screws. Care is taken to avoid putting the knee into valgus. Results usually give the patient a good 5–10 years of comfort prior to a total joint replacement.

The procedure allows more vigorous sports participation and impacting than after a total joint replacement, because the natural femoral and tibial surfaces are still intact.

Operative complications should be discussed realistically with the patient (Petrie, 1996).

- Eleven percent of patients need revision at 7.5 years (Simurda, 1994)
- Nonunion occurs in 8% percent of cases
- Vascular injury may occur
- Intra-articular fracture occurs in 5–10%
- Peroneal nerve injury occurs in 6–10%
- Compartment syndrome may occur
- Deep venous thrombosis may occur

TOTAL KNEE ARTHROPLASTY

This procedure basically gives the patient a new knee. The patient ends up with a metal cap on the femur, a metal and polyethylene replacement of the proximal tibia, and a polyethylene cap on the patella. It is a good, well-engineered operation. The indications are the same as for an osteotomy: inability to function well on the job or in sports.

Usually the patients have to be over age 60 because the prosthesis only lasts 10–15 years depending on the amount it is used. Often the opposite or good knee and hip become painful from overuse and this provokes the patient to seek the surgery. The procedure, hospitalization, and physiotherapy are all much more prolonged than with an HTO.

TABLE 21-2 Complications of Arthroplasty

Intrinsic	Principles to avoid
Loosening	Overload of joint
Sepsis	Repetitive strain
Occult fracture	Impact more than body
Prosthesis failure	weight
Extrinsic	Lack of conditioning
Spine pathology	**Failure**
Bursitis tendinitis	Loss of implant fixation
Nonunion of osteotomy	Chronic pain
Neurologic lesions	Swelling of leg

The patient is hospitalized for 3–5 days on anticoagulants and antibiotics and may require an additional week of rehabilitation care. A continuous passive motion machine is used, although scientific results do not indicate significant long-term benefit. The first 2 days are quite painful in spite of a nerve block and use of patient-controlled analgesia. Complications are the same as in HTO plus loss of implant fixation and chronic pain and swelling of the leg (Table 21-2).

Postoperative manipulation under anesthesia is required in 15–21% of cases up to 8 weeks postoperatively. Indications include less than 75° flexion in 10 days and less than 110° flexion in 6 weeks. Patients can return to sedentary work in 6 weeks, moderately hard work in 10 weeks (i.e., orthopaedic surgery), and heavier work in 12 weeks.

The ultimate goal with activity is mild pain, mild swelling, no NSAIDs, no bracing, and range of flexion of 100–130° with a normal knee (good leg) flexion of 140°.

Patients with arthroplasty should be given antibiotics for all dental and surgical procedures, similarly to prosthetic heart valve patients. Physiotherapy in a clinic or at home should be done for 6 months. Strength improves up to 1 year. Home programs are effective up to 48 months after total hip or knee replacement. Return to sports depends on the preoperative fitness level of the patient (Table 21-3). Principles to avoid are:

TABLE 21-3 Categories of Sports for the Osteoarthritic Patient

Very good	With care—ask doctor
Stationary bike	Low-impact aerobics
Golf	Weight lifting (free or
Dancing	machines)
Walking	Stair master (quick short
Swimming	steps)
Good	Tennis doubles
Bowling	**Bad**
Cross-country skiing	All contact sports
Speed walking (4 mph)	Baseball, basketball,
No jogging or running	football, hockey,
Skilled sports	soccer, squash
Bicycling (street)	**Extreme**
Ice skating	Mountain bike riding
In-line rollerskating	Ski racing
Horseback riding	Horse jumping
	Dog sled racing
	Marathon cycling

- Overloading of joint
- Repetitive straining
- Impact more than body weight
- Lack of conditioning

Thus no running and jumping are allowed, because the load on the joint above the impact strength of the polyethylene leads to increased wear. Stress analyses indicate that the thickest polyethylene component possible be used.

REFERENCES

Jackson R. What works and what doesn't. *Pract Arthroscop.* 1995;1:33.

Petrie D. *Pract Arthroscop.* 1996;2:60.

Rudan JF, Simurda A. Valgus high tibial osteotomy. A long-term follow-up study. *Clin Orthop.* 1991;July:157–160.

Stiehl JB, de Amdrade JR, Activities after replacement of the hip and knee. *Ortho Spec Ed.* 1995;1.1:32.

22 | Knee Bracing

Neeru A. Jayanthi and Douglas B. McKeag

QUICK LOOK

- Five general classes of braces: Patellofemoral, prophylactic, functional, rehabilitative, and off-loading
- Evidence of efficacy is variable with some braces
- Patellofemoral braces provide some subjective improvement in anterior knee pain without significant objective findings (Finestone et al., 1993; Paluska et al., 1999b)
- Prophylactic bracing has not been effective for prevention of medial collateral ligament injuries (American Academy of Orthopedic Surgeons, 2002; Martin et al., 2001)
- Functional bracing can reduce translation at subphysiologic loads, but has not been consistently effective in clinical studies (Branch et al., 1989; Liu et al., 1995)
- Postoperative rehabilitative braces after ACL reconstruction have better knee rating scores at 3 months than nonbraced individuals, but also have increased thigh muscle atrophy (Risberg et al., 1999)
- Biomechanical gait studies demonstrate appropriate unloading of unicompartmental osteoarthritis in off-loading braces, but do not demonstrate postural control (Komistek et al., 1999)

INTRODUCTION

Injuries to the knee joint are common occurrences in athletes and numerous braces have been designed to prevent or modify injuries to the knee. Knee braces were originally introduced for postpolio patients during the first half of the century. Bracing also consisted of cumbersome knee-ankle-foot orthotics primarily used for severe degenerative or paralytic extremities (Wirth et al., 1990). Functional knee bracing for sports activities initially became popular in the late 1960s after a Lennox-Hill derotation brace was designed for Joe Namath after a serious knee injury. The emphasis on early return to play and prevention of knee injuries has grown exponentially over the years. Injuries to the knee are often minor, but a serious knee ligament injury can end an athlete's season and sometimes career. The American Academy of Orthopedic Surgeons (AAOS) held a consensus meeting regarding knee bracing in 1984 and categorized braces into prophylactic, functional, or rehabilitative (AAOS, 2002). Since then patellofemoral bracing has become more popular, and more recently osteoarthritis off-loading braces have entered the market. In this chapter, we will examine the biomechanical evidence for each type of brace, and the injuries each are intended to treat. We will also discuss appropriate evaluation of patients and clinical evidence regarding use of these braces (Table 22-1). Finally, red flag situations and practical tips as well as newer injury prevention programs will be presented.

PATELLOFEMORAL BRACING

Pathophysiology, Biomechanics, and Injuries

Patellar stability is achieved through a combination of three factors: dynamic stabilization, static stabilization, and geometric constraints. Dynamic stabilization is maintained by muscles such as the quadriceps, hamstrings, and

285

TABLE 22-1 Biomechanical and Clinical Evidence of Knee Brace Efficacy

Brace type	Biomechanical evidence	Clinical evidence
Patellofemoral	No change in patellar alignment seen radiographically PTO demonstrated improved alignment on kinematic MRIs	No decrease in patellofemoral symptoms Effective in prevention of anterior knee pain during high-intensity training
Prophylactic	No reduction in abduction angle in cadaveric studies Limited protection with surrogate knee model	No significant differences or decrease in MCL injuries for linemen, linebackers, and tight ends Increase in injuries in skill positions
Functional	Reduction in abduction angle in cadaveric studies Reduction in anteroposterior and rotational forces at subphysiologic loads	Subjective improvement in stability Ineffective in decreasing ACL strain in some studies
Rehabilitative (postoperative ACL)	Decreased anteroposterior translation and varus/valgus rotation	Improved knee ratings at 3 mo s/p ACL reconstruction No differences compared to nonbraced group at 2 y Increased thigh muscle atrophy with bracing
Off-loading braces	Increased intercondylar separation during heel-strike of gait	Improvements in 2-year outcome if BMI <25 and lower grade of osteoarthritis

Data taken from Albright et al, 1994a; Albright et al, 1994b; Baker et al, 1987; Barnes et al, 2002; Bengal et al, 1987; Cawley, 1990; Cawley, 2002; Cherf et al, 1990; Finestone et al, 1993; France et al, 1987; Hoffman et al, 1984; Jonsson et al, 1989; Komistek et al, 1999; Liu et al, 1995; Paluska, 1999b; Risberg et al, 1999; Ward et al, upcoming; Wojtys et al, 1996.

those that cross the knee joint. Static stabilization involves soft tissue structures such as the patellar retinaculum. Finally, geometric constraints related to bony anatomy hold the patella in its track. It is a common perception in the sports medicine community that lateral patellar tracking abnormalities contribute to patellar instability as well as patellofemoral pain (Arroll et al., 1997; Bockrath et al., 1993) Bracing has been designed to decrease the lateral tilt in static fashion, and more recently in a dynamic fashion, with a patellar tracking orthosis (PTO). Traditional patellofemoral braces have little biomechanical or radiographic evidence supporting their effectiveness (Paluska et al., 1999b). The goal of the PTO is to provide some patellar stability in its most vulnerable positions of 10–20° of knee flexion, as well as to decrease the contact forces of the patellar facets to reduce pain. In a recent unpublished study, kinematic MRIs on women with a history of patellar subluxation were performed while these individuals were wearing a PTO from 0–30° of knee flexion (Ward et al., upcoming). The PTO significantly reduced lateral patellar displacement as well as lateral patellar tilt as compared to controls and a more traditional patellofemoral brace.

The design of patellofemoral braces most commonly has a patellar cutout and lateral buttresses (Fig. 22-1). The newer patellar tracking orthoses

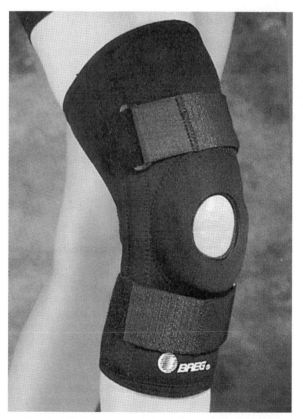

FIG 22-1   Patellofemoral brace with lateral buttress support. (Courtesy of Breg Inc., Vista, CA.)

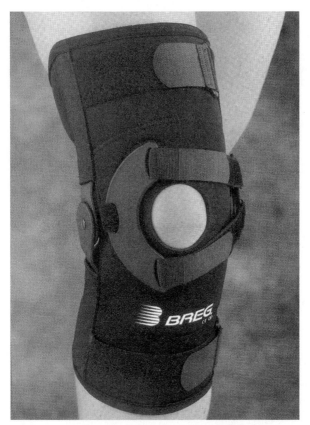

FIG 22-2   Patellar tracking orthosis (PTO). (Courtesy of Breg Inc., Vista, CA.)

include a single-hinge system to allow bilateral application of the brace and to control varus/valgus rotation (Fig. 22-2). They also incorporate a shell system, straps, undersleeve with lateral buttresses, and a hyperextension block to prevent subluxation as the knee approaches extension (Cherf, 1990). The greatest benefit of these braces is for patients who have demonstrable lateral tilt and displacement as well as increased patellar mobility.

Evaluation and Management

The clinical evaluation of a patient who has a history of patellofemoral pain with or without patellar instability primarily revolves around patellar alignment. Lateral patellar tilt, lateral patellar tracking with a positive J sign, and patella alta may increase patellofemoral symptoms and place an athlete at risk for lateral patellar instability. One should also look for genu valgum and recurvatum, excessive femoral anteversion, increased Q angle, hamstring tightness, iliotibial band tightness, hip-flexor tightness, SI joint dysfunction, and mobile pes planus, as they may all contribute to patellar instability and worsening anterior knee pain. Radiographic evaluation involves standing posteroanterior, lateral, and Merchant's views of the knee with evaluation for lateral patellar tilt, a shallow trochlear groove, and patella subluxation. A lateral knee radiograph taken with about 60° of flexion and additional hyperextension views may also demonstrate patella alta or patella baja.

An athlete who presents with classic patellar instability and/or patellofemoral knee pain should first be treated with the appropriate activity and training error modifications, regular icing, short course anti-inflammatory drugs for pain, and correction of biomechanical predispositions via devices such as foot orthoses for pes planus. Appropriate rehabilitation should include closed kinetic chain exercises and stretching for flexibility about the knee. Lastly, for athletes who develop symptoms only during activity, McConnell taping may be an inexpensive alternative for weight-bearing exercise periods. Although there has been much anecdotal success from patellar taping, there is still a lack of convincing biomechanical and clinical evidence (Bockrath et al., 1993).

If these treatments are not adequate, patellofemoral bracing may be a consideration as adjuvant treatment if there are patellar malalignment issues. Unfortunately, clinical evidence supporting the effectiveness of treatment of patellar instability or anterior knee pain with bracing has not been seen (Finestone et al., 1993). Bengal and colleagues (1987) found a knee brace with a silicon patellar support ring to be effective in *prevention* of anterior knee pain in athletes involved in a strenuous physical training course. This prospective trial with nonbraced individuals as controls demonstrated that the incidence of anterior knee pain increased as the intensity of exercise increased, and that a reduction in the incidence was achieved statistically by males who wore braces. Clinical studies involving the PTO are still in progress. If the decision is made to wear a patellofemoral brace or PTO, it may be worn during sports and other activities, and also during normal weight-bearing daily activities if still symptomatic. Additional reported benefits are increased proprioception and warmth by compression (Paluska et al., 1999b). Surgical alternatives such as medial realignment procedures for recalcitrant patellofemoral pain and patellar instability do exist. These should be reserved for those patients who have been compliant with the above treatment plans and are still symptomatic, but yet did attain some temporary relief with medially directed forces by taping or bracing.

PROPHYLACTIC BRACING

Pathophysiology, Biomechanics, and Injuries

There is a 44–64% chance of knee injury over 4 years for college football players, with the MCL being by the far the most commonly injured part of knee anatomy (Hewson et al., 1986). Medial collateral ligament injuries may take up to 12 weeks to heal, which may be a significant portion of a player's season, while an anterior cruciate ligament injury quite often ends a season for most players. The original design of prophylactic braces was to prevent MCL injuries from a valgus force on the knee and to support the cruciate ligaments from rotational forces. The large lever arm would prevent excess joint line opening during valgus stress, and subsequent injury to the medial collateral ligament (Fig. 22-3). This concept has not been supported in biomechanical studies. Baker and associates (1987) demonstrated that abduction forces at 0°, 15°, and 30° of knee flexion applied to cadaver knees with

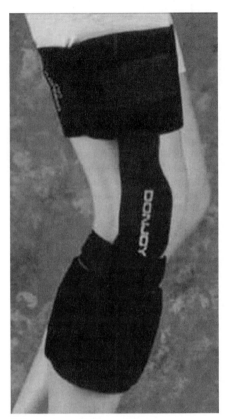

FIG 22-3 Prophylactic brace.

prophylactic braces did not demonstrate a reduction in the abduction angle. A cadaveric study by Paulos and coworkers (1987) showed similar results with no significant protection documented using two different types of prophylactic braces. Part II of this study demonstrated that MCL protection was provided by lateral knee bracing on a surrogate knee model in limited situations (France et al., 1987).

Evaluation and Management

The determination of those athletes who would benefit the most from this type of bracing is problematic. The intent of these braces is to decrease the incidence or severity of knee injuries during sport without impairing the athlete's performance. Greene and associates (2000) demonstrated that prophylactic braces did not affect speed and agility, but were prone to slippage.

Despite some continued enthusiasm for prophylactic knee bracing in the sports of American football and motocross racing, a definitive study showing its efficacy has yet to be conducted. In 1979 Anderson and colleagues (1979) described the use of a lateral hinged knee brace to prevent further injury in an athlete who had suffered a medial collateral ligament injury.

They termed this brace *the stabler*, and since then the use of prophylactic lateral hinged braces to prevent knee injuries in American football had become increasingly popular. However, studies to determine the effectiveness of this type of bracing failed to show conclusively a reduction in the number, incidence, or severity of injuries. Hewson and coworkers (1986) found no difference in the knee injury rate using a prophylactic knee brace in intercollegiate-level football players. Grace and associates (1988) found that players wearing single-hinged braces had a higher incidence of injury, as well as an increased number of injuries of the ankle and foot.

More recently a multicenter study by Albright and Powell (1994a, 1994b) on NCAA Division I college football players, demonstrated a decrease in injury incidence for all offensive and defensive positions during practice situations and for line positions, linebackers, and tight ends during both practices and game situations. In this 3-year prospective study involving all the Big Ten teams, they also noticed an increase in the incidence of injury in players in skilled positions (backs and kickers) during game situations using unilateral hinged prophylactic bracing.

In 1997, the AAOS position statement on prophylactic bracing stated that their routine use has not been proven effective in reducing the number or severity of knee injuries, and that in some circumstances such braces may also have the potential to increase injury (AAOS, 2002). Thus it would appear that if used, prophylactic knee bracing can only be recommended for defensive line positions and linebackers in American football, and they should be avoided in skill positions. Functional knee braces have been increasingly utilized in a prophylactic fashion instead. In fact, some major brace manufacturers do not even make the traditional prophylactic brace anymore. When contemplating the use of prophylactic knee bracing, it is important to consider the effect the brace may have on the performance of the player and the possible harmful effect the brace may have on opposing players.

FUNCTIONAL BRACING

Pathophysiology, Biomechanics, and Injuries

The initial goals for these braces were to provide knee joint stability for athletes who suffered serious knee ligament injuries and continued to participate in activities that required rapid direction changes. Traditional functional braces can be classified into two basic designs: the hinged post strap and the hinged post shell brace. Some feel that this basic description is too confining and numerous variants of these two basic design types now exist (Fig. 22-4). The intent of the brace is to reduce anteroposterior translation, by reducing rotational instability, and by reducing varus and valgus stresses. One must understand that to truly control internal and external rotary instability, bracing should theoretically also incorporate the hip and ankle joints. An additional benefit is to modify the muscular control of the knee by affecting the neural impulses. Biomechanical analyses of functional knee bracing can be divided into those involving the use of cadaver models and those involving in vivo analyses of brace function.

Cadaver studies constitute a large body of the present knowledge of the effect of functional knee bracing on knee stability. Unfortunately, the involvement of muscle action in knee stability and brace function has been difficult to reproduce in the cadaver setting. Baker and colleagues (1987) studied the effect of prophylactic and functional knee braces on strain in the

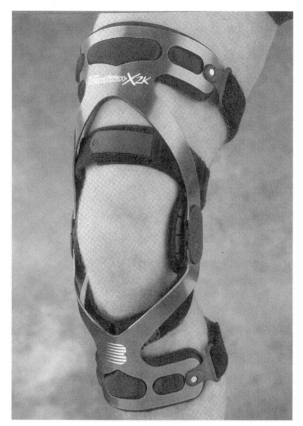

FIG 22-4 Tradition X2K functional brace. (Courtesy of Breg Inc., Vista, CA.)

MCL and ACL during application of a valgus force to the foot, and found that functional knee braces are more effective than prophylactic braces in resisting abduction and rotational stresses in both flexion and extension.

Wojtys and associates (1996) tested cadaveric specimens under axial load near full extension and demonstrated that the braces were effective in constraining knees to anteroposterior and rotational forces, but at force levels that must be considered subphysiologic. Some of the braces tested actually appeared to overconstrain the knee when tested in axial rotation, and one must be aware of the possible negative effect this could have on an athlete's performance in the in vivo setting.

Another group of studies employed the use of instrumented knee ligament testing, or radiographic stereophotogrammetric techniques in evaluating tibial translations and rotation during applied external forces. Jonsson and Karrholm (1989) assessed the constraint afforded by functional knee orthoses in the anterior cruciate ligament–deficient knee using these radiographic techniques. Their analyses revealed that these braces did reduce anterior tibial translation, but not to normal levels. Their studies also showed a reduction in external tibial rotation, but not internal tibial rotation. However, the loads exerted on these braced limbs did not approach physiologic levels. Cawley and associates (1991) commented on the use of knee ligament arthrometers when assessing the effectiveness of functional knee braces, and pointed out that the loads exerted by these devices are subphysiologic, and concluded that the data obtained from these types of studies are of little clinical use.

Of greater validity in determining the effect of knee bracing on the unstable knee are studies performed in the in vivo setting. Knutzen and coworkers (1984) assessed the effect of a functional knee brace on a reconstructed anterior cruciate ligament–deficient knee. They found no statistical difference between the braced and unbraced knees when tested for tibial rotation at 90° of flexion, but stated that there appeared to be a slight trend toward reduction of internal rotation in the braced subjects.

Evaluation and Management

The selection of the appropriate patient for a functional brace has been variable. Its original intent was to reduce knee instability following anterior cruciate ligament injuries. Athletes who had torn their ACL but still wished to participate in activities that required rapid direction changes were the target for marketing of these types of braces. The reliability and success rates of the original ACL reconstructions at that time were not very good. Rehabilitation was quite often not predictable with unacceptable rates of arthrofibroses (Shelbourne et al., 1994). Contraindications to functional bracing are listed in Table 22-2. A reliable surgery, and aggressive, consistent rehabilitation has now allowed most athletes to choose ACL reconstruction therapy over a trial of conservative treatment with bracing (Shelbourne et al., 1990).

Another area where functional bracing has seen use was that of the skeletally immature athlete. In the 1980s, ACL reconstruction in children with open physes was generally avoided by many orthopedic surgeons for fear of growth arrest. Allowing these young athletes to play sports activities, possibly with some bracing, seemed to be a viable option. However, the results of nonoperative treatment of ACLs in young athletes has been terrible, with significant premature meniscal and articular cartilage damage (Aichroth et al., 2002; McCarroll et al., 1988). Furthermore, McCarroll and colleagues (1988) demonstrated that growth arrest is an unlikely event after ACL reconstruction with an open physis. Almost all of the patients in this series returned to previous athletic activities without any significant problems.

The middle-aged athlete who defers ACL reconstruction but wishes to continue in his or her sport, already has some arthritis, or is reducing the level of his or her activity intensity, may be a more appropriate candidate for a functional knee brace. The brace should be worn in conjunction with a comprehensive rehabilitation program with attention toward closed kinetic chain exercises for quadriceps as well as hamstrings.

TABLE 22-2 Contraindications to Functional Bracing

Higher level or young athlete with isolated ACL
Lateral sided injuries with instability
Multiple ligament injuries/knee dislocations
Subluxations or instability despite bracing

Clinical studies have demonstrated that functional knee braces may cause a subjective improvement in stability in ACL-deficient patients (Marans et al., 1991). Romash and associates (1989) also found subjective improvements with marginal objective improvements in braced ACL-deficient subjects. An unpublished study demonstrated neurosensory improvements in motor control after 1 month of bracing (Howard et al., 1996). With more objective measures, other studies were less supportive of these braces. Wojtys and associates (1994) found that six custom functional knee braces on five ACL-deficient patients helped to control anterior tibial displacement, but did not improve isokinetic strength and delayed muscle reaction time. Beynnon and coworkers (1995) placed transducers on ACLs at the time of an arthroscopy to measure in vivo ACL strain patterns. They found that only two of the functional braces studied gave any strain-shielding effect to the ACL, even during activities of daily living.

Despite the lack of evidence, the use of functional braces has extended past providing stability for ACL-deficient patients. Following ACL reconstruction, some surgeons feel the functional brace can be used either immediately or soon after continuing some activities (Risberg et al., 1999). Some have used them in a temporary manner from the time of injury to the time of surgery so that patients develop more confidence during rehabilitation and normal everyday activities.

REHABILITATIVE BRACING

Pathophysiology, Biomechanics, and Injuries

Temporary bracing following ACL reconstruction is one of the more common uses for knee bracing. This brace is designed with bilateral hinges, post, and shell, with lockouts on motion to help protect intra-articular structures following surgery (Fig. 22-5). There is a theoretical concern for the graft as it may have as little as 10% of the strength of the native ACL at 4 weeks (Cawley, 2002). Although there is widespread use of postoperative bracing, the biomechanical studies supporting its use are sparse. Available studies have demonstrated decreased anteroposterior translation and rotational stability while wearing the brace, as well as less strain on the ACL. Cawley and colleagues (1898) did find that postoperative braces that integrated and functioned as a single unit were more effective at controlling rotations and translations at the knee. Controlling postoperative range of motion still seems to be one of the primary goals of these braces.

Evaluation and Management

There is variability with postoperative rehabilitation and management of many orthopedic surgeries. Bracing after ACL reconstruction is generally more of a personal decision for the surgeon, as there is little clinical evidence to date supporting its routine use. One prospective study does suggest improved Cincinnati knee rating scores at 3 months after using the brace for 2 weeks, followed by a functional knee brace (Risberg et al., 1999). However, no significant differences between braced and nonbraced groups were noted with regard to knee joint laxity, ROM, muscle strength, functional tests, or pain. Additionally, increased thigh atrophy was noted as a result of their use. The conclusions were also that there is no convincing evidence that there is increased morbidity such as an increased risk to the

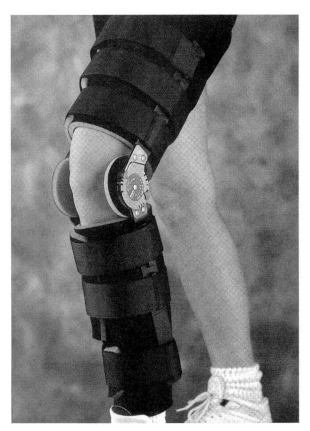

FIG 22-5   Postoperative rehabilitative brace. (Courtesy of Breg Inc., Vista, CA.)

meniscus or cartilage as a result of not using postoperative bracing after ACL reconstruction.

OSTEOARTHRITIS OFF-LOADING BRACES

Pathophysiology, Biomechanics, and Injuries

Patients who suffer from unicompartmental osteoarthritis often suffer with daily pain when ambulating. Off-loading braces were designed to correct the alignment abnormalities in early to moderate unicompartmental disease of the knee (medial or lateral). The brace itself is designed with bilateral adjustable hinges across the joint line (Fig. 22-6). The brace is adjusted to the symptomatic osteoarthritic compartment. The objective is to open the joint space in the affected compartment to provide some reduction in joint surface contact during weight-bearing activities. An in vivo analysis of the effectiveness of the osteoarthritic knee brace during heel-strike of gait demonstrated intercondylar separation of 2.0 mm in the 80% (12/15) of the patients who reported pain relief with the brace (Komistek et al., 1999). The

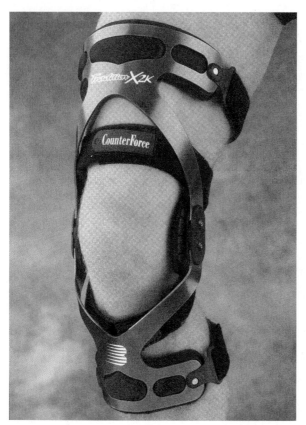

FIG 22-6 Counterforce osteoarthritis off-loading brace. (Courtesy of Breg Inc., Vista, CA.)

three patients who did not demonstrate intercondylar separation between the tibia and femur were judged to be obese (>20% of ideal body weight), and therefore had difficulty with fitting of the brace. In another study, proprioception was minimally improved following application of similar braces for medial compartment osteoarthritis (Bockrath et al., 1993). In the same study, postural control was not changed with the bracing, suggesting that the likely benefits of this type of bracing are more mechanical than neuromuscular.

Evaluation and Management

After appropriate oral medications, activity modifications, physical therapy, injections, and viscosupplementation, the nonoperative options available are generally few. Variable results have been seen with heel wedges and forefoot insoles in attempts to correct alignment abnormalities. The efficacy of the newer off-loading braces is dependent on appropriate patient selection. Clinical evaluation involves observing for an antalgic gait, noting the size of the patient, and also assessing tibial alignment. Patients with varus alignment tend to develop medial compartment osteoarthritis, which in turn worsens their tibial alignment. Valgus alignment is associated with a higher development of lateral compartment osteoarthritis (Sharma et al., 2001). Assessing for knee effusion, range of motion including flexion contractures, and flexibility and strength about the knee are also important components of the exam. Foot pronation and its biomechanics probably plays a minor role as well.

Choosing a brace for the right type of patient depends mostly on the level of symptoms and the presence of unicompartmental disease. A 2-year study used a Counterforce brace (Breg Inc., Vista, CA) on 30 symptomatic patients with unicompartmental osteoarthritis. After 8 weeks of use, the majority of patients noted reduction in pain, and at an average follow-up of 2.7 years, 41% of 29 patients were still using the brace, and only 24% had undergone arthroplasty. Patients who are not obese, and whose osteoarthritis is less severe seem to have the most predictable long-term improvements. Off-loading braces may not be a viable option in advanced unicompartmental osteoarthritis to prevent surgery, but they may be considered in earlier disease in appropriately selected patients.

SIDELINE TIPS

It is very important to remember that braces are meant to provide comfort or stability for very specific conditions. With regard to functional bracing, there may be some benefit for those isolated chronic ACL patients who choose nonoperative treatment, and are involved in activities of decreased intensity. Combined ligament injuries should not be braced for stability and return to play. ACL injury with a high-grade MCL has been treated with serial casting to provide absolute immobilization until the MCL heals (Jari et al., 2001). Hinged braces or unhinged knee immobilizers that stabilize the knee and allow weight bearing can also be used to avoid the pitfalls of prolonged casting, with range of motion exercises several times a day. Either an ACL or a PCL injury with a lateral-sided injury is also an inherently unstable situation. If significant lateral instability is noted, urgent surgical referral is necessary to reattach the lateral capsule and other posterior lateral-sided structures. Knee dislocations generally have multiligamentous involvement including the ACL and PCL, and should not be braced for stability as well. In fact, the natural history of improvements noted with isolated PCL injuries (Shelbourne et al., 1999), and the inherent difficulty of bracing should preclude the need for a functional brace.

Another important set of tips involve the proper ways to obtain and fit a brace. The most important aspects of choosing the proper brace are accurate diagnosis of the injury, and an appropriate explanation to the patient regarding the proven potential benefits of the brace, as well as its limitations. In general, bracing is more effective in stabilizing a knee with low-grade linear instability rather than high-grade rotational instability. A brace is most effective in stabilizing against varus and valgus instabilities and stresses and is less effective against abnormal anterior or posterior motion. It is least effective in stabilizing against rotational instability.

In choosing a brace, the patient must be willing to use the brace and be compliant if it is to be effective. Functional braces are either of hinge-post-shell design, which is molded and more rigid but more effective, and the hinge-post-strap design, which is more comfortable, but less effective in reducing instability. Most braces are suspended by the superior calf strap.

The adequate function of this strap is dependent on an adequate superior calf muscle definition. Instances of poor muscle definition in this area, and the presence of the inverted conically shaped leg, present a particularly difficult fitting problem for the orthotist. Under these circumstances braces are prone to slippage and malrotation. Caution should be exercised in undertaking fitting of patients with these types of limbs.

Adequate brace performance also depends on the proper application of the brace. It is incumbent on the brace fitter, or orthotist, to instruct the patient in appropriate application of the brace and the appropriate tensioning of the brace straps. Careful attention should be paid to positioning of the hinges over the femoral condyles so that it crosses the joint line appropriately. The longer the lever or hinge is, the more effective a brace will be in absorption of forces while sacrificing comfortability.

Use of a functional, or prestressed, knee brace can lead to loss of muscle strength and the brace wearer should be encouraged to maintain muscle strength in the quadriceps, hamstring, and surrounding muscles by the performance of daily muscle strengthening exercises and rehabilitation. The timing of brace fitting is important. Most braces will accommodate 10–15% changes in thigh girth, and less than 5% changes in calf girth while still functioning adequately. It is important at the time of time brace fitting to take into account adequate rehabilitation of thigh and calf musculature. Some patients are not sure whether to choose readily available off-the-shelf bracing or to order custom fitted braces. Studies have demonstrated no difference between the efficacy of these two types (Beynnon et al., 1997; Paluska et al., 2000; Wojyts et al., 1996). If there is no anticipated significant change in thigh girth, or abnormal limb contour, and a brace is still comfortable, an off-the-shelf brace may be a viable, more inexpensive alternative.

New symptoms of instability or pain in a braced individual may be an indication that: (1) the brace hinges or other moving parts have worn out, or the straps are no longer adequately fitting; (2) the patient's musculature may be deficient and the patient may need a further rehabilitation program; (3) the patient has developed new intra-articular pathology; (4) the patient's degree of instability has increased due to meniscal lesions or loosening of the secondary constraints about the knee, or (5) the patient is noncompliant with use or application of the brace.

Certain sports usually do not require the use of a brace as they do not involve pivoting or lateral movement. These sports are cycling, running on level ground, swimming, and cross-country skiing. Some sports-governing bodies prohibit the use of braces fabricated with rigid material as they feel this may constitute a danger to the other participants in the sports (eg, rugby, soccer, and wrestling). Certain sports are better suited to brace use as they involve participation with the knee in a flexed position; sports such as downhill skiing, skating, and hockey are examples.

A brace, particularly one fitted with a patellar cup, may also provide protection in contact sports such as football, hockey, or motocross racing.

CONFOUNDING CONDITIONS

Although there may be certain situations in which brace use is reasonable, pitfalls still exist. Despite proper fitting, slippage of the brace through higher-level activities is still possible. Frequent adjustments may be necessary in order for the brace to be effective. Use of braces has been shown to be associated with thigh muscle atrophy as well as decreased strength (Risberg et al., 1999). The potential for muscle fatigue and decreased performance is an important concern for competitive athletes. Some studies show no difference indicating that selected prophylactic braces do not significantly reduce speed or agility, but show a variable tendency towards migration (Greene et al., 2000). Sforzo and colleagues (1989) demonstrated that quadriceps peak torque and anaerobic power in prophylactically braced athletes were not significantly different, and did not necessarily impair performance.

Expense also becomes a real factor for those deciding about using a particular brace. Prices may range from US$35 for simple patellofemoral sleeves to over US$1200 for custom-made functional braces (Paluska et al., 2000). Insurance plans are still quite variable on reimbursement for durable medical equipment such as braces. Another concern is the possibility of injury to other athletes. This possible danger makes the rigid braces illegal in soccer, wrestling, and rugby, and is a legitimate concern in other sports such as football and hockey. Last, the psychological effects of bracing are still not completely understood. Psychologically, it is felt that those who wear functional braces feel they have more confidence in their knee (Cawley, 2002). Of 73 ACL reconstructed patients, the braced patients were more aggressive in their approach to physical therapy, more compliant, and more confident in their resistive exercises. The negative effects of that are increased risk-taking behavior, especially in the ACL-deficient patient. Finally, some patients become dependent on the brace for all activities, and ignore the importance of a comprehensive rehabilitation program.

PREVENTION

Prevention of serious knee injuries has been an important goal for most anyone involved in the care of competitive athletes. As discussed earlier, efficacy of prophylactic bracing is suspect. Methods other than bracing have been receiving more attention in prevention of serious knee injuries. The Vermont Ski Program appeared to be successful in prevention of knee injuries for those who saw an instructional video on common mechanisms leading to ACL tears and proper ways to fall. This prospective study demonstrated a decrease in serious injuries to the ACL by 62% in ski area employees (Ettlinger et al., 1995). Another area of recent interest is the prevention of ACL tears in female athletes. It is well known that the rate of tears is significantly higher in women. Theories for this discrepancy include the size of the notch, and presumably the size of the ACL (Shelbourne et al., 1998), hormonal influences (Hewett et al., 1999), or intrinsic anatomic differences in alignment (Hewett et al., 1999). Some feel that neuromuscular imbalances exist and landing techniques are deficient in women (Hewett et al., 1996; Huston et al., 1996). Studies have demonstrated that a preseason program involving plyometrics and proper jumping and landing techniques may decrease serious knee injuries (Hewett et al., 1999). More research and less time-consuming programs still need to be developed, but there seems to be some promise in prevention of knee injuries that ultimately may obviate the need for certain types of knee braces.

SUMMARY

There has been a decline in the overall interest in researching the effects of knee bracing, as well as their overall use by orthopedic and sports medicine physicians. We should be careful not to uniformly advocate nor discourage the use of knee braces, but rather to look at each situation individually. There are some early promising data regarding patellofemoral bracing. Certainly there are few risks associated with their use if other conservative measures have been ineffective. Unilateral hinged prophylactic braces have not been found to be effective in prevention of MCL or serious ligament injuries. Functional knee braces have found their way into this prophylactic role for some college and professional football teams. Cost issues and risk/benefit analysis should be considered before employing such brace use at other levels. Functional knee braces after serious knee ligament injuries such as to the ACL should be reserved for older athletes who are able to reduce their level of their previous activity, and are involved in a rehabilitation program as well. Rehabilitative bracing, especially after ACL reconstruction, may not be necessary to prevent morbidity. However, if used in the short-term, appropriate range of motion and strength goals should still be met. Functional knee braces have also entered this postoperative market as patients transition into their activities. There still is no convincing evidence that not wearing a brace postoperatively leads to clinical failure of ACL reconstructions. This as well as cost issues should be considered when deciding about the adjuvant use of braces during the postoperative period. Finally, in an attempt to provide some palliative symptom relief, and possibly delay arthroplasty, the newer off-loading braces have also shown some early promise. Patients who are not obese and have a lower grade of osteoarthritis seem to be the ones that obtain long-term benefit from these braces. Although it is impossible to ignore personal anecdotal successes and failures, the orthopedist or sports medicine physician should incorporate the body of evidence available in making decisions about knee bracing. Most importantly, the patient should be well-educated regarding the benefits, limitations, and importance of compliance with the brace if there is to be any notable improvement in their symptoms.

REFERENCES

Aichroth PM, Patel DV, Zorillz P. The natural history and treatment of rupture of the anterior cruciate ligament in children and adolescents. *J Bone Joint Surg.* 2002;84-B:38–1.

Albright JP, Powell JW, Smith W. Medial collateral ligament knee sprains in college football. Effectiveness of preventive braces. *Am J Sports Med.* 1994a;22:12–18.

Albright JP, Powell JW, Smith W. Medial collateral ligament knee sprains in college football. Brace wear preferences and injury risk. *Am J Sports Med.* 1994b;22:2–11.

American Academy of Orthopedic Surgeons. The use of knee braces. Accessed September 2002 fromURL: http://www.aaos.org/wordhtml/papers/position/kneebr.htm

Anderson G, Zeman SC, Rosenfeld RT. The Anderson knee stabler. *Phys Sports Med.* 1979;7:125.

Arroll B, Ellis-Pegler E, Edwards A, et al. Patellofemoral pain syndrome: A critical review of the clinical trials on nonoperative therapy. *Am J Sports Med.* 1997;25:207–212.

Baker BE, VanHanswyk E, Bogosian S, et al. A biomechanical study of the static stabilizing effect of knee braces on medial stability. *Am J Sports Med.* 1987;15:566–570.

Barnes CL, Cawley PW, Hederman B. Effect of CounterForce brace on symptomatic relief in a group of patients with symptomatic unicompartmental osteoarthritis: A prospective 2-year investigation. *Am J Orthop.* 2002;31:396–401.

Bengal S, Lowe J, Mann G, et al. The role of the knee brace in the prevention of anterior knee pain syndrome. *Am J Sports Med.* 1987;25:118–122.

Beynnon BD, Fleming BC, Johnson RJ, et al. Anterior cruciate ligament strain behavior during rehabilitation exercises in vivo. *Am J Sports Med.* 1995;23:24–34.

Beynnon BD, Johnson RJ, Fleming BC, et al. The effect of functional knee bracing on the anterior cruciate ligament in the weightbearing and nonweightbearing knee. *Am J Sports Med.* 1997;25:353–359.

Birminghan TB, Kramer JF, Kirkley A. Knee bracing for medial compartment osteoarthritis: Effects on proprioception and postural control. *Rheumatology.* 2001;40:285–289.

Bockrath K, Wooden C, Worrell T, et al. Effects of patella taping on patella position and perceived pain. *Med Sci Sports Exerc.* 1993;25:989–992.

Branch TP, Hunter R, Donath M. Dynamic EMG analysis of anterior cruciate deficient legs with and without bracing during cutting. *Am J Sports Med.* 1989;17:35–41.

Cawley PW, France P, Paulos LE. Comparison of rehabilitative knee braces. *Am J Sports Med.* 1989;17:141–146.

Cawley PW. Post-operative knee bracing. *Clin Sports Med.* 1990;9:763–770.

Cawley PW, France P, Paulos LE. The current state of functional knee bracing research. *Am J Sports Med.* 1991;19:226–233.

Cawley PW. Bracing: Science or psychology? In: Ellenbecker TS, ed. *Knee Ligament Rehabilitation.* New York: Churchill Livingstone; 2002;252–261.

Cherf J, Paulos LE. Bracing for patellar instability. *Clin Sports Med.* 1990;9:813–821.

Colville MR, Lee CL, Ciullo JV. The Lenox Hill brace, an evaluation of effectiveness in treating knee instability. *Am J Sports Med.* 1986;14:257–261.

Deakon RT, Zarnett R. Knee braces. In: Bull RC, ed. *Handbook of Sports Injuries.* New York: McGraw-Hill; 1998;785–794.

Ettlinger CF, Johnson RJ, Shealy JE. A method to help reduce the risk of serious knee sprains incurred in alpine skiing. *Am J Sports Med.* 1995;23:531–537.

Finestone A, Radin EL, Levy B, et al. Treatment of overuse patellofemoral pain. Prospective randomized clinical trial in a military setting. *Clin Orthop.* 1993;293:208–210.

France PE, Paulos LE, Jayaraman G, et al. The biomechanics of lateral knee bracing. Part II: Impact responses of the braced knee. *Am J Sports Med.* 1987;15:430–438.

Grace TG, Skipper BJ, Newberry JC, et al. Prophylactic knee braces and injury to the lower extremity. *J Bone Joint Surg.* 1988;70A:422.

Greene DL, Hamson KR, Bay RC, et al. Effects of protective knee bracing on speed and agility. *Am J Sports Med.* 2000;28:453–459.

Hewett TE, Stroupe AL, Nance TA, et al. Plyometric training in female athletes. Decreased impact forces and increased hamstring torques. *Am J Sports Med.* 1996;24:765–773.

Hewett TE, Lindenfeld TN, Riccobene JV, Noyes FR. The effect of neuromuscular training on the incidence of knee injury in female athletes. *Am J Sports Med.* 1999;27:699–705.

Hewson GF, Mendini RA, Wang JB. Prophylactic knee bracing in college football. *Am J Sports Med.* 1986;14:262–266.

Hoffman AA, Wyatt RW, Boyne MH, et al. Knee stability in orthotic knee braces. *Am J Sports Med.* 1984;12:371–374.

Howard ME, Cawley PW. The effect of functional knee bracing on motor control performance in a group of ACL-deficient subjects. Presented at the American Academy of Orthopedic Surgeons Annual Meeting, Atlanta, GA, Feb. 24, 1996.

Huston LJ, Wojtys EM. Neuromuscular performance characteristics in elite female athletes. *Am J Sports Med.* 1996;24:427–436.

Jari S, Shelbourne KD. Non-operative or delayed surgical treatment of combined cruciate ligaments and medial side knee injuries. *Sports Med Arthrosc Rev.* 2001;9:185–192.

Jonsson H, Karrholm J. The stabilizing effect of the knee braces after ACL rupture. *Acta Orthop Scand*. 1989;231:29.

Knutzen KM, Bates BT, Hamil J. Knee brace influences on the tibial rotation and torque patterns of the surgical limb. *J Orthop Sports Phys Ther*. 1984;6:116.

Komistek RD, Dennis DA, Northcut EJ, et al. An in vivo analysis of the effectiveness of the osteoarthritic knee brace during heel-strike of gait. *J Arthroplasty*. 1999;14:738–742.

Kowall MG, Kolk G, Nuber GW, et al. Patellar taping in the treatment of patellofemoral pain. *Am J Sports Med*. 1996;24:61–66.

Liu SH, Mirzayan R. Current review, functional knee bracing. *Clin Orthop Rel Res*. 1995;317:273–281.

Marans HJ, Jackson RW, Piccinin J, et al. Functional testing of braces for anterior cruciate ligament-deficient knees. *Can J Surg*. 1991;34:167–172.

Martin TJ, and the Committee on Sports Medicine and Fitness, The American Academy of Pediatrics. Technical report: Knee brace use in the young athlete. *Pediatrics*. 2001;108:503–507.

McCarroll JR, Rettig AC. Anterior cruciate ligament injuries in the young athlete with open physes. *Am J Sports Med*. 1988;16:44–47.

Paluska SA, McKeag DB. Do preventative knee braces keep their promise? *Your Patient Fitness*. 1999a;13:20–24.

Paluska SA, McKeag DB. Using patellofemoral braces for anterior knee pain. *Physician Sports Med*. 1999b;27:81–82.

Paluska SA, McKeag DB. Knee braces: Current evidence and clinical recommendations for their use. *Am Fam Physician*. 2000;61:411–418.

Paulos LE, France P, Rosenberg TD. The biomechanics of lateral knee bracing. Part I: Response of the valgus restraints to loading. *Am J Sports Med*. 1987;15:419–429.

Risberg MA, Holm I, Steen H, et al. The effect of knee bracing after anterior cruciate ligament reconstruction. *Am J Sports Med*. 1999;27:76–83.

Romash MM, Henningsen HJ, Claybaugh J. Knee braces—Comparative functional testing. *Orthop Trans*. 1989;13:501.

Sharma L, Song J, Felson DT, et al. The role of knee alignment in disease progression and functional decline in knee osteoarthritis. *JAMA*. 2001;286:188–195.

Shelbourne KD, Nitz P. Accelerated rehabilitation after anterior cruciate ligament reconstruction. *Am J Sports Med*. 1990;18:292–299.

Shelbourne KD, Johnson GE. Outpatient surgical management of arthrofibrosis after anterior cruciate ligament surgery. *Am J Sports Med*. 1994;22:192–197.

Shelbourne KD, Davis TJ, Klootwyk TE. The relationship between intercondylar notch width of the femur and the incidence of anterior cruciate ligament tears, a prospective study. *Am J Sports Med*. 1998;26:402–408.

Shelbourne KD, Gray T. Natural history study of athletes with PCL-deficient knees. *J Sport Rehabil*. 1999;8:279–288.

Sforzo GA, Chen NM, Gold CA, et al. The effect of prophylactic knee bracing on performance. *Med Sci Sports Exerc*. 1989;21:254–257.

Ward SR, Powers CM. Preliminary review of Stanford kinematic MRI PTO investigation. Unpublished and to be presented at American College of Sports Medicine Annual Meeting.

Wirth MA, DeLee JC. The history and classification of knee braces. *Clin Sports Med*. 1990;9:731–741.

Wojtys EM, Kothari SU, Huston LJ. When should anterior cruciate ligament braces be used in sports? *Orthop Trans*. 1994;18:748–749.

Wojtys EM, Kothari SU, Huston LJ. Anterior cruciate ligament functional brace use in sports. *Am J Sports Med*. 1996;24:539–546.

23 | Soft Tissue Injuries: Overuse Syndromes

Christopher T. Daley and William D. Stanish

Overuse injuries of soft tissue are common in the athlete and nonathlete alike. In our fitness-conscious society, individuals seem motivated by a heightened awareness of the beneficial aspects of exercise. This has resulted in more people than ever exercising regularly and participating in sports. Although individuals seem aware of the cardiorespiratory and associated health benefits of exercise, they also need to be aware that these activities also bring problems with injury.

Regardless of whether the sporting individual is an elite world-class competitor, a weekend novice, or an "aging warrior," tendinitis and other overuse injuries can and do occur. Although the incidence of overuse injuries is not exactly known, they have been estimated to account for 35–65% of all sports injuries (Renstrom, 1994).

It is difficult, if not impossible, to determine the true incidence because frequently, overuse injuries are never brought to the attention of a physician. Despite this, such injuries account for over 50% of the injuries seen in a primary care setting (Herring, 1987) and are the most frequently encountered athletic injury.

Independent of whether muscle, tendon, cartilage, or hard tissue is involved, injury results from a simple mismatch between stress on a given tissue and the ability of that tissue to withstand the stress. There are two basic mechanisms behind tissue trauma: single-impact macrotrauma and repetitive microtrauma (damage at the microscopic or molecular level). Overuse, therefore, can be defined as the level of repetitive microtrauma sufficient to overwhelm the tissue's ability to adapt (Renstrom, 1994) or, in other words, its healing capacity. Overuse injuries of soft tissue include damage to tendons (from paratenonitis to tendinosis), muscles, bursa, and nerves. They include impingement and snapping syndromes, apophysitis, friction syndromes, and compartment syndromes.

When reviewing past published research results, it appears that the term overuse injury was first coined by Slocum (1968). These types of injuries received recognition years before, and several examples are cited in other major texts (Renstrom, 1988, 1994). In the past, treatment regimens included mandatory rest and/or immobilization, which resulted in predictable musculoskeletal atrophy with impaired function. In addition, the treatment and rehabilitation programs were aimed at the acute problem without much emphasis on the etiology of the injury. The result was methods of treatment that often fell short of the athlete's expectations. Many experienced sports medicine physicians can, no doubt, cite a poststeroid injection tendon rupture as evidence of another pitfall of the treatment regimens of the past.

In the past several decades, much greater emphasis has been placed on basic research of the pathophysiology and etiology of overuse injuries. We do know that these maladies most frequently result from repetitive microtrauma and overload secondary to extrinsic factors (such as training errors) and intrinsic factors (such as decreased flexibility). We know that relative rest with early movement, not forced immobilization, with later emphasis on a graduated exercise program is more physiologic and will likely return the athlete to his or her premorbid activity level sooner. We are also aware

303

that this group of disorders remains a great diagnostic and therapeutic challenge for sports medicine clinicians because our understanding of overuse problems is still somewhat limited.

PATHOLOGY AND PATHOMECHANICS

Pathomechanics of Microtrauma

Prior to exploring specific overuse injuries, it is necessary to have an adequate understanding of how repetitive microtrauma affects tissues. The most basic principle in the etiology of an overuse injury is that tissue is exposed to a force that can provoke damage (Curwin, 1984). A single episode of excessive stress may cause microtrauma, but usually it results from repetitive loading at a force well within the physiologic range (Renstrom, 1994). Injury from overuse results from a mismatch between stress on a given tissue and the ability of that tissue to withstand the stress. The failure pattern of tendons is representative of the disruption observed in most tissues with a high collagen content and serves as an excellent model for demonstrating microtrauma (Renstrom, 1994). As a tendon is elongated, its collagen fibers are stretched from a relaxed, resting configuration to a taut, straight cord. If the tensile force causing elongation is removed after the initial 4% of elongation, then the fibers return to their natural resting state. If, however, sufficient tension is maintained to achieve 4–8% elongation, microtrauma occurs as the molecular bonds and cross-links are disrupted, allowing the collagen fibers to deform. Beyond this degree of elongation, individual collagen fibers eventually fail along with the remaining structural elements, leading to complete macroscopic failure of the tendon (Curwin, 1984).

Inflammatory Healing Response to Injury

The response to the microtrauma sustained in overuse is usually in the form of inflammation that progresses through distinct pathologic phases (Nirschl, 1986). Immediately after injury, the inflammatory cascade is activated, and vasoactive substances (including prostaglandins synthesized from arachidonic acid) are released, resulting in increased capillary permeability and fluid transudation. These, in turn, activate the complement system. Neutrophils, monocytes, and eosinophils are attracted to the injured area, where these cells release degradative enzymes that can destroy tissue. Fibroblasts and endothelial cells migrate to the area to aid in the healing process. If no further injury occurs, the inflammatory phase will run its course in 48 hours to 6 days (Curwin, 1994). If further injury occurs, this phase can last much longer and be more intense. Pain, swelling, and tenderness are hallmarks of this stage. Tissues adjacent to the injured tissue can become enveloped by this process so that localizing the exact site of injury is difficult. It becomes obvious that even though inflammation is necessary for healing to occur, treatment needs to minimize this inflammatory process to avoid a chronic situation leading to tissue destruction and eventual fibrosis. Nonsteroidal anti-inflammatory drugs (NSAIDs) are important because they are able to block the synthesis of the vasoactive prostaglandins via the cyclooxygenase-mediated pathway. This will help to control the whole inflammatory cascade at a very early step. Ice, elevation, and compression help limit inflammation, but relative rest with avoidance of the provocative activity remains the most important treatment modality.

TABLE 23-1 Effects of Exercise and Disuse

Exercise		Disuse
↑	Collagen synthesis	↓
↓	Collagen degradation	↑
↑	Collagen cross-linking	↓
↑	Metabolic enzymes	↓
↑	Collagen fibril size	↓
↑	Collagen tensile strength	↓
↑	White muscle fiber vascularization and conversion	↓
↑	Tissue strength and endurance	↓

The second, or proliferative, phase begins the third day after injury and usually lasts 1–2 weeks, producing collagen and ground substance. At this stage, these early products of repair are immature and disorganized, so applied stress must be low enough to avoid disruption and triggering of another inflammatory response. Gradual introduction of stress allows collagen cross-linking and fibril size to increase while preventing progressive musculoskeletal atrophy.

Beginning at approximately 20 days after injury, the remodeling and maturation stage occurs, during which, collagen cross-linking continues, slowly returning the damaged structure to its preinjury strength (Renstrom, 1994). It is during this phase that the healing of tendons and ligaments will be increased if progressive, controlled stress is applied on the tissues. If excessive stress is applied, resulting in injury, the inflammatory response will be restarted.

These three stages are a continuum and are essentially occurring in waves at about the same time. In addition to these three pathologic stages, the pathway common to all tissues likely involves a direct or indirect effect on the microvasculature with subsequent oxygen deprivation (Archambault, 1995).

Effects of Disuse

It is well established that all musculoskeletal tissues atrophy under conditions of deprivation load (Akeson, 1980). The tissues become weaker both structurally and materially as collagen degradation exceeds synthesis, resulting in a net decrease in collagen. In athletes undergoing strength and endurance training who receive proper rest and nutrition, the vascularization of the white (fast-twitch) muscle fibers and the reversion to red (slow-twitch) fibers gradually improve, which increases strength and endurance of the muscle. In prolonged disuse, the fiber conversion is reversed, and the muscle loses strength and endurance with resulting atrophies. The effects of disuse are shown in Table 23-1.

Because most musculoskeletal tissues adapt to increased loads by becoming larger or stronger, the concept of using early motion with gradual stress application has been used in treating overuse injuries (Curwin, 1984).

ETIOLOGY

Given that repetitive stress can traumatize tissue, the potential for injury is enhanced by a wide variety of predisposing factors. These risk factors can be divided into extrinsic and intrinsic factors (Table 23-2). Exercise and the challenge of sport expose even subtle anatomic imperfections.

TABLE 23-2 Risk Factors Associated with Overuse Injury in Sports

Intrinsic
    Malalignment: foot pronation, cavus foot, arthritis, femoral neck
      anteversion, genu valgum/varum, previous malunion fractures
    Leg-length discrepancy
    Poor flexibility
    Muscle weakness and imbalance
    Neuromuscular coordination defect
    Ligamentous laxity
    Female gender
    Youth/elderly
    Obesity
    Type O blood group
Extrinsic
    Training errors: distance, intensity, frequency, hill work,
      technique, slope running
    Playing surface
    Footwear: improper fit, inadequate cushioning,
      excessively stiff sole, poor heel counter
    Environmental conditions
    Poor equipment

Extrinsic Risk Factors

Extrinsic factors play a large part in preventing many runners from participating fully in their sport because they predispose the athlete to injury. Of these injuries, 60–80% are associated with extrinsic factors, such as training errors and changes in running activities (Renstrom, 1993). The most important risk factor for injury is a training error, such as excessive mileage, sudden change in intensity, and running on sloped surfaces. In track and field athletes, overuse injuries are more common in middle- and long-distance runners than in sprinters, hurdlers, and jumpers (Bennell, 1996), presumably because they are associated more with endurance training. Hill work, especially downhill running, can give rise to patellofemoral disorders, popliteus tendinitis, and iliotibial band friction syndrome. Running on banked surfaces can lead to the "short-long syndrome," and the athlete may suffer from iliotibial band friction syndrome or trochanteric bursitis. For cyclists, riding with too much pedal resistance is a major cause of injury, illustrating poor technique as a cause for overuse problems. Tennis players who perform on surfaces such as all-weather concrete suffer more commonly from injury than do those who play on a less rigid, lower-friction clay surface. Overuse injuries are more common in soccer played on artificial turf than in that played on grass or gravel. Proper footwear, including supportive and cushioning insoles, has been shown to decrease the incidence of overuse injuries in military recruits and in running athletes.

Most injuries that occur during cold weather are due to rigorous exercise without warm-up. Under such conditions, as found in fall football and winter skiing, the muscle and connective tissue viscosity is not optimal (increased tissue stiffness and inter tissue resistance), thus, predisposing to injury on muscle contraction because the elastic component cannot absorb the forces. An increase in temperature is observed for optimal muscle functioning. Excessive elevation in muscle temperature, however, also needs to be avoided because it impairs circulatory thermoregulation and contributes to the destruction of tissue proteins with water loss.

Intrinsic Risk Factors

Intrinsic factors are also common in running athletes, especially malalignments such as excessive pronation and cavus foot deformity (Renstrom, 1993). Excessive pronation is associated with injuries such as medial tibial stress syndrome, Achilles tendinitis, tibialis posterior tendinitis, plantar fasciitis, patellofemoral disorders, and iliotibial band friction syndrome. Leg-length discrepancy, poor flexibility, muscle weakness and imbalance, deficit in neuromuscular coordination, and ligamentous laxity also can cause running injuries (Renstrom, 1993). Although pronation of the foot can lead to medial injuries, a cavus foot predisposes to injuries of the lateral side of the lower extremities, such as iliotibial band friction syndrome, trochanteric bursitis, Achilles tendinitis, metatarsalgia, and stress fractures.

Some athletes can manifest malalignments known as "miserable malalignment syndrome" that predisposes to significant risk in activities such as distance running. The combination of malalignments includes excess femoral neck anteversion, genu valgum, squinting patellae, excessive Q angle, functional equinus, and foot pronation (Renstrom 1994). The clinician therefore needs to assess the lower extremity as a complete functional unit. Posture has been shown to be important in patients with shoulder overuse problems.

Age itself is a risk factor, because the elderly have been reported to have an increased incidence of overuse injuries. Increasing age in track and field (Bennell, 1996) and other running activities predisposes to Achilles tendinitis and other overuse syndromes. Young athletes also are at increased risk. All too frequently, promising young athletes are being exposed to high-intensity training at a very young age without awareness by coaches and parents that the immature musculoskeletal system is unable to cope with excessive repetitive biomechanical stress. Sites of overuse injury reflect the sites of rapid musculoskeletal development, as evidenced by such injuries as Osgood-Schlatter disease and Little Leaguer elbow. The risk of injury in adolescents is most pronounced during the rapid growth spurt when other factors, such as muscle tightness, also become important in the etiology of sports injury (Dalton, 1992).

Gender may be a factor, because there seems to be a higher incidence of overuse injuries among women. Females with menstrual irregularities are at a higher risk for certain injuries, especially stress fractures (Bennell, 1996; Drinkwater, 1986; Rubin, 1991). Women have less muscle mass per body weight (23%) than do equally trained men (40%; Drinkwater, 1986). Women also have a lower bone mass than men. During running activities, the repetitive loads of the activity will be forced on the weaker musculoskeletal system in women (as compared with a man of equal body weight), thus predisposing to injury of the lower extremity.

A significant association has been reported between the blood group O and chronic Achilles peritendinitis and tendon rupture (Renstrom, 1994). This suggests a genetic linkage between ABO blood groups and tendon structure.

CLINICAL EVALUATION

The presentation of overuse injuries is usually of an insidious nature because they arise from repetitive activity. Occasionally, there may have been an acute injury or strain, but this will be the exception rather than the norm. As a group, overuse injuries have similar clinical features in that they often present with a history of nonspecific pain that can be temporally experienced either before, during, or after sport and exercise. Often, there is not a lot of

TABLE 23-3 Functional Class of Pain Relating to Activity

Level	Description of pain	Level of sports performance
1	No pain	Normal
2	Pain only with extreme exertion	Normal
3	Pain with extreme exertion and 1–2 hours afterward	Normal or slightly decreased
4	Pain during and after any vigorous activities	Somewhat decreased
5	Pain during activity and forcing termination	Markedly decreased
6	Pain during daily activities	Unable to perform

(*Source: From Curwin S. Stanish WD: Tendinitis: Its Etiology and Treatment. Lexington, MA, DC Heath & Co, 1984, p 64, with permission.*)

swelling except if the joint itself has experienced overload. Nonlocalized tenderness and heat are apparent, whereas thickening or crepitus may be palpable in the patient with tenosynovitis. The diagnosis is based to a great degree on the clinical experience of the treating physician, although a sound and complete history followed by an accurate, thorough physical examination should offer at least a short list of differential diagnoses.

History

The importance of obtaining a detailed history from the athlete regarding these injuries must be stressed because the diagnosis and treatment will be based to a great extent on the functional inquiry. The history essentially becomes the way for the clinician to delineate the extrinsic risk factors for injury that exist with the particular athlete in question. The clinician must first ascertain the nature of the presenting problem with a specific time frame as to the onset of symptoms, their duration and intensity, and associated symptoms. It may be helpful to categorize the pain in a functional way (Curwin, 1984) as it relates to the aggravating or inciting activity (Table 23-3). Pain that is chronic and unremitting is typically found with chronic tendinitis associated with fibrosis and degeneration. It is important to determine if the pain is associated with any swelling, clicking, grating, popping, or locking. Identify any specific relieving factors for the pain aside from rest or medication. The athlete's training program needs to be explored for recent changes in intensity of training, distance, hill work, cross-training, and number of workouts, for example. The types of stretching, strength training, and endurance training need to be identified, plus the location of the activity and the type of playing surface and equipment used, including footwear. Does the athlete usually wear out his or her footwear in a peculiar pattern? The clinician should explore the general health and nutrition of the athlete and identify if he or she has been fatigued more than usual. Perhaps the patient uses an orthotic, a brace, or taping. It is important to discover how the athlete achieves a warm-up and for how long, especially in cold weather.

It is important for the physician treating overuse injuries to be aware of the biomechanics of the particular activity in question to be able to analyze the demands placed on the individual and determine whether excess stress is being placed on the tissues from poor technique or equipment.

Physical Examination

The physical examination likewise requires thoroughness because the objective is not only the diagnosis of the involved tissues(s) but also identification of the physical etiologic risk factors and biomechanical imbalances that hopefully can be modified effectively in the treatment plan. A basic understanding of the biomechanics of the extremities including stresses and joint reactive forces that occur during sport can greatly aid in proper diagnosis and management. There are major textbooks devoted solely to aspects of physical examination of the musculoskeletal system, and it is entirely beyond the scope of this chapter to present any more than limited aspects of the examination of a patient with an overuse injury. First, remember that the human body is a masterfully orchestrated machine with a motor system designed to resist gravity and provide purposeful movement via complex neuromuscular mechanisms. Normal learned movements, and gaits in particular, are highly efficient, with considerable preservation of energy, work, and effort. Second, injuries that are a source of pain induce change in muscle function through reflex inhibition via neural feedback loops. This will be manifest clinically by subtle changes from the normal efficient gait movements. These reflex changes may go unrecognized, however, because of the body's ability to substitute alternative muscles for those inhibited. Thus in upper extremity problems, the clinician needs to specifically look for weakness of the scapular stabilizers and rotator cuff muscle. Dysfunction of these muscles, coupled with loss of glenohumeral rhythm, is the functional basis for the extremely common anterior shoulder impingement syndrome. After lower extremity injuries, weakness of the primary hip stabilizers ensues, which will manifest as subtle changes in gait. This is not to say that the athlete is not capable of excellent performance but that inevitably, secondary injuries will occur because of loss of efficiency.

It has been stated that the five components of good physical performance are strength, endurance, speed, coordination, and flexibility (Cooper, 1978). Poor flexibility, or the inability of a joint to move through a normal range of motion, is a major factor in the development of overuse injuries. Any time a motion segment in the body is restricted, the adjacent motion segments must increase their relative motion, which increases stress in the associated supporting structures. Tight muscles can cause significant postural adaptations that detract from efficiency of movement. The testing of passive muscle length, therefore, becomes very useful in examination for flexibility. Imbalance of quadriceps and hamstring strength and flexibility is believed by many to be the fundamental cause of knee dysfunction during running; thus the clinician should examine both passively. Other musculotendinous units that are important to examine are the iliopsoas (Thomas test) and the iliotibial band (Ober test).

Analyzing coordination of movement, such as observing walking and running, is subjective but should be performed as part of the routine assessment of the athlete. Gait laboratories (or a gait belt) are not at the disposal of most clinicians examining athletes, but a trained eye and clinical examination of isolated postural muscles can enable a clinician to recognize abnormalities. In performing screening examinations of postural muscles, iliopsoas (hip flexor test), gluteus medius (hip abduction test), vastus medialis obliquus (tested at terminal knee extension), and tibialis posterior (ankle inversion test), it is not the overall strength of the maneuver that is important but ascertaining whether the normally triggered muscle is doing the work or is a substituting muscle. This is exemplified in testing terminal extension of the knee and has long been a pearl of knowledge passed on to junior colleagues by the senior author (WDS). In a healthy patient, there will be a good balance of size of the vastus medialis obliquus (VMO) compared with the rest of the quadriceps. In an injured patient, the strength of terminal extension may not be affected, but often there will be a discernible lack of bulk in the VMO because atrophy occurs more rapidly than in the rest of the quadriceps.

The clinician, aware that poor postural alignment will bring abnormal stresses on joints and muscles and recruit secondary muscles into counteracting the effects of gravity, should include a quick screen for posture in the examination of athletes. This can be done by observing standing posture in the frontal and sagittal planes, posture during gait, and sitting posture. Proper standing posture in the frontal plane is judged by a plumb line drawn from the center of the occiput following equally between the scapulae and through the anal crease. In the sagittal plane, the line should pass through the ear, the center of the shoulder, the center of the hips, and slightly anterior to the center of the knee and ankle.

While standing, the back and overall alignment of the lower extremities should be examined. When sitting, in addition to noting the posture, the patient's knee alignment, ankle motion and stability, and foot alignment can be examined. While in the prone position, the sole of the patient's foot can be examined for anatomic abnormalities and callus pattern, the Achilles can be palpated, and the foot-thigh-leg alignment can be viewed. With the patient supine, range of motion of the hip, knee, ankle, and subtalar joints should be examined.

Imaging and Arthroscopy

An x-ray examination often is indicated in the investigation of soft tissue overuse injuries because x-rays can detect or rule out numerous skeletal problems, such as fractures, subluxations, diastasis, epiphyseal damage, apophyseal irregularities, spondylolisthesis, and dysplasia. Using a 36-in. cassette, the physician can determine the anatomic and mechanical axes of the lower extremities or postural abnormalities of the spine. Plain radiographs are less helpful for soft tissue pathology but can be used successfully in detecting intratendinous calcific deposits (rotator cuff tendinitis), calcified ligament (Pellegrini-Stieda disease), joint effusions, and some soft tissue swellings. Localized edema and thickening on a soft tissue x-ray strongly suggest a partial tendon rupture.

Computed tomography (CT) provides excellent bony visualization, and when used with contrast material, the CT-arthrogram can offer an improved view of articular cartilage, muscle, and soft tissues in the hips, shoulders, knees, and spine. CT is also valuable in detecting soft tissue calcification, including myositis ossificans.

Technetium bone scanning can be very useful in detecting an occult stress fracture when plain films or CT is normal. It can help in the diagnosis of medial periostitis where it may be positive in the subacute stage. In soft tissue lesions such as tendinitis and bursitis, the uptake is positive during the early period and is normal in the late period (Byers, 1996). Bone scanning has been used successfully in identifying insertional iliotibial band injury in an endurance athlete.

Ultrasound examination is a useful and reliable diagnostic tool that provides an inexpensive method to examine muscles and tendons in athletes. It can be used to detect intrinsic muscular defects, such as a partial tear, areas of calcification, and fibrous and cystic degeneration. Ultrasound also has been used to detect muscular herniation, but some muscles, such as the biceps femoris, are difficult to examine. High-resolution sonography provides valuable diagnostic information about tendons, including rotator cuff rupture, lateral epicondylitis, and tenosynovitis (or nodular tendinitis) of the fingers and wrist. Ultrasound is useful in differentiating tendinitis from partial rupture in achillodynia, and iliopsoas tendinitis, and it also assists in guided local injection of steroids.

Magnetic resonance imaging (MRI) is an extremely valuable diagnostic modality in evaluating soft tissue overuse injuries. It achieves excellent resolution of soft tissue structures and is sensitive in detecting edema and hemorrhage. In conditions such as tennis elbow (especially if refractory to treatment), not only can MRI results be used to evaluate tendon pathology, but they also can help the physician to determine whether other disorders are present that could give rise to symptoms that are similar to lateral epicondylitis. Examples include entrapment of the posterior interosseous nerve at the arcade of Frohse, synovitis, anconeus or extensor muscle compartment syndrome, lateral ligament incompetence, and degenerative arthritis. With MRI, it is possible to delineate the extent of tendon degeneration that must be surgically corrected. In the investigation of other ligament and tendon pathology, MRI has proved extremely valuable.

MRI is currently the optimal noninvasive diagnostic tool to accurately evaluate the status of muscle strains in athletes. It can accurately identify the location and extent of injury to the musculotendinous unit and help identify whether the injury requires surgical intervention to repair a fascial herniation, anastomose a complete muscle tear, or evacuate a hematoma.

MRI is also proving to have an important role in nerve injuries. In cubital tunnel syndrome, for example, repetitive valgus stress may cause inflammation of the ulnar nerve as it passes through an anatomic tunnel posterior to the medial humeral epicondyle. With MRI images, inflammation of the nerve can be seen as areas of thickening and high signal intensity. MRI can delineate the exact position of the ulnar nerve and evaluate the morphology of the perineural soft tissue, osseous structures, and space-occupying lesions such as a ganglion cyst.

Electromyography also has a role in the diagnosis of soft tissue overuse injuries. Decreased activity will be evident in muscles innervated distal to the level of nerve entrapment, whereas increased activity is seen on the injured side of an athlete with an Achilles tendon injury.

Arthroscopy is used both in diagnosis and in treatment. Operative arthroscopy is discussed later in this chapter. For soft tissue overuse injuries, arthroscopy is used mainly in the evaluation of the shoulder for signs of internal impingement, instability, rotator cuff damage, and labral tears. It has a similar role in other joints, including elbow, ankle, knee, and wrist, in the assessment of joint overload and synovitis. The condition of the tissues found at the time of arthroscopy helps dictate the therapeutic course for the athlete in question.

GENERAL CLASSIFICATION OF SOFT TISSUE OVERUSE INJURIES

All major tissues in the musculoskeletal system are subject to overuse injuries. Most commonly, overuse problems develop in the muscles and tendons. Although it is convenient to divide these muscles and tendons for ease of presentation, it is important to realize that they function together as a unit—the musculotendinous unit. Other soft tissues, including the bursa, fascia, synovium, and nerves, are also affected by overuse.

Muscle Overuse Injuries

Muscle Strains

The majority of musculotendinous injuries are acute muscle strains, or "pulls." A muscle strain occurs when there is disruption of muscle fibers, either partial or complete. It has been demonstrated that rapid, repetitive cyclic exercise above a rate of 1.0 cycle per second constitutes a high-risk condition. At this frequency of movement, the regulating and stabilizing effects of proprioception and joint antagonist muscle are grossly compromised. Muscle strains occur near the muscle-tendon junction regardless of the amount or rate of deformation of the muscle and regardless of the muscle shape or structure. Partial injuries heal with significant fibrosis, as do intramuscular hematomas. The fibrotic tissue is unyielding and may give rise to a significant inelastic region lying adjacent to normal tissue. This heterogeneity in the muscle may predispose to chronic overuse injuries unless prevented through the use of regular strengthening and stretching.

Muscle Soreness

Three types of muscle soreness are known to be associated with prolonged periods of sustained or intermittent forceful contraction. The first type, and most common, is *delayed-onset muscle soreness* (DOMS), which is experienced 12–48 hours after exercise by the athlete as diffuse muscle tenderness, stiffness, and soreness. This discomfort has been experienced by many athletes returning to exercising after a period of inactivity or after a very rigorous workout. It is often experienced in the beginner athlete as well. The phenomenon has been reported in the literature since 1902, when the theory of microrupture was proposed. Initially supported, this hypothesis gave way to the idea that soreness is due to muscle spasms elicited by the P-substance: noxious elements that are produced after strenuous exercise. The constituents of this substance, directly or indirectly (via osmotic induced changes), result in edema and produce the soreness. Regardless of the mechanism, there is little doubt that muscle damage is incurred, as evidenced by increased levels of urinary myoglobin and hydroxyproline. This type of soreness seems related to eccentric work.

The second type of muscle soreness is *acute soreness*. This is experienced only during the exercise period and disappears after exercise because it is a reflection of circulation. It can be experienced both by the beginner and by the experienced athlete. It is related to isometric contractions that induce ischemia and lead to anaerobic metabolism with lactic acid production.

The third type is *injury-related pain,* which is experienced during high-speed, repetitive exercise and is analogous to a pulled muscle.

Chronic Compartment Syndrome

All muscles are contained within a fascial sheath that acts as a constraint to exercise-induced muscle hypertrophy or increased intramuscular pressure from strong contractions. Either blood inflow or the exit of metabolites becomes impeded, leading to fluid accumulation within the interstitial space, increasing intracompartmental pressures. These syndromes occur most commonly in the anterior or peroneal compartments of the leg, and a diagnosis is suspected with a history of exercise-induced leg pain and associated tightness of the compartment that is palpable. Diagnosis is confirmed with documented intramuscular pressure criteria of one or more of the following: (1) preexercise pressure greater than 15 mm Hg; (2) a 1-minute postexercise pressure greater than 30 mm Hg, and (3) a 5-minute postexercise pressure of greater than 20 mm Hg. Initial treatment includes a modification of training (including limitation of running), a modification of athletic footwear or orthotic use, and NSAIDs. Surgical decompression by way of fasciotomy is often required to achieve permanent improvement, especially in the anterior compartment (see Chapter 24).

Tendon Overuse Injuries

Painful areas of tendon traditionally have been diagnosed by physicians as tendinitis, implying an inflammatory nature of the lesion. It is not clear whether inflammation is truly present in all forms of the pathology, especially in more chronic situations, where the histologic picture is more in keeping with a degenerative condition (Patten, 1995). These states, from a pathologic point of view, are probably best designated as tendinosis. The problem with the orthopedic literature is that there has been a lack of agreement on the use of these terms. Some researchers question whether tendinitis is appropriate to use at all and have designated conditions solely as tendinosis (Teitz, 1997). Other researchers have given tendinitis an all-inclusive definition of being a syndrome of pain and tenderness, including inflammation of sheath and tendon, and associated with degenerative changes in structure (Curwin, 1994).

In keeping with anatomic pathology, four conditions of the tendon have been described: paratenonitis, paratenonitis with tendinosis, tendinosis, and tendinitis (Puddu, 1976). For many clinicians, it may be easier and more practical to classify the injury based on the clinical entity observed: paratenonitis, tendinitis, tendinosis, or tenoperiostitis (Table 23-4), including whether there is clinically a partial or complete rupture.

Because clinically, it is often impossible to determine the exact source of pain around a tendon (i.e., palpation, as well as contraction, involves both tendon and sheath), we to reiterate the usefulness of the functional classification presented earlier (see Table 23-3).

Joint Overuse Involving Soft Tissues

Any joint that is subjected to abnormal loads, ranges of motion, or activity is prone to develop a reactive synovitis. This reaction does not necessarily have to be associated with articular surface damage and does not preclude developing arthritis but involves reactive effusion and thickening of the synovial membrane. Most commonly, this occurs in the knee, where anterior knee pain is derived from periarticular tendinitis, bursitis, fat pad impingement, plica syndrome, and chondromalacia patellae. Other joints can be affected, including the facet joints in the lumbar and cervical spine.

Overuse Injuries of Nerves

Nerve Entrapment Syndromes

These maladies may develop as a consequence of reactive swelling in the surrounding soft tissue secondary to overuse. The median nerve can be

TABLE 23-4 Classification of Tendon Overuse Injuries

	Definition	Clinical findings	Clinical example
Paratenonitis	Inflammation of paratenon sheath	Swelling, heat, tenderness, crepitation	de Quervain tenosynovitis
Tendinitis	Inflammation of tendon	Swelling, heat, tenderness, redness	Rotator cuff tendinitis
Acute	Symptoms present 2 weeks		
Subacute	Symptoms present 2–6 weeks		
Chronic/refractory	Symptoms present 6 weeks		
With partial rupture		Dramatic limitation in active motion	Partial tear rotator cuff
With complete rupture		Inability to perform active motion	Drummer boy palsy
Tendinosis	Tendon degeneration, no inflammation	Tender, palpable deformity	Achilles tendinosis
Assoc. with paratenonitis			
Assoc. with partial rupture		Distinct palpable tenderness, swelling	Partial Achilles tear
Assoc. with complete rupture		Palpable defect in continuity	Achilles rupture
Tenoperiostitis	Inflammation of insertion/origin of tendon or muscle into bone	Point tenderness over insertion, pain against resistance during active motion	Adductor longus tenoperiostitis Osgood-Schlatter disease
Skeletally mature			
Skeletally immature			

entrapped (carpal tunnel syndrome) under the flexor retinaculum; also, the ulnar nerve in Guyon canal is sometimes symptomatic for cyclists; tennis players may experience posterior interosseous nerve entrapment; and any running athlete may get entrapment of the medial and lateral plantar nerves. Soccer players may experience nerve entrapments in the groin area.

Neuritis and Neuromas

A nerve can be injured by stretching, friction, compression, or intermittent entrapment. This can lead to an inflammatory state, as in ulnar neuritis secondary to valgus overload of the elbow in pitchers, or to a neuroma, as can be located interdigitally in a Morton neuroma, which is bothersome for some runners.

Overuse Injuries of the Bursa

The bursa can be injured by direct trauma or repeated trauma, leading to the development of an adventitious bursa or hemobursa. This often occurs in bursae overlying the elbow or knee. Such a hemobursa can lead to a chronic bursitis with calcification and loose bodies that are bothersome to athletes. Bursae can be injured by friction, as in the subacromial bursa on the shoulder, the bursa around the Achilles tendon (retrocalcaneal or superficial), the pes anserine bursa of the knee, and the trochanteric bursa of the hip. Trochanteric bursitis often occurs after prolonged running on a banked surface and can be very difficult to treat. Treatment includes rest, compression, protection, NSAIDs, and occasional corticosteroid injections. Surgery is reserved for chronic symptomatic bursitis.

Treatment Philosophy of Overuse Injuries

From the outset, it should be stated that overuse injuries and chronic tendon problems can be very difficult to treat. The impact on an athlete's career can be profound because such injuries have forced many athletes to change their conditioning and training programs, prevented many from returning to competition at an elite level, and have forced some to give up athletic competition completely (Renstrom, 1988; Welsh, 1992). The following are 12 fundamental principles that guide management of these injuries.

Principle 1: Initiate Treatment Early with Focus on Both Symptoms and Etiology(s)

The treatment of soft tissue overuse injuries should be started as early as possible. If seen early and treated appropriately, injuries such as tendinitis respond quickly. When injuries become chronic, they are more difficult to treat both from a physical and a psychological point of view. The athlete who is suffering from a chronic injury that prevents active participation is often frustrated and looking for a "quick fix" to get back to competition. Once this stage is reached, the athlete requires even more counseling to remain patient with what will no doubt be a lengthy course of treatment.

Appropriate management entails treatment directed toward both cause (intrinsic and extrinsic factors) and effect (the symptoms). The initial treatment of pain, swelling, and inflammation is of paramount importance, and therefore, initial management should include the components of rest, protection, ice, compression, and elevation. The injury should be protected and rehabilitated in parallel with the healing process (Renstrom, 1994). The injured tissue needs to be stressed to activate collagen remodeling and alignment but also protected from overstress, which will cause reinjury and incite a further inflammatory response. Taping and bracing can be helpful for providing protection (Perrin, 1995). Ice is useful for treating pain, hemorrhage, and edema. It induces vasoconstriction, which results in a decrease in local blood flow. Ice acts as a topical anesthetic agent to control pain and decrease reflex muscle spasms by reducing the conduction velocity in peripheral nerves. Ice bags compared with cold gel packs elicit the greatest decrease in tissue temperature over the longest period of time, and application for 15–20 minutes is recommended. Treatment may be repeated every 1–2 hours in acute cases. In lowering the temperature, ice decreases metabolism and enzymatic function; furthermore, it slows down the inflammatory process. It is useful during the first 48 hour in acute cases and in chronic cases can be applied postactivity for 30 50 minutes.

Compression in concert with cold therapy helps to reduce the swelling. When properly applied, an elastic wrap provides effective compression without causing a tourniquet effect. Elevation decreases edema by aiding lymphatic and venous return. In acute ankle sprains, elevation has been shown to be the most effective method of reducing swelling.

Without treating the cause of the injury, relapse and recurrence are not only possible but predictable. Once the overuse injury occurs, activity must be modified. Training routines and conditioning programs need to be analyzed and changed, if necessary, because continuation of the provocative activity will cause further aggravation of the injured tissue. Participation in sport is allowed within the limits of pain. Often, the only modification necessary may be a decrease in duration, frequency, or intensity of participation to achieve effective control of symptoms. For some athletes, the particular provocative activity will have to be eliminated entirely. A swimmer, for example, who specializes in the butterfly and is suffering from shoulder impingement may have to switch to the breast stroke for a brief period.

Malalignment needs to be corrected if possible. Foot orthotics are helpful in treating some malalignment conditions (i.e., excessive pronation) that, when combined with overtraining, create excessive or unusual stress on various tissues. The purpose of the molded orthotic is to adjust the subtalar joint in its neutral position during the midstance phase of running. It also provides support for the medial longitudinal arch of the foot. Pronation occurs when the plane of the forefoot shifts so that the medial side drops below the neutral plane. It is the physiologic result of weight on the foot. Orthotics function to shorten the duration of pronation during the stance phase of running. It is important not to overcorrect, and it is always safest to aim for a slight undercorrection. Pronation can be made worse. Overcorrection can cause lateral ligament pain of the ankle and result in peroneal tendinitis. There are advocates for and against the use of orthotics. Most athletic orthotics prescribed are of the semirigid variety and have been shown to reduce loads and balance forces that are creating strain on the musculoskeletal system (Bull, 1989), although in a competing study in U.S. Marines no beneficial effect was found (see Chapter 27).

A good athletic shoe can provide support and shock absorption, both of which are important for the athlete. The shoes should be flexible in the forefoot, provide support to the medial longitudinal arch, and have a well-fitted heel counter. Modern athletic shoes are marketed as being well designed to provide this cushion and support but have not been shown scientifically to be better than the shoes of yesteryear.

Other intrinsic risk factors, such as leg-length discrepancy, poor flexibility, and muscle weakness, also need to be addressed in treating the causes of these injuries.

Principle 2: Treatment Type Depends on the Stage of Healing

The treatment of a particular overuse injury should be chosen based on the stage of healing of the damaged tissue of the musculoskeletal system (Renstrom, 1993). There are essentially three phases of healing: (1) inflammation, (2) proliferation of new collagen and ground substance, and (3) scar remodeling and maturation.

In stage 1, the objective is to treat the initial symptoms with the techniques discussed earlier to prevent prolonged inflammation and avoid new tissue disruption. In addition, measures of relative rest are used to protect the tissues from further injury. In stage 2, the objective is to gradually introduce stress and apply modalities to increase collagen production, size, cross-linking, and alignment. The rate of collagen fiber formation is directly related to the functional state of the affected area (Curwin, 1984). The collagen fibers reorient themselves in line with the tensile force applied to the tissue. In stage 3, the objective is to make the collagen as elastic as possible and decrease the formation of scar tissue. Progressive stress is placed on tissue to promote an increase in collagen fibril size and to increase cross-linking in tissues. Flexibility training is needed to decrease cross-linking in the joint capsule.

Principle 3: Specific Treatment Requires an Exact Diagnosis

It is of paramount importance that the clinician makes an exact diagnosis before specific treatment is started. An aggressive exercise program, for example, will not be the most appropriate initial treatment for a compartment syndrome, complete tendon rupture, or nerve entrapment.

Principle 4: Active Rest Is Better Than Immobilization

Immobilization is not innocuous. Prolonged immobilization of joints may result in loss of collagen ground substance and elastin. Immobilization of newly formed collagen results in a decrease in the number, size, and proper orientation of the fibers (see Table 23-1). It takes 15–18 weeks for ligaments and tendons to regain strength after immobilization has ended. Absolute rest should only be used for 1–2 days until the inflammation response has settled or in the most severe, chronic cases of tendinitis, after active rest has failed.

Active rest means that the injured area can be used, but it should be protected from significant stress, which may cause further damage(Renstrom, 1988). Active rest can be accomplished by decreasing the frequency or intensity of the activity, cross-training (i.e., biking instead of running), altering the biomechanics of the activity by decreasing body reactive forces (i.e., pool running), increasing mechanical advantage (i.e., larger grip size or racket head), or changing the athletic techniques (i.e., change in delivery of pitching). It is important as well to maintain cardiorespiratory fitness through nonaggravating exercise.

Principle 5: Physical Therapy Is the Cornerstone of Treatment; Other Modalities Are Adjunctive

Exercise and physical therapy are the keys to a successful rehabilitation program if they are timely and properly applied. Injured joints need to be fully mobilized, and tissues acting around those joints need to be conditioned to optimal levels. It is important to begin an exercise program carefully, gradually increasing the intensity and load within the limits of pain. A properly devised physical conditioning program that emphasizes flexibility and strength is most appropriate for eliminating the cause of an overuse injury. The use of medication and physical modalities is excellent for relieving symptoms and may greatly facilitate a conditioning program.

Nonsteroidal anti-inflammatory drugs (NSAIDs) are useful in the treatment of acute overuse injuries, especially if used early, when they can decrease the production of arachidonic acid derivatives in the inflammatory pathway. They are probably best prescribed at maximum dose for 10–14 days, and if no benefit is noted in the first 3 days, then likely there will be little benefit in continuing their use (Welsh, 1992). They probably do not have a major anti-inflammatory role in the treatment of chronic injuries because there is scant histologic evidence of a true inflammatory reaction (Puddu, 1976; Teitz, 1997). They are widely prescribed but have not been shown conclusively to shorten recovery time. NSAIDs used here may still be of benefit, however, for their analgesic effects in allowing patients to comply with physical therapy.

Corticosteroids are very potent anti-inflammatory drugs, and they are occasionally indicated in a few chronic overuse syndromes. Injections should never be given into the tendon because they can lead to tissue breakdown and degeneration, which can predispose the tendon to rupture. Because these injections result in decreased tensile strength, decreased production of collagen and ground substances, and may lead to circulatory stasis, the patient needs to decrease his or her physical activity for 5–10 days after injection (Renstrom, 1988, 1994). Tendon sheath injections, in contrast, are quite effective in treating tenosynovitis of the ankle or wrist. Intrabursal injections, for example, in impingement syndrome, can be effective when care is taken to remain in the bursal space and not to enter tendon or muscle. Local steroid side effects include depigmentation of the skin (particularly in black athletes) and subcutaneous fat dissolution. Steroid injections also can be given intra-articularly when there is significant reactive synovitis with an effusion. Corticosteroids may be administered topically and driven through the skin by the use of ultrasound (phonophoresis) or electricity (iontophoresis).

Ice as a modality in the treatment of acute symptoms has been mentioned, and it also may play an important role once exercise programs have begun. Ice should then be used at the end of each exercise session to help prevent recurrence of inflammation and swelling.

Heat is effective 48 hours after the acute phase and in the chronic phase. It is not used acutely in the first stage of healing because the aim is to minimize the inflammatory process. Later in the healing process, heat is used to improve blood flow, relieve muscle spasm, and decrease tissue stiffness, allowing greater ease of deformation. Heat can be applied in different ways. Neoprene sleeves help to retain heat during exercise, whereas superficial heat modalities, such as infrared lamps, heating pads, and chemical heat bags, increase heat to a depth of 1 cm (Renstrom, 1988). The most beneficial form of deep heat is ultrasound, because the high-frequency waves render the tissues less stiff and more susceptible to remodeling by applied tensile forces (Curwin, 1984). Ultrasound also increases local circulation and has been shown to speed wound healing. Lasers are another modality that has positive effects on wound healing, but unlike ultrasound, they also decrease inflammation.

Two types of electrical stimulation are used in treatment. Transcutaneous nerve stimulation (TENS) is used for pain relief and can be a useful adjunctive modality (Gleck, 1987). High-voltage galvanic stimulation (HVGS) not only produces heat in the tissues but also has been reported to be effective in retarding the formation of edema.

Lastly, deep friction massage is a modality used by physiotherapists to prevent the formation of adherent scars early in healing and later break down scar tissue. It should be avoided in the first couple of days after injury because it can produce microtrauma, induce inflammation, and have a deleterious effect on healing.

Principle 6: Develop Tissue Strength (Incorporating Eccentric Contractions)

A strength-training program should start as early as possible while being very careful to use incremental increases in load below the threshold of pain. Initially, isometric exercises are recommended and should be performed without a load. Gradually increasing loads can then be applied, but contractions should be done at levels below the "70% maximum voluntary contraction level" and should be held for less than 1 minute because they do induce ischemia. Isometric contractions can be augmented with the use of electrical muscle stimulation. When isometric exercise can be performed without pain, then active motion (isotonic or dynamic) exercises are initiated. Dynamic exercise correlates better with improved functional performance (Renstrom, 1994). These dynamic exercises include both concentric (muscle-shortening) and eccentric (muscle-lengthening) contractions. Concentric exercises, such as flexing the elbow while holding a weight, may begin relatively early in the rehabilitation program as soon as they can be performed without pain. Eccentric contractions attain significantly greater tension in the muscle-tendon unit. This increased tension and force production are the result of the noncontractile connective tissues working together with the contractile tissues. This is to say, concentric contractions stress only muscle tissue, whereas eccentric contractions stress both muscle and connective tissues (Welsh, 1992). Eccentric exercises should be avoided early when there is an increased risk of overloading the newly formed collagen. When they are started, they should be carried out initially without pain or discomfort.

It is vital that eccentric exercises be included in the physical-conditioning program because the tissues need to be strengthened to withstand the greatest stress they will endure—eccentric loading. Overuse injuries are commonly the result of cumulative trauma from repetitive eccentric loading (Puddu, 1976).

A proven effective eccentric exercise program (Fig. 23-1) has been devised (Curwin, 1984).

1. *Stretch:* Hold a static stretch for 15–30 seconds, and repeat three to five times.
2. *Eccentric exercise:* Progress from slow on days 1 and 2, moderate on days 3–5, and fast on days 6 and 7. Then, increase the external resistance and repeat the cycle. Three sets of repetitions should be performed.
3. *Stretch:* As in step 1.
4. *Ice* for 5–10 minutes.

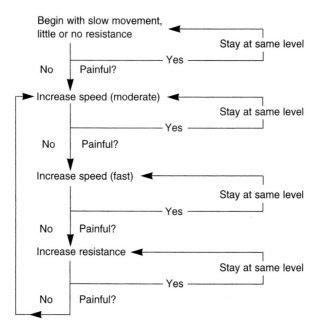

FIG 23-1 General outline of eccentric exercise program. (*Reprinted with permission from Curwin S, Stanish WD. Tendinitis: Its Etiology and Treatment. Lexington, Mass: Heath; 1984, p 65.*)

If athlete is performing the series correctly, pain should be experienced only in the last set of 10 repetitions. The pain indicates that slight overloading of the tissues is occurring, which will increase its strength. If pain is felt during all sets, then it is a sign that too much force is being applied, which in fact, may worsen the injury. If there is no pain, this indicates insufficient loading, and the patient is not working hard enough to effect benefit or improvement in symptoms. A key factor in this program is not only the progressive use of resistance load but also progressive increase in the speed of the contraction (velocity of the exercise).

Isokinetic exercise is another type of dynamic exercise in which mechanical exercise equipment provides resistance at a controlled velocity. Resistance is increased, but no acceleration is allowed. Isokinetics can be initiated early, within the limit of pain, and like any exercise, should be preceded by the application of heat and then stretching and followed by stretching and ice application.

Principle 7: Flexibility Training Must Accompany Strength Training

Strength training alone decreases joint flexibility but is counteracted when combined with flexibility training (Renstrom, 1988). The flexibility of a joint is limited primarily by tightness of the bridging connective tissues. Flexible tissue is better able to adapt to the load placed on it without suffering structural damage, and therefore, a flexibility program is essential.

Flexibility can enhance athletic performance and aid in preventing or treating injury. There are different methods of flexibility training. These methods include ballistic stretching (utilizes quick movement characterized by bobbing or rebound motions), slow static stretching (involves slowly stretching the muscle as far as possible and then holding the position for 20–60 seconds), contract-relax stretching (includes principles of proprioceptive neuromuscular facilitation in which slow stretch is followed by a maximum isometric contraction and then relaxation and another stretch), and the 3S, or scientific stretching for sport technique (muscle is passively stretched and then exposed to an isometric contraction while another person maintains the stretch).

In general, slow static stretching is the most widely used method for treatment of overuse injuries. Contract-relax stretching is popular as well. Stretching should precede and follow training or competitive athletics and is best done after a brief warm-up. Stretching should last 5–10 minutes and be repeated prior to vigorous activity. The most effective permanent change in connective tissue deformation has been accomplished with increased tissue temperature and slow static stretching.

Principle 8: Sport-Specific Training Needed Prior to Full Return to Sport

Sport-specific training involves training of the muscles and tendons involved in the athlete's specific sport. This is important and should be carried out before a full return to the particular sport, because this is essentially another phase of eccentric conditioning because it is in sporting activities that the trauma is sustained. Whether deceleration is occurring on an upper extremity while pitching or a lower extremity while stopping from a run, significant and specific eccentric loads are placed on the musculotendinous tissues.

Functional activities bridge the gap between rehabilitation of the physical components and full return to sport (Welsh, 1992). Although conditioning programs offer a controlled method of loading soft tissue, the joint movement is restricted to a single axis of rotation. When a person participates in athletic endeavors, however, well-coordinated and purposeful movement occurs about multiple axes of rotation. Therefore, even in gifted natural athletes, sport-specific training is mandatory to enable the muscle strength and endurance gains to be integrated in a functional manner. Functional training in a basketball player after knee injury, for example, might involve jogging at first, then running straight, then figure-of-eight drills, and then jumping and pivots. This would be followed by a brief time on the floor playing ball and gradually increasing the length and intensity of participation.

Additionally, it is important to incorporate proprioceptive training into the program by using exercises that require balance, weight shift, and maintenance of center of gravity. This type of training is more important for injuries such as chronic ankle pain and instability.

Principle 9: Treatment Best Involves a Team Approach

To be assured of the best chance for success, a multidisciplinary approach to the injury should be adopted. The need for the physician and therapist to work as a team is obvious, but equally important are the coach, the athletic trainer, and perhaps the family, because they can be instrumental in ensuring compliance with the directed treatment and rehabilitation. In addition, the more active the individual is in the treatment plan, the more informed and educated he or she will become with regard to preventative measures.

Principle 10: Treatment Must Be Individualized

This point cannot be overemphasized. No two athletes are exactly alike, nor will their bodies respond in the exact same fashion to an identically prescribed treatment program. One structured program is not the cure-all for all overuse injuries, and the clinician and therapist must tailor the program to the individual needs of the athlete. The only true guide that the clinician can follow is the patient's subjective complaint of pain. Respect for the individual athlete's report of pain should be a prevailing factor when designing and redesigning the treatment program.

Principle 11: Avoid Surgery Until Nonoperative Treatment Fails

With proper diagnosis and recognition of contributing risk factors, most cases of overuse injury can be treated successfully using the nonoperative methods discussed. Only after conservative methods have failed should surgery be employed (unless there is frank rupture), and only then, in a limited, yet well-defined, role.

For conditions such as lateral epicondylitis or chronic partial tears of the Achilles, adductor longus, or rotator cuff tendons, excision of scar and degenerative tissues can give good results. Release of a tight fascial compartment may be required in conditions such as de Quervain tenosynovitis and similar involvement of the peroneal tendons. Myofascial release may be required to decompress a tense compartment in the lower extremity, as with anterior exertional compartment syndrome. Carpal tunnel or Guyon canal nerve compression injuries respond well to surgical release.

Arthroscopic surgery of the knee joint in joint overload conditions to lightly debride irritated synovium and a redundant fat pad often allows an early return to sport. Arthroscopic subacromial decompression for impingement problems of the shoulder and use in repairing or debriding lesions of the labrum and rotator cuff are performed capably. Arthroscopy is also used in ankle and elbow pathology in treating synovitis or retrieving loose bodies.

Of all surgery on the body for overuse injuries, the most common is for chronic Achilles tendon pathology, accounting for almost 25% of all surgeries in one study (Orava, 1991). Surgery on tendons and tendon sheaths accounted for over 30% of operations, with over 90% of operations performed on the lower extremity.

Principle 12: Prevention Is Easier Than Treatment

Many factors, both intrinsic and extrinsic, contribute to the production of an overuse injury. The time invested by the athlete in recognizing, minimizing, or eliminating these contributing factors will be rewarded in helping to prevent initial injury and will decrease the risk of recurrence. Physicians and therapists need to stress preventive techniques to the athlete and caution against training sessions that cause fatigue. Fatigue causes imbalances and increased strain on structures less well protected than they would normally be (Welsh, 1992). It is essential that the athlete to preserve a high level of cardiorespiratory fitness, strength, and flexibility.

CONCLUSION

Overuse injuries are the result of repetitive microtrauma to the musculoskeletal system. They are common in recreational and elite athletes. Treatment protocols are based on the stage of the healing process that is active at the time of diagnosis. Most overuse injuries resolve quickly after activity modification. However, they are not always so innocuous, and some leave prolonged symptoms. With the modern-day focus on prevention with identification of risk factors and pathomechanics of injury, many of the overuse injuries can be avoided with scientific coaching and contemporary sports medicine.

REFERENCES

Akeson WH, Amiel D, Abel ME, et al. Effects of immobilization on joints. *Clin Orthop.* 1980;219:28, 1980.

Anderson RB. Ankle and foot: reconstruction. In: Kasser JR, ed. *OKU5 Home Study Syllabus.* Rosemont, Ill; American Academy of Orthopaedic Surgeons; 1996:532.

Archambault JM, Wiley JP, Bray RC. Exercise loading of tendons and the development of overuse injuries: A review of current literature. *Sports Med.* 1995;20:77.

Bennell KL, Crossley K. Musculoskeletal injuries in track and field: Incidence, distribution and risk factors. *Aust J Sci Med Sports.* 1996;28:69.

Blazina ME, Kerlan RK, Jobe FW, et al. Jumper's knee. *Orthop Clin North Am.* 1973;4:665.

Bull RC. Orthotic devices: Indications. In: Torg J, Welsh P, Shephard RD, eds. *Current Therapy in Sports Medicine*, vol 2. Philadelphia: Decker; 1989:214.

Byers GE, Berquist TH. Radiology of sports-related injuries. *Curr Probl Diagn Radiol.* 1996;25:1.

Coonrad RW. Tendonopathies at the elbow. In: Tullos HS, ed. *Instructional Course Lectures*, vol XL. Park Ridge, Ill: American Academy of Orthopaedic Surgeons; 1991:25.

Cooper DL, Fair J. Developing and testing flexibility. *Phys Sports Med.* 1978;6:137.

Curwin SL, Stanish WD. *Tendinitis: Its Etiology and Treatment.* Lexington, Mass: Collamore Press, DC Heath; 1984.

Curwin SL. The aetiology and treatment of tendinitis. In: Narries M, Williams C, Stanish WD, Micheli LJ, eds. *Oxford Textbook of Sports Medicine.* New York: Oxford University Press; 1994:512.

Dalton SE. Overuse injuries in adolescent athletes. *Sports Med.* 1992;13:58.

Drinkwater BL. *Female Endurance Athletes.* Champaign, Ill: Human Kinetics; 1986.

Fernandez PF, Rivas S, Mujica P. Achilles tendinitis in ballet dancers. *Clin Orthop.* 1990;257:257.

Gill TJ 4th, Micheli LJ. The immature athlete: Common injuries and overuse syndromes of the elbow. *Clin Sports Med.* 1996;15:401.

Gleck JH, Saliba EN. Application of modalities in overuse syndromes. *Clin Sports Med.* 1987;6:427.

Herring SA, Nilson KL. Introduction to overuse injuries. *Clin Sports Med.* 1987;6:225.

Kavlsson J, Sward L, Kalebo P, Thomee R. Chronic groin injuries in athletes: Recommendations for treatment and rehabilitation. *Sports Med.* 1994;17:141.

Lentz SS. Osteitis pubis: A review. *Obstet Gynecol Surv.* 1995;50:310.

Mayfield GW. Popliteus tendon tenosynovitis. *Am J Sports Med.* 1977;5:31.

Michael RH, Holder LE. The soleus syndrome. *Am J Sports Med.* 1985;13:87.

Micheli LJ, Fehlandt AF. Overuse injuries to tendons and apophyses in children and adolescents. *Clin Sports Med.* 1992;11:713.

Nirschl RP. Shoulder tendinitis. In: Pettrore FA, ed. *Symposium on Upper Extremity Injuries in Athletics.* St. Louis: Mosby; 1986:322.

Orava S, Leppilahti J, Karpakka J. Operative treatment of typical overuse injuries in sport. *Ann Chir Gynaecol.* 1991;80:208.

Patten RM. Overuse syndromes and injuries involving the elbow: MR imaging findings. *Am J Radiol.* 1995;164:1205.

Perrin DH. *Athletic Taping and Bracing.* Champaign, Ill: Human Kinetics; 1995.

Puddu G, Ippolito E, Postacchini F. A classification of Achilles tendon disease. *Am J Sports Med.* 1976;4:145.

Pyne JIB, Adams BD. Hand tendon injuries in athletics. *Clin Sports Med.* 1992;1:833.

Renstrom AF. Mechanism, diagnosis, and treatment of running injuries. In: *Instructional Course Lectures,* vol 42. Champaign, Ill: American Academy of Orthopaedic Surgeons; 1993:225.

Renstrom P. An introduction to chronic overuse injuries. In: Haries M, Williams C, Stanish WD, Micheli LJ, eds. *Oxford Textbook of Sports Medicine.* New York: Oxford University Press; 1994:531.

Renstrom P. Diagnosis and management of overuse injuries. In: Dirix A, Knuttgen HG, Tittel K, eds. *The Olympic Book of Sports Medicine.* Oxford: Blackwell Scientific; 1988:446.

Rubin CJ. Sports injuries in the female athlete. *N Engl J Med.* 1991;88:643.

Safran MR. Elbow injuries in athletes: A review. *Clin Orthop.* 1995;310:257.

Schaberg JE, Harper MC, Allen WC. The snapping hip syndrome. *Am J Sports Med.* 1984;12:361.

Slocum DB, James SL. Biomechanics of running. *JAMA.* 1968;205:720.

Teitz CC, Garrett WE Jr, Miniaci A, et al. Tendon problems in athletic individuals. *J Bone Joint Surg.* 1997;79A:138.

Thomas DR, Plancher KD, Hawkins RJ. Prevention and rehabilitation of overuse injuries of the elbow. *Clin Sports Med.* 1995;14:459.

Welsh RP, Woodhouse LJ. Overuse syndromes. In: Shephard RJ, Astrand PO, eds. *Endurance in Sport.* Oxford: Blackwell Scientific; 1992:505.

24 | Chronic Exertional Compartment Syndrome

Mark R. Hutchinson and Mary Lloyd Ireland

QUICK LOOK

- Defined as exertional leg pain secondary to elevated intracompartmental pressures.
- Anterior-lateral leg pain is the most common presentation. Palpable compartment tenseness and occasional peripheral numbness is also possible.
- Diagnosis is confirmed with pre- and post-exertional intracompartmental pressure testing. Elevated pressures at rest over 15 to 20 mm Hg and after exertion of over 25 to 30 mm Hg are considered positive.
- The differential diagnosis of leg pain in athletes is broad. If all other diagnoses are ruled out, conservative treatment for CECS is rarely successful. Definitive treatment is surgical release of the compartment with elevated pressure.

INTRODUCTION

Leg or calf pain can be a debilitating problem for athletes in a variety of sports but especially impact and endurance sports. Diagnosis-based treatment is frequently delayed as the athlete's self-diagnosis is "shin splints" and simply tries to tough it out. The delay in diagnosis can create chonic problems that are more difficult to treat or respond more slowly to standard conservative treatment. The differential diagnosis of chronic leg pain in the athlete is extensive but commonly includes muscle strains, stress fractures, diffuse medial tibial periostitis, and chronic exertional compartment syndrome (CECS) (Table 24-1). The "waste-basket" diagnosis of shin splints should be avoided and a more specific diagnosis should be offered to assist in targeting treatment. This chapter presents the specific diagnosis and presentation of one of the most common causes of leg pain in athletes, chronic exertional compartment syndrome. Clinical pearls that can be used to rule out other diagnoses of leg pain in athletes, the pathophysiology of acute and chronic compartment syndromes, tests to confirm CECS, conservative and

---

TABLE 24-1 Differential Diagnosis of Leg Pain in Athletes

Chronic exertional compartment syndrome
Muscle herniation
Chronic muscle strain and tendinopathies
Stress fractures
Medial tibial periostitis (shin splints)
Popliteal artery entrapment
Vascular claudication
Others
  Referred pain (spine, hip, knee)
  Malalignment (knee, leg, ankle, foot)
  Tumors (primary, malignant, metastatic, benign)
  Metabolic issues (rickets, hyperparathyroidism)
  Systemic issues (sickle cell, sarcoid)
  Nutritional (hydration, electrolytes, supplements)
  Infection
  Trauma, postsurgical adhesions, abuse

---

surgical treatment of CECS including prognosis and outcomes, and finally, brief mention of other body compartments that can suffer exertional compartment syndrome also are discussed.

EPIDEMIOLOGY AND CLINICAL PRESENTATION

Historically, some sports medicine professionals failed to consider or denied the existence of CECS. Most clinicians will readily admit the potential orthopeidic emergency of an acute compartment syndrome but not all will recognize the differences in presentation of CECS (Table 24-2). Fortunately, with accurate and readily available testing devices as well as successful surgical techniques that target specific anatomy, chronic exertional compartment syndrome is becoming increasingly recognized and treated as a cause of exercise-induced leg pain in athletes. Exertional leg pain is a common complaint in athletes and may afflict up to 15% of runners (Bates, 1985). The key in narrowing the diagnosis of CECS from the broad differential of leg pain in athletes is special attention to clinical presentation associated with a targeted physical examination. CECS is predominantly a problem of endurance athletes. Sprinters and anaerobic athletes are less likely to have CECS. Athletes with CECS present with *exertional* leg pain. Pain at rest or pain with first impact are more indicative of stress fractures, muscle strains, or medial tibial periostitis. Focal pain to palpation on the tibia is indicative of a stress fracture. Diffuse pain to palpation along the posterior medial border is commonly seen in medial tibial periostitis. Focal pain in the muscle belly or at the muscle tendon junction is more commonly seen in muscle strains or tendinopathy. Night pain should raise concern of bone tumors. Associated paresthesias are possible with CECS but are absent at rest and usually resolve with cessation of activities. Palpable soft tissue masses are indicative of tumors, cysts, or muscle herniations, and not CECS. With exertion, athletes with CECS frequently complain of progressive tightness about a specific compartment. Palpation may reveal increased tenseness compared to other compartments. The anterior and lateral leg compartments are most commonly involved but the deep and superficial posterior compartments have occasionally been implicated (Fig. 24-1). If athletes present with exertional pain in the posterior compartments and proximal posterior calf, consideration should be given to the diagnosis of popliteal artery entrapment syndrome.

With these clinical clues, the astute physician can narrow the differential diagnosis and document associated factors. It is possible for an athlete to have findings consistent with CECS in association with any of the other

TABLE 24-2 Compartment Syndromes

Traumatic	Exertional
• Secondary to fracture, crush, and reperfusion injuries	• Consistently exercise-induced
• Surgical emergency	• Generally occurs in endurance athletes
• Skin and fascia may both contribute to compartmental restriction and increased pressure	• No pain at rest; pain consistently relieved with cessation of sport
• Nonphysiologic swelling secondary to trauma	• Attributed to restriction of muscle swelling secondary to tight fascial compartments
	• Diagnosed with pre- and post-exercise pressure measurements

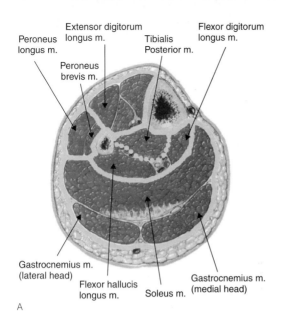

A

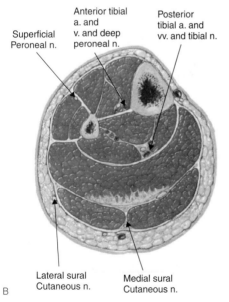

B

FIG 24-1   Cross-sectional anatomy just above the middle of the leg revealing all four compartments and the nerves at risk for ischemia A. Muscles. B. Nerves. Eighty percent of CECS involve the anterior or lateral compartments. (*Source*: From Davey J, Rorabeck C, Fowler P. The tibialis posterior muscle compartment. *Am J Sports Med*. 1984;12:391–397. © CIBA-Geigy.)

listed diagnoses. When the associated diagnosis is treated, the CECS complaints and pressure elevations can diminish. Nutritional factors, including hydration, electrolyte abnormalities, supplements, and anabolic steroid use, can increase the risk of CECS. Creatine or other nutritional supplements can increase fluid retention and cause an athlete at risk for CECS to become symptomatic. Anabolic steroids can cause an increase in muscle mass without an accompanying expansion of the fascia, leading to restriction and increased incidence of CECS. Correcting nutritional abnormalities and ceasing supplement use can return the athlete to physiologic balance and, in turn, a resolution of the CECS complaints. CECS has been reported in all adult age groups and as young as a 12-year-old female rhythmic gymnast (Hutchinson, 1998). The latter introducing unique questions regarding not only pathophysiology but of the potential of the immature growing skeleton to develop past or grow out of the complaints of CECS. Those questions remain unanswered.

PATHOPHYSIOLOGY

The pathophysiology of acute compartment syndrome is well understood (Hoffmeyer, 1987; Matsen, 1989; Mubarak, 1982; Sheridan, 1975). An increase in muscle tissue pressure can occur due to blunt or crush injury, hemorrhage, ischemia, or revascularization after arterial injury. Swelling and increased pressure within a noncompliant restrictive envelope, including fascial compartment, skin, dressings, or casts, limit arterial perfusion to the muscle, which in turn, leads to the release of inflammatory mediators and increased swelling. The downward spiral results in further ischemia, and muscle necrosis and neurovascular injury can result.

This acute pathophysiologic process, however, cannot necessarily be extrapolated to explain CECS. CECS is chronic and generally less severe in nature. Many etiologies of CECS have been proposed (Fleckenstein, 1988; Hill, 1948; Hoffmeyer, 1987; Hoing, 1981; Jacobsson, 1964; Sejersted, 1986). One widely accepted theory is pain due to ischemia from increased compartment pressure. It is known that muscle responds to exertion with increased blood volume, increased intramuscular pressure, muscular edema, and hypertrophy. Expansion may be limited by abnormal unyielding fascia, and arterial pressure may become insufficient to transport oxygen and nutrients to the muscle capillary beds. Pain and diminished performance result. No experimental model, however, has demonstrated this sequence of events. Furthermore, recent MRI and nuclear medicine blood flow studies have not been able to clearly show postexercise ischemia in patients with documented CECS, as evidenced by elevated compartment pressure measurements (Amendola, 1990; Qvarforft, 1983; Styf, 1986). Using nuclear magnetic resonance (NMR) spectroscopy to reliably evaluate muscle metabolism, ischemia has not been shown to be a significant component of CECS (Balduini, 1993; Chenton, 1986; Inch, 1986). The pathophysiology of CECS is, needless to say, complex, and future research at the cellular level may help elucidate its cause.

CONFIRMING THE DIAGNOSIS AND ADVANCED TESTING

The working differential diagnosis of leg pain in athletes is extensive and the specific diagnosis can occasionally be complicated by concurrent diagnoses. After a thorough history and physical, the work-up should target the most likely diagnoses based on the working differential created from the history and physical. Physical examination should include a lumbar spine examination, knee examination, and a weight-bearing foot and ankle examination to rule out radicular complaints, referred pain, knee pathology leading to a Baker cyst or other problems referred to the leg, alignment abnormalities, pes planus, or cavus feet. The examiner should carefully palpate all anatomic landmarks including tibia, fibula, fascia, and muscle tendon units.

Two radiographic views of the entire lower leg are routinely obtained. Although they are commonly interpreted as normal, they are a cost-effective and efficient tool in ruling out fractures, systemic bone disease, and tumors. Oblique views, soft tissue windows, and "coned-down" images can expose subtle changes related to stress fractures or periostitis. In athletes with focal bone pain, use of a hot-lamp while carefully inspecting the entire cortex of the tibia and fibula can reveal subtle radiolucencies indicative of stress fractures that may be missed on cursory inspection and review of the films. If radicular pain from the spine is present, lumbar spine films should also be obtained. Tomography and CT scans are uncommonly used as part of the initial work-up in leg pain. They are usually reserved for better delineation of fracture patterns and evaluation of benign and malignant bone tumors. Recently, high-resolution, spiral CT scans have been advocated for some soft tissue processes.

After radiographs are reviewed, additional studies should target the most likely diagnosis. If the athlete has negative radiographs with focal or diffuse bone pain, technetium bone scan can confirm the presence of stress fractures or medial tibial periostitis. Magnetic resonance imaging is sensitive for stress fractures but can also reveal a number of soft tissue pathologies leading to leg pain including Baker cysts, ganglion cysts, soft tissue tumors, myositis, muscle herniation, tenosynovitis, and tendinopathy. Pre- and post-exertion MRI has also been advocated to diagnosis CECS; however, the added cost precludes exertional MRI scanning as the initial test to confirm a likely diagnosis of CECS (Amendola, 1990; Pedowitz, 1990; Styf, 1989). Athletes who present with exertional pain referred primarily to the posterior calf and not the anterior-lateral leg, should raise suspicion of popliteal artery entrapment syndrome. Work-up should include Doppler studies or arteriograms with the knee in both a flexed and extended position, as well as with and without active muscle contraction. If the artery is entrapped by a fascial band, treatment is a local release of the band and not compartment releases. In athletes who present with bilateral neurologic symptoms, paresthesias that do not resolve with rest, and persistent motor weakness, in depth work-up of a potential nerve injury should be performed including electromyographic nerve conduction studies with advanced imaging of the lumbar spine.

In athletes who present with exertional leg pain and no other complicating factors, the initial work-up should target the diagnosis of chronic exertional compartment syndrome. The "gold standard" for diagnosis of CECS is both pre- and post-exertion intracompartmental pressure measurements. (Fig. 24-2) Historically, measurement techniques have included: Whiteside; indwelling slit catheters; wick catheters; and microcapillary infusion techniques. Each is minimally invasive and requires a percutaneous needle stick to deliver a fluid column or a wick catheter into the compartment. The catheter or needle is then attached with tubing to an

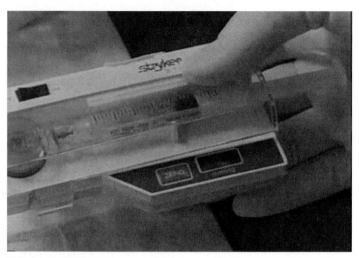

FIG 24-2 Diagnostic criteria of chronic exertional compartment syndrome with picture of Stryker portable intracompartmental pressure testing device. Intracompartmental pressure measurements are key to diagnosis. *Normal:* 0–10 mm Hg. *Abnormal:* Resting, >15 mm Hg; post-exertion, >30 mm Hg; delayed, >20 mm Hg. (*Source:* From Pedowitz et al., 1990.)

external transducer. Each technique requires a skin prep to assure sterility. Use of subcutaneous lidocaine or topical ethylene chloride can make it a less painful test.

The Whiteside technique has the distinct advantage that it can be done in any hospital room or emergency room with readily available equipment; intravenous tubing, a three-way stopcock, and a wall blood pressure gauge. (Table 24-3) This is an injection technique where the intracompartmental pressure is measured via a fluid column. Pressure is gradually increased by depressing a syringe that is connected by intravenous tubing to a mercury manometer and a hollow needle placed in the patient's compartment. When the pressure in the fluid column equilibrates with the pressure applied (by evaluating the fluid meniscus), the examiner reads the concurrent pressure off of the manometer. The advantage of the Whiteside technique is that it is inexpensive and readily available. The disadvantage is that it is a bit cumbersome and requires some finesse.

The wick catheter technique uses a specially prepared catheter with fibrous material in the lumen. The catheter is connected to a pressure transducer with tubing filled with heparinized solution to prevent clotting. The catheter is placed in the skin through a larger inserting canula. The advantage of the catheter technique is that the catheter can be left in place and multiple readings can be performed. This avoids serial needle sticks. The disadvantage is that specialized apparatus is required, including the catheter and transducer. In addition, the catheter may clot requiring flushing, or the catheter may be displaced completely with activity, necessitating replacement.

TABLE 24-3 Whiteside Technique: Step-by-step

1. Identify compartment to be measured and perform a sterile preparation of the skin with Betadine.
2. Inject 1 to 3 cc of 1% lidocaine into the subcutaneous skin. Avoid entering the fascial compartment.
3. Connect an 18-gauge needle to intravenous tubing. The opposite end of the tubing should be connected to a three-way stopcock. On one of the remaining portals of the three-way stopcock, attach a 30-cc syringe filled with air. On the final portal connect a wall blood pressure manometer; a connector and intravenous tubing may be necessary.
4. Using the syringe draw a column of sterile saline into the tubing between the needle and the stopcock.
5. Close the stopcock and insert the needle into the compartment to be measured.
6. Open the stopcock to all portals and observe the air–fluid level in the lumen of the intravenous tubing. The fluid meniscus will bubble away (convex) from the compartment with elevated fluid pressure.
7. Gradually increase pressure on the syringe and observe the air–fluid meniscus. When the bubble switches from convex to concave (the meniscus inverts), the pressure being placed on the syringe (and that is being read on the manometer) is equal to the pressure in the compartment.
8. Read the pressure on the wall manometer and record.

The continuous infusion technique uses an ordinary needle or intravenous catheter connected to one port of a pressure transducer while the other port is connected to a syringe infusion pump. Patency of the catheter is maintained by continuous infusion. Tissue pressure is read from the transducer monitor. A variation of this technique can easily be performed in the operating room making use of equipment commonly used for arterial lines, such as the pressure transducer. There is some risk of infusing too much fluid into the compartment, which leads to local edema and an abnormal pressure reading. However, it is quick and continuous.

Commercially available, battery-operated, hand-held units are now available, which make measurement of compartment pressures simple, quick, accurate, and reproducible (Stryker Corp, Kalamazoo, MI 49001) (Table 24-4). These devices are most popular for use in the emergency room or private office. A disposable, saline-filled syringe with a needle is attached via a diaphragm pressure transducer to the base unit. A simple push of a button zeros the unit and it is ready for insertion into the compartment. These units now offer the user a selection of direct needle and slit catheter techniques.

The authors' preferred technique is the portable, hand-held intracompartmental pressure monitor available from Stryker (Stryker Corp, Kalamazoo, MI 49001). It is simple and reproducible and requires little additional equipment. Even if the athlete complains of pain in a single compartment, all four compartments are routinely measured both pre-exertion and immediately post-exertion (Fig. 24-3). Delayed measurements at 15-minutes post-exertion have been recommended by some (Rorabeck, 1983); however, in our hands, they have not usually helped to clarify the diagnosis and we have discarded their routine use.

TABLE 24-4 Stryker Intracompartmental Pressure Monitor System: Step-by-step Technique

1. Identify compartment to be measured and perform a sterile preparation of the skin with Betadine.
2. Inject 1 to 3 cc of 1% lidocaine into the subcutaneous skin. Avoid entering the fascial compartment.
3. Connect the prefilled syringe, the diaphragm transducer, and the prepackaged needle in series. Clip into place on the Stryker intracompartmental pressure monitor system device.
4. Turn unit on. Make sure that a fresh battery has been installed.
5. Press the syringe so that a small drip of saline exudes from the needle tip. This will prime the diaphragm and ensure a solid column of fluid from the needle tip to the transducer.
6. Press the "zero" button to zero the Stryker intracompartmental pressure monitor system device.
7. Place needle into the compartment through the preanesthetised area of skin.
8. Inject a small amount of saline to assure a solid fluid column.
9. Wait for the reading to equilibrate.
10. Record the reading and remove the needle.

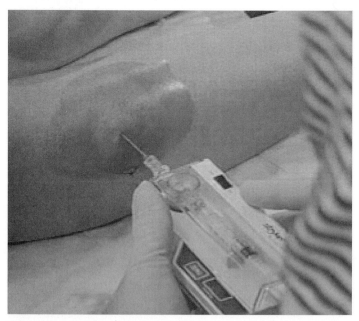

FIG 24-3 The patient is undergoing intracompartmental pressure testing of the anterior and lateral compartments, after a betadine prep, using a Stryker portable intracompartmental pressure monitor.

DIAGNOSTIC CRITERIA

In acute compartment syndrome, diagnostic criteria have included absolute pressure measurements of 40 to 60 mm Hg, relative pressure measurements within 20 mm Hg of diastolic blood pressure, and/or delta P (a calculated ratio evaluating pulse pressure and intracompartmental pressure measurements). In CECS, pressures rarely approach those seen in acute compartment syndrome (Pedowitz, 1990; Styf, 1989). Normal intracompartmental pressure measurements should be below 10 mm Hg (Fig. 24-3). In CECS, resting pressures that exceed 15 to 20 mm Hg are considered positive. Immediate post-exertion pressures that elevate over 10 mm Hg from resting or are greater than or equal to 30 mm Hg are considered diagnostic. Delayed testing 15 minutes after exertion that remains elevated above normal is also considered positive. If the resting or delayed pressures are borderline and the post-exertion testing is not diagnostic, additional work-up for other sources of leg pain is indicated.

Even with the use of local anesthetics, intracompartmental testing is a relatively painful procedure secondary to the need for relatively large bore needles, which hurt as they penetrate the fascia or skin. Future diagnostic tools will hopefully be less invasive but still accurate. Phosphorous spectroscopy (^{31}P-NMR) has provided information in the research of CECS pathophysiology and, in the future, may assist in diagnosis. (Bates, 1985; Balduini, 1993; Chenton, 1986; Inch, 1986; Styf, 1986). Near-infrared spectroscopy can evaluate oxygenation of deep tissues and has been used to monitor tissue ischemia related to both acute and chronic exertional compartment syndrome (Garr, 1999; Giannotti, 2000; Ota, 1999). It has the exciting potential of being a non-invasive and continuous testing tool. Unfortunately, currently available devices are prohibitively expensive for standard office use. Modified bone scan protocols have also been proposed as potential diagnostic tools to confirm CECS (Hayes 1995; Owens, 1999). Unfortunately, most of the non-invasive diagnostic tools are currently prohibitively expensive or not readily available.

MANAGEMENT

The management of chronic leg pain in athletes is diagnosis specific. With the diagnosis of CECS confirmed by elevated compartment measurements, the clinician should once again rule out other factors that could lead to increased pressures within the compartment such as; space occupying lesions, diffuse periostitis, stress fractures, and supplement use. If no other factors are present, nonoperative treatments such as rest, immobilization, physiotherapy, massage, cryotherapy, anti-inflammatory medication, and foot orthoses may be attempted, but, unfortunately, frequently they do not provide permanent relief of complaints. Fasciotomy has been shown to be very effective by many investigators (Almdahl, 1989; Matsen, 1989; Pedowitz, 1990; Qvarforft, 1983; Styf, 1986) and is recommended if the patient is not interested in ceasing the offending sport activity. When fasciotomy is done properly in the presence of an accurate diagnosis, excellent results can be achieved, with 90% of athletes returning to sport. Micheli (1999) suggested that the success might be slightly less in female athletes.

Anterior symptoms are most common and have been noted to comprise 70% of CECS patients (Amendola, 1990). Patients with anterior or lateral symptoms and elevated pressures should undergo a release of both the anterior and lateral compartments. The two are easily accessed through the same anterior-lateral incision/s. Medial and deep posterior complaints should be carefully screened for medial tibial periostitis or popliteal artery entrapment syndrome. Release of the deep and superficial compartments are released via a medial approach by elevating and releasing the fascial attachment off of the posterior medial border of the tibia. Historically, some investigators advocated releasing all four compartments if any single compartment was elevated. The belief was that it would reduce the risk of recurrence or missing a quiescent deep posterior compartment. However, since the most common surgical complication is post-operative bleeding and cellulitis secondary to injury of the saphenous vein during the posterior medial surgical approach and fascial release, it is wiser to be selective regarding which compartments are released. If the posterior compartment pressures are elevated with pre- and post-exertion testing, all four compartments should be released. If not, only the anterior and lateral compartments are released. As a rule, the posterior compartments should not be released without releasing the anterior compartments at the same time.

SURGICAL TECHNIQUES

The goal of surgery is to safely and effectively release the restrictive fascia of the offending compartments, which will, in turn, bring long-term symptomatic relief to the athlete. For acute compartment syndrome, the standard of care includes extensive skin incisions in association with the fascial release because the skin itself can be a restrictive layer. In CECS, only the fascia is restrictive, and extensive skin incisions are unnecessary. A majority of the anterior and lateral compartment fascia can be released through a single, mid-leg vertical incision or two separate small incisions placed proximally and distally over the raphe between the anterior and lateral compartments. The deep and superficial compartments can be addressed in a similar fashion with a medial incision placed just posterior to the posterior medial border of the tibia. The benefit of these smaller incisions is improved cosmesis and quicker recovery. However, when optimal visualization is compromised, there is an increased risk of surgical complications. When releasing the lateral compartment, the superficial peroneal nerve is at risk for injury as it penetrates from beneath the fascia to a subcutaneous position 3 to 8 cm proximal to the lateral malleolus. More proximally, the common peroneal nerve could be at risk as it wraps around the neck of the fibula. Fortunately, this is rarely injured secondary to the depth of the nerve and by maintaining a superficial direction of the fasciotome during fascial release. When releasing the deep and superficial posterior compartments through a medial incision, the most common structures injured are saphenous vein or branches of it. Special care should be made when performing deep and superficial posterior compartments to identiify and control bleeders at the time of the surgery to avoid the complication of post-operative hematomas and cellulitis. Indeed, we do not inflate the tourniquet at the time of surgery so we can identify and control each bleeder as it occurs.

Historically, blind percutaneous fascial releases have been described and reported to be effective. A minimal skin incision is made and a fasciotome is inserted and pushed blindly (Hutchinson et al., in press; Leversedge, 2002) proximally and distally to release the fascia. The advantage would be the minimal incision and the quickness of the procedure. Comparative studies in cadaveric specimens between percutaneous and endoscopically assisted techniques have revealed an unacceptably high rate of nerve and vessel injuries when this procedure is performed precutaneously and blindly. In addition, the fasciotome may slip off of the fascial edge leading to an incomplete fascial release. We would discourage this technique secondary to the risk of injury.

Two-incision fascial releases for the anterior and lateral compartments are commonly used and allow for improved visualization of structures and, therefore, reduced risk of post-operative complications (Rorabeck, 1988). Larger single mid-tibia incisions or using an endoscope through a small mid-tibia incision can also accomplish the goal of improved visualization. The anterior intermuscular septum is identified superficially between the lateral border of the tibia and medial border of the fibula. The 2- to 3-cm incisions are centered on the intermuscular septum, which can be visualized quite easily in non-obese limbs. The septum and superficial peroneal nerve are identified, and the nerve is protected. The nerve is released if its exit from the fascia is felt to be tight. Using subcutaneous finger dissection, the entire fascia adjacent to the intermuscular septum can be palpated from the knee to the ankle. Small longitudinal fascial incisions are made into the anterior and lateral compartments 1 cm on either side of the intermuscular septum. Using extended (12 in.) Metzenbaum scissors, the fasciotomies are completed subcutaneously. Care to point the scissor tips away from the nerve is important in reducing the risk of injury. Complete release of both compartments is confirmed by palpation.

A one-incision technique is used for release of the deep posterior and tibialis posterior compartments. The incision is located 1 cm posterior to the posteromedial subcutaneous border of the tibia. It is centered at the level of the distal gastrocnemius curve and is 8 to 10 centimeters long. The greater saphenous nerve and vein are easily identified and protected. Dissection down to fascia will identify the medial intermuscular septum and the periosteal-fascial junction of the tibia. This plane is then carefully developed proximal and distal to the incision. In the distal aspect of the incision, the tibialis posterior muscle and tendon are identified on the posteromedial border of the tibia. Proximally, the flexor digitorum longus occupies this position. A small vertical incision is made at the osseofascial junction. Then, using Metzenbaum scissors and staying directly on the posterior border of the tibia, the fascia is released to the level of the tibialis posterior tendon. Finger dissection is used to ensure a complete release distally. The release is then extended proximally. The soleus will then be encountered in the proximal third of the tibia at the soleus bridge. Release of this stout structure must be complete because it also represents the proximal confluence of the flexor hallucis longus and flexor digitorum longus fascia. This completes the release of the deep posterior compartment. A blunt periosteal elevator, such as a Bristow elevator, is then used to release the tibialis posterior muscle off the tibia, completing the release of the tibialis posterior compartment. Remaining on the posterior aspect of the tibia ensures avoidance of the posterior tibial neurovascular bundle. The posterior release also must be confirmed by digital palpation.

Single rather than dual incision releases of the anterior and lateral compartments can also be performed; however, visualization can be more difficult, especially as one looks more distally to try to protect the superfical peroneal nerve. Ota et al (1999) presented a single case report of an endoscopically assisted release of the anterior and lateral compartment through a single midleg incision. Since 1996, we have performed over 50 compartment releases using minimal incision and endoscopic assistance for visualization of all at-risk structures. Compartment releases are performed without a tourniquet and any bleeding is controlled immediately with an arthroscopic bovie. The superficial peroneal nerve is visualized penetrating the fascia prior to advancing the fascial release. If these guidelines are carefully followed, risk of post-operative bleeding, cellulitis, and nerve injury can be minimized. Due to the increased risk of injury to branches of the saphenous vein, even with endoscopic assistance, we continue to approach the deep and superficial posterior compartments through a larger medial approach with direct visualization. Indeed, for this reason, we abandoned routinely releasing all four compartments with any positive testing, and now selectively release only the anterior and lateral compartments if the deep and superficial posterior compartment pre- and post-exertional pressure tests are normal.

Surgery is performed as an outpatient. Some researchers recommend the use of a postoperative drain, which remains in place for several hours in the postanesthetic care room and is removed prior to discharge. We have found if careful attention to bleeding is performed intraoperatively without the use of a tourniquet, that this is not necessary. Training on crutch ambulation and the postoperative therapy protocol are given by the physiotherapist. The first few days consist of rest, ice, compression, and elevation. We have found that the use of cryotherapy devices are quite helpful at reducing both pain and swelling. Perhaps the most important instruction post-operatively is immediate ankle range of motion and stretching three to five times per day. A towel or cord can be used to assist the athlete in attaining full dorsiflexion. If the athlete is allowed to stay immobile with the foot plantar flexed, post-operative adhesions and stiffness will occur that slow rehabilitation and reduce the optimal outcome. When comfortable, we encourage the athlete to begin to massage the leg both proximal and distal to the incision to reduce the risk of subcutaneous adhesions. When comfortable, usually by the third to fourth post-operative day, the patient commences progress to walking and cycling once weaned off crutches. At 2 weeks, the wounds are checked, and formal physiotherapy for stretching and functional return to sport-specific activity is begun. A gradual return to running and impact activities is stressed, with appropriate warm-up and stretching.

OTHER COMPARTMENTS AT RISK

As noted previously, the most common anatomic region at risk for exertional compartment syndrome is the leg and, more specifically, the anterior and lateral compartments. Nonetheless, the sports clinician should be aware that any fascially restrictive muscle compartment is at risk for compartment syndrome and chronic exertional compartment syndrome (Hutchinson, 1994; Table 24-5). Fortunately, most of these are excedingly rare, with the possible exception of forearm exertional compartment syndromes in gymnasts.

TABLE 24-5 Upper and Lower Extremity Compartments with Associated Muscles, Arteries and Nerves

Region	Muscles	Artery	Nerve
Deltoid	Deltoid	Posterior humeral Circumflex	Axillary
Anterior arm	Biceps	Brachial	Musculocutaneous
	Brachialis		Median, Ulnar, Radial
	Coracobrachialis		Lateral antebrachial cut.
Posterior arm	Triceps	Profunda brachii	Radial, ulnar
Volar forearm	FCU, FCR, FDS	Radial, ulnar	Median, ulnar
	Pronator teres, FDP FPL, EPL, EPB		Anterior interoseous
Dorsal forearm	EDC, ECU		Radial
	Abductor pollicus longus		Posterior interoseous
	Extensor pollicus longus and brevis		
Mobile wad	Brachioradialis ECRB, ECRL		
Central hand	Lumbricals	Digital	Digital
	Flexor digitorum superficialis and profundus		
Thenar	Opponens pollicus	Digital	Digital
	Abductor pollicus brevis		
	Flexor pollicus brevis		
Hypothenar	Abductor digiti minimi		
	Opponens digiti minimi		
Interossei	Interossei muscles		
	Adductor pollicus		
Gluteal	Tensor fascia lata	Gluteals	Sciatic
	Gluteus maximus, medius, minimus		
Iliacus	Iliacus	Femoral	Femoral
	Psoas major and minor		
Anterior Thigh	Quadratus	Femoral	Femoral
	Sartorius		Saphenous
Posterior Thigh	Biceps femoris	Deep femoral	Obturator
	Semimembranosis		Sciatic
	Senitendinosis		
	Adductor magnus, brevis, longus		
Anterior leg	Tibialis anterior	Anterior tibial	Deep peroneal
	Peroneus tertius	Peroneal	
	Extensor digitorum longus		
	Extensor hallucis longus		
Lateral leg	Peroneus longus		Superficial peroneal
	Peroneus brevis		
Superficial	Gastroc-soleus		Sural

—cont.

TABLE 24-5 Upper and Lower Extremity Compartments with Associated Muscles, Arteries and Nerves (*Continued*)

Posterior leg	Plantarus		
Deep	FDL, FHL	Tibial	Tibial
Posterior leg	Tibias posterior		
Medial foot	Abductor hallucis	Digital	Digital
	Flexor hallucis brevis		
Lateral foot	Flexor digiti minimi brevis	Digital	Digital
	Abductor digiti minimi		
Central foot	Adductor hallucis	Digital	Digital
	Quadratus platae	Digital	Digital
	Interossei		

Abbreviations: FCU, flexor carpi ulnaris; FCR, flexor carpi radialis; FDS, flexor digitorum superficialis; FPL, flexor pollicis longus; EPL, extensor pollicis longus; EPB, extensor pollicis brevis; ECU, extensor carpi ulnaris; ECRB, extensor carpi radialis brevis; ECRL, extensor carpi radialis longus; FDL, flexor digitorum longus; FHL, flexor hallucis longus.

CONCLUSION

Chronic exertional compartment syndrome is commonly encountered as causes of exercise-induced leg pain. The understanding of the complex pathophysiology is improving through recent clinical and basic research. Accurate diagnosis and proper treatment are required to achieve successful results and to allow the patient to return to the demanding levels of sports activities.

ACKNOWLEDGMENT

We would like to acknowledge Doctors Ned Amendola and David Bell, (33) the authors of the original chapter on stress fractures and exertional compartment syndrome in the first edition of *Bull's Handbook of Sports Medicine*, who allowed us to update and addend their original, excellent offering.

REFERENCES

Almdahl SM, Samdal F. Fasciotomy for chronic compartment syndrome. *Acta Orthop Scand.* 1989;60:210–211.

Amendola A, Rorabeck CH. Chronic exertional compartment syndrome. *Curr Ther Sports Med.* 1990;2:250–253.

Amendola A, Rorabeck CH. The use of magnetic resonance imaging in exertional compartment syndromes. *Am J Sports Med.* 1990;18:29–34.

Amendola N, Bell D. Stress fractures and exertional compartment syndrome. In: Bull CR, ed. *Handbook of Sports Injuries.* New York: McGraw-Hill; 1998:245–263.

Balduini FC, Shenton DW, O'Connor KH, et al. Chronic exertional compartment syndrome: Correlation of compartment pressure and muscle ischemia utilizing 31P-NMR spectroscopy. *Clin Sports Med.* 1993;12:151–165.

Bates P. Shin splints: A literature review. *Br J Sports Med.* 1985;19:132–137.

Chenton DW, Heppenstall RB, Chance B, et al. Electrical stimulation of human muscle studied using 31P-NMR spectroscopy. *J Orthop Res.* 1986;4:204–211.

Fleckenstein JL, Conby RC, Parkey RW, et al. Acute effects of exercise on MR imaging of skeletal muscle in normal volunteers. *Am J Res.* 1988;151:231–237.

Garr JL, Gentilello LM, Cole PA. Monitoring for compartmental syndrome using near-infrared spectroscopy. *J Trauma.* 1999;46:613–618.

Giannotti G, Cohn SM, Brown M, et al. Utility of near infrared spectroscopy in the diagnosis of lower extremity compartment syndrome. *J Trauma Injury Crit Care.* 2000;48:396–401.

Hays AA, Bower GD, Pitstock KL. Chronic exertional compartment syndromes of the legs diagnosed with thallous chloride scintigraphy. *J Nuclear Med.* 1995;36:1618–1624.

Hill AV. The pressure developed in muscle during contraction. *J Physiol.* (Lond) 1948;107:518–526.

Hoffmeyer P, Cox JN, Fritschy D. Ultrastructural modifications of muscle in three types of compartment syndrome. *Int Orthop.* 1987;11:53–59.

Hoing CR. *Modern Cardiovascular Physiology.* Boston: Little, Brown; 1981:225–262.

Hutchinson MR, Bederka B, Koppelin M. Anatomic structures at risk during minimal incision, endoscopically-assisted, fascial compartment releases of the legs. *Am J Sports Med* (in press).

Hutchinson MR, Briner W. Leg pain in a rhythmic gymnast: A case report. *Med Sci Sports Exerc* 1998;30:S185.

Hutchinson MR, Ireland ML. Compartment syndromes in athletes: Treatment and rehabilitation. *Int J Sports Med.* 1994;17:200–208.

Inch WR, Serebrin B, Taylor AW, et al. Exercise muscle metabolism measured by magnetic resonance spectroscopy. *Can J Appl Sports Sci.* 1986;11:60–65.

Jacobsson S, Kjellmer I. Accumulation of fluid in exercising skeletal muscle. *Acta Physiol Scand.* 1964;60:286.

Leversedge FJ. Endoscopically assisted fasciotomy: Description of technique and in vitro assessment of lower leg compartment decompression. *Am J Sports Med.* 2002;30:272–278.

Matsen FA, Rorabeck CH. Compartment syndromes. In: *Instructional Course Lectures,* vol 38. Park Ridge, Ill: American Academy of Orthopedic Surgeons; 1989:463–472.

Micheli L, Solomon R, Solomon J, et al. Chronic exertional compartment syndromes. *Am J Sports Med.* 1999;27:197–201.

Mubarak SJ, Gould RN, Lee YF, et al. The medial tibial stress syndrome: A cause of shin splints. *Am J Sports Med.* 1982;10:201–205.

Ota Y, Senda M, Hashizume H, et al. Chronic compartment syndrome of the lower leg: A new diagnostic method using near-infrared spectroscopy and a new technique for fasciotomy. *Arthroscopy.* 1999;5:439–444.

Owens S, Edward P, Miles K, et al. Chronic compartment syndrome affecting the lower limb: MIBI perfusion imaging as an alternative to pressure monitoring: Two case reports. *Br J Sports Med.* 1999;33:49–51.

Pedowitz RA, Hagens AR, Mubarak SJ, Gershrine DH. Modified criteria for the objective diagnosis of chronic compartment syndrome of the leg. *Am J Sports Med.* 1990;18:35–40.

Qvarforft P, Christenson J, Eklof B, et al. Intramuscular pressure, muscle blood flow and skeletal muscle metabolism in chronic anterior tibial compartment syndrome. *Clin Orthop.* 1983;179:284–290.

Rorabeck CH, Bourne RB, Fowler PJ, et al. The role of tissue pressure measurement in diagnosing chronic anterior compartment syndrome. *Am J Sports Med.* 1988;16:146.

Rorabeck CH, Bourne RB, Fowler PJ. The surgical treatment of exertional compartment syndrome in athletes. *J Bone Joint Surg.* 1983;65A:1245–1251.

Sejersted OM, Hargens AR. Regional pressure and nutrition of skeletal muscle during isometric contraction. In: Hargen AR, ed. *Tissue Nutrition and Viability.* New York: Springer-Verlag; 1986:263–283.

Sheridan GW, Matsen FA. An animal model of the compartmental syndrome. *Clin Orthop.* 1975;113:36–42.

Styf J, Korner LM. Microcapillary infusion technique for measurement of intramuscular pressure during exercise. *Clin Orthop.* 1986;207:253–262.

Styf J. Chronic exercise-induced pain in the anterior aspect of the lower leg. *J Sports Med.* 1989;7:331–337.

25 | Stress Fractures

Peter G. Gerbino

QUICK REFERENCE

- Stress fractures occur in bones, physeal cartilage, apophyseal cartilage, and articular cartilage.
- Stress fractures occur from abnormal loads in healthy bone or normal loads in deficient bone.
- Many risk factors exist that predispose to stress fracture.
- Look for point tenderness.
- Treat with relative rest, strengthening around it, and modification of risk factors.

Stress fractures can occur in almost any bone in the body. They have been called *fatigue fractures, insufficiency fractures, march fractures*, and *pseudofractures*. A stress fracture in bone is best described as the variable extent of microcracks caused by the cyclic loading of that bone. The microcracks may or may not lead to a fatal crack, resulting in bone failure (Jepsen, et al., 2001).

In sports medicine, stress fractures occur in normal bones subjected to excessive loading (cycles, forces, or both) or in deficient bone subjected to normal loads (sometimes called *insufficiency fractures*). Managing stress fractures involves understanding both the loads placed on the bone and the particular strength and calcium homeostasis of that bone.

The forces that cause stress fractures can occur as compression, tension, or torsion. These forces are responsible for the majority of bone stress fractures and for all of the cortical bone stress fractures (Jepsen, et al., 2001). Cyclic compression of cortical bone causes oblique shear microcracks at approximately 30–40° to the loading axis (Jepsen, et al., 2001). Tensile loading damage occurs at lower stresses. The microcracks occur perpendicular to the stress axis. Torsional loads lead to interlamellar and cement line cracks in a radial pattern (Jepsen, et al., 2001). In trabecular bone, compression can lead to complete fracture, microcracks along lamellae, microcracks across lamellae or to diffuse damage (Jepsen et al., 2001).

Loading a bone strengthens that bone. *Wolfe's law* states that bone responds to stress in such a way as to strengthen the bone to resist that stress (Wolff, 1892). The mechanism by which bone becomes stronger is *remodeling*. This process is a balance between osteoclastic bone resorption and osteoblastic bone creation. When cyclic stresses exceed the ability of the bone to remodel, fracture begins. If repeated cyclic loading occurs without adequate healing, the cracks propagate.

A stress fracture can occur with repeated loading until failure during a single session. More commonly, the first microcracks occur at one event and propagate during subsequent stresses. In vitro femoral specimens stressed at 5000 lb/in^2 failed at one million cycles and tibiae at two million cycles (Evans, 1957).

Stress fractures occur in all age groups and can occur in cartilage as well as in bone. In children, *growth cartilage stress fracture* is common. Apophysitis including Osgood-Schlatter syndrome, Severs syndrome, and Little League Elbow are all likely due to stress failure of apophyseal cartilage. Little League Shoulder is a stress fracture to the proximal humeral

341

physis from excessive throwing. Articular cartilage can fail from repeated stress. Wear-induced chondrolysis is a type of fatigue failure to the articular cartilage matrix and can occur at any age.

LOCATIONS OF STRESS FRACTURES

As one might expect, most stress fractures occur in the load-bearing lower extremities. In military recruits, a group subjected to a sudden increase in athletic activity, virtually all stress fractures are in the lower extremities. Fifty-one percent of these fractures have been found to occur in the metatarsals, 26% the calcaneus, 17% the tibia, 4% the femur, and 2% fibula or pelvis (Morris and Blickenstaff, 1967). These areas are the most common sites of injury in athletes as well. Some stress fractures occur most often in athletes with specific risk factors. Dancers, for example, sustain far more sesamoid stress fractures than other athletes.

RISK FACTORS FOR STRESS FRACTURE

Previous studies have found multiple host and environmental risk factors contributing to the development of a stress fracture. The most frequent and universal risk factor is *training error*, sometimes referred to as "too much, too soon" (McBryde, 1985; Misrahi et al., 2000). In general, anything that increases cyclic loading or increases the load level to the bone leads to more stress fractures. Variables that lead to decreased bone density or strength increase the risk of stress fracture as well.

Youth is an independent risk factor for stress fracture (Milgrom et al., 1994). Likewise, fitness level (Beck et al., 2000; Gilbert and Johnson, 1966; Jones et al., 1993a), thigh muscle size (Beck et al., 2000; Jones et al., 1993b), and tibia thickness (Beck et al., 2000) are inversely related to numbers of tibia stress fractures. A table of risk factors for stress fracture is provided (Table 25-1). Poor or deficient bone nutrition is a major risk factor for bone weakness and stress fractures.

NUTRITION

Bone nutrition is a complex metabolic process balancing osteoblastic bone synthesis and osteoclastic bone resorption. Disproportionate resorption leads to osteopenia and osteoporosis. Dual energy x-ray absorptiometry studies assess bone density. A major determinant for bone strength is calcium mineralization; adequate calcium intake is imperative. The present guideline for calcium intake is 1200–1300 mg/d. Vitamin D, necessary to incorporate calcium into bone, should be consumed at the rate of 200–400 IU/d (National Academy of Sciences, Institute of Medicine, 2002). Decreased caloric intake (Arendt, 2000), eating disorders and disordered eating (Nattiv et al., 1994), and isolated oligo- or amenorrhea all contribute to bone density deficiency (Barrow and Saha, 1988; Bennell and Brukner, 1997; Frusztajer et al., 1990; Kadel et al., 1992; Marcus et al., 1985). Low estrogen levels in females, for whatever reason, is a separate (independent) risk factor for bone demineralization and stress fracture (Bennell and Brukner, 1997a, 1997b; Bennell et al., 1995; Cline et al., 1998; Drinkwater et al., 1990). The *Female Athlete Triad* includes bone health, amenorrhea, and nutrition risks in the constellation of the syndrome; stress fracture is often the first sign of problems in girls and young women. In summary,

TABLE 25-1 Risk Factors for Stress Fracture in Bone

Risk factor	Reference(s)
Overtraining	McBryde, 1985; Mizrahi et al., 2000
Abrupt load change	Beck, 1998
Fatigue	Mizrahi et al., 2000
Female gender	Arendt, 2000; Hulkko and Orava,1987; Jones et al., 1993b; Pester and Smith, 1987; Protzman and Griffis, 1977
Previous stress fracture	Korpelainen et al., 2001
Anatomic malalignment	Giladi et al., 1991; Matheson et al., 1987
Younger age	Milgrom et al., 1994
Low bone density	Arendt, 2000; Bennell et al., 1996; Drinkwater et al., 1990; Myburgh et al., 1990
Low estrogen level	Bennell et al., 1995, 1996; Brukner and Bennell, 1997; Cline et al., 1998; Drinkwater et al., 1990
Poor footwear	Anderson, 1990; Hulkko and Orava, 1987; McKenzie et al., 1990; Milgrom et al., 1985
Hard running surface	Hulkko and Orava, 1987
Increased foot pronation	Matheson et al., 1987; Sullivan et al., 1984
Reduced ankle dorsiflexion	Hughes, 1985
Leg length discrepancy	Clement et al., 1981; Friberg, 1988
Narrow tibia	Finestone et al., 1991; Giladi et al., 1987
Thin tibial cortex	Beck et al., 1994
Smaller thigh muscles	Beck et al., 1994; Jones et al., 1993b
Lower fitness level	Beck et al., 1994; Gilbert and Johnson, 1966; Jones et al., 1993a
Increased jumping	Arendt, 2000
Calcium deficiency	Myburgh et al., 1990
Vitamin D deficiency	Arendt, 2000
Inadequate caloric intake	Arendt, 2000
Eating disorder	Barrow and Saha, 1988; Frusztajer et al., 1990; Nattiv et al., 1994
Oligo- or amenorrhea	Barrow and Saha, 1988; Bennell and Brukner, 1997; Kadel et al., 1992; Marcus et al., 1992

proper bone nutrition requires adequate amounts of calories, estrogen, calcium and vitamin D.

DIAGNOSIS

History

Pain brought on by athletic activity and relieved by rest is typical for stress fractures. Night pain at the site can occur. There is usually a history of recent increase in volume or intensity of training. Questioning should be focused on identifying specific risk factors.

Physical Examination

Point tenderness at the site of the stress fracture is the most consistent finding. Comparison to the contralateral side may be necessary. For tibial and other long bone stress fractures, indirect three-point bending away from the fracture usually reproduces the pain (Fig. 25-1).

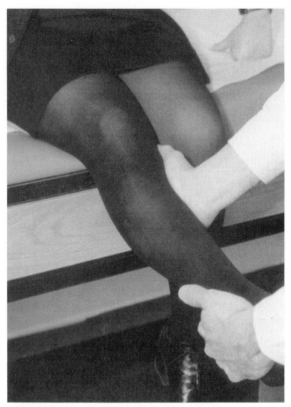

FIG 25-1 Three-point bending of the tibia applying pressure at sites away from the fracture will reproduce pain if stress fracture is present.

Imaging

Initially, plain radiographs are normal. Once healing has begun in 3–4 weeks, periosteal reaction can be seen at the fracture site (Fig. 25-2). Unfortunately, 50% of stress fractures never show radiographic evidence of their presence (Savoca, 1971). The radionucleotide bone scan is the most commonly used technique to prove the existence of a stress fracture (Roub et al., 1979) (Fig. 25-3). The bone scan also has the advantage of identifying other areas of impending stress fracture, the *stress reactions*.

Magnetic resonance imaging (MRI) can detect and perhaps even grade stress fractures (Fredericson et al., 1995). As MRI improves, it may become the study of choice when image confirmation is required to document stress fracture. It cannot supplant the bone scan for confirming metabolic activity at the site.

TREATMENT

Once a stress fracture has occurred, minimizing motion at the fracture site, providing adequate nutrients, and time allow the break to heal. Because the same deforming forces that strengthen a bone can fracture it, determining

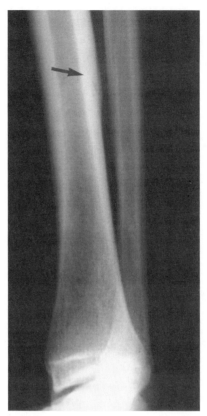

FIG 25-2 Plain radiograph of a tibia demonstrating localized periosteal reaction (arrow) consistent with a healing stress fracture.

the precise amount of micromotion necessary to optimize healing is difficult. It is probably impossible to determine for each fracture exactly the correct amount of rest and time for healing. It is generally accepted that so long as the fracture is pain free, healing is taking place. Conversely, persistent pain indicates prolonged healing or worse, enlarging fracture.

Decreasing the loads to the damaged bone is done in a number of ways. For the tibia, a pneumatic leg brace (Whitelaw et al., 1991) or simply stopping running or jumping may be adequate. Casting or crutches might be necessary, at least for a short period of time. Certain tibia stress fractures may require intramedullary nail fixation to achieve healing (Barrick and Jackson, 1992; Chang and Harris, 1996). Bone stimulators can be used to shorten healing time (Benazzo et al., 1995; O'Brien et al., 1995). The bone-building drugs, such as alendronate, calcitonin, parathyroid hormone, and estrogen, are sometimes used when there is osteoporosis and a high risk of refracture. Many of these drugs have not yet been approved for the premenopausal woman. Addressing the particular risk factors implicated in a stress fracture shortens healing time and prevents recurrence. Other techniques such as water training can maintain fitness while the fracture heals.

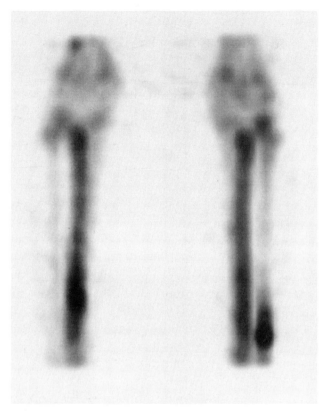

FIG 25-3 Radionucleotide bone scan demonstrating right tibia and left fibula stress fractures in the same athlete.

Prevention entails identifying potential risk factors for stress fractures in a particular individual and sport. From diet to training techniques to protective equipment, identifying and eliminating the risk factors decreases injury numbers. A meta-analysis evaluating the prevention and treatment of stress fractures found that shock-absorbing insoles and decreasing running and jumping intensity are preventative for lower extremity stress fractures. The study found that pneumatic braces decreased healing time (Gillespie, 2002). Another study concluded that specific conditioning techniques can be used to toughen bones and make them resistant to stress fractures (Milgrom et al., 2000). Intelligent training schedules that only increase activity duration or intensity by 10% per week probably protect against stress fracture better than any other intervention.

CONCLUSION

Stress fracture in bone is a predictable physical phenomenon resulting from cyclic loading at certain loads. A stronger bone is more resistant to stress fracture. Many variables can be modified to reduce cycles, reduce loads, or enhance bone strength. After fracture has occurred, damaged bones are protected to allow healing. Risk factors are addressed to reduce recurrence.

REFERENCES

Anderson E. Fatigue fractures of the foot. *Injury*. 1990;21:275–279.

Arendt EA. Stress fractures and the female athlete. *Clin Orthop*. 2000;372:131–138.

Barrick EF, Jackson CB. Prophylactic intramedullary fixation of the tibia for stress fracture in a professional athlete. *J Orthop Trauma*. 1992;6:241–244.

Barrow G, Saha S. Menstrual irregularity and stress fractures in collegiate female distance runners. *Am J Sports Med*. 1988;16:209–216.

Beck B. Tibial stress injuries. An etiologic review for the purposes of guiding management. *Sports Med*. 1998;26:265–279.

Beck TJ, Ruff CB, Shaffer RA, et al. Stress fracture in military recruits: Gender differences in muscle and bone susceptibility factors. *Bone*. 2000;27:437–444.

Benazzo F, Mosconi M, Beccarisi G, et al. Use of capacitive coupled electric fields in stress fractures in athletes. *Clin Orthop*. 1995;310:145–149.

Bennell K, Brukner P. Epidemiology and site specificity of stress fractures. In: Mandelbaum B, Knapp T, eds. *Clinics in Sports Medicine*, vol 16. Philadelphia: Saunders: 1997;179–196.

Bennell K, Malcom S, Thomas S, et al. Risk factors for stress fractures in female track-and-field athletes: A retrospective analysis. *Clin J Sport Med*. 1995;5:229–235.

Brukner P, Bennell K. Stress fractures in female athletes. Diagnosis, management and rehabilitation. *Sports Med*. 1997;24:419–429.

Chang PS, Harris RM. Intramedullary nailing for chronic tibial stress fractures. *Am J Sports Med*. 1996;24:688–692.

Clement D, Taunton J, Smart G, et al. A survey of overuse running injuries. *Physician Sportsmed*. 1981;9:47–58.

Cline A, Jansen G, Melby C. Stress fractures in female army recruits: Implications of bone density, calcium intake, and exercise. *J Am Coll Nutr*. 1998;17:128–135.

Drinkwater B, Bruemmer B, Chestnut C, et al. Menstrual history as a determinant of current bone density in young athletes. *JAMA*. 1990;236:545–548.

Evans FG. *Stress and Strain in Bones: Their Relation to Fractures and Osteogenesis*. Springfield: Thomas; 1957.

Finestone A, Shlamkovitch N, Eldad A, et al. Risk factors for stress fractures among Israeli infantry recruits. *Mil Med*. 1991;156:528–530.

Fredericson M, Bergman AG, Hoffman KL, et al. Tibial stress reaction in runners: Correlation of clinical symptoms and scintigraphy with a new magnetic resonance imaging grading system. *Am J Sports Med*. 1995;23:472–481.

Friberg O. Leg length asymmetry in stress fractures. A clinical and radiological study. *J Sports Med Phys Fitness*. 1982;22:485–488.

Frusztajer N, Dhupar S, Warren M, et al. Nutrition and the incidence of stress fractures in ballet dancers. *Am J Clin Nutr*. 1990;51:779–783.

Giladi M, Milgrom C, Simkin A, et al. Stress fractures and tibial bone width: A risk factor. *J Bone Joint Surg*. 1987;69B:326–329.

Giladi M, Milgrom C, Simkin A, et al. Stress fractures. Identifiable risk factors. *Am J Sports Med*. 1991;19:647–652.

Gilbert RS, Johnson HA. Stress fractures in military recruits: A review of 12 years experience. *Mil Med*. 1966;131:716–721.

Gillespie W. Interventions for preventing and treating stress fractures and stress reactions of bone of the lower limbs in young adults. *The Cochrane Database of Systematic Review*. 2002;2.

Hughes L. Biomechanical analysis of the foot and ankle predisposition for developing stress fractures. *J Orthop Sports Phys Ther*. 1985;7:96–101.

Hulkko A, Orava S. Stress fractures in athletes. *Int J Sports Med*. 1987;8:221–226.

Jepsen KJ, Davy DT, Akkus O. Observations of damage in bone. In: Cowin SC, ed. *Bone Mechanics Handbook*, 2nd ed. Boca Raton, Fla: CRC Press; 2001:17-9–17-10.

Jones BH, Bovee MW, Harris JM 3d, Cowan DN. Intrinsic risk factors for exercise-related injuries among male and female army trainees. *Am J Sports Med.* 1993b;21:705–710.

Jones B, Cowan D, Tomlinson J, et al. Epidemiology of injuries associated with physical training among young men in the army. *Med Sci Sports Exerc.* 1993a;25:197–206.

Kadel NJ, Tietz CC, Kronmal RA. Stress fractures in ballet dancers. *Am J Sports Med.* 1992;20:445–449.

Korpelainen R, Orava S, Karpakka J, et al. Risk factors for recurrent stress fractures in athletes. *Am J Sports Med.* 2001;29:304–310.

Marcus R, Cann C, Madvig P, et al. Menstrual function and bone mass in elite women distance runners. *Ann Intern Med.* 1985;102:158–163.

Matheson G, Clement D, McKenzie D, et al. Stress fractures in athletes: A study of 320 cases. *Am J Sports Med.* 1987;15:46–58.

McBryde AM. Stress fractures in runners. *Clin Sports Med.* 1985;4:737–752.

McKenzie D, Clement D, Taunton J. Running shoes, orthotics, and injuries. *Sports Med.* 1985;2:334–347.

Milgrom C, Finestone A, Shlamkovitch N, et al. Youth is a risk factor for stress fracture: A study of 783 infantry recruits. *J Bone Joint Surg.* 1994;76B:20–22.

Milgrom C, Giladi M, Katshan H, et al. A prospective study of the effect of a shock absorbing orthotic device on the incidence of stress fractures in military recruits. *Foot Ankle.* 1985;6:101–104.

Milgrom C, Simkin A, Eldad A, et al. Using bone's adaptation ability to lower the incidence of stress fractures. *Am J Sports Med.* 2000;28:245–251.

Mizrahi J, Verbitsky O, Isakov E. Fatigue-related loading imbalance on the shank in running: A possible factor in stress fractures. *Ann Biomed Engineering.* 2000;28:463–469.

Morris JM, Blickenstaff LD. *Fatigue Fractures: A Clinical Study.* Springfield: Charles C Thomas; 1967:12.

Myburgh K, Bacarach L, Lewis B, et al. Low bone density is an etiologic factor for stress fractures in athletes. *Ann Intern Med.* 1990;113:754–759.

National Academy of Sciences, Institute of Medicine. *Daily Reference Intakes Table.* 2002. Accessed February 12, 2003, from URL: www.iom.edu.

Nattiv A, Agostini R, Drinkwater B, et al. The female athlete triad: The interrelatedness of disordered eating, amenorrhea, and osteoporosis. *Clin Sports Med.* 1994;13:405–418.

O'Brien T, Wilcox N, Kersch T. Refractory pelvic stress fracture in a female long-distance runner. *Am J Orthop.* 1995;24:710–713.

Pester S, Smith P. Stress fractures in the lower extremities of soldiers in basic training. *Orthop Rev.* 1992;21:297–303.

Protzman R, Griffis C. Comparative stress fractures incidence in males and females in an equal training environment. *Athletic Training.* 1977;12:126–130.

Renker K, Ozbourne S. A comparison of male and female orthopedic pathology in basic training. *Mil Med.* 1979;144:532–536.

Roub LW, Gumerman LW, Hanley EN. Bone stress: A radionucleotide imaging perspective. *Radiology.* 1979;132:431–438.

Savoca CJ. Stress fractures: A classification of the earliest radiographic signs. *Radiology.* 1971;100:519–524.

Sullivan D, Warren R, Pavlov H, et al. Stress fractures in 51 runners. *Clin Orthop.* 1984;187:188–192.

Whitelaw GP, Wetzler M, Levy AS, et al. A pneumatic leg brace for the treatment of tibial stress fractures. *Clin Orthop.* 1991;270:301–305.

Wolff J. *Das Geset der Transformation der Knochen.* Berlin: Verlag August Hirschwald; 1892

26 | Foot and Ankle Injuries

Stephen M. Simons and Robert Kennedy

ANATOMY

The ankle joint, which is shaped like a carpenter's mortise, is formed by the distal end of the tibia (tibial plafond and the medial malleolus), the distal end of the fibula (lateral malleolus), and the dome of the talus. The anterior tibiofibular ligament and the posterior tibiofibular ligament hold the fibula securely in the sigmoid notch of the tibia. The dome of the talus is held under the mortise by the deltoid ligament medially, and anterior talofibular ligament, calcaneofibular ligament, and posterior talofibular ligament laterally. In general, the ankle has approximately 15–20° of dorsiflexion and 35–40° of plantarflexion. With normal walking, the ankle joint has an arc of motion ranging from 20–36°, with an average of 24° (Berry, 1952; Ryker, 1952). Abduction–adduction is 10° and internal–external rotation about 15–20° (Swain and Holt, 1993; Wilkerson, 1992).

Beneath the ankle joint is the subtalar joint. It is formed by the talus and the calcaneus. These two bones are held together by several ligaments: cervical, interosseous, lateral talocalcaneal, posterior talocalcaneal, and medial talocalcaneal (Sarrafian, 1993). The subtalar joint is one of the most important joints of the foot and ankle because it acts like a mitered hinge. It converts rotation of the vertical axis (ankle joint) into rotation of the horizontal axis (calcaneocuboid and talonavicular joints). The total arc of motion from inversion to eversion can vary from 20–60° (Isman and Inman, 1969).

The talonavicular and calcaneocuboid joints together are also known as the *transverse tarsal joint*. The significance of the transverse tarsal joint is that it transmits the motion that occurs in the subtalar joint into the forefoot. When the subtalar joint is in an everted position, the transverse tarsal joint is unlocked and the forefoot is supple, ready to make contact with the ground. When the subtalar joint is in an inverted position, the transverse tarsal joint is locked and the forefoot becomes a rigid lever arm ready for powerful push-off.

The navicular articulates with the three cuneiforms (medial, middle, and lateral). Each of the cuneiform bones, in turn, articulates with a metatarsal bone (first, second, and third). Usually, minimal motion occurs between the navicular–cuneiform articulation and between the cuneiform–metatarsal articulation. Occasionally, there is an increased laxity in the navicular–medial cuneiform joint and medial cuneiform–first metatarsal joint, which can lead to problems in these joints. The cuboid articulates with both the fourth and the fifth metatarsals. These two joints are more mobile compared to the three medial tarsometatarsal joints. Most commonly, there are three phalanges (proximal, middle, and distal) in each toe except for the great toe, where there are two phalanges (proximal and distal).

The tendons around the ankle joint can be divided into four compartments. The *medial compartment* contains the posterior tibial, flexor digitorum longus, and flexor hallucis longus tendons. The *lateral compartment* includes the peroneus brevis and longus tendons. The Achilles tendon and the plantaris tendon, if present, are in the *posterior compartment*. Finally, the tibialis anterior, extensor hallucis longus, extensor digitorum longus, and the peroneus tertius tendons are located in the *anterior compartment*. The tendons in the foot include the extensor digitorum brevis, extensor hallucis brevis, flexor digitorum brevis, flexor hallucis brevis, abductor hallucis, adductor hallucis, abductor digiti minimi, flexor digiti minimi brevis, quadratus plantae, interossei, and lumbricals.

There are five major nerves supplying the foot and ankle: tibial, saphenous, superficial peroneal, deep peroneal, and sural. The tibial nerve divides into two main branches while coursing through the tarsal tunnel: medial plantar nerve and lateral plantar nerve. Prior to entering the tarsal tunnel, posterior tibial nerve gives off the medial calcaneal nerve, which provides sensation to the posterior heel. The medial and lateral plantar nerves innervate the muscles that originate in the foot and provide sensation on the plantar aspect of the foot. The first branch of the lateral plantar nerve (also known as Baxter's nerve) travels under the heel to supply motor function of abductor digiti minimi. The saphenous nerve supplies sensation to the medial side of the ankle and foot. Superficial peroneal nerve innervates peroneus longus and brevis muscles in the lower leg. It then divides into two branches in the distal leg: intermediate cutaneous and dorsal medial. Dorsal medial branch provides sensation to the medial aspect of the great toe and lateral aspect of the second toe. The intermediate cutaneous branch supplies sensation to the medial and lateral aspects of the third and fourth toes. Deep peroneal nerve innervates extensor hallucis longus, tibialis anterior, extensor digitorum longus, peroneus tertius and extensor digitorum brevis muscles, and sensation to the first web space.

DIAGNOSIS

Making the diagnosis of a sports-related injury frequently requires the following: some understanding of the sport and the mechanism of the injury, performing a detailed physical examination, and obtaining the appropriate diagnostic studies, if necessary. The foot and ankle injuries that are discussed in this chapter include the following:

- Lateral and medial ankle sprain
- Syndesmosis sprain
- Achilles tendinopathies
- Achilles rupture
- Midfoot sprain
- Peroneal tendinitis and rupture
- Peroneal tendon subluxation and dislocation
- Posterior tibial tendon injuries
- Turf toe
- Osteochondral lesions of the talus

Each injury is reviewed in detail, along with mechanism of injury, physical findings, diagnostic studies, and treatment.

LATERAL AND MEDIAL ANKLE SPRAINS

Quick Look

- Lateral ankle sprain is defined as injury to lateral ligament complex, usually by inversion.
- Medial ankle sprain is much less frequent and is injury to the deltoid ligament.
- Initial management is protection, rest, ice, compression, and elevation (RICE).

- Early mobilization improves short-term disability if the joint is protected with an external support.
- Rehabilitation should progress from range of motion to weight bearing, strengthening, and proprioception training.

Epidemiology

The ankle sprain is the most common injury in sports. Of all ankle injuries, 80–90% are to the lateral side. It is estimated that there is 1 ankle sprain per 10,000 people per day (Katcherian, 1994). Athletes in jumping sports including volleyball, basketball, soccer, and football are most prone to ankle injuries. Risk factors for ankle sprains include previous injury to the same ankle. For example, basketball players with previous ankle injury are five times more likely to sustain a sprain (McKay et al., 2001). Taller and heavier people are also more likely to be injured.

Pathophysiology

One sustains a lateral sprain when the foot is plantarflexed and inverted. The anterior talofibular ligament (ATFL) is the first and often the only ligament affected. The ATFL lies in a horizontal plane and becomes taut when the foot plantarflexes. The calcaneofibular (CFL) and posterior talofibular ligaments are the other components of the lateral ligament complex. The CFL extends inferiorly and posteriorly from the fibula and is taut only in extreme inversion. The CFL is involved in approximately 25% of lateral ankle injuries, but never alone. The posterior talofibular ligament is only injured with frank dislocation of the ankle.

Medial ankle sprains are much less common than lateral for two main reasons. First, the fibula extends further distally than the tibia, providing a bony impediment to ankle eversion. Second, the deltoid ligament is stronger than the lateral ligaments. The deltoid ligament is the conglomeration of the posterior tibiotalar, tibionavicular, and tibiocalcaneal ligaments. These injuries occur by pronation and eversion injuries.

Injuries

Lateral ankle sprains are classified into three grades. *Grade I* injuries are mild. Swelling may be absent and tenderness is localized over the ATFL. Because the ligaments are only stretched, there is no joint laxity. Moderate sprains are termed *grade II*. With this, the ATFL and the CFL may be partially torn. Pain and tenderness are evident over the involved ligaments. Although some laxity is present, a firm endpoint can be found on ligament stress testing. Swelling and ecchymosis will develop. *Grade III* is defined as complete rupture of the ATFL and CFL and may involve the PTFL. The ankle is unstable, the patient usually cannot bear weight, and no firm endpoint is found with ligament testing. Medial sprains can be graded similarly.

Evaluation

History should be directed at the mechanism of injury, ability to bear weight or continue activity, and previous ankle injuries. The first distinction must be whether the inversion or eversion occurred. Inversion injuries with a pop felt or heard or a feeling of giving way imply more severe ligament damage.

Immediate swelling is also concerning. Additional medical history is important for any condition that may cause an insensate foot. Examination involves inspection of the ankle for swelling and bruising. Ecchymosis indicates a more severe injury or fracture and may collect in a gravity-dependent manner. Direct palpation of each of the three lateral complex ligaments helps to determine involvement. Palpation of the posterior aspect of each malleolus, fifth metatarsal, and navicular is important owing to the possibility of fractures in these areas during ankle injuries. Further, the fibular head should be palpated to rule out a Maisonneuve fracture. Range of motion is likely restricted, especially with plantarflexion, inversion, and internal rotation. These motions may also be painful. Special tests of the ankle include the anterior drawer and talar tilt tests. The *anterior drawer* tests the ATFL integrity. It is performed with the ankle in a neutral position by applying an anterior force to the posterior calcaneus while stabilizing the lower leg. The laxity should be compared to the uninjured ankle. A positive *talar tilt test* indicates injury to the CFL. This is performed by stabilizing the lower leg and then inverting and everting the calcaneus. Again, the laxity is compared to the unaffected side.

The *Ottawa ankle rules* determine the necessity of x-rays for people ages 15–55 years. The patient requires ankle x-rays if there is (1) inability to bear weight immediately and at some later evaluation (four steps), *or* (2) tenderness over posterior tip of the lateral malleolus, *or* (3) tenderness over the posterior edge of the medial malleolus. Foot x-rays are required if the patient either (1) cannot bear weight at all immediately and for less than four steps at later evaluation, *or* (2) has bony tenderness at the navicular, *or* (3) has bony tenderness at the base of the fifth metatarsal. These rules reduce use of radiography and cost, yet no fractures are missed and patient satisfaction is unchanged (Steill et al., 1994).

Management

In general, pain primarily guides ankle rehabilitation. Immediate management requires rest, ice, compression, and elevation (RICE). The goal is to protect the joint integrity and reduce pain and swelling. Cooling of the joint combined with compression leads to less swelling than either alone (Sloan et al., 1988). Ice should be applied for 15–20 minutes three to four times daily. Nonsteroidal anti-inflammatory drugs (specifically diclofenac and diflunisal) provide some benefit for pain and inflammation (Ogilvie-Harris and Gilbart, 1995). Pain-free range of motion exercises including cycling and foot motions to trace letters should begin within the first day. Depending on the amount of pain, the patient begins weight bearing as soon as possible while using an external support. At least partial weight bearing should commence within the first day. A semi-rigid brace or lace-up brace is preferable to an elastic bandage, showing a tendency toward earlier return to sport or work (Kerkhoffs et al., 2002).

Ankle strengthening with inversion, eversion, plantarflexion, and dorsiflexion exercises begins as soon as the patient's pain allows. This is usually within 2 days for a grade I or II injury. Elastic tubing can be used for resistance. Weight bearing heel raises and body weight transfers follow the open kinetic chain exercises. Finally, proprioceptive and functional training are very important. Proprioception therapy using one leg balancing and progressing to a biomechanical ankle platform system (BAPS board) improves return to sport and long-term stability. Randomized controlled trials have failed to demonstrate a significant benefit to ultrasound therapy (Van Der Windt et al., 2002). The rehabilitation advances to the next treatment when the previous is accomplished pain free.

When able to walk without pain, the patient may begin light jogging, progressively increasing the intensity as tolerated. As the patient returns to activity, cryotherapy can be restricted to after exercise. Strengthening exercises should progress to unilateral, injured side heel raises and body weight transfers with resistance. Straight-line running advances to figure-of-8 running with progressively smaller circles and cariocas. When the athlete performs these tasks pain free, he or she may return to sport. Additional ankle support from taping or bracing is used to reduce the chance of repeat injury.

Grade III injuries return to sport or work faster with early mobilization than with casting and immobilization (Konradsen et al., 1991). Long-term functional results are similar with either treatment. Early mobilization using a functional brace to allow plantar/dorsiflexion while restricting eversion/inversion is maintained at all times for at least 6 weeks. Essentially, treatment and progression of a grade III sprain is the same as less severe sprains, but the time course is prolonged and more joint protection is necessary.

Acute management of medial sprains parallels that of lateral ankle sprains with RICE. Generally allow twice as long as a lateral sprain for progression through rehabilitation and return to sport.

Confounding Injuries

History and examination should evaluate for other possible acute ankle injuries. These include a syndesmosis sprain, subtalar sprains, osteochondral defect of the talus, peroneal tendon injury or dislocation, and tibialis posterior tendon injury or dislocation. Fractures to consider include those of the lateral and posterior processes of the talus, distal fibula, distal tibia/medial malleolus, and base of the fifth metatarsal. A fracture of the proximal fibula, the Maisonneuve fracture, occurs when there is some disruption of the tibiofibular joint and forces are transmitted proximally along the syndesmosis.

For apparent ankle sprains that do not improve, one must consider a broader differential diagnosis. Chronic instability, peroneal weakness, sinus tarsi syndrome, chronic synovitis, and complex regional pain syndrome are some soft tissue causes. Aside from the above-mentioned fractures, a fracture to the anterior process of the calcaneus is possible. Finally, anterior and posterior impingement syndromes can cause chronic ankle pain. If the pain has persisted for 3 months or more all the above maladies must be considered. Evaluation of these conditions can start with MRI if available. Otherwise, consider a bone scan to help delineate bony from soft tissue injury.

Prevention

A Cochrane review found good evidence for the beneficial effect of ankle bracing such as semi-rigid orthoses or air-cast braces to prevent ankle sprains during high-risk activities (Handoll et al., 2002). Those with a history of previous ankle should use these supports during at risk activities. There may be a slight decrease in performance with these supports, but this has been inconsistently demonstrated (Thacker et al., 1999). Following a typical ankle sprain a brace should be used for sports activities for at least 6 months to help prevent further injury.

Sideline Tips

After the initial evaluation, ice should be applied as soon as possible. The numbing effect should begin within the first 5 minutes. Often an ankle injury is mild enough to allow continued participation. The athlete must be able to run, cut, and jump effectively. This can be tested with straight-line sprints, figure-of-8 running, and vertical leaping five times. The ankle should be reinforced with tape or a brace prior to return. Moderate and severe sprains will likely require crutches for exit from the sidelines.

Summary

The ankle sprain is the most common injury in sports, seen especially in basketball, volleyball, football, and soccer. The ATFL is most commonly involved and may be either stretched, partially torn, or ruptured. Regardless, rest, ice, compression, elevation, and protection are the staples of early treatment. Thereafter pain guides return to range of motion, weight bearing, strengthening, and proprioception training. Because a previous ankle injury is a significant risk factor for future sprains, a brace or air cast should be used during future athletic endeavors.

SYNDESMOSIS SPRAINS

Quick Look

- Injury to anteroinferior tibiofibular ligament with or without interosseous membrane tear.
- Often confused with severe lateral ankle sprain and may be concomitant with lateral and/or medial sprains.
- Healing time is about double a severe lateral ankle sprain.

The distal tibiofibular joint is stabilized by the syndesmotic ligaments—the anterior inferior tibiofibular ligament (AITFL), posterior inferior tibiofibular ligament (PITFL), transverse tibiofibular ligament, interosseous ligament and interosseous membrane. This structure keeps the mortise intact throughout plantarflexion and dorsiflexion talar movements. The *syndesmosis sprain* is also known as the *high ankle sprain*. Acutely they are almost always extremely painful, preventing immediate return to sport. Recovery time is at least twice that of a lateral ankle sprain and full recovery may take months.

Epidemiology

The exact incidence is difficult to discern because syndesmosis sprains are often mistaken for severe lateral ankle sprains and treated accordingly. These tend to occur in high-velocity collisions—when the foot is jammed into the ground or during a kicking motion. Skiing and football are the primary sports for this injury. High ankle sprains are less common in basketball or volleyball, despite their relatively high rates of other ankle sprains.

Pathophysiology

The mechanism produces an injury to the anterior inferior tibiofibular ligament. More severe injuries cause tibia and fibula separation and therefore tearing of the syndesmosis. Interosseous membrane rupture begins distally and progresses proximally. Syndesmosis sprains occur because, in dorsi-flexion and external rotation, the widest diameter of the talus abuts the mortise. Additional pressure to this contact forces the tibia and fibula apart. However, other mechanical stresses can lead to a syndesmosis sprain, including inversion with internal rotation (Taylor and Bassett, 1993).

Injuries

Syndesmosis sprains are graded from 1 through 3. *Grade 1 injuries* are a stretching of the ligaments and show only tenderness over these structures. *Grade 2 injuries* encompass a wide range of incomplete ligament tears and partial joint instability. *Grade 3 sprains* involve a complete disruption of the ligaments with frank instability and diastasis.

Evaluation

Again, the history should focus on the mechanism of injury. These injuries generally involve a rotation action, typically external but possibly internal rotation. Inspection reveals some degree of swelling over the lateral ankle, which makes this difficult to separate from a lateral ankle sprain. The swelling is generally less impressive and more anterior and proximal. Palpation over the AITFL and syndesmosis should reveal pain; the lateral ligament complex is pain free in an isolated syndesmosis injury. However, lateral and/or medial sprains accompany approximately one half of syndesmosis sprains. Pain restricts dorsiflexion range of motion. Syndesmosis-specific tests include the squeeze test and external rotation test. The squeeze test involves squeezing the tibia and fibula together in the midcalf and is positive if pain is elicited over the distal tibiofibular junction. Syndesmosis sprain is also suggested by pain with dorsiflexion and external rotation of the ankle. Evaluating this may be best done with the patient prone and knee at 90° flexion. In severe injuries, this test also elicits separation of the tibiofibular joint. Weight bearing AP, lateral, and mortise radiographs may aid in evaluation of diastasis of the syndesmosis, demonstrated by widening of the ankle mortise. Stress views with external rotation of the ankle are occasionally required. Later plain films may show ossification in the interosseous membrane. This has little clinical significance unless synostosis is seen, which confers a higher risk of long-term disability.

Management

Principles of treatment parallel those for other ankle sprains. Rest, ice, compression, and elevation comprise initial management. Weight bearing should be advanced as pain allows, but crutches are required initially for grades 2 and 3. The use of semi-rigid orthoses or taping help to stabilize the injury. As pain allows, strengthening and proprioceptive therapies should begin. If diastasis is present, surgical referral is necessary for stabilization.

Confounding Injuries

Other ligamentous injuries must be considered and may complicate the evaluation. Fractures are of additional concern. Avulsion of the posterior tibial tubercle, distal fibula fractures, and Maisonneuve fractures are most commonly associated with a similar mechanism of injury.

Sideline Tips

As with lateral ankle sprains, starting ice and compression quickly is helpful. On the sideline it may be difficult to differentiate a grade 1 syndesmosis sprain from a moderate lateral ankle sprain. Pain is an appropriate guide and often syndesmosis sprains are too painful to allow continued participation.

Summary

Syndesmosis or high ankle sprains can be difficult to discern from lateral ankle sprains initially. On examination, the squeeze test and pain with external rotation are most diagnostic. Initial management should consist of RICE; pain guides progression through weight bearing and functional rehabilitation. These sprains are typically disabling for a longer period time than lateral ankle injuries. Diastasis of the tibiofibular joint on examination or stress radiograph requires surgical intervention for stabilization.

ACHILLES TENDINOPATHIES

Quick Look

- Achilles tendinopathies include tendinosis, insertional tendinitis, paratenonitis, and retrocalcaneal bursitis.
- These maladies are overuse problems seen primarily in runners.
- History and examination can make the diagnosis, with tenderness over the tendon and pain with plantarflexion activities.
- Rest from the offending activity is the primary management.

The Achilles tendon, also known as the calcanean tendon, is the largest tendon in the body. It is formed by the confluence of the gastrocnemius and soleus muscles and attaches to the posterior calcaneus. It transmits the forces of the primary plantarflexors of the foot. Overuse injuries commonly, called *tendinitis*, should be referred to more generically as *tendinopathies*, because there is often no true inflammation. Instead, the tendon develops altered fiber structure and partial tears. The tendon insertion, paratenon, and retrocalcaneal bursa may become inflamed and contribute to Achilles-area symptoms.

Epidemiology

Achilles tendinosis is an overuse injury associated with runners. It primarily affects middle-aged athletes and men more than women. The injury is more common with a sudden increase in running distance and hill training. Other factors that predispose patients to Achilles injuries include excessive pronation, a cavus foot, improper footwear, calf weakness and lack of flexibility, and history of previous running injury or Achilles trauma.

Pathophysiology

Biopsy of tender tendon areas demonstrates abnormal fiber structure, hypercellularity, and vascular proliferation. Partial tendon rupture is seen in about one in five symptomatic patients (Astrom and Rausing, 1995). Aging naturally causes tendon degeneration. The tendinosis ensues following microtrauma. The paratenon is a single cell layer that surrounds the tendon. *Paratenonitis* is an irritation of the paratenon, often from friction between it and the underlying Achilles tendon. *Insertional tendinitis* is the only true inflammation within the tendon and occurs at the calcaneal insertion.

Injuries

Achilles tendinopathies include tendinosis and partial rupture, paratenonitis, insertional tendinitis, retrocalcaneal bursitis, and complete rupture. Tendinosis typically occurs in the mid-third of the tendon due to the high stresses and limited blood supply. Paratenonitis causes a diffuse swelling and tenderness in the Achilles area and crepitation is often felt with ankle movement. Palpable nodules occasionally form in the paratenon. Insertional tendinitis causes localized pain over the calcaneal insertion. It has the same risk factors as tendinosis. This condition is also associated with retrocalcaneal bursitis. The retrocalcaneal bursa is compressed between the Achilles tendon and calcaneus when the ankle is dorsiflexed so it becomes particularly susceptible to irritation when running steep gradients. Haglund's deformity is a prominence of the posterosuperior lateral calcaneus that can irritate the bursa. Achilles rupture is covered in a subsequent section.

Evaluation

The history should elucidate any of the above-mentioned factors that predispose to Achilles injury. The pain may appear gradually in a trained athlete or hours after a burst of activity in an otherwise sedentary individual. There is a feeling of stiffness in the morning that subsides with continued walking. The pain typically worsens with activity, especially with the initiation of activity. Examination should start with observation of the feet and lower leg both prone and weight bearing. Tendon swelling or enlargement indicates the likely area of affliction. One should palpate the entire tendon to determine points of tenderness, tendon thickening, irregularities or step-off, and if nodules are present. The retrocalcaneal bursa can be palpated between the tendon and calcaneus. Maximum tenderness here implies bursitis. Active and passive range of motion further evaluate biomechanical predisposing factors as well as posterior impingement. Heel raises and one-footed hops elicit the pain.

Typically, imaging is not required. However, if conservative therapy is progressing more slowly than expected or if further definition of the anatomy is desired, ultrasound or MRI clarify the exact nature of the injury. MRI is performed more often in the United States than ultrasound and is particularly helpful for preoperative management.

Management

Initial management include rests from the offending activity and ice with compression. The amount of rest is dependent on the amount of pain. Pain that does not limit performance may only require relative rest (decrease training by 25–50%), whereas pain that limits performance or does not wane with rest requires tendon rest until pain free. Adding heel lifts to the shoes reduces tendon tension. Nonsteroidal anti-inflammatory medicines should only be used acutely to help with the pain and not chronically to mask the pain during continued activity.

Chronic management includes calf muscle stretching, ultrasound, and transverse friction massage. Correction of mechanical problems with orthotics can be helpful. Strengthening is also very important. Heavy load eccentric muscle training results in decreased pain with activity and faster return to preinjury strength (Alfredson et al., 1998a). This is accomplished by starting on toes on a step and performing heel drop with the affected leg in a controlled manner. The healthy leg then assumes body weight and raises to the original position. This should be done for three sets of 15 repetitions twice daily with knee flexed and extended. Icing for 10–15 minutes after activity helps with pain. When this exercise becomes pain free, weight is added in the form of a backpack. Injectable corticosteroids are generally avoided due to the risk of rupture. However, steroids may be used to inject the retrocalcaneal bursa in refractory bursitis.

Surgery is indicated for the 25% of patients that fail at least 6 months of appropriate conservative therapy. Surgical intervention achieves a satisfactory outcome for approximately 80% of patients. Postoperatively, mobilization should begin in 2 weeks with physical therapy, but recovery is slow (Alfredson et al., 1998b).

Confounding Injuries

Aside from the distinct pathologies already discussed, complete rupture of the tendon must be ruled out with the Thompson's test or ultrasound. Sever's disease (calcaneal apophysitis) causes posterior calcaneal pain in adolescents. Posterior impingement syndrome causes pain with passive plantarflexion and may have radiographic evidence of bony abnormalities. Finally, systemic arthropathies should be considered if the clinical picture is clouded.

Prevention

There is no evidence regarding prevention of Achilles tendinopathies, but based on the mechanism of disease, certain recommendations can be made. Training regimens should be structured to provide a gradual increase in running for those starting a program, especially those over age 25. Further, hill training should be increased slowly. A program that allows for days of rest or an alternate activity (cycling, swimming) are best. Stretching and strengthening of the calf are also advantageous. If pronation is identified, custom orthotics are advisable.

Summary

Achilles tendinopathies encompass multiple entities caused by the same basic overuse mechanism. These are seen primarily in runners, associated with mechanical problems, and directly related to exercise regimens. Rest is the primary treatment; stretching and strengthening are important for rehabilitation.

ACHILLES TENDON RUPTURE

Quick Look

- Incidence of complete rupture of the Achilles tendon is increasing and has a peak occurrence in middle age.
- Examination includes Thompson's test and palpating for a gap in the tendon.

- Controversy exists regarding surgical versus conservative management.
- Most athletes choose surgical intervention due to reduced rerupture rates and quicker return to sport.

Epidemiology

Tendon rupture is most often seen in male weekend warriors ages 30–40. There is a second peak prevalence in the 70s (Moller et al., 1996). Males outnumber females by approximately five to one. The left is more commonly ruptured. The incidence is increasing from 2 per 100,000 in 1979–1986, to 12 in 1987–1994, to 18 in 1994 (Leppilahti et al., 1996). Ruptures occur most frequently in ball and racquet sports. Fluoroquinolones have been implicated in Achilles ruptures, especially in adolescents.

Pathophysiology

The injury occurs when the foot is suddenly plantarflexed against resistance or foot is forcefully dorsiflexed. Only 15–20% of patients have a prodrome of regional pain. The rupture occurs most frequently 5–6 cm proximal to the insertion due to the relatively poor blood supply in this area.

Evaluation

History often reveals a pop felt or heard and many believe they have been kicked in the heel. The acute onset generally occurs during sport. Physical examination often demonstrates a palpable step-off in the contour of the tendon. Laying the patient prone and squeezing the gastrocnemius performs the Thompson's test. If the foot does not plantarflex, the test is positive, indicating rupture. If the diagnosis is uncertain, MRI or ultrasound can be helpful. Ultrasound has an overall sensitivity of 94% and a specificity of 100% for partial ruptures (Kalebo et al., 1992).

Management

There are two treatment options, operative and nonoperative. Each option has relative advantages. Surgical intervention offers a significantly lower rerupture rate and a higher likelihood of return to sport at the same level. Conservative management eliminates the risk of wound infection and surgical scar, and is less expensive. Conservative treatment has been advocated only for those with limited functional needs and an inability to tolerate surgery (Schepsis et al., 2002). Postoperative rehabilitation can be safely started with full weight bearing and a removable walker, leading to earlier return of strength than previous regimens of casting (Speck and Klaue, 1998). However, there is no difference in coordination with an aggressive or conservative rehabilitation (Kaurenen et al., 2002). Nonoperative rehabilitation has traditionally been accomplished with casting in plantarflexion for 4 weeks followed by a walking cast or boot, and increasing weight bearing over the ensuing 4 weeks. Early mobilization with a functional brace greatly hastens return to work, provides the same strength as casting, and may be comparable to operative outcomes (DeHaven, 2000; McComis et al., 1997).

Confounding Injuries

Partial rupture of the tendon may cause a palpable defect in the tendon but allow function albeit with pain.

Sideline Tips

An athlete with a ruptured Achilles should initially be splinted in plantarflexion and should be non-weight bearing pending the decision regarding operative versus nonoperative management.

Summary

Achilles tendon rupture is most frequently seen in middle-aged men during a sporting event. They will often report a popping sensation or the feeling of being kicked or shot in the heel. Examination shows signs consistent with a loss of the continuity of the tendon. A decision must be made between operative and nonoperative management. In either case, functional bracing and early mobilization seem to provide improved immediate function without loss of future strength.

MIDFOOT SPRAINS

Quick Look

- A midfoot sprain is defined as an injury to the tarsometatarsal joints.
- A high index of suspicion and early identification is necessary for successful treatment.
- Tenderness, swelling, and weight bearing pain are most often located medially at the tarsometatarsal joint.
- Weight bearing and stress radiographs are necessary to determine stable versus unstable injury.
- Cast or boot immobilization needed for 6–8 weeks for stable injuries.
- Early surgical treatment for unstable injuries is preferred.

Midfoot sprains occur at the tarsometatarsal joints. Fortunately these potentially career-ending injuries are rare, but the true incidence is unknown. Considering the diagnosis is often missed or overlooked, it is reasonable to assume any published results probably underestimate the injury incidence. Based on published case reports it is safe to say midfoot sprains are more likely to occur in sports such as gymnastics and football. Offensive linemen are at greatest risk (Meyer et al., 1994).

The tarsometatarsal joints form a curvilinear connection of the midfoot to the forefoot. The second metatarsal base is recessed into a mortise formed by the cuneiforms. This recessed relationship provides the key to the Lisfranc joint. The Lisfranc ligament tethers the second metatarsal base to the medial cuneiform. It is this ligament that is vulnerable to sprains.

An indirect injury to Lisfranc ligament occurs by two mechanisms. In the first, while the player's knees are down, the foot is in direct line with the ground and toes are dorsiflexed, a force is applied to the heel. This may be another player falling directly onto the heel and applying a force in line with the axis of the foot. The second mechanism places the foot in extreme plantarflexion, such as a ballet dancer en pointe. A force is then applied directly along the long axis of the foot thereby disrupting the weaker dorsal ligaments and buckling the foot.

Examination reveals swelling and midfoot tenderness. Medial tenderness is associated with the longest time to recovery. The examiner should observe for an acutely flattened medial longitudinal arch. An antalgic gait and perhaps even inability to bear weight on the injured foot suggest a more severe injury.

Initial radiographs are either inadequate or misinterpreted 20–35% of the time. Weight bearing anteroposterior, lateral, and 30° internal oblique views of both feet should be obtained. The medial border of the second metatarsal and the medial border of the middle cuneiform should be aligned, although a widened intermetatarsal space is an unreliable indicator of injury presence (Mantas and Burks, 1994). A weight bearing lateral view has been suggested to evaluate these injuries (Faciszewski et al., 1990). On a lateral weight bearing film, the lower border of the medial cuneiform is normally positioned above the plantar border of the fifth metatarsal base. The collapsed medial longitudinal arch from a midfoot sprain reverses this relationship. Chiodo and Myerson (2001) suggest this lateral weight bearing view is most useful for evaluating the chronic injury, before and after reconstruction. These same authors encourage stress radiographs if there is persistent tenderness over the tarsometatarsal joint but no radiographic evidence of fracture or dislocation. MRI is used to assess subtle ligamentous injuries.

Nonoperative treatment is possible for the stable midfoot sprain. Immobilization is done in a cast or boot coupled with weight bearing as tolerated. Repeat radiographs are necessary to demonstrate no instability. Immobilization is continued for 6–8 weeks. Return to sport depends on the severity of the sprain. This may take as long as 6–12 weeks (Curtis et al., 1993). Orthotic support of the medial longitudinal arch is advised. Early operative treatment must be performed on all unstable midfoot injuries. Surgical planning is beyond the scope of this handbook. The surgeon should refer to many excellent treatises on this subject.

PERONEAL TENDINITIS AND RUPTURE

Quick Look

- Peroneal tendinitis is most often due to overuse.
- Weight bearing pain to the lateral aspect of the foot and ankle is common.
- Swelling, tenderness, and pain with passive inversion or active eversion of the foot should raise suspicion.
- Radiographs are not helpful, but MRI is diagnostic.
- RICE plus immobilization is the initial treatment.
- Surgical debridement or reconstruction is necessary for chronic injury.

Peroneal tendinitis is most often caused by overuse and may be an overlooked cause of lateral ankle pain. Frank tendon rupture is rare, but longitudinal tears are probably more common than previously appreciated (Alanen, 2001). Running, basketball, volleyball, and dancing can place considerable repetitive loads to the peroneal tendons. Abrasive injury or possibly subtle ischemia makes the tendon vulnerable at the fibular and cuboid grooves.

The athlete presents with weight bearing pain on the lateral side of the ankle or foot. Examination reveals local swelling, tenderness along the tendon course, possible tendon crepitus, and pain with passive inversion or active eversion of the foot. Standard radiographs are not helpful for peroneal tendon injury diagnosis, but are necessary to evaluate for other causes of ankle or foot pain. Clinical examination cannot distinguish tendinitis, tendon tears, or rupture. MRI or ultrasonography is necessary for cases not responding to conservative care.

Treatment begins with rest from the offending activity, ice, NSAIDS, and a stretching and strengthening program. Temporary immobilization can be helpful for chronic cases. Ankle bracing during sport participation can reduce tendon stress. Corticosteroid injections are not recommended (Sammarco, 1994).

Surgical treatment is undertaken when chronic pain and disability persist. Tendon sheath and tendons are debrided for tendinitis. Primary repair for tendon ruptures is preferable, but a proximal tenodesis to the adjacent tendon is performed if the tendon is not reparable.

PERONEAL TENDON SUBLUXATION AND DISLOCATION

Quick Look

- Peroneal tendon subluxation or dislocation may accompany an ankle sprain.
- The patient experiences pain and possible popping sensation to the lateral ankle.
- Subluxation can be provoked by asking the patient to dorsiflex the foot and then evert against resistance.
- Imaging is not very helpful, although dynamic sonography can confirm the clinical suspicion.
- Nonoperative care by cast immobilization is successful in only 50% of cases.
- Operative care is necessary based on the patient's functional impairment.
- Soft tissue repair or creation of a bone block is determined by surgeon's experience.

Peroneal tendon subluxation and dislocation are uncommon conditions. Originally described in dancers, skiing is now the activity most associated with these peroneal injuries (Earle et al., 1972). Any sport with propensity to injure the ankle is also fodder for peroneal tendon displacement. The peroneal tendons course through a fibroosseous tunnel posterior to the lateral malleolus. The superior peroneal retinaculum retains the tendons in this tunnel that is deepened by a groove on the posterior aspect of the malleolus. The usual mechanism of injury is sudden passive dorsiflexion on the everted foot coupled with a strong reflex contraction of the peroneals. The retinaculum tears at the lateral malleolus or midsubstance, allowing the tendons to course anteriorly. Certain tendon anomalies such as an accessory tendon or split peroneus brevis may predispose to subluxation.

This diagnosis is often overlooked or delayed because the patient's symptoms are attributed to chronic ankle sprain. The patient usually reports a single traumatic event. Symptoms include pain proximal to the joint line and posterior to the malleolus, swelling, disability, and ecchymoses acutely. A popping noise is noted by some. Physical examination is crucial to distinguish this entity from ankle sprain. The subluxing peroneal tendons are tender posterior and proximal to the malleolus. This is contrary to the ankle sprain, which shows anterior tenderness. The patient may have swelling or crepitus along the tendon and they may also have pain or apprehension to resisted eversion. Provocative testing is done by positioning the foot in dorsiflexion and asking the patient to evert against resistance. Safran et al. (1990) suggest performing this examination while the patient is prone and the knee is positioned at 90°. The foot is actively dorsiflexed and plantarflexed while everted against resistance.

Radiographs are not usually helpful unless a small avulsion fracture is visible on the lateral malleolus. MRI may help with a differential diagnosis and assessing copathologies to the tendon. Sonography may provide a dynamic imaging study to assess tendon displacement from the fibular groove.

Treatment for acute injuries is somewhat controversial. If the diagnosis is evident acutely, then nonoperative care in a short leg non-weight bearing cast for 4–6 weeks is an option. The foot is placed in plantarflexion and inversion to retain the tendons posteriorly. This has a reported success rate of only 50%. Operative care is gaining preference for the acute tendon dislocations.

The patient's symptoms and functional impairment determine chronic tendon subluxation or dislocation management. Efforts to buttress the tendons by ankle bracing can be attempted but are usually unsuccessful. If the patient has minimal pain and disability then observation is all that is necessary.

Surgical treatment for the acute retinacular tear or chronic subluxation generally produces quite good results (Kollias and Ferkel, 1997; Mason, and Henderson, 1996; McLennan, 1980). There are a variety of procedures available. These include retinaculum repair, bone anchors to retain the retinaculum, groove-deepening procedures, and bone block. A concomitant ankle stabilizing procedure can be undertaken if indicated. A modification of the Chrisman-Snook procedure has been recommended for the skeletally immature (Forman et al., 2000). There are no large series comparing operative with nonoperative treatments and no series comparing the various procedures. The procedure performed should be at the discretion of the surgeon's experience.

POSTERIOR TIBIAL TENDON INJURIES

Quick Look

- Posterior tibial tendon (PTT) injuries are uncommon in athletes.
- Overuse is responsible for most PTT injuries.
- The patient experiences pain and swelling to the medial side of the ankle.
- Examination reveals tenderness along the course of the tendon between the medial malleolus and the insertion in the medial longitudinal arch.
- The patient has difficulty performing a single limb heel rise.
- Plain radiographs do not assess the tendon but may reveal associated pathologies such as an accessory navicular or tarsal coalition.
- MRI can be diagnostic for PTT injury.
- Early diagnosis is necessary to prevent medial longitudinal arch collapse.
- Rest, immobilization, arch support with orthotics, and strengthening are necessary.
- Surgical care is reserved for those with progressive arch collapse and intractable symptoms.

Posterior tibial tendon (PTT) injuries are fortunately uncommon in athletes. Numerous case studies are published but incidence data are lacking (Simpson and Gudas, 1983; Woods and Leach, 1991). PTT tendinopathy or rupture is a common, often undiagnosed affliction of the middle aged or elderly with aggravating conditions such as obesity, diabetes, hypertension, rheumatoid arthritis, and steroid use. PTT injury has been associated with tarsal coalitions; these tarsal fusions usually cause a rigid flat foot thereby applying tremendous tensile loads to the PTT. Athletes acquire PTT most often from overuse. The pathomechanics of the foot and the tendon's poor vascularity just distal and inferior to the medial malleolus contribute to this site of injury (Frey et al., 1990). The PTT dynamically stabilizes the heel against eversion forces on contact and midstance. Tensile eccentric loading and compression under the medial malleolus contributes to tendon pathologic changes at this location.

Historical information varies but, often includes medial ankle pain, midarch pain, swelling, inability to push-off or jump, and progressive loss of the medial longitudinal arch. Examination shows tenderness along the course of the tendon between the medial malleolus and the navicular attachment. Inversion weakness or pain with resisted inversion may be present although this manual muscle testing can be insensitive in an athlete. Weight bearing collapse of the longitudinal arch appears late but comparison to the contralateral foot can detect this arch failure at an earlier stage. The patient is unable to perform a single limb heel raise as described by Johnson (1983).

PTT injuries are most often clinical diagnoses but recently imaging advances assist the diagnosis. Plain radiographs can identify an accessory navicular or tarsal coalition, conditions that may contribute to PTT pathology. MRI and sonography can visualize abnormal intrasubstance tendon changes, longitudinal tears, tendon thickening, and complete rupture (Fessell and van Holsbeeck, 1999). The arch collapse and mechanical stresses to the foot can also cause MR signal abnormalities in the sinus tarsi. Any abnormal signal in the sinus tarsi should prompt a review of the PTT (Anderson, 2000).

Management is directed by the patient severity at presentation. Early diagnosis is imperative to good clinical outcome. Initial care includes rest, ice, NSAIDs, and supportive footwear or orthoses. Immobilization by cam walking boot or short leg cast can be necessary for particularly painful cases. Corticosteroid injections should be avoided due to the high eccentric loads placed on the PTT and subsequent risk of tendon rupture. Surgical debridement is performed for chronic cases failing conservative care. Surgical reconstruction with tendon transfer becomes necessary for complete tendon rupture and severe arch collapse.

TURF TOE

Quick Look

- Turf toe is injury to the first metatarsophalangeal joint (MTP).
- Athletes are more susceptible to this injury when playing on artificial surfaces.
- There is usually a single traumatic episode.
- The athlete experiences pain, swelling, ecchymoses, and joint motion restriction.
- Diagnosis is largely based on clinical examination, but radiographs can be done to rule out associated fractures.
- Initial management includes RICE principles and using a stiff-soled shoe or walking boot.
- Orthotic support or a stainless steel forefoot plate may reduce the stress at the MTP when returning to sport.
- Return to sport time varies from near immediate for a grade 1 sprain to 6 weeks or more for a grade 3 sprain.

Injury to the first MTP is commonly known as *turf toe*. American football players participating on artificial turf sustained this injury at higher rates than when playing on grass surfaces. Turf toe occurs commonly when the first MTP is forcibly dorsiflexed. This causes a stretch injury to the plantar capsule of the joint and occasional compression injury to the dorsal articular cartilage of the joint.

Artificial turf becomes harder and stiff with time. This surface with its higher coefficient of friction coupled with more flexible shoes predisposes the athlete to injury. Players wearing stiffer shoes have fewer turf toe injuries (Clanton et al., 1986). Athletes with pes planus foot structure may be predisposed to turf toe as more valgus stress is applied to the medial side of the joint (Rodeo et al., 1990).

The athlete usually reports a single traumatic episode initiating pain. The MTP exhibits swelling, ecchymoses, motion restriction, and pain. A *grade 1* sprain shows minimal swelling, medial tenderness, and minimal joint motion restriction. *Grade 2* sprains show more diffuse swelling and tenderness, moderate ecchymoses, and mild to moderate motion restriction. *Grade 3* sprains have severe pain, tenderness, swelling, and ecchymoses. Motion is also severely restricted and the patient has difficulty weight bearing.

Imaging is not usually necessary. Severe or chronic cases may deserve evaluation to assess for other potential injuries such as sesamoid, metatarsal, or phalangeal fractures. This can be best done with MRI.

Treatment is with RICE initially. A stiff-soled or surgical shoe is used to reduce MTP motion. A few days non-weight bearing can be helpful for severe cases. Early range of motion efforts can reduce the return to play time. Upon return to play, a stiff athletic shoe with a stainless steel forefoot plate or a custom orthosis with a Morton's extension reduce the stress at the MTP. Return to play times vary with the injury severity. Grade 1 sprains may return to the field nearly immediately. Grade 2 sprains may return in 1–2 weeks as pain resolves and range of motion is restored. Athletes should have minimal pain and skillfully push off the affected side without difficulty to return to play. Grade 3 sprains range from 3–6 weeks for recovery.

OSTEOCHONDRAL LESIONS OF THE TALUS

Quick Look

- Osteochondral lesions of the talus follow some form of ankle trauma.
- Peak age is 22.
- Symptoms of chronic ankle pain, occasional swelling, and possible locking.
- MRI provides the best imaging.
- Stable lesions deserve a trial of conservative treatment consisting of non-weight bearing or cast immobilization.
- Surgical excision is performed for those patients with obstructive symptoms or those failing conservative care.

Osteochondral lesions of the talus (OLT) usually form after ankle trauma. Sports that involve frequent stopping and starting predispose to OLT. It is a common reason for chronic ankle pain although prevalence data are sorely lacking. The pathophysiology is controversial, but the most accepted theory proposes a subtle transchondral fracture followed by subsequent spontaneous bone necrosis. Peak age of awareness is approximately age 22. Lesion location appears nearly equal medially and laterally. More specifically the lesions tend to be posteromedial and anterolateral. The anterolateral lesions tend to be shallower and more wafer-like in shape whereas the posterior-medial lesions are more cup-like.

Most patients recall an ankle sprain, although the original injury may have been relatively trivial. They typically present with chronic ankle pain and if the lesion has progressed to fragmentation there may be mechanical symptoms such as locking, catching, clicking, or popping. Examination is non-specific. Swelling may or may not be present and the examiner should palpate the talocrural joint for tenderness to the talar dome. This can best be accomplished with the foot fully plantarflexed. Examination for associated ankle instability is warranted.

Plain radiography is performed first although radiographs of the ankle reveal only 50% of all OLTs (Anderson et al., 1989). Bone scintigraphy is very sensitive but nonspecific. CT scan can be insensitive to detecting stage I subchondral fractures, but may be used to document progression of more advanced lesions. MRI can provide a detailed look at the extent of OLT involvement. Berndt and Harty (1959) developed a classification scheme based on radiographs that until recently was widely used.

Stage I	Localized trabecular compression
Stage II	Incomplete separated fragment
Stage III	Undetached, undisplaced fragment
Stage IV	Separated and displaced fragment

Recently, Shearer et al. (2002) suggested another, Stage V lesion that was not described by Berndt and Harty. These stage V lesions are described in chronic OLT as radiolucent defects detected by CT or tomography. In a series of 220 OLT, 77% were stage V lesions.

Treatment strategies depend on the diagnosis and stage assignment. If the OLT is found after an acute injury then non-weight bearing cast or boot immobilization can be initiated. Usually these lesions are identified after some chronic ankle pain remote from the original injury. Stable lesions deserve a trial of conservative therapy again utilizing prolonged non-weight bearing immobilization. Shearer et al. (2002) detail the results of nonoperatively managed stage V lesions as follows:

- non-surgical management of stage V OLT is a viable option with little or no risk of developing significant osteoarthritis;
- most lesions remain radiographically stable;
- there is a poor correlation between changes in lesion size and clinical outcome; however, the few patients with lesions that decrease in size tend to do well and those with lesions that increase significantly in size do poorly;
- the development of mild radiographic changes of osteoarthritis does not correlate with clinical outcome;
- the general course of stage V OLT is benign with over half of the patients improving to good or excellent results with nonsurgical management;
- lateral lesions tend to do better than medial ones;
- adult-onset lesions tend to do better than juvenile-onset lesions.

Several surgical treatments are available including excision of the fragment, excision and curettage with drilling, excision and curettage without drilling, cancellous bone grafting, osteochondral transplantation, or internal fixation of the fragment. There are no randomized controlled trials comparing the different types of treatment (Tol et al., 2000). After surgery, depending on the size and location of the lesion, a period of non-weight bearing in a cast or a brace followed by a period of weight bearing in a brace is the general postoperative care.

ACKNOWLEDGMENTS

The authors acknowledge contributions by Wen Chao and William G. Hamilton from the first edition of this book.

REFERENCES

Alfredson H, Pietila T, Jonsson P, Lorentzon MD. Heavy-load eccentric calf training for the treatment of chronic Achilles tendinosis. *Am J Sports Med.* 1998a;26:360–366.

Alfredson H, Pietila T, Ohberg L, Lorentzon R. Achilles tendinosis and calf strength. *Am J Sports Med.* 1998b; 26:166–171.

Alanen J. Peroneal tendon injuries. Report of thirty-eight operated cases. *Ann Chir Gynaecol.* 2001;90:43–46.

Anderson IF, Crichton KJ, Grattan-Smith T, Cooper RA, Brazier D. Osteochondral fractures of the dome of the talus. *J Bone Joint Surg Am.* 1989;71:1143–1152.

Anderson MW. Association of posterior tibial tendon abnormalities with abnormal signal intensity in the sinus tarsi on MR imaging. *Skeletal Radiol.* 2000;29:514–519.

Astrom M, Rausing A. Chronic Achilles tendinopathy. A survey of surgical and histopathologic findings. *Clin Orthop.* 1995;316:151–164.

Berndt AL, Harty M. Transchondral fractures (osteochondritis dissecans) of the talus. *J Bone Joint Surg Am.* 1959;41A:988–989.

Berry FR Jr. Angle variation patterns of normal hip, knee and ankle in different operations. *Univ Calif Prosthet Devices Res Rep.* 1952;11(21).

Chiodo CP, Myerson MS. Developments and advances in the diagnosis and treatment of injuries to the tarsometatarsal joint. *Orthop Clin North Am.* 2001;32:11–20.

Clanton TO, Butler JE, Eggert A. Injuries to the metatarsophalangeal joints in athletes. *Foot Ankle.* 1986;7:162–176.

Curtis MJ, Myerson M, Szura B. Tarsometatarsal joint injuries in the athlete. *Am J Sports Med.* 1993;21:497–502.

DeHaven KE. Functional bracing of Achilles tendon rupture. *Sports Med Arth Rev.* 2000;8:102–104.

Earle SA, Moritz JR, Tapper EM. Dislocation of the peroneal tendons of the ankle: An analysis of 25 ski injuries. *Northwest Med.* 1972;71:108–110.

Faciszewski T, Burks RT, Manaster BJ. Subtle injuries of the Lisfranc joint. *J Bone Joint Surg.* 1990;72:1519–1522.

Fessell DP, van Holsbeeck MT. Musculoskeletal ultrasound: Foot and ankle sonography. *Radiol Clin North Am.* 1999;37:831–858.

Forman ES, Micheli LJ, Backe LM. Chronic recurrent subluxation of the peroneal tendons in a pediatric patient, surgical recommendations. *Foot Ankle Int.* 2000;21:51–53.

Frey C, Shereff M, Greenridge N. Vascularity of the posterior tibial tendon. *J Bone Joint Surg Am.* 1990;72A:884–888.

Handoll HHG, Rowe BH, Quinn KM, de Bie R. Interventions for preventing ankle ligament injuries (Cochrane Review). In: *The Cochrane Library*, Issue 3, 2002. Oxford: Update Software.

Isman RE, Inman VT. Anthropometric studies of the human foot and ankle. *Bull Prosthet Res.* 1969;97:10–11.

Johnson KA. Tibialis posterior tendon rupture. *Clin Orthop.* 1983;177:140–147.

Kalebo P, Allenmark C, Peterson L, Sward L. Diagnostic value of ultrasonography in partial ruptures of the Achilles tendon. *Am J Sport Med.* 1992;20:378–381.

Katcherian DA. Soft-tissue injuries of the ankle. In: Dutter LD, Mizel MS, Pfeffer GB, eds. *Orthopaedic Knowledge Update: Foot and Ankle.* Rosemont, Ill: American Academy of Orthopaedic Surgeons; 1994;241–253.

Kauranen K, Kangas J, Leppilahti J. Recovering motor performance of the foot after Achilles rupture repair: A randomized clinical study about early functional treatment vs. early immobilization of Achilles tendon in tension. *Foot Ankle Int.* 2002;23:600–605.

Kerkhoffs GMMJ, Struijs PAA, Marti RK, Assendelft WJJ, Blankevoort L, Dijk van CN. Different functional treatment strategies for acute lateral ankle ligament injuries in adults (Cochrane Review). In: *The Cochrane Library*, Issue 3, 2002. Oxford: Update Software.

Kollias SL, Ferkel RD. Fibular grooving for recurrent peroneal tendon subluxation. *Am J Sports Med.* 1997;25:329–335.

Konradsen L, Holmer P, Sondergaard L. Early mobilization treatment for grade III ankle ligament injuries. *Foot Ankle.* 1991;12:69–73.

Leppilahti J, Puranen J, Orava S. Incidence of Achilles tendon rupture. *Acta Orthop Scand.* 1996;67:277–279.

Mantas JP, Burks RT. Lisfranc injuries in the athlete. *Clin Sports Med.* 1994;13:719–730.

Mason RB, Henderson JP. Traumatic peroneal tendon instability. *Am J Sports Med.* 1996;24:652–658.

McComis GP, Nawoczenski DA, DeHaven KE. Functional bracing for rupture of the Achilles tendon. *J Bone Joint Surg Am.* 1997;79A:1799–1808.

McKay GD, Goldie PA, Payne WR, Oakes BW. Ankle injuries in basketball: Injury rate and risk factors. *Br J Sports Med.* 2001;35:103–108.

McLennan JG. Treatment of acute and chronic luxations of the peroneal tendons. *Am J Sports Med.* 1980;8:432–436.

Meyer SA, Callaghan JJ, Albright JP, Crowley ET, Powell JW. Midfoot sprains in collegiate football players. *Am J Sports Med.* 1994;22;392–401.

Moller A, Astrom M, Westlin NE. Increasing incidence of Achilles tendon rupture. *Acta Orthop Scand.* 1996;67:479–481.

Ogilvie-Harris DJ, Gilbart M. Treatment modalities for soft tissue injuries of the ankle: A critical review. *Clin J Sport Med.* 1995;5:175–186.

Rodeo SA, O'Brien S, Warren RF, et al. Turf-toe: An analysis of metatarsophalangeal joint sprains in professional football players. *Am J Sports Med.* 1990;18:280–285.

Ryker NJ Jr. Glass walkway studies of normal subjects during normal walking. *Univ Calif Prosthet Device Res Rep.* 1952;11(20).

Safran MR, O'Malley DO, Fu FH. Peroneal tendon subluxation in athletes: New exam technique, case reports, and review. *Med Sci Sports Exerc.* 1990;31:S487–S492.

Sammarco, GJ. Peroneal tendon injuries. *Orthop Clin North Am.* 1994;25:135–145.

Sarrafian SK: *Anatomy of the foot and ankle: Descriptive, topographical and Functional.* 2nd ed. Philadelphia: Lippincott; 1993.

Schepsis AA, Jones H, Haas AL. Achilles tendon disorders in athletes. *Am J Sports Med.* 2002;30:287–305.

Shearer C, Loomer R, Clement D. Nonoperatively managed Stage 5 osteochondral talar lesions. *Foot Ankle Int.* 2002;23:651–654.

Simpson RR, Gudas CJ. Posterior tibial tendon rupture in a world class runner. *J Foot Surg.* 1983;22:74–77.

Sloan JP, Giddings P, Hain R. Effects of cold and compression on edema. *Phys Sport Med.* 1988;16:116–120.

Speck M, Klaue K. Early full weightbearing and functional treatment after surgical repair of acute Achilles tendon rupture. *Am J Sports Med.* 1998;26:789–793.

Stiell IG, McKnight RD, Greenberg GH, et al. Implementation of Ottawa Ankle Rules. *JAMA.* 1994;271:827–832.

Swain RA, Holt WS. Ankle injuries. Tips from sports medicine physicians. *Postgrad Med.* 1993;3:91–100.

Taylor DC, Bassett FH. Syndesmosis ankle sprains diagnosing the injury and aiding recovery. *Phys Sport Med.* 1993;21:39–46.

Thacker SB, Stroup DF, Branche CM, Gilchrist J, Goodman RA, Weitman EA. The prevention of ankle sprains in sports. A systematic review of the literature. *Am J Sports Med*. 1999;27:753–759.

Tol JL, Struijs PAA, Bossuyt PMM, Verhagen RAW, vanDijk CN. Treatment strategies in osteochondral defects of the talar dome: A systematic review. *Foot Ankle Int*. 2000;21:119–126.

Van Der Windt DA, Van Der Heijden GJ, Van Den Berg SG, Ter Riet G, De Winter AF, Bouter LM. Ultrasound therapy for acute ankle sprains. *Cochrane Database of Systematic Reviews*. (1):CD001250, 2002.

Wilkerson LA. Ankle injuries in athletes. *Sports Med*. 1992;19:377–392.

Woods L, Leach RE. Posterior tibial tendon rupture in athletic people. *Am J Sports Med*. 1991;19:495–498.

27 | Orthotics

Lloyd Nesbitt

QUICK LOOK

- Orthotics can control the biomechanics of the foot.
- Orthotics function is optimum with a neutral subtalar joint.

INTRODUCTION

The successful use of orthotic devices to control abnormal foot biomechanics has focussed attention on podiatric sports medicine. However, in recent years, there has been increasing overutilization of orthotics and orthotic devices are often recommended when other treatment modalities may suffice. Overutilization is due in part to the many allied health personnel and retailers who have jumped onto the orthotics bandwagon. Indeed, some providers are dispensing basic arch support inserts for a shoe and calling it an "orthotic." The difference is that arch supports, which have been around for over 50 years, simply push up against the arch during static stance, whereas biomechanical orthotics, when properly prescribed and fabricated, precisely control the gait cycle from heel contact through midstance and toe-off.

The key to understanding the effective use of orthotics lies in the basics of foot biomechanics. An overview of foot and gait biomechanics will help the reader to ascertain which problems can best be treated with orthotics and the preferred methodology to use in their fabrication.

HISTORY OF PODIATRIC BIOMECHANICS AND ORTHOTICS

Prior to 1970, mechanical foot problems, such as flat feet, were usually addressed from a static point of view. That is, arch supports were used to provide support for the foot by pushing up against the arch when a patient was standing. In some cases, these arch supports would provide some degree of relief for common problems like foot fatigue. Shoe modifications such as "arch cookies," heel wedges, and metatarsal pads were also commonly used to alter the position of the foot slightly, but were nonspecific from a biomechanical point of view. The treatment was basically hit-and-miss. Common advice for flat feet in the 1950s was to "wear good shoes."

In the late 1960s, biomechanics researchers at the California College of Podiatric Medicine in San Francisco were analyzing the various segments of the gait cycle to better understand the forces affecting the foot. Motions of the foot during heel contact, midstance, and toe-off were analyzed to assess the subtalar and midtarsal joint function during the weight-bearing phases of walking and running. The researchers discovered that controlling abnormal subtalar and midtarsal joint motion during weight bearing successfully treated many foot problems. The subtalar (talocalcaneal) joint has triplane motions of adduction and abduction, inversion and eversion, dorsiflexion and plantarflexion (Sgarlato, 1971). The subtalar joint allows the foot to adapt to the supporting surface. Therefore, pronation during the first 25% of the gait cycle is a normal and necessary component of walking as the subtalar joint allows the foot to absorb shock by abducting, everting, and dorsiflexing all at the same time.

During the midstance phase, the foot resupinates to become a rigid lever for propulsion. The subtalar joint then adducts, inverts, and plantarflexes.

The subtalar joint, when held in its neutral position, allows for normal foot stability during the midstance phase of the gait cycle (Hlavac, 1967). The "neutral position" is that position where the subtalar joint is neither pronated nor supinated. From the neutral position, the subtalar joint can supinate twice as much as it can pronate.

Forefoot imbalances lead to rear foot compensation. For example, forefoot varus is a common problem that results in subtalar joint pronation. Forefoot varus is an inverted relationship of the forefoot (metatarsals 1 to 5) in relationship to the vertical bisection of the calcaneus. Therefore, when the heel is vertical, the forefoot would be inverted and basically off the ground. The foot then compensates as the patient bears weight, and the forefoot comes down to the ground and the subtalar joint pronates (Fig. 27-1; Root, 1977). If the forefoot and rearfoot imbalances can be corrected, then the subtalar joint remains neutral and is, hence, more stable.

A non-weight-bearing plaster cast of a patient's foot can accurately capture the inherent angular imbalances between the forefoot and rearfoot. With the patient sitting on the examination table with the legs extended, the subtalar joint is placed in a neutral position and a dorsal direction loading force is applied to the plantar surface of the fourth and fifth metatarsal heads to fully pronate the forefoot at its oblique midtarsal joint axis to mimic the reactive force of gravity and achieve the optimum stable position of the foot (Kominsky, 1996). The cast would then be slipped off the patient's foot and sent off to a podiatric biomechanics laboratory along with the orthotic prescription.

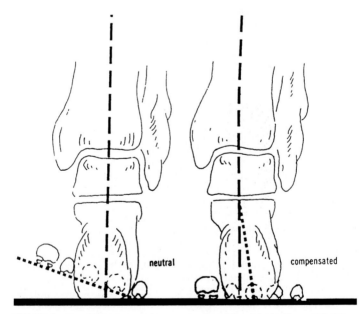

FIG 27-1   Forefoot varus and compensation. (*Reprinted with permission from Subotnick S. Podiatric Sports Medicine. Mt. Kisco, NY: Futura; 1975, p 40.*)

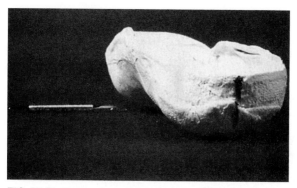

FIG 27-2 Forefoot varus as seen in neutral cast. Note that when heel is vertical, the forefoot is inverted, causing compensation at subtalar joint with weight bearing.

The orthotic laboratory uses the cast of the foot as a "negative" to form a mold of the patient's foot by laboratory technicians. A vertical line bisecting the posterior aspect of the heel demonstrates the forefoot varus when the heel model is vertical (Fig. 27-2). The orthotic device is fabricated to the patient's corrected foot position by balancing or angulating the orthotic with forefoot or rear foot varus posts. These posts bring the ground up to meet the foot so that the forefoot or rearfoot do not have to compensate away from the neutral subtalar position (Fig. 27-3). Subtalar joint motion is controlled and the foot is maintained in its most stable structural position, resulting in normal adaptation to the supporting surface at heel strike followed by resupination of the foot at midstance as it becomes a rigid lever for toe-off. In the early 1970s, Rhoadur, a rigid plastic material, was being used for orthotic devices. Over time, more shock absorbing materials as well as more flexible plastics were used in the fabrication of orthotic devices for enhanced

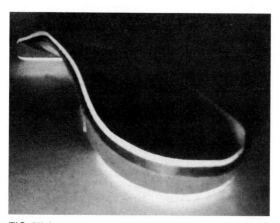

FIG 27-3 Forefoot varus on orthotic matches forefoot varus of cast. Rear foot varus post is also shown, which prevents pronation but allows 4 degrees of motion at heel strike for normal shock absorption.

comfort. Biomechanical problems that were previously unresponsive to treatment were responding to correction with orthotics (Subotnick, 1975).

RUNNING BOOM

By the mid-1970s many Canadians and Americans were running for fitness and were not willing to accept the commonly prescribed "aspirin and rest" as a treatment. Physicians treating runners found that the typical treatment protocols; rest, anti-inflammatories, ice, stretching, strengthening, and physiotherapy treatments, were ineffective over time, providing only temporary relief from pain. Articles in running magazines were steering runners to podiatrists for the treatment of running-related foot and leg overuse syndromes. In 1975, Dr. George Sheehan, a prominent cardiologist and runners' guru, wrote in his book that under the care of a podiatrist with the use of orthotic devices, he was again able to run for prolonged periods of time. His anecdotal report convinced thousands of runners to consult with podiatrists. With symptoms improved using podiatrists' orthotics, the word spread and podiatrists became an integral part of the sports medicine team.

By the 1980s, orthotics were well established as an effective treatment modality for biomechanically related foot problems (Rinaldi, 1980).

ORTHOTICS OVERUTILIZATION

In the late 1980s, there were many people taking an interest in foot care. Some practitioners were more skilled than others in assessing and treating the athlete's biomechanical problems. As a result, the efficacy of treatment was quite varied, and many people thought orthotics were useless since they did not work for them. The question in these cases must address how the orthotic devices were fabricated. For example, a weight-bearing foam impression of a pronated foot will capture the foot in its deviated, unstable position. A plaster cast of the foot in its neutral, subtalar joint position is preferred to obtain a corrected or neutral foot position for the laboratory. Often, orthotics made from a foam impression of the foot are based on off-the-shelf, stock items. Those using this type of orthotic, who have had some cursory courses on biomechanics, may have elected to add some forefoot or rear foot varus posting to the devices. This helps somewhat, but foam "casting" should be avoided if true biomechanical correction is to be achieved.

Although some patients may have symptoms improve with various types of inserts placed in their shoes, the key is optimum control of the biomechanics of the foot through each phase of the gait cycle.

INDICATIONS FOR THE USE OF ORTHOTICS

Biomechanical Analysis

The evaluation of foot biomechanical imbalance begins with visual inspection. Calluses inferior to the second and third metatarsal heads are indicative of shearing forces of pronation during the gait cycle. As the foot pronates, the metatarsal heads undergo valgus rotation, resulting in friction and hyperkeratosis (Root, 1977). Rolling off the medial aspect of the hallux during toe-off produces calluses and is also indicative of pronation.

Callus formation inferior to the first and fifth metatarsal heads usually indicates a rigid pes cavus foot. When the first metatarsal of a pes cavus foot is plantarflexed, the weight-bearing areas are inferior to the first and fifth metatarsal heads as well as the heel (Root, 1977; Sgarlato, 1971).

Stance

In the standing position, it is easy to distinquish a normal foot from an excessively pronated or rigid pes cavus foot. In a pronated foot, the arches are flattened, the ankles roll in medially toward each other, and from the posterior aspect, a vertical bisection of the calcaneus appears everted. To see this more clearly, draw a line on the posterior aspect of the heels in the prone position, and have the patient stand. Also with excessive foot prona-tion, the hallux is often in abduction with valgus rotation.

A rigid pes cavus foot type is easily distuinquished by a high arch at the medial aspect of the foot and a plantarly prominent first metatarsal head (Fig. 27-4A). The posterior view demonstrates inverted heels, which is reflected in casts of a pes cavus foot as well (see Fig. 27-4B and C).

Calluses

Calluses are a protective skin mechanism for the underlying boney struc-tures. Those located inferior to the metatarsal heads 2, 3, or 4 are caused by shearing forces during pronation or plantarflexed metatarsals. Calluses located under the first or fifth metatarsal heads are usually associated with a rigid cavus foot. Debridement, padding, and cushioning of calluses pro-vide temporary relief, but unless the foot mechanics are treated, calluses recur.

Gait Analysis

Observing the foot motion while walking reveals eversion of the calcaneus in a pronated foot (Fig. 27-5). The talus is adducted and prominent medi-ally. The patient usually has an apropulsive gait, rolling off the medial aspect of the hallux and the arch is flattened in mid stance.

Conversely, with a pes cavus foot type, the patient has an inverted position to the rear foot with excessive supination, resulting in an inverted forefoot appearance in relation to the rear foot. The first metatarsal is prominantly plantarflexed in the pes cavus foot, and as the forefoot bears weight, the plantarflexed first metatarsal forces the rear foot into inversion. Patients with abnormal foot types may benefit from an orthotic device designed to specif-ically control each phase of the walking cycle.

When patients present with lower extremity and foot complaints and no history of trauma, think of abnormal biomechanics. Inspect the stance and gait, put the ankle and subtalar joints through the ranges of motion, and eval-uate the first metatarsal for abnormal dorsiflexion or plantarflexion in rela-tion to the other metatarsals. By routinely examining the biomechanics of the foot, the clinician will often be able to determine the cause of the patient's problem, resolve the symptoms, and prevent recurrence of the prob-lem. Weight-bearing x-rays also reveal abnormal biomechanics (Fig. 27-6).

ASSESSING ORTHOTICS

If a patient presents with orthotics that are not working or uncomfortable, the orthotics may not fit properly or may not be suitable for the patient. Orthotics that are uncomfortable or causing knee, hip, or back problems are

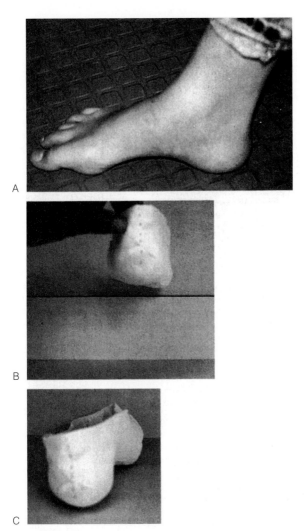

A

B

C

FIG 27-4 **A.** Rigid pes cavus foot type. Excessive pressure inferior to first metatarsal head, which is plantarflexed, can be easily visualized when the patient is standing. **B.** Forefoot valgus/plantarflexed first ray as seen in neutral case. When heel is vertical, the medial side of this left foot is plantarflexed or in valgus. This cannot be accurately captured in a foam box impression. **C.** When the cast is placed on a table, one can see how the compensated or weight-bearing position of the forefoot causes the rear foot to invert. Therefore, forefoot valgus posting is required on orthotic along with 0-degree rear foot post.

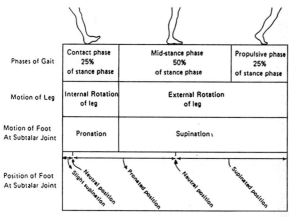

Phases of Gait	Contact phase 25% of stance phase	Mid-stance phase 50% of stance phase	Propulsive phase 25% of stance phase
Motion of Leg	Internal Rotation of leg	External Rotation of leg	
Motion of Foot At Subtalar Joint	Pronation	Supination	
Position of Foot At Subtalar Joint	Slight supination / Neutral position	Pronated position / Neutral position	Supinated position

FIG 27-5 *(Reprinted with permission of the author from Hlavac HF. The Foot Book. Mountain View, Calif: World Publications; 1977, p 90.)*

most likely over correcting the biomechanical deficit (Subotnick, 1983). Inspect the device for fit that seems excessively high under the arch, as the medial correction can be decreased. Reducing the posting height or enhancing the flexibility will improve the tolerance of the orthotic device. Four degrees of motion has to be available at heel strike, so the orthotic should rock or tilt medially with downward pressure when placed on a table. Orthotics that do not work at all may not have enough correction and the height of the arch or the posting has to be increased. This is a common problem with orthotics made from a foam impression. If the patient stepped into a foam box or the orthotics were "made from a computer," they may not be providing proper biomechanical control.

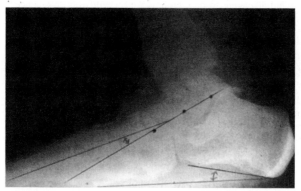

FIG 27-6 Pronated foot as seen on weight-bearing x-ray. Bisection of talus should normally bisect long axis of first metatarsal, but with pronation, this bisection falls plantarly. Also note the decrease of the calcaneal inclination angle. This demonstrates why weight-bearing x-rays should always be taken of the foot.

COMPUTERIZATION AND ORTHOTICS

In recent years, we have seen the development of some very sophisticated gait analysis machines. Patients can take a few steps over a pressure pad and a digital readout of the foot pressure points is projected on a screen. As a research tool it is excellent, but it is not a substitute for biomechanical knowledge when it comes to treating foot imbalances. An astute clinician should be able to determine where the pressure points are on the foot by simple examination, as indicated earlier in this chapter. Orthotic devices that are dispensed after computer analysis may be no more than off-the-shelf prefabricated devices with varying arch heights for each size of the foot that do not specifically control the biomechanics of the gait cycle. There are digital computer scanners that allow a direct scan of the non-weight-bearing foot held in a neutral position providing a biomechanically correct mold of the foot. The digital image is used to direct the cutting tools that produce the orthotic device.

Laser Foot Scanners

Non-weight-bearing, three-dimensional laser scanners have been developed that can capture the contours of the foot in a corrected non-weight-bearing, neutral subtalar joint position. This digital image of the foot can then be e-mailed to a laboratory and the orthotic device fashioned from the three-dimensional digital "cast." The difference between laser imaging and weight-bearing computer impressions is that with a weight-bearing view, the foot is in a deviated or uncorrected, pronated position.

New Techniques for the Fabrication of Orthotics

Langer Biomechanics Laboratories has developed a "castless measurement system" (CMS) that utilizes a 9-point parameterized digital assessment of the patient's foot, instead of plaster casts. A biomechanical examination of the foot is required to develop the prescription for fabrication of the orthotics. The CMS data is entered into the laboratory computer to determine the morphology of the patient's foot. Since this methodology is just being introduced, it remains to be seen how well it will work in practice.

ABNORMAL FOOT BIOMECHANICS AND THE USE OF ORTHOTICS

There are a number of clinical entities related to abnormal foot biomechanics that respond to biomechanical control. At the same time, symptoms can be treated with stretching and strengthening exercises; massage therapy; application of ice, rest, compression, and elevation; and possibly, nonsteroidal anti-inflammatories (NSAIDs). Wearing soft-soled, laced walking shoes or running shoes may enhance comfort. Modification of activity, such as a runner shortening the stride, eliminating hills or speed work, or reducing running mileage, may help. Often, lessons from a sport-specific coach will correct improper techniques that can contribute to overuse syndromes. When assessing and treating symptoms, always address the biomechanics to find the cause of the problem.

Patellofemoral Pain Syndrome

When a patient presents with chronic symptoms in the peripatellar area with no history of trauma, consider patellofemoral pain syndrome (PFPS) in the differential diagnosis. Look at the feet when the patient is standing. A pronated foot will result in internal rotation of the lower leg and increase the Q -angle of the knee. Abnormal patellar tracking is often associated with pronated feet (Gordon, 1986; Valmassy, 1996). Biomechanical treatment of the feet for excessive pronation often helps relieve symptoms.

Shin and Lower Leg Pain

Shin pain is usually caused by periostitis, myositis, or tendonitis of the anterior or posterior tibial muscles or tendons that supinate the foot. If the foot is pronated, then ongoing stretching of the tendons and muscles results in anterior and/or posterior tibialis muscle strain. Stretching exercises for tight Achilles tendons may lessen the forces required to dorsiflex the foot during the swing phase of the gait cycle, along with strengthening exercises for the anterior lower leg muscles. Rest, ice, and activity modification are helpful. However, the reduction of symptoms with stretching and strengthening therapy will likely result in a return of symptoms when activity is resumed if the foot remains pronated. Excessive use of the posterior tibial muscle to supinate or elevate the foot into its proper position can also play a role in compartment syndrome, which confounds the diagnosis of posterior tibialis muscle strain (Subotnick, 1975).

There are also patients with shin pain who have rigid pes cavus feet that lack shock absorption from heel strike through the mid stance phases of running. The continual jarring from a rigid pes cavus foot type requires enhanced shock absorption that is afforded by a flexible, well-cushioned orthotic device that redistributes the weight-bearing areas.

Plantar Fasciitis and Heel Spur Syndrome

Heel pain, due to plantar fasciitis, is one of the most common foot complaints seen in athletes who have closed calcaneal apophyses. Typically, these patients have pain on weight bearing the first thing in the morning from the contraction of the plantar fascia that occurs with the foot in an equine position while asleep. Weight bearing pulls on the plantar fascia. Abnormal foot mechanics definitely play a role. A rigid pes cavus foot type has a high calcaneal inclination angle and there is excessive jarring that takes place at heel strike. The normal 4 degrees of motion at heel strike is absent and the heel strike forces are transmitted to the plantar posterior aspect of the heel. At the same time, there is excessive tension on the plantar fascia during the mid stance phase of the gait cycle.

The pronated foot is an even more common cause of heel pain. The ongoing stretching of the plantar fascia at its origin results in the development of a calcaneal spur as calcium is deposited at the site of plantar fascia inflamation and tissue damage, usually at the medial tuberosity of the calcaneus (Fu, 1994). Controlling the abnormal biomechanical forces with a neutral position orthotic device relieves the strain on the plantar fascia and allows the area to heal (Valmassy, 1996). Enhanced cushioning will help the cavus foot, and more control is beneficial for the pronated foot. Well-cushioned heel pads, low-dye fashion taping, ice, massage, and wearing of soft-soled shoes is often beneficial for immediate pain relief. Stretching exercises for the plantar fascia can aggravate the acute problem.

An anti-inflammatory injection can be used when these heel spur syndromes are not responding to more conservative care or when the pain is in an acute stage. A medial approach to the plantar fascia origin is safer than a plantar approach as there is less leaching of steroid into the fat pad of the heel. A 27-gauge, 1.25-in. needle can be used and is far less painful for the patient. Extracorporal shock wave therapy is available for treatment of plantar fasciitis and is effective in 80–95% of cases after 3 to 5 treatments.

In adolescence, calcaneal apophysitis should be differentiated from plantar fasciitis. In these cases, ice, rest, heel pads, and taping are usually all that is required and the symptoms settle with reduced activity.

Neuromas

The typical history for a neuroma is an intermittent burning pain in the forefoot that sometimes radiates to the toes. The pain is often relieved by stopping activity, removing the shoe, and massaging the foot. The pain can occur when non-weight bearing for no apparent reason. Neuromas are often associated with a pronated foot, where the valgus rotation of the metatarsals results in impingement of the intermetatarsal nerve, most commonly between the third and fourth metatarsal heads (Kominsky, 1995). Ice will help relieve the pain and wearing soft-soled shoes with a wide toe box will decrease some of the pressure on the intermetatarsal head spaces. A metatarsal pad placed proximal to the affected metatarsal heads may relieve pain in some athletes, but generally is not effective.

Correcting the foot mechanics with orthotics can dramatically reduce symptoms associated with a neuroma. In fact, athletes with neuromas who go without their orthotics often find that their symptoms recur. Resuming orthotic use will frequently resolve the symptoms. Painful neuromas can be injected with anesthetic and corticosteriod using a dorsal approach utilizing a 27-gauge, 1.25 in. needle. This is less painful than a plantar approach to the interdigital space. The usual injection solution is a corticosteroid combined with xylocaine and marcaine. Cyanocobalamin (vitamin B_{12}) can be added and seems to have a sclerosing effect on the neuroma. A series of up to three injections spaced 2 to 4 weeks apart (maximum of three injections in a year) along with orthotics is enough to circumvent surgery in the majority of cases.

Hallux Abducto Valgus and Associated Bunion Deformity

Patients present with bunions in various stages of deformity. Mild to moderate bunion deformities are often asymptomatic, but are worth treating to avoid progression of the deformity. Bunions in mild to moderate stages respond well to orthotics. Mild symptoms often subside and the problem no longer progresses. In most cases, patients will have pronated feet and demonstrate forefoot varus, as described earlier in this chapter. As the inverted forefoot bears weight, the subtalar joint compensates with increased pronation so the forefoot can touch the ground. The patient rolls off the medial aspect of the hallux forcing the hallux into abduction. This increases the pressure on the first metatarsal head area, eventually causing a bursitis to develop (Gerbert, 1981). Left untreated, an exostosis develops at the medial aspect of the first metatarsal head as the hallux is forced into abduction. The first metatarso-phalangeal joint deviates in a bunion deformity, and in an advanced stage, subluxes.

As bunions become more severe, the hallux is forced into a greater degrees of abduction. A retrograde force of the hallux pushes the first metatarsal medially, compounding the bunion deformity (Gerbert, 1973). Although orthotic devices will allow a patient to propel off the plantar aspect of the hallux rather than the medial aspect, advanced bunion cases cannot be resolved with orthotic devices alone. Therefore, surgical correction with an osteotomy to realine the first metatarsal and the proximal phalanx of the hallux is necessary to correct the anatomic deformity and relieve the pain. Postoperative orthotic devices reduce pressure to the surgical site allowing speedier recovery and reduce recurrence by shifting the forces of the toe-off phase of gait to propel off the plantar aspect of the hallux.

Stress Fractures

Stress fractures are common overuse injuries caused by excessive and repetitive trauma to a specific area of the foot or lower leg. Faulty foot mechanics often contribute to stress fractures. Tibial stress fractures are frequently associated with a rigid pes cavus foot type. A rigid pes cavus foot type can also be associated with stress fractures in the foot because of excessive jarring. Abnormal foot pronation places excessive strain on the metatarsals and increases valgus rotation of the metatarsals, which results in stress fractures commonly found in the second, third, or fourth metatarsals. X-rays within 1 to 2 weeks of the pain onset are often normal, but bone callus formation is usually present 4 to 6 weeks after the onset of pain. Relative rest, analgesics for pain, and orthotics will improve comfort during healing and correcting biomechanics, proper nutrition, and training errors will reduce recurrence.

Tarsal Tunnel Syndrome

This less common condition involving pain, numbness, or tingling at the medial aspect of the foot inferior to the medial malleolus is often associated with a pronated foot. As the foot pronates, the tibial nerve is compressed inferior to the laciniate ligament, and pain or paresthesia may radiate either proximal or distal from the site of nerve impingement. Nerve conduction studies may be abnormal and confirm the disorder. Anti-inflammatory injections are sometimes used to reduce swelling and relieve pain, although often simply treating the mechanics of the foot will reduce symptoms. A rear foot varus post on the orthotic will limit pronation and decrease the nerve compression. Surgical releases are rarely necessary.

Sesamoiditis

Inflammation of the sesamoids located inferior to the first metatarsal head is relatively common in athletes. Palpation may pinpoint a tibial or fibular sesamoid tenderness. A rigid, plantarflexed first metatarsal is associated with sesamoiditis, and pronation can increase pressure on the tibial sesamoid during the toe-off phase. Orthotics can accommodate the area of excessive pressure, provide enhanced cushioning, and limit the biomechanical forces that create the problem.

TYPES OF ORTHOTICS

Orthotics used in the early 1970s were primarily made of Rhoadur material. This rigid plastic worked well in maintaining a neutral subtalar joint foot position allowing the necessary 4 degrees of pronatory motion at heel strike required for mobile adaptation to the supporting surface. Despite their rigidity, patients were able to run marathons with them. Currently, there are a number of materials that allow more flexibility and shock absorption. Flexible, polypropylene 1/16-in. plastic works well with a PPT or Poron top cover for added shock absorption. An orthotic device that is too well-cushioned bottoms out and will not provide the degree of support required for the athlete. For a rigid pes cavus foot type, a Spenco top cover provides additional cushioning.

SPORT-SPECIFIC ORTHOTICS

Often one orthotic can be used for a number of activities and will work well in controlling the mechanics of the foot. However, the needs of the patient have to be accurately assessed and the end-product orthotic should satisfy the patient's requirements in terms of sport. For example, a patient with a rigid pes cavus foot type who is playing basketball, tennis, or other lateral motion sports requires orthotics with deep heel cups and 0-degree rear foot posts to enhance stability and prevent inversion sprains with sudden stops. The clinician should be careful when using rear foot varus posting to raise the orthotic rear segment medial aspect to control pronation, as too much rear foot posting may result in lateral ankle sprains in sports where there are sudden lateral motion stops.

In contrast, a long-distance runner with a rigid cavus foot type requires maximum shock absorption at heel strike. The athlete with pain at the ball of the foot, a neuroma, calluses, or a plantarflexed metatarsal may require accommodative extensions distal to the orthotic to balance the forefoot and allow for more cushioning. This is especially helpful for those sports where a lot of time is spent on the ball of the foot, such as tennis.

WHEN ONE PAIR OF ORTHOTICS CAN BE USED AT ALL TIMES

Often, patients can use the same orthotics for their sport shoes and dress shoes. The orthotics can be made with a shallow heel cup, with no top covers and they can allow for good control in sport shoes and at the same time, they will fit easily into dress shoes. Intrinsic forefoot or rear foot posting can be used so that the orthotic is not bulky and so that the patient's heels do not flip out of the shoe (a common problem with posted or bulky orthotics). Some people recommend orthotics specifically for sport shoes and others for dress shoes; however, in many cases, one pair of orthotics will work for both (unless the patient is a female wearing dress pumps or similar shoes).

HOW TO AVOID USING EXPENSIVE ORTHOTICS

An athlete with a mild biomechanical imbalance demonstrating slight pronation and mild symptoms may respond to an over-the-counter arch support found at a local pharmacy, shoe repair shop, or sporting goods store. Try using a rear foot varus pad that can be fabricated out of 1/4 in. felt by thinning it down laterally so that it raises the heel at the medial side to reduce calcaneal eversion by a few degrees. PPT materials can be used with adhesive felt placed along the medial segment to provide temporary support.

Athletes with a rigid cavus foot type may respond to a well-cushioned sports insole, such as Spenco, Viscoped, or Sorbathane. Inspect the running shoes for excessive wear. More supportive or simply new shoes may resolve mild problems. Reducing pressure points on the plantar aspect of the foot with 1/8 adhesive felt pads used in a biplane fashion can often accommodate a sore spot by placing pressure around the sore spot.

DOING WHAT IS BEST FOR THE PATIENT

Foot problems can be complex. There are 26 bones in each foot and considering that the average person walks over 100,000 miles in a lifetime, our feet do an amazing job of getting us from place to place. Very often, biomechanical abnormalities are associated with orthopedic or structural problems that may then produce dermatologic manifestations of the underlying pathology. Neurologic or vascular involvement can further complicate the picture.

Orthotic devices are not a panacea for foot problems. When indicated, however, they work well in reducing symptoms and treating the cause of problems as well as preventing further deforming forces. Unfortunately, there is such a broad range of inserts being placed in patient's shoes that are being referred to as "orthotics" that often, neither the patient nor the practitioner knows where to turn to achieve optimal results. Plaster casting techniques are preferred and a combination of flexible plastics and shock-absorbing materials can be used to optimize foot function and comfort (Hunter, 1995). Follow-up visits are important to evaluate the athlete's progress with orthotics. Modifications or adjustments can be done to the orthotic that will enhance patient compliance or improve correction. Orthotics alone are often not adequate for athletes and consideration has to be given to other therapeutic modalities.

REFERENCES

Donatell R, Hurlbert C, Conaway D, et al. Biomechanical foot orthotics: A retrospective study. *J Orthop Sports Phy Ther.* 1988;10:205–212.

Fu FH, Stone DA. *Sports Injuries.* Baltimore: Williams & Wilkins; 1994:573–574, 994–995.

Gerbert J, Mercado OA, Sokoloff TH, et al. *The Surgical Treatment of the Hallux Abducto Valgus and Allied Deformities.* Mt, Kisco, NY: Futura; 1973:19–28.

Gerbert J, Sokoloff TH. *Textbook of Bunion Surgery.* Mt. Kisco, NY: Futura; 1981:46–54.

Gordon GM. Knee, ankle, and foot problems in the preadolescent athlete. *Clin Podiatric Med Surg.* 1986;3:742–744.

Hlavac HF. Differences in x-ray findings with varied positioning of the foot. *J Am Podiatry Assoc.* 1967;57:465.

Hunter S, Dolan M, Davis J, et al. *Foot Orthotics in Therapy and Sport.* Champaign, Ill: Human Kinetics; 1995:76–80.

Kominsky J, Jay RM, Silvani SM, et al. *Advances in Podiatric Medicine and Surgery.* St. Louis: Mosby; 1996:1–13.

Rinaldi RR, Sabio ML. *Sports Medicine 1980: Part I.* Mt. Kisco, NY: Futura; 1980:19–20.

Root ML, Orien WP, Weed JH. *Normal and Abnormal Function of the Foot.* Los Angeles: Clinical Biomechanics; 1977:313–314, 319–321, 344–345.

Sgarlato TE. *A Compendium of Podiatric Biomechanics.* San Francisco: College of Podiatric Medicine; 1971:60–66, 237–245.

Subotnick SI. Foot orthoses: An update. *Phys Sports Med.* 1983;11:108.

Subotnick SI. *Podiatric Sports Medicine.* Mt. Kisco, NY: Futura; 1975:79–81, 87–88, 181–187.

Valmassy RL. *Clinical Biomechanics of the Lower Extremeties.* St. Louis: Mosby; 1996:67–68, 75–76.

28 | Heat and Cold Injuries

William O. Roberts

QUICK LOOK

Exertional Heat Stroke

- Defined as rectal temperature >104°F with CNS changes.
- Look for ashen sweaty skin; if skin is red, hot, and dry, hypothalamic failure is present and the prognosis is worse.
- Treatment is immediate cooling in an ice water tub or packing the groin, neck, and axillary area with ice.
- Cool on site if stable.

Cold injury

- Frostbite is treated with water immersion at 104°–106°F.
- Severe hypothermia is rare in athletic competitions but can occur with training accidents and in recreational activities.
- Transfer then rewarm in hospital.

Exercise and muscle work produce excess heat energy that must be removed from the body to maintain a normal core body temperature. In extreme environments—hot and humid or cold and wet—it can be nearly impossible to remove excess heat or maintain adequate core heat. However, conditions that lead to both hyperthermia and hypothermia are often not extreme and both conditions can occur with ambient temperatures in the 60°–70°F range. The effective environmental thermal stress is a function of ambient temperature, humidity, sun exposure, wind, and rain. The final core temperature is dependent upon multiple intrinsic and extrinsic factors that may affect an athlete adversely. Both heat stroke and hypothermia can lead to permanent injury and death.

HEAT-RELATED AND HEAT-INDUCED INJURY

The maladies that occur in athletes can be viewed as heat-induced and heat-associated problems. Activity in the heat forces the body to utilize energy stores to remove heat from the system and can fatigue the athlete earlier in the time course of activity compared to the same work load in lesser heat stress conditions. *Exertional heat stroke* and *exertional hyperthermia* are heat-induced problems in athletes caused by metabolic heat production in environments that overwhelm the body's cooling systems. Exercise (heat) exhaustion or fatigue, exercise-associated muscle (heat) cramps, and exertional hyponatremia occur more frequently in hot conditions but may also occur in cool conditions. The energy demand of thermostasis and large-volume sweat losses in unacclimatized athletes are important contributing factors.

Epidemiology

Heat stroke is the cause of death for 1–5 athletes per year in the United States, usually in the first 2–3 days of preseason football practice, and occasionally in summer road races. Fatal exertional hyponatremia seems to be on the rise, but it usually occurs in slower endurance athletes who drink large volumes of fluid beyond the amount of fluid lost from sweating. Other forms of heat-related illness occur with more regularity, but the actual incidence is difficult to determine because nonfatal forms of heat illness are not often reported.

There are several risk factors that contribute to the onset of heat-related problems. Three of the most important factors are environment heat stress, level of acclimatization to heat, and ability to maintain appropriate hydration. Other factors include clothing and equipment (including helmets and hats) that impact heat exchange, sunburn damage to the skin, health status, acute and chronic illness, conditioning, sleep volume, nutrition, salt intake, medications, supplements, obesity (decrease in surface to mass area and thick fat layer making it more difficult to eliminate heat), inflammatory muscle damage, age, alcohol use, and recreational drug use. Athletes who have sickle cell trait are at risk for sudden death associated with heat exposure. Children are more at risk than adults because they are more dependent on conduction and convection to remove the heat generated by exercise, they absorb more heat from the environment, and they perspire less for the same amount of work as an adult.

Pathophysiology

Body temperature is regulated by heat transfer through sensors in the hypothalamus and in the skin. Elevation of skin and core blood temperatures induces vasodilatation to increase transfer of heat to the body surface or shell and sweating to facilitate heat loss through evaporation. Heat transfer to maintain core temperature during exercise occurs by conduction, convection, radiation, and evaporation. However, the control systems can be overwhelmed by conditions that do not support heat loss or conservation, resulting in hyperthermia or hypothermia, respectively.

Conduction is the transfer of heat by direct contact. Air is a poor conductor of heat, and conversely a good insulator. Water has a thermal conductivity that is 32 times greater than air, so ice water immersion is a rapid form of heat transfer for cooling a hyperthermic athlete; and cold rain, cool water swimming, or sweaty clothes can drain the body of the heat necessary to maintain a normal core temperature. *Convection* is the transfer of heat to or from an object by moving air or fluid. The most common example for athletes is *wind chill*, which quantifies the effective cooling rate of moving air across exposed skin, but hot wind can add to body temperature if the air temperature is greater than skin temperature. *Radiation* is the electromagnetic transfer of heat from warmer to cooler objects. The radiant energy of the sun affects athletes, especially in hot conditions. *Evaporation* transfers heat through the latent heat of vaporization at a rate of 0.58 kcal/mL of water vaporized and is the most powerful of the heat loss mechanisms in dry air conditions. Heat transfer is inhibited by equipment and uniforms that block conduction, convection, and evaporation.

At ambient air temperatures lower than 35°C (94°F), conduction, convection, and radiation contribute to the loss of heat from the body. At higher air temperatures, evaporation becomes the sole means of heat loss and is hampered by increasing relative humidity. Above 94°F and 100% relative humidity, the body has no effective heat transfer mechanisms and the core temperature can rise even at rest. Exercise in favorable temperature and humidity conditions for 30 minutes in full football pads increases core temperature about 1°F more than the same exercise in shorts alone. Potentially more significant is the separation of core temperatures after 30 minutes of rest where the core temperature of the shorts only group was nearly back to baseline, while the core temp of the full pads group was almost 2°F higher. Repeated exercise sessions produce a greater separation of the shorts and full gear groups, increasing the risk of hyperthermia and exertional heat stroke in the full football uniform.

In hot humid environments, especially when equipment and clothing inhibit heat transfer, some measure of heat stress must be used to protect the athletes from exertional heat stroke. Ambient temperature and relative humidity charts, wet bulb globe temperatures (WBGT) scales, and heat index charts are common tools used to evaluate the relative heat stress during exercise. The temperature–humidity charts are probably the easiest to use and the most recent chart based on physiologic responses to exercise in three uniforms; shorts and T-shirt, helmet and shoulder pads, and full football pads (Fig. 28-1). The *heat index* gives an estimate of how the combination of heat

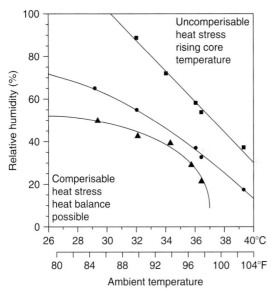

FIG 28-1   Mean critical heat balance limits for exercise at 35% $\dot{V}O_2$ max in a full football uniform, a practice uniform (shorts instead of football pants with pads), and in shorts and t-shirt only. Combination of temperature and humidity below and to the left of each line represent zones of compensable heat stress, in which heat balance is possible. Areas above and to the right of each line are zones of uncompensable heat stress for each uniform configuration. In these environments, heat gain exceeds heat loss and core temperatures would be predicted to rise continuously. As players wear more clothing, each line becomes more curvilinear as ambient humidity has relatively less effects or maximal sweating rates are approached. ■ Shorts only. ● Practice uniform. ▲ Full football uniform. (*Reproduced with permission from: Kulka TJ, Kenney WL. Heat balance limits in football uniforms: How different uniform ensembles alter the equation. Phys Sportsmed. 2002;30:29–39.*)

and humidity feels to the body. This is not a helpful guide for activity recommendations because it does not predict uncompensible heat loss while wearing shorts and T-shirts and is even less predictive with equipment that blocks heat transfer. The WBGT was developed for activity wearing khaki pants and a T-shirt. It is the only index that includes the radiant heat of the sun and is good for activity in light clothing like running and soccer. Even at mild ambient temperatures, a high relative humidity can elevate the heat stress to dangerous levels and adolescents have died of exertional heat stroke with ambient temperatures in the 70°F range. The recommendations based on WBGT that are outlined in Table 38-1 are difficult to administer in some geographic regions where the heat stress is always in the very high-risk ranges, and practice or competition could be prohibited for months at a time. Therefore, other factors including acclimatization, fitness status, health status, nutrition, hydration, sleep hygiene, and access to air conditioning away from practice and at night for sleeping must be used to guide practice and competition. An interesting study on Israeli soldiers demonstrated that sleep deprivation was a very significant factor in the frequency of heat stroke. In hot conditions, the intensity and duration of practices can be shortened and rest breaks increased to allow cooling and fluid replacement. In games like soccer, substitution can be increased, rest breaks can be mandated within the usual playing time, games lengths shortened, and half time lengthened to decrease heat production and increase heat loss (Table 28-1).

Heat production during exercise can be extremely high, generating as much as 1000 kcal/h of heat during intense exercise that the body must eliminate to maintain a normal core temperature. The radiant heat of the sun during outdoor sporting events can increase the body heat load by an additional 150 kcal/h.

The body cooling mechanism relies heavily on evaporation of sweat and circulatory system transfer of heat to the body surface. Unreplaced fluid losses create a deficit that reduces sweating and decreases intravascular volume, adversely affecting heat transfer from active muscles to the shell. Maintaining fluid status is critical, and dehydration negates the positive effects of acclimatization to heat by decreasing sweat output, cardiac output, cardiac stroke volume, and gastric emptying, all of which increase the risk of developing hyperthermia, even in conditions that are below the usual event cancellation levels. A 1% loss of fluid from the body increases the body core temperature another 0.1–0.4°C and increases the heart rate 8 beats per minute. A simple rule to maintain adequate hydration is to replace a

TABLE 28-1 Wet Bulb Globe Temperature (WBGT)* and
Risk of Heat Illness

Range				
°F	°C	Risk	Flag color	Soccer
<64	<18	Low	Green	Normal play
64–73	18–23	Moderate	Yellow	Quarter breaks
73–82	23–28	High	Red	Unlimited subs and/or shorten games
>82	>28	Hazardous	Black	Move mid-day games to AM or PM
>90	>32	Military—cancel all training activities		

*WBGT = $(0.1 \times$ dry bulb temp) + $(0.7 \times$ wet bulb temp) + $(0.2 \times$ globe temp).

volume of fluid that approximates the sweat losses every 15–20 minutes of athletic activity, and replace 150% of the deficit at the end of activity in equal volumes every 20–30 minutes over 2–4 hours. Scheduled volume replacement during activity based on average fluid needs of a 70-kg man of 8–12 ounces every 15–20 minutes underhydrates athletes who sweat profusely and can dangerously overhydrate smaller athletes with low sweat rates who participate in long duration events. Ingesting 4–6 ounces of fluid every 20 minutes during activity is safe for most athletes in road races. However, football athletes can lose up to 25 lb (12 kg) in a 2-hour practice and should be given scheduled and mandatory fluid breaks with large volume replacement during practices. When athletes use thirst to initiate fluid intake, there is already a fluid deficit present. Fluid that is flavored and cooled is usually better tolerated for replacement and is therefore more likely to be consumed during competition. Fluids with high carbohydrate concentrations like carbonated sodas and fruit drinks are slowly absorbed and make poor fluid replacements during competition. It is not advantageous to consume electrolyte/carbohydrate replacement fluids during competitions that last less than 1 hour; however, electrolyte/carbohydrate fluid replacements improve performance in events of longer duration. When appropriate fluid is available, the rate-limiting step is generally oral intake rate, so it is critical to encourage athletes to consume fluids throughout competition.

Dehydration

- 1 lb of fluid loss = 1 pint of fluid
- 2% weight loss impairs mental and work performance

Replacement Fluids are Tolerated Best when

1. Cooled
2. Flavored
3. Low carbohydrate

- Do not wait for thirst.
- Schedule sweat volume replacement at regular intervals.
- Do not restrict fluids during activity.
- Weigh athletes before and after activity.
- Replace 150% of fluid deficit at end of activity.

Heat Injuries

Heat-induced injury includes exertional syncope, exertional hyperthermia, and exertional heat stroke; heat-associated injury includes exercise (heat) exhaustion or exercise-associated collapse, exercise-associated muscle (heat) cramps, and exertional hyponatremia. Unfortunately the most severe heat problem, exertional heat stroke, can progress to total system failure and death if it is not recognized and treated immediately.

Exertional syncope is a simple fainting episode that occurs early in exposure to the heat. Vasodilatation at the skin level steals blood volume and results in a fainting episode that clears rapidly once the head is positioned below the rest of the body. This occurs more frequently in athletes with high sweat volume losses early in the acclimatization process. Treatment is simply leg elevation until the sensorium clears followed by fluid replacement and salt supplementation until the athlete can maintain adequate blood pressure, remain upright, and return to activity. The orthostatic syncope usually disappears once an athlete is acclimated to the heat, and can be blunted with salt supplementation in the acclimatization process.

Exertional hyperthermia, defined as a rectal temperature greater than 104°F, occurs in short-duration, high-intensity activity when the body cannot remove the heat generated by muscle work. The elevated core and muscle temperatures manifest as weakness and malaise. Central nervous system (CNS) function and mental status remain intact, and symptoms clear with cooling and rest. Exertional hyperthermia combined with moderate to severe dehydration can insidiously progress into exertional heat stroke; extreme vigilance is required to identify these athletes.

Heat stroke is the most serious condition associated with excess body heat, and can be fatal if not recognized and treated in the golden hour. *Exertional heat stroke* (EHS) is defined as a rectal temperature greater than 104°F associated with CNS disturbance that results in multiple system failure if the elevated core temperature in not reversed immediately. Body temperature elevated to 104°F and beyond causes severe tissue damage affecting multiple organs within 1 hour, and there is a grave prognosis for athletes who have rectal temperatures above 108°F for more than 1 hour. Although heat stroke is common in hot weather conditions, it can also occur in cool-to-moderate environments (45–82°F). EHS seemingly occurs without warning in many cases because the CNS changes can be very subtle, and athletes seem on casual evaluation to be functioning well. However, close observation and attention to an athlete's variations from usual behavior patterns signal impending problems and athletes must be monitored closely in heat stress conditions. The first few days of heat exposure for unacclimatized athletes pose the greatest risk for heat stroke and most of the football deaths occur in the first 2–3 days of practice, especially if the full uniform is used before the athletes have partially acclimatized to heat.

There is confusion over the presence of dry skin versus continued perspiration with exertional heat stroke. Athletes with exertional heat stroke continue to perspire, presenting with cool wet skin despite dangerously high rectal temperatures, until the hypothalamus overheats and shuts down the sweating mechanisms. The athlete then presents a classic heat stroke picture with hot and dry skin. When the thermal load shuts down the hypothalamus, the prognosis for full recovery is poor. Therefore, it can be deadly to wait until the skin is hot and dry before evaluating a collapsed athlete for heat stroke (Table 28-2).

Exercise (heat) exhaustion is simply the inability to continue exercise with a core body temperature between 97°F and 104°F and is characterized by fatigue, malaise, dizziness, nausea, and headache. It is often associated with dehydration due to excessive sweating in the first few days of heat exposure. Exercise exhaustion can occur in any environment when athletes push the limits of their physical capacity, but occurs more frequently in the heat due to the energy cost of cooling the body while exercising. Exercise exhaustion that occurs in hot environments is generally called *heat exhaustion* and is considered a precursor to exertional heat stroke. Heat exhaustion that is detected and treated is not a serious medical problem unless it is associated with large body fluid deficits. Heat exhaustion is hallmarked by increasing core body temperature and dehydration of 2% or greater; if athletes are dehydrated more than 7%, there is nearly 100% incidence of heat exhaustion. Mental performance and physical ability suffer as core temperatures and fluid deficits rise. The main difference between exertional heat

TABLE 28-2 Symptoms and Signs of Exertional Heat Stroke

Symptoms	Signs
Fatigue	Hyperthermia
Impaired judgment	Hyperventilation
Weakness	Blood pressure low
Flushing	Pulse elevated (100–120 bpm common)
Chills	Profuse sweating
Headaches	Skin pale and sweaty
Nausea	CNS depression
Irritability	Confusion
Dizziness	Vomiting
	Diarrhea
	Bizarre behavior
	Memory loss from time of body temperature elevation
	Contact sports mistaken for head injury
	Staggering gait (Loss of lower limb function)
	Collapse to ground
	Seizure
	Coma

stroke and severe heat exhaustion is the absence of mental status changes and a rectal temperature below 104°F in heat exhaustion. If exercise is continued and core temperature continues to rise, heat exhaustion can progress to exertional heat stroke and potential brain injury. Once exercise is stopped and the athlete is moved out of the sun, the rise in core temperature should decline as the metabolic heat source is removed.

Mild exercise exhaustion is associated with minimal dehydration and poor acclimation to the environment. This produces a generalized malaise and fatigue, and may lead to mild decreases in mental and physical performance. This condition is often noticed in early training or associated with seasonal changes in the spring or summer as temperature and humidity increase heat strain and stress in the unacclimatized athlete.

Evaluation and Management

Mental status changes and associated rectal temperature elevations are the simplest ways to distinguish heat stroke from heat exhaustion. Waiting for vomiting, confusion, disorientation, collapse, or unconsciousness puts the athlete at unnecessary risk; proactive intervention prior to the onset of severe symptoms can be lifesaving. When any of these signs appear, stop the athlete from participating, check the rectal temperature, and begin cooling the body with immersion in cool water or ice packs applied to the neck, axilla, and groin. In hot conditions, any athlete who falls out or exhibits any symptoms of heat exhaustion or exertional heat stroke should be evaluated and not allowed to return to practice until a normal rectal temperature and normal fluid volume can be documented.

EHS is life threatening and it is critical to cool the athlete immediately to bring the core temperature into the normal range as rapidly as possible. The core temperature is measured rectally to confirm the diagnosis. Other measurement sites—tympanic membrane or aural canal, oral, and axillary— are in the shell of the body and can be spuriously cool despite an elevated core temperature. As quickly as possible, move the athlete to a cool area, remove the equipment and clothing, and begin on-site cooling therapy. Immersion in a tub of ice water is the most rapid means of cooling an athlete because water has a high thermal conductive capacity compared to air. Fluid immersion is much more effective at reducing body temperature than fans, mists, or ice packs. Ice packs and cold towels placed in the highest heat loss areas (neck, axilla, groin) reduce the body temperature at about half the rate of immersion therapy in a tub. During cooling therapy, it is important to monitor the respiratory and cardiac status. Placing a child's wading pool or livestock feeding tub in a cool shaded place is a simple precaution that facilitates rapid cooling in an emergency. Replacing any fluid deficit is the second step in managing these athletes, and intravenous normal saline solution with or without 5% dextrose is the fluid of choice, if oral fluids cannot be safely ingested.

The emergency management plan should be instituted as soon as the problem is recognized and emergency medical transportation should be summoned. If the medical condition permits, it is best to treat the hyperthermia on site to lessen the tissue exposure to dangerous hyperthermia, and then transport for further evaluation. If there is cardiorespiratory arrest, there is no choice but immediate transfer for more sophisticated life support measures than can be delivered in the field. As a general rule of thumb for an athlete who is not in acute cardiovascular collapse, the athlete should be cooled first and transported later.

Heat exhausted athletes have normal temperatures and fluid replacement is best administered orally; however, if there is any neurologic impairment, the intravenous route is required. Removing clothing on the field improves heat loss. Athletes who experience moderate to severe heat exhaustion should be held from practice until fluid and energy deficits have been fully replaced, core temperature and orthostatic blood pressure are normal, and malaise, vomiting, and other symptoms are fully cleared.

Field Treatment

- Initiate emergency CPR if necessary.
- Remove from heat.
- Contact EMS.
- Measure rectal temperature.
- Initiate immersion or other cooling therapy.
- Initiate fluid replacement—orally if alert; IV if severe.
- If stable treat first, then transfer.

Exercise-associated muscle (heat) cramps receive a lot of attention during competition and can have a major impact on the athletic performance of teams and individuals. The cramps are related to muscle fatigue, energy depletion, low sodium levels, and dehydration. Athletes can develop cramps in any temperature environment if the work capacity of the muscle is exceeded. Cramping may vary from a solitary muscle cramp, particularly in the calf muscle, to entire body cramps, and can remove an athlete from competition. Although fluid status plays a very powerful role, electrolyte status, glycogen stores, anxiety, and acclimation all impact cramping. Football athletes in early season workouts can lose as much as 10 g of sweat sodium during a 2-hour practice. Sodium replacement appears to be helpful in the first few weeks of acclimation when cramping appears most frequently, and is often associated with dehydration. Athletes can increase sodium intake by salting their food and eating salty food products during the first few weeks of practice, using sports drinks that contain sodium, and for repeat crampers, adding extra salt to sports drinks. Anecdotally, supplementation with potassium does not seem to reduce cramping, although some athletes seem to benefit from magnesium supplementation. Carbohydrate replacement following strenuous exercise can reduce the incidence of cramping in the first few weeks of increasing strenuous activity.

When isolated to a solitary muscle, a prolonged stretch to full length resolves most cramps, especially if salted fluids are ingested during the stretching treatment. When cramping involves multiple muscle groups and salted oral fluids fail to resolve the cramps, IV fluid replacement may be necessary. Dextrose 5% in normal saline or normal saline work well to replace fluid, sodium, and energy stores. If cramping persists after IV fluid replacement, low doses of IV diazepam are usually effective (off-label indication). Endurance athletes with persistent cramping, especially if not relieved by prolonged stretch to full length, should have a serum sodium level checked prior to administering large volumes of oral or IV fluids.

Exertional hyponatremia is an emerging problem in endurance activity that is related to two basic mechanisms: ingesting fluids at a rate greater than sweat losses and losing sweat that has high salt concentrations with hypotonic fluid replacement that often does not match the fluid losses. Both forms dilute the extracellular space causing a flow of water into cells that results in cellular swelling in the brain and lungs manifesting as cerebral and pulmonary edema. Although it is most likely a survival mechanism for the kidney to hold on to water in the face of heat and exercise, renal water clearance should not be inhibited when the exercise losses are replaced. During competition, fear, excitement, stress, and other nonosmotic factors may stimulate the inappropriate release of arginine vasopressin that prevents the kidney from clearing excess free water. Athletes must be educated to replace, but not overreplace fluids; slow runners in marathons and other long duration events are at risk for water intoxication. In even longer events like the Ironman triathlon, the salt-loss form of hyponatremia is seen when athletes switch from salt-containing fluids to gain variety.

Confounding Conditions

In contact and collision sports, concussion can be confused with heat stroke and heat exhaustion, especially in football. In a collapsed athlete, consider cardiac arrest, exertional heat stroke, exertional hyponatremia, head injury (collision sports), and exercise-associated collapse as the most likely causes. Check for breathing and pulses, rectal temperature, serum sodium, and mental status to rapidly assess the athlete. Exercise-associated collapse is the diagnosis of exclusion and is treated with supine rest and leg elevation.

Return to Play

Heat exhaustion and heat stroke are both serious medical illnesses and therefore require rest and recovery before returning practice and competition. Practice and competition are limited following heat exhaustion and most athletes return to practice the next day for mild cases and may require 1–2 days away from activity for more severe cases. All cases of exertional heat stroke miss several days to weeks of practice and need to be carefully monitored and evaluated before returning to competition.

Remove from Activity for

- Loss of coordination
- Hyperventilation
- Vomiting
- Profuse sweating
- Pale appearance
- Severe cramping
- Visual disturbance
- Hallucination

Prevention

Although heat illness is said to be a preventable illness it still may occur, even with extreme caution and preparation. Heat injury increases above 65°F and 50% relative humidity. It is important to have a plan to reduce the frequency and severity of injuries as well as a plan to recognize and treat the problems as quickly as possible. The risk of heat stroke and exercise-induced heat exhaustion is reduced in well-hydrated, well-fed, well-rested, well-conditioned, and acclimatized athletes. An ongoing illness, respiratory infection, diarrhea, vomiting, or fever should serve as a warning to postpone exercise in the heat. The two most important factors in preventing heat illness are acclimation and hydration. Fluid status can be monitored by weighing athletes before and after practice to detect and correct fluid imbalance prior to the next practice. As an athlete becomes more dehydrated urine color becomes darker. Athletes should be taught to monitor for dehydration, and their urine should look like pale lemonade rather than dark apple juice.

In normal circumstances, people naturally react to core heating with protective behavioral changes, and stop physical activity voluntarily. Athletes suspend their normal behavioral adaptations, and depend on coaches and event administrators to suspend activity when it is too hot. The responsibility for athlete safety usually rests with the head coach with advice from the medical team, and athletes hang in the balance when this responsibility is ignored. Physiologic acclimatization improves heat tolerance and performance, and is induced by repeated exposure to hot conditions over 10–14 days and maximizes in 3–4 weeks. Heat acclimatization is most safely accomplished by gradually increasing the duration and intensity of exercise training during the initial days of heat exposure, and requires daily exposure of at least 30 minutes. Once-a-day exposure induces acclimatization faster than every-other-day exposure, but there are no data to extrapolate to twice-a-day exposure speeding acclimatization. Twice-daily exposure also carries a greater risk of cumulative dehydration and fatigue. Even after athletes are acclimatized, the most strenuous workouts should be conducted during the cooler morning hours to reduce the risk of heat injury. Acclimation to extremes of heat induces several physiologic changes including an increase in intravascular fluid volume to accommodate the large fluid losses associated with perspiration; increases in the distribution, rate, onset, and Na^+ concentration of sweat production; and decreased heart rate. Body system responses to adaptation include decreased core body temperature at comparable work and heat loads, increased exercise tolerance time, and decreased perceived exertion. Early in heat exposure, athletes can lose large volumes of fluid and several grams of sodium in their sweat. Aggressive fluid replacement and salt supplementation speed acclimatization. An athlete can lose heat acclimation rapidly during periods of no training; therefore, during injury it is important to incorporate heat exposure into the rehabilitation program prior to returning athletes to their previous level of activity. Acclimatization can be induced and maintained in cool environments by wearing heavy clothing during training.

Scheduling practice time is also helpful during acclimation. It is best to begin practice periods when the extremes of the environment are minimized, particularly in the early morning and later evening when possible. This helps avoid practicing in the hottest part of the day by eliminating peak sun exposure. Scheduling more frequent breaks for cooling and fluid replacement increases the rest-to-work ratio and improves fluid intake, especially during the period of acclimatization. The breaks can be manipulated depending on the heat stress and the acclimatization of the athletes. Never withhold fluids during practice, and have the fluids available and easily accessible during practice. The intestinal tract can be trained to absorb more fluid by drinking during exercise and has potential to absorb 1–2 L/h.

Clothing and equipment have an impact on the ability of the body to exchange heat. Maintaining maximum skin exposure to allow for evaporation helps heat exchange, but solar radiation can damage the skin. Therefore it is best to wear lightweight, light-colored, loose-fitting, mesh-type clothing that allows for better heat dissipation in hot conditions. Lighter colors also decrease the heat absorbed from solar radiation. Athletes with extra tape and equipment decrease the exposed surface area for heat exchange. During breaks in the shade it is helpful to remove head gear. In football, the uniform blocks heat transfer and shorts should be substituted for pants in moderate conditions, and the entire uniform should be removed in high-risk conditions. Athletes should be encouraged to remove their helmets at every opportunity, and conditioning drills should be conducted with pads off when it is hot. Athletes should be moved to the shade and cooled with fans during rest breaks (Table 28-3) (Fig. 28-2).

Other factors to consider as preventative measures include health status, medications, supplements, obesity, and age. Obese athletes are a high-risk group, especially early in the season when there is limited acclimatization. Obesity is a reflection of decreased conditioning and represents a decrease in surface area to mass ratio making it more difficult to eliminate heat. The excess fat layer at the skin surface also inhibits heat transfer.

Health status impacts heat injury. A recent febrile illness can reset the hypothalamic set point that regulates body temperature, increasing the risk

TABLE 28-3 Prevention

Monitor heat stress.
Program acclimatization.
Maintain hydration.
Schedule time for breaks and fluid replacement.
Increase rest to work ratio in hot conditions.
Wear loose-fitting, light-colored clothing.
Take off helmet and pads whenever possible.
Monitor weight before and after practice.
Increase salt intake first few weeks of exercise.
Eat carbohydrates after exercise.
Get adequate sleep.
Be aware of medications, supplements, and illness.

COMPETITION INDEX FOR HEAT

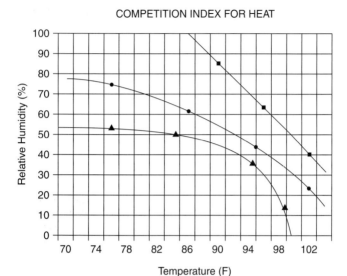

FIG 28-2 MSHSL Heat Guideline. ▲ Regular practices can be conducted for conditions that plot to the left of this line. ■ Cancel all practices when the temperature and relative humidity plot to the right of the ■; practices may be moved into air conditioned spaces. *Between* ■ *and* ●. Increase rest to work ratio with breaks every 20 minutes and all protective equipment should be removed to practice in shorts only when the temperature and relative humidity plot between the ■ and ● lines. *Between* ● *and* ▲. Increase rest to work ratio with breaks every 30 minutes and wear shorts with helmets and shoulder pads only when the temperature and relative humidity plot between the ● and ▲ lines. Heat risk rises with increasing heat and relative humidity. Fluid breaks should be scheduled for all practices and increases as the heat stress rises. Add 5° to the temperature between 10 AM and 4 PM from mid-May to mid-September on bright, sunny days. Practices should be modified to reflect the conditions for the safety of the athletes. ■ Shorts only. ● Light pads. ▲ Full pads. (*Adapted from Kulka and Kenney, 2002.*)

of heat injury for the next several days. Recent gastroenteritis with vomiting and decreased fluid intake or increased fluid loss can greatly impact heat tolerance during exercise. Diarrhea increases fluid losses and interferes with fluid absorption over the next several days.

Medications and supplements can decrease heat tolerance and increase metabolic rate. In particular, supplements used by athletes to gain a competitive edge may contain substances like ephedra, which are known to predispose to heat illness. Medications can interfere with fluid and electrolyte balance, and the central thermoregulation centers. Athletes should be required to disclose all medication and supplement use.

Children are more at risk than their adult counterparts. They are more dependent on convection for removal of heat and in higher temperatures absorb more heat from the environment. Children perspire at a slower rate for the same amount of work as an adult. Therefore, it is especially important to include more frequent breaks, increase fluid intake, and avoid the heat of day with practice.

Sideline Tips

- Preparation
- CPR training
- Cool water immersion tub
- Telephone
- Sunscreen
- IV setups
- D5 normal saline
- IV valium

Summary

Exertional heat stroke is deadly and can be prevented. Be prepared to treat heat stroke on site and set up protocols to promote the safety of the athlete. The most effective prevention strategy for heat stroke is to cancel or markedly curtail training and conditioning in the high-risk conditions.

COLD-RELATED INJURIES

Cold weather exposure can lead to chilblains, frostbite of the skin and deeper tissues, and hypothermia that can depress core temperature to fatal levels. A cold, dry environment can trigger bronchospasm and exercise-induced asthma exacerbations are frequent in cold weather athletes. Very cold dry air can induce bronchospasm in athletes who normally fare well during exercise. Exercise-induced bronchospasm should be treated with medications, but care must be taken to use medications that are both effective and not restricted for use during competition. Athletes still sweat in cold conditions and hydration is a critical factor in optimum performance and injury reduction.

Epidemiology

The common cold injuries are chilblains, frost nip, frostbite, and hypothermia. Frost nip and frostbite occur when the ambient temperature is below 31°F, and both chilblains and hypothermia can occur with ambient temperatures well above freezing, especially if clothing is wet. *Wind chill* is the convective effect of air moving across the skin and can markedly increase the risk of cold-related injuries. Cold-related injuries occur more frequently in recreational sporting activities, but hypothermia can occur in prolonged cool weather activities where participants do not generate enough muscle heat to maintain the core temperature. For example, 10% of casualties in World War II were secondary to cold injuries, especially chilblains.

Pathophysiology

The same pathways activated to remove heat also assist with heat conservation in cold conditions. The skin and central sensors induce vasoconstriction to contract the body core and conserve heat, while the central sensors also stimulate shivering for muscle heat generation. Skin that is near freezing alternately vasoconstricts, to conserve heat, and vasodilates, to postpone freezing.

Cooling of body tissue slows cell metabolism and preserves cells until the freezing point is reached. Freeze injuries start at the skin level and progress into the underlying tissues, often resulting in tissue and possible limb loss. Exposed skin is at greatest risk for frostbite and frost nip, but unexposed appendages in tight or blood flow-restricted garments can also freeze.

Heat is lost from the body during exercise through the same heat transfer mechanisms as heat stress: evaporation, conduction, radiation, and convection. *Respiratory evaporative heat losses* can be significant in dry cold air. *Sweating* that wets clothing next to the skin conducts heat to the surface of the clothing and greatly enhances the removal of heat from the body; lowering body temperature. Therefore, the ability to keep clothing next to the skin dry is of utmost importance in maintaining insulation and core body temperature in cold conditions. As the Eskimos say, "sweat kills." *Heat conduction* through cold water immersion is up to 32 times faster than air and cold water swimming or falling out of a boat or kayak can lower core temperature rapidly.

Radiation heat loss occurs through the skin into the cold environment and can be decreased by covering exposed areas, especially the head and hands. *Convection* occurs when the body heat is removed by wind (wind chill factor). The warm air trapped next to the skin and in the clothing can be maintained by protecting the skin with a wind-resistant shell as the outer layer.

Cold Injuries

Chilblains or *pernio* are caused by chronic exposure to damp cold conditions and is characterized by red papules and nodules that occur on the toes or dorsum of the feet and hands. Long distance runners are at an increased risk of developing pernio or chilblains if their running shoes are not properly insulated. Chilblains are quite painful and can also occur on the ears and face. Chilblains are treated with vasodilators like dipyridamole 25 mg three times a day or nicotinamide 100 mg three times a day. Nifedipine from the calcium channel blocker class is also effective. It is important to avoid prolonged immersion in warm water for treatment as this leads to itching, burning, and redness of the skin. Preventative measures include wearing synthetic or wool socks in cool conditions and drying the feet thoroughly once to twice per day. Occlusive footwear combined with cotton socks that are soaked in sweat or wet footwear in cool conditions lead to chilblains. Antiperspirants that decrease foot sweating decrease the risk of chilblains in athletes who have chronic exposure to cool conditions.

Frostbite and frost nip are the freeze-related skin injuries. *Frost nip* is a very mild and superficial freezing of the skin surface that is easily treated with application of a warm hand or some other gentle heat source or covering the area with insulated clothing. It should be treated as soon as it is discovered to prevent the progression to frostbite. Covering ears with warm hands and warming feet by placing them next to a heat source or simply moving them inside dry shoes may help restore heat and circulation. Frost nip may cause surface numbness, skin whiteness, and may even go unnoticed.

Frostbite can be very destructive leading to permanent injury and limb loss. The areas at greatest risk for freeze injury include the ears, nose, hands, fingers, feet, toes, and genitalia. Frostbite is a deeper freeze than the superficial layer of the skin and can extend to the bone in the most severe cases. The tissue is damaged by ice crystal formation and cell expansion during the freeze, and the inflammatory response and free radical formation during the thaw. A refreeze of thawed tissue is even more destructive. As tissue freezes, it initially feels cold, then becomes painful and finally numb. Thawing frostbite causes pain and burning, and should not be done when there is a risk of refreezing.

Frostbite presents with white, cold, firm or hard tissue; there are vascular changes and inflammation with rewarming due to free radical oxidative stress tissue damage. Frostbite is classified based on the initial examination as *superficial*, with mobile subcutaneous tissue, or *deep*, with deep tissue that is hard, immobile, and remains cool and insensitive postthawing. The frostbite severity rating is determined several days after the injury based on the following criteria in addition to erythema and edema.

First Degree

- Numbness

Second Degree

- Clear, fluid-filled blisters

Third Degree

- Hemorrhagic blisters

Fourth Degree

- Tissue mottled and lifeless
- Injury to bone and muscle

The preferred treatment is to immerse the frozen tissue in hot water in the range of 104°–108°F. Do not massage the frozen tissue for thawing because it physically damages the tissue. Blisters may develop but should not be opened because of the risk of serious infection. Frozen tissue may develop a black eschar which, should be left in place because it eventually falls off. Once a clear line of viable tissue is evident, amputation of the nonviable tissue can be done.

Treatment of Freeze Injuries

Frost Nip

- Rapid warming
- Protection from reinjury

Frostbite

- Thaw in hot water (104°–108°F)
- Thaw only if no risk of refreezing
- Use pain medicine liberally
- Pharmacologic interventions
- Topical aloe vera (70% aqueous extract)
    - Dermaide aloe cream
- Oral ibuprofen 400 mg bid

Do Not

- Remove blisters or blackened skin
- Massage

Hypothermia is the reduction of core temperature below 97°F. Unlike heat injury, cooling without freeze injury is cell protective and the slowed cell metabolism can withstand prolonged hypothermia if the organ systems do not fail from other causes. The severity of hypothermia increases as the body temperature varies from normal. Hypothermia can have a powerful role in athletics, reducing physical ability and judgment. When the body temperature decreases below 36°C (95°F), athletes should be removed from competition and cold exposure.

Symptoms and signs of hypothermia are usually gradual and progressive including confusion, drowsiness, slowed slurred speech, frequent stumbling, trembling hands, withdrawn or bizarre behavior, shallow breathing, decreased blood pressure, weak pulse, paradoxical removal of clothing, decreased coordination, unconsciousness, and altered vision. Mental status is often quickly impaired with even mild hypothermia, and may be the first clue that the athlete is in danger. Hypothermia often occurs between 30°F and 50°F during prolonged runs or walks as people underestimate the impact of wet, windy conditions on a fatigued and energy-depleted athlete.

As with heat illness, cold tolerance is greatly dependent on hydration status. Maintaining adequate hydration remains critical to thermoregulation in both hot and cold weather extremes. Dehydration reduces circulation and leads to increased risk of frostbite injuries of the extremities. Adequate nutrition is also necessary to generate the heat energy required to maintain core temperature.

When core temperature is maintained by physical activity, an athlete who stops to rest or is unable to continue secondary to fatigue or injury is at high risk of hypothermia. Body temperature may drop rapidly following competition as heat production from activity is decreased. Fatigue is a particular concern in athletes, and cold fatigued athletes should be moved to a warm environment as quickly as possible to prevent the rapid fall in temperature that can occur with continued exposure.

Hypothermia

Type	Body Temperature	Recovery
Mild	93°–97°F	Good
Moderate	86°–93°F	Fair, permanent injury possible
Severe	<86°F	Poor, permanent injury probable

Hypothermia can be classified as mild, moderate, or severe. *Mild hypothermia* is present when body temperature is reduced but maintained above 93°F. The person feels chilled with numb sensation in the skin; stiff, clumsy fingers; and slowed, improper responses to normal stimuli develop. If core temperature drops below 93°F, temporary amnesia may occur. Shivering to maintain an adequate core temperature is a warning sign that basal temperature is decreasing and should never be ignored. Shivering can increase basal heat production by up to three times. When your body begins to lose heat faster than it produces heat, you may spontaneously exercise to increase heat production. When this fails to maintain the temperature, shivering begins.

What to Watch for

- Shivering
- Cessation of shivering

- Poor judgment
- Exercising to keep warm
- Skin discoloration

Moderate hypothermia is a drop in core temperature to the 86°–93°F range, and is associated with decreasing muscular coordination, stumbling, confusion, decreased cooperation, and lethargy. Cardiac irritability increases and standing becomes difficult with a core temperature of less than 90°F.

Severe hypothermia occurs when core temperature is below 86°F. Shivering stops because there is depletion of energy stores, and there is progressive mental deterioration, incoherence, and irrational behavior. Exposed skin may be pale blue.

Prevention

As mentioned, even mild and moderate hypothermia produce impaired cognitive performance and poor decision making, so the buddy system improves safety in cold conditions. The best prevention is preparing with adequate nutrition, fluids, and clothing.

- Maintain hydration status
- Wear appropriate clothing
- Keep hands, feet, head all well protected
- Protect all exposed areas
- Get to warm environment at first sign of cold injuries
- Keep dry and protected from wind
- Have a companion with you
- Avoid alcohol

Clothing is a critical factor in preventing hypothermia. Clothing should be worn in layers, and the layer closest to the skin should wick moisture away from the body. Clothing that provides insulation, retains heat, and limits water absorption is preferred in cold conditions. Wool and synthetic fabrics (pologuard, polypropylene, fiberfill, quollofil) have good wet characteristics, limit conductive losses, and are good base layers. Cotton and down provide little thermal protection when wet, and lose most of their insulating value. In the cold, "cotton is rotten." Wind, either real or apparent, quickly removes heat from the body so an outer wind-resistant, but water vapor permeable, layer helps to conserve heat. A tremendous amount of body heat is lost from the exposed head, so a cap or hood can help conserve body temperature. The thermoregulatory system is greatly influenced by the hands and feet, and appropriate socks, footwear, and mittens or gloves need to be considered with the same principles mentioned. It is imperative that shoes and socks fit appropriately and not minimize insulation or restrict blood flow. Clothing that is too tight can decrease the blood flow and greatly increase the risk of freeze injuries. This is often seen with ski boots that are too tight around the ankles and toes, causing frostbite damage to the feet. It is wise to bring extra clothing to change into after activity to decrease the amount of heat loss from evaporation.

Clothing

- Synthetic wicking material next to skin
- Insulating middle layer(s)
- Outer wind- and water-resistant breathable shell layer

- Hat that covers exposed areas well
- Well-fitted shoes, boots, and socks
- Gloves or mittens

Do Not

- Wear cotton in the cold
- Allow wet clothing next to skin
- Use tight or compressive clothing or footwear

In emergency situations when a person is unprepared for cold weather, it is wise to take advantage of surrounding material and sources of heat. For example, insulation can be removed from car seats in an accident or a vehicle trapped in severe weather. Sharing a sleeping bag with another person can help to minimize heat loss. Creating a shelter to avoid wind and water exposure also cuts down on risk of hypothermia. Do not encourage hypothermia victims to exercise to generate metabolic heat unless the body temperature is >95°F. Cooled blood returning from the extremities may cause an afterdrop in temperature and trigger cardiac arrhythmias in an irritable heart.

As with heat injury, risk of cold injury increases with medical illness, and ill athletes should not participate in cold weather activities. Many medications impact circulation, judgment, and fluid balance, and make a difference in cold tolerance. Alcohol consumption increases blood flow to the skin enhancing heat loss and decreases awareness of skin surface temperature changes in addition to impairing decisions. Children and the elderly are also at increased risk. The elderly generate less metabolic heat and children have larger body surface to mass ratio. In contrast to heat injury, increased body fat is somewhat protective. Larger, fatter people are less affected by cold exposure; the thicker the fat layer, the greater the insulation.

Diuretics and vasoconstriction of any kind can decrease available fluids to the skin and increase the risk of hypothermia and skin injuries. Smoking causes vasoconstriction and increases the risk of cold injuries. Training or traveling alone in severe weather is risky because injuries or exhaustion may prevent return to shelter and lead to hypothermia. At least let another person know the route of travel and anticipated time of return when training in the cold.

Treatment

The keys to hypothermia treatment are drying and warming. It is important to remember, however, to thaw frozen tissue only if there is no chance of refreezing. In the field, remove the injured individual from cold and dry the skin. Do not rub the skin with snow or anything else as this may further damage the tissue. It is critical to remove all wet clothing and then begin rewarming. If the individual is mentally aware, drinking warmed fluids can be helpful, as well as warm packs next to the skin, particularly next to the major arteries. Sharing body contact with another person can increase body temperature if other sources are not available. To thaw frozen skin, hot water immersion is most effective with temperatures between 40° and 45°C (104° and 108°F). Water warmer than this risks burn injury.

Treatment

- Remove person from cold and wet environment and clothing.
- Warm and dry body as rapidly as possible.
- Hot water immersion is best for extremities.

- Give warmed IV or oral fluids depending on mental status.
- Use other heat sources as available for warming (other body heat).

Do Not

- Use exercise to rewarm a hypothermic patient.

If a person is suffering from cold exposure and mental status is affected, try to keep the person awake. Warm IV fluids, if available, can be very helpful to rewarming. The chance of permanent injury greatly increases with decreasing core temperatures. With mild hypothermia, recovery is usually very good with little permanent risk. However, moderate hypothermia commonly produces some permanent injury and in cases of severe hypothermia, many people do not survive.

Cold water immersion is also important to consider. Water at temperatures below 60°F can rapidly decrease body temperature. Obviously, body temperature can best be maintained by removal from the exposure. Do not try to swim, however, unless you can easily reach safety because swimming will increase body heat loss and speed the decline in core temperature. Keep your head out of water as much as possible and huddle with others if present.

In summary, exercise takes place in dry subzero temperatures, on wet and windy days, and in stifling heat and humidity. When environmental conditions cannot be controlled, athletes must adapt and learn when to "say no" to prevent severe injury. Prevention is key and a plan to manage heat and cold related injuries quickly and effectively is essential to athlete safety.

REFERENCES

American College of Sports Medicine. Position statement on exercise and fluid replacement. *Med Sci Sports Exerc.* 1996;28:i–vii.

American College of Sports Medicine. Position statement on heat and cold illnesses during distance running. *Med Sci Sports Exerc.* 1996;28:i–vii.

Armstrong LE, Crago AE, Adams R, Roberts WO, Maresh CM. Whole-body cooling of hyperthermic runners: Comparison of two field therapies. *Am J Emerg Med.* 1996;14:355–358.

Armstrong LE, Maresh CM, Crago AE, Adams R, Roberts WO. Interpretation of aural temperatures during exercise, hyperthermia, and cooling therapy. *Med Exerc Nutr Health.* 1994;3:9–16.

Armstrong LE, Maresh CM. The induction and decay of heat acclimatisation in trained athletes. *Sports Med.* 1991;12:302–312.

Barthel HJ. Exertion-induced heat stroke in a military setting. *Military Med.* 1990;155:116–119.

Bouchama A, Knochel JP. Heat stroke. *N Engl J Med.* 2002;346:1978–1988.

Brengelman GL. The dilemma of body temperature measurement. In: Shiraki K, Yousef MK, eds. *Man in Stressful Environments: Thermal and Work Physiology.* Springfield: Thomas, 1987.

Brodeur VB, Dennett, SR, Griffin LS. Exertional hyperthermia, ice baths, and emergency care at The Falmouth Road Race. *J Emerg Nurs.* 1989;15:304–312.

Channa AB, Seraj MA, Saddique AA, Kadiwal GH, Shaikh MH, Samarkandi AH. Is dantrolene effective in heat stroke patients? *Crit Care Med.* 1990;18:290–292.

Costrini AM. Emergency treatment of exertional heat stroke and comparison of whole body cooling techniques. *Med Sci Sports Exerc.* 1990;22:15–18.

Coyle EF, Montain SJ. Benefits of fluid replacement with carbohydrate during exercise. *Med Sci Sports Exerc.* 1992;24:S324–S330.

Deschamps A, Levy RD, Cosio MG, Marliss EB, Magder S. Tympanic temperature should not be used to assess exercise induced hyperthermia. *Clin J Sports Med.* 1992;2:27–32.

Elias S, Roberts WO, Thorson DC. Team sports in hot weather: Guidelines for modifying youth soccer. *Phys Sportsmed.* 1991;19:67–80.

Hubbard RW, Matthew CB, Durkot MJ, Francesconi RP. Novel approaches to the pathophysiology of heatstroke: The energy depletion model. *Ann Emerg Med.* 1987;16:1066–1075.

Knochel JP. Catastrophic medical events with exhaustive exercise: "White collar rhabdomyolysis." *Kidney Int.* 1990;38:709–719.

Knochel JP. Heat stroke and related heat stress disorders. *Dis Mon.* 1989;35:301–377.

Kulka TJ, Kenney WL. Heat balance limits in football uniforms: How different uniform ensembles alter the equation. *Phys Sportsmed.* 2002;30:29–39.

McCann DJ, Adams WC. Wet bulb globe temperature index and performance in competitive distance runners. *Med Sci Sports Exerc.* 1997;29:955–961.

Nadel ER. Recent advances in temperature regulation during exercise in humans. *Fed Proc.* 1985;44:2286–2292.

Noakes TD. Dehydration during exercise: What are the real dangers? *Clin J Sport Med.* 1995;5:123–128.

Noakes TD, Berlinski N, Solomon E, Weight L. Collapsed runners: Blood biochemical changes after IV fluid therapy. *Phys Sportsmed.* 1991;19:70–82.

Noakes TD, Myburgh KH, du Pliessis J, et al. Metabolic rate, not percent dehydration, predicts rectal temperature in marathon runners. *Med Sci Sports Exerc.* 1991;23:443–449.

O'Toole ML, Douglas PS, Laird RH, Hiller WDB. Fluid and electrolyte status in athletes receiving medical care at an ultradistance triathlon. *Clin J Sport Med.* 1995;5:116–122.

Richards D, Richards R, Schofield PJ, Ross V, Sutton JR. Management of heat exhaustion in Sydney's *The Sun* City-to-Surf fun run. *Med J Aust.* 1979;2:457–461.

Roberts WO. Assessing core temperature in collapsed athletes. *Phys Sportsmed.* 1994;22:49–55.

Roberts WO. A twelve year profile of medical injury and illness for the Twin Cities Marathon. *Med Sci Sports Exerc.* 2000;32:1549–1555.

Roberts WO. Environmental concerns. In: Kibler WB, ed. *ACSM's Handbook for the Team Physician*. Baltimore: Williams and Wilkins; 1996.

Roberts WO. Exercise associated collapse in endurance events: A classification system. *Phys Sportsmed.* 1989;17:49–55.

Roberts WO. Managing heatstroke: On-site cooling. *Phys Sportsmed.* 1992;20:17–28.

Roberts WO. Mass participation events. In: Lillegard WA, JD Butcher, KS Rucker, eds. *Handbook of Sports Medicine: A Symptom Oriented Approach*, 2nd ed. Newton, Mass: Butterworth Heinemann; 1998.

Sawka MN, Young AJ, Latzka WA, Neufer PD, Quigley MB, Pandolf KB. Human tolerance to heat strain during exercise: influence of hydration. *J Appl Physiol.* 1992;73:368–375.

III | SPORT-SPECIFIC ISSUES

29 | Ice Hockey

Shauna Martiniuk

Ice hockey is theoretically Canada's national sport, with an average annual participation rate of over 500,000 registered amateur players. Although Canada is considered to be the birthplace of ice hockey, the sport is extremely popular in the United States and in Europe. The McGill report states that the first match took place in March of 1875 in Montreal, although a more nostalgic account records the first game as having occurred on Christmas day in either 1855 or 1866 in Halifax. There were reports of 20 men on each side. The game lasted for 6 hours and 20 minutes. The match was between two garrison teams from the Canadian Royal Rifles, one from Halifax and one from Kingston. No victor was recorded (Schlerer, 1978). The number of individuals playing hockey has increased during this century, and the inclusion of the best professional players in the world and women's hockey at the 1998 Winter Olympics provided a tremendous boost to the sport. No finer moment in Canadian hockey was experienced than in the 2002 Winter Olympics in Salt Lake City, with both the Men's and Women's Canadian Hockey teams winning Gold.

Ice hockey is an intensely physical sport that demands both aerobic and anaerobic fitness in combination with great skill execution due to the speed at which it is played. It is a fast and rough game, with varying degrees of aggressive and contact play. In a professional game of three 20-minute periods, a player generally plays for 45–60 seconds at one time (Cos et al., 1995). The intense play periods add up to 16 minutes of playing time on average (Cox et al., 1995). Physiologically, both anaerobic and aerobic energy pathways are used for both the intense bursts of activity and endurance and power. Overall, 80% of injuries are due to trauma and 20% from overuse (Daly et al., 1990). Most injuries occur in the third period, with fewest in the first.

The mechanisms of injury in hockey are several. They involve high skating speeds of 24 km/h (Sim and Chao, 1978), plus sticks, pucks, blades, quick changes in direction without stopping, boards, goalposts, and other players. A hockey puck's maximal impact force has been measured at 567.5 kg (Stuart and Smith, 1995). The hockey stick's speed has been measured at angular velocities of 100–200 km/h, and the puck's speed has been measured at up to 192 km/h in professional hockey.

Several studies have been performed to elicit the type and number of injuries. Variable reports exist because of different reporting characteristics and protective equipment such as visors. A study of elite international Swedish hockey players found an incidence of 79.2 injuries resulting in player absence per 1000 player-hours and 70.8 per 1000 for facial lacerations. All injuries were traumatic in nature. Stick injuries accounted for 82.3% of the facial lacerations, and many would have been prevented by wearing a visor. Only 40% of players were wearing a visor (Lorentzon et al., 1988a). Another study of elite Swedish hockey players found that contusions made up 33% of traumatic injuries, with strains (17%), sprains (16%), and fractures (13%) being next most common (Lorentzon et al., 1988b). The lower limb was most affected (54%), with the upper limb (24%), back (16%), and head (6%) following. The most common mechanisms of injury for traumatic injuries were checking (33%), player contact (25%), puck (14%), and stick (12%). Cutting and skate contact accounted for less than

10% of injuries. Overuse injuries only made up 20% of the study, most commonly adductor and patellar tendonitis. Eight major injuries occurred in their study, with five of these being total tears of the medial collateral ligament, working out to between one and four ligamentous tears in each elite hockey team per season.

A 1995 study of injuries in Junior A hockey found an incidence of 96.1 injuries per 1000 player-hours in games (Stuart and Smith, 1995). Of all injuries, 51% were caused by collision, with the most commonly injured area the face and then the shoulder. A study of intercollegiate ice hockey injuries reported knee injuries to be most common (19%) and then the face (18%) (Pelletier et al., 1993). A full 45% of the injuries were caused by legal body checks. Not surprisingly, in ice hockey for youths under 11 years of age, where body checking is illegal, many fewer injuries occur (Stuart et al., 1995).

One concern in youth hockey is the size difference between players of similar ages. One study showed a 357% difference in force of impact during simulated body checking between the weakest and strongest players.

A 2000 review of injuries between the 1970s and the 1990s in the Finnish National Hockey League (NHL) provides evidence that there has been an increase over the latter years of contusions, sprains, and strains (Molsa et al., 2000). Areas affected include the knee, ankle, back, groin, shoulder, and hip. Notably, body checking and collisions with players or boards have increased during this time, which may explain the injury pattern. They also refer to the increasing mass, weight, strength, and speed of players as a contributing factor to a significant rise in this type of injury.

In addition to the more common injury patterns mentioned, occasionally more sinister events occur. According to Dr. Robert Cantu, ice hockey is "the most dangerous sport in the United States for nonfatal catastrophic injury." However, fatalities do occur. One paper published in 1995 outlined case reports of sudden cardiac arrest from blunt chest injury (Maron et al., 1995). In these case reports, four sudden deaths occurred in hockey players, two from puck injuries, one from a body collision with another player, and one by the heel of a hockey stick during slashing. The cause of death in most blunt chest injuries such as these is likely ventricular dysrythmia. The body sites most frequently injured in ice hockey are as follows:

Head and neck	20–30%
Upper body	15–20%
Trunk	15–25%
Arm	8–20%
Leg	20–30%

These percentages are based on a composite of studies.

The injury rates by player position in ice hockey are as follows:

Forward	49–60%
Defense	35–48%
Goalie	3–8%

HEAD AND NECK INJURIES

Head

In a study of elite players, 5.3% of all traumatic injuries in hockey were head concussions (Lorentzon et al., 1988a). Death from head injury also has

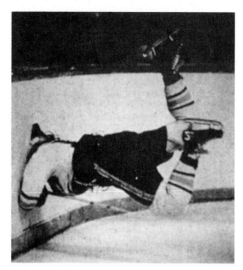

FIG 29-1 The sports practitioner should watch the play at all times. This is a true emergency, and you must be prepared. Your team should be ready to manage this serious concussion and cervical spine injury.

occurred in hockey (Cox et al., 1995). One can expect a range of head injuries to occur in hockey, from superficial hematomas to epidural hematomas requiring surgical treatment (Fig. 29-1).

Concussions

Concussions are the most common head injury in sports, and concussion occurs most commonly in ice hockey when a player strikes the boards head first. A concussion may be a consequence of a direct blow to the head, but also may occur when the neck suffers a whiplash injury with enough force being applied to the brain (Kelly and Rosenberg, 1997). In ice hockey, approximately 0.27 concussions occur for every 1000 athlete exposures (Dick, 1994), a number larger than that found for football (0.25 per 1000) and for sports without helmets such as soccer (0.25 per 1000) (Dick, 1994). A review of brain injuries in hockey from 1966 to 1997 found the most common head injury to be concussion (Honey, 1998). Rates for concussion ranged from 0.0–0.8 for players 5–14 years old, 0.0–2.7 for high school players, 0.2–4.2 for university players, and 0.0–6.6 for elite players. Concussion rates may be decreased by several initiatives, including rules on player contact as well as equipment requirements. A study of male players in the Canadian Inter-University Athletics Union found the use of a full face mask instead of a half mask significantly decreased player time lost due to concussion (Benson et al., 2002).

The First International Symposium on Concussion in Sport was held in Vienna in 2001 (Summary and Agreement Statement, 2002). They define *concussion* as a complex pathophysiologic process affecting the brain, caused by direct or transmitted forces to the head. It results in short-lived impairment of neurologic function that resolves spontaneously. The clinical symptoms are graded and occur with or without loss of consciousness. Neuroimaging studies reveal grossly normal structure, and symptom resolution follows a sequential course. The Concussion Protocol involves the following:

1. *Clinical history:* Previous number and symptoms of concussion; previous head, face, and neck injuries; any disproportionate impact and symptom severity; any loss of consciousness; and postconcussive symptoms including type and duration of amnesia. No single system for grading concussions was endorsed, and they concluded that combined measures of recovery should provide an index to injury severity and thus guide return to play activity.

2. *Evaluation:* The signs and symptoms of concussion include being unaware of the current period, opposition, score of game; confusion; amnesia; loss of consciousness; being unaware of time, date, place; headache; dizziness; nausea; unsteadiness/loss of balance; feeling stunned or dazed; seeing stars or flashing lights; tinnitus; diplopia; and subjective feeling of slowness or fatigue. Physical signs include loss of consciousness/impaired conscious state; poor coordination or balance; seizure; gait unsteadiness; slowness to answer questions; poor concentration; inappropriate emotions; nausea/vomiting; slurred speech; personality changes; inappropriate playing behavior; and significantly decreased playing ability.

3. *Neuropsychological assessment postconcussion:* This testing is a very important aspect of concussion evaluation and contributes significantly to management of the individual. Several different paradigms are in current use including pen and paper tests, protocols administered by neuropsychologists, and computerized test platforms. Baseline testing is recommended to maximize these tests clinically.

4. *Neuroimaging:* Brain CT or MRI contributes little to management of concussion, and should only be employed to evaluate any structural concerns. These occasions include seizure activity, focal deficits, and prolonged symptoms. Newer modalities such as positron emission tomography may be useful in the future.

5. *Management and rehabilitation:* If there are any signs of concussion, the player must not return to play or be left alone, and requires medical evaluation. Return to play must follow a medically supervised stepwise approach. For optimal injury recovery and safe return to play, a rehabilitation protocol must be followed. Rehabilitation must only begin after completely normal neurologic and cognitive evaluations. The return-to-play protocol is as follows: (1) complete rest until asymptomatic; (2) light aerobic exercise; (3) sport-specific training; (4) noncontact drills; (5) contact training after medical clearance; and (6) game play. Each level should take at least 24 hours. If any postconcussive symptoms arise, the player must drop back to the previous asymptomatic level for at least an additional 24 hours.

The physician also must be aware of an even more dangerous scenario called the *second impact syndrome.* In this situation, a second concussion occurs while the player is still symptomatic from the first. Consequently, the brain loses cerebrovascular autoregulation, leading to brain swelling and increased intracranial pressure (Kelly and Rosenberg, 1997). Articles have been written about hockey players dying from second impact syndrome (Cantu and Voy, 1995; Fekete, 1968). In addition, the effects of concussion may be cumulative, and chances of getting a second concussion may be four times higher than in athletes without a previous concussion (Leblanc, 1994). The number of concussions a player has accumulated in his or her career must be taken into consideration when discussing future play. Unfortunately, we are still without standards for how many concussions are too many and when an athlete should retire. When considering the diagnosis of concussion, always include in the differential diagnosis the following: epidural hematoma, subdural hematoma, intracerebral hematoma, intracerebral contusion, subarachnoid hemorrhage, cerebral concussion, malignant brain edema syndrome, second impact syndrome, and cervical spine injury. Epidural hematomas occur most commonly with a tear to the middle meningeal artery. This may be the result of a high-velocity impact, such as from a hockey stick or a puck, especially to the temporoparietal region.

On-ice treatment of a suspected head or neck injury begins with not attempting to move the player from the ice. Maintain an airway using jaw-thrust maneuvers with proper cervical spine precautions. The helmet may be removed only if adequate protection of the cervical spine is maintained. A neurologic examination may then be done, including assessment of consciousness, pupils, arm and leg movements, and strength. Sideline or off-ice testing mental status should include the following:

Area	What To Do
Orientation	Check for orientation to person, place, and time
Attention	Repetition of digits or months of the year, in backward order. Spell *world* backwards.
Retrograde amnesia	Memory of previous plays, what player was doing at the time of injury and just before, game site, score, score of last game, who scored last, who assisted, period of play, season record.
Anterograde amnesia	Memory of three objects immediately and after 5 minutes.
General appearance	Dazed look, incoherent speech, any changed behavior.

Barriers to the evaluation of neuropsychological testing include

- Lack of understanding of the evaluation process
- Apprehension about test results by both athletes and medical staff
- Time constraints placed on the athlete
- Financial considerations
- High rewards compared with low perceived risk
- English as a second language, long road trips, trained physicians not traveling with teams
- Difficulty in evaluating patients rink side

Dental Injuries

Dental injuries are permanent and can lead to later complications, most commonly root resorption, peri-apical lesion, pulpal obliteration, and loss of vitality (Lanti et al., 2002). A Finnish study found the most common injury to be a noncomplicated crown fracture, 70% occurring in games (Lanti et al., 2002). The mechanism was usually a blow from the stick, with an incidence three times higher in games than in practice. Only 10% of injured players were wearing a face guard, and full face shields combined with a dental mouth guard decrease the incidence of noncomplicated crown fracture.

Facial and Eye Injuries

To adequately protect the face and eyes from injury in this high-risk sport, certified protective full face visors should be worn at all times, including during games, practices, and shinny. One prospective study of injuries in adult recreational leagues revealed that only 35% of players wore some form of face shield (Voaklander et al., 1996). It is likely that the role models in professional leagues who do not wear face masks are a negative influence on recreational players. Prior to the use of face masks, lacerations were the major injury. Facial fractures also occur, but with the use of face masks, the incidence is likely much lower. Helmets with face masks have reduced the number of facial injuries by 70% (Pashby, 1987). Minor league hockey associations in Canada have required that players wear approved face masks and helmets since 1978. A prospective study of a National Collegiate Athletic Association (NCAA) Division I team with mandatory use of face masks found an incidence of 14.9 facial lacerations per 1000 player-hours (LaPrade et al., 1995). This incidence was lower than that found in other studies, where the use of face masks was not required.

Concerns that full face masks may increase the incidence of head and neck injuries have not been substantiated. A recent study investigating the use of full face masks found a decreased incidence of facial and dental injuries in those wearing full masks without an increase in neck injuries or concussions (Benson et al., 1999). Another study comparing the use of no, partial, or full face masks in elite amateur hockey players found full and partial face protection significantly reduced the number of eye and facial injuries without increasing the incidence of neck injuries or concussions (Stuart et al., 2002).

Pashby, a Toronto ophthalmologist, researched eye injuries in hockey, and it was his work that brought in a rule requiring full face masks in 1976 for players in the Minnesota State High School League. This requirement is now universal in North American youth and high school hockey and has virtually eliminated eye and facial injuries (Pashby, 1979). The most common eye injuries prior to face mask use were periorbital soft tissue trauma, followed by hyphema and iris damage. Injuries are caused mostly by sticks and pucks. The number of blinded eyes in ice hockey has been recorded by Dr. Pashby since 1972. Of 309 blinded eyes, 8 occurred while wearing a half mask and none while wearing a full visor. It is not known how many players wearing the half visor were wearing it correctly; it is often worn too high on the forehead (Juhn et al., 2002).

Female ice hockey players must wear full facial protection. Injury studies have revealed similar anatomic distribution of injuries to other leagues where full facial protection is mandatory (Hart and Walker, 2001). Most hockey players in the National Hockey League do not use facial protection for various reasons, although more are wearing half shields than ever before (Juhn et al., 2002). An interesting study was performed using sports goggles and a hockey visor to see if visual impediment was a substantial factor in the resistance to wear protective eyewear (Ing et al., 2002). Snellen acuity and contrast sensitivity was not affected by protective eyewear. The central 30° field of vision was minimally decreased with use of the visor but the far temporal field was more significantly decreased with both the goggles and visor.

Eye Injuries

A player can return from an eye injury with the following three-step protocol:

1. The ocular tissue has healed sufficiently to sustain a blow to the head or body that produces a Valsalva maneuver and thereby increases the pressure inside the eye.
2. The eye is comfortable with adequate return of vision. Appropriate, well-fitting eye protectors must be worn.
3. Immediate return to play after injury during a game depends on the complaint.

Danger signs and symptoms of potentially serious eye injuries include a sudden decrease in or loss of vision, loss of visual field, pain with eye movement, photophobia, diplopia, protrusion of the eye, lightening flashes, floaters, and irregularly shaped pupil, a foreign body sensation, and red eye or blood in the anterior chamber. Always obtain an adequate history and determine the force and direction of the blow. Assess visual acuity, visual fields, pupils, and fundi.

Facial Fractures

Always observe and palpate for facial asymmetry, point tenderness, bony steps, mobility, ecchymosis, and paresthesia. Occlusal (bite) discrepancy, pain, and limitation of mouth opening suggest a jaw fracture. Fracture of the nasal bone and cartilage is common, and findings include bleeding, nasal airway obstruction, nasal asymmetry, crepitus over the nasal bridge, periorbital and subconjunctival ecchymoses, and septal hematomas. Treatment includes controlling the airway and bleeding, protecting from further injury, and transporting for definitive diagnosis. Malar fractures are common, with loss of opacity of the maxillary sinus a good clue to this type of fracture. Mandibular fractures are also fairly common in hockey.

Neck

The most common mechanism responsible for fracture of the cervical spine is axial loading in a slightly flexed position, which flattens the normal cervical lordosis (Fig. 29-2). This occurs most commonly when a helmeted player strikes the boards. When the neck is flexed approximately 30°, the cervical spine becomes straight. From the standpoint of force, energy absorption, and the effect on tissue deformation and failure, the straightened cervical spine in axial loading acts as a segmented column. This injury is seen commonly when a player hits the boards head on. According to Tator (1987), sliding is also a common mechanism of neck injury. This may be attributed to the difficulty of changing position or direction while sliding. Rotational forces also manifest in the upper cervical spine, especially at C1, C2, and C3, and whiplash forces are transmitted to the C5–C6 area of the neck.

A study of major spinal cord injury from 1980 to 1996 in Finland found 16 cases with permanent disability (Molsa et al., 1999). In 50% of cases, the mechanism was body checking from behind followed by a blow to the head from the boards. In 69% of cases, the vertebral injury was fracture and/or luxation between C5 and C7. This type of injury could be avoided by rule prohibiting checking near the boards.

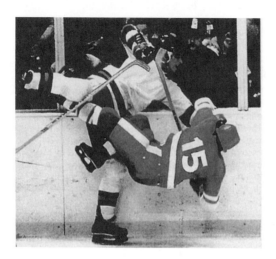

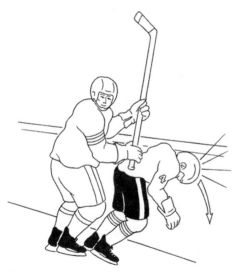

FIG 29-2 A sudden collision into the boards or a check from behind caused most neck injuries, although the stick is also a major culprit. The mechanism is usually active flexion. The cervical spine is more readily broken in flexion than in hyperextension.

Tator's most recent publication on spinal injuries occurring in hockey includes the period from 1966 to 1996 (Tator et al., 2000). Two hundred forty-three injuries have been recorded in Canada during this time with 85% at the cervical level. Burst fractures and fracture-dislocations were the most common injury types. A push or check from behind was the mechanism in 40% of cases, and the boards were the object of impact in 77% of cases.

Most injuries occurred in games and in men (only six cases in women). Despite being illegal, checking from behind still occurs. Articles are published that recommend greater penalties for this act, which can result in serious injury (Juhn et al., 2002).

The management of any suspected cervical spine injury requires neck immobilization until radiologic evaluation of the injury is undertaken. The helmet of the player should not be removed, but the face mask may be cut off to enable access to the airway if needed. The player should not be moved from his or her position, including turning the patient over or straightening the head.

Regarding return to play advice, a player with permanent neurologic damage should not return to competition (Maroon and Bailes, 1996). A player with a stable fracture according to flexion-extension views with no spinal cord injury may return to normal daily activities. A player with any unstable fracture or dislocation (that requiring a halo brace or surgery) should not return to contact sports because he or she does not have enough spinal strength. Despite healing of the bone, there is loss of normal motion in the segments above and below the injury that predisposes to future injury (Maroon and Bailes, 1996).

Since the introduction of mandatory helmet use, some investigators have suggested a possible link to increased serious cervical spine injury.[3] This increase may be related to players' perception of invincibility as well as referee leniency with rules if the consequences of actions such as high sticking are less obvious (Murray and Livingston, 1995). The incidence of illegal use of the stick has increased (Murray and Livingston, 1995). A helmet decelerates the head, with the neck decelerating the torso. Other factors have also contributed to the increase in neck and spinal injuries, such as increased speed and muscle mass in players and increased play along the boards as skaters use more ice surface with an improved fitness level (Murray and Livingston, 1995). The main mechanism of spinal cord injuries is a check from behind, and it is important that players and coaches realize this and take it into consideration when battling for the win.

Laryngeal fractures can be life threatening. Symptoms include loss of airway, hemoptysis, crepitus, and loss of the Adam's apple prominence. The need for a cricothyroidotomy has to be considered. This injury is basically impossible to protect against. Crosschecks over the neck or garroting from behind should be decreased by proper application of the rules (Fig. 29-3). Treatment consists of rest, humidification, and no hockey for 6–12 weeks.

Stinger Syndrome

The stinger syndrome is a common injury in hockey that presents as a burning pain down the arm, either acute or chronic. This injury is caused by traction on the brachial plexus or nerve root impingement within the cervical neural foramen (Cantu, 1997). The brachial plexus mechanism is commonly a forceful blow to the side of the head, although head extension or shoulder depression may also occur. Nerve root impingement results from the player's head being forced down toward the shoulder pad. The C5 and C6 dermatomes are most commonly affected. The injury is unilateral, typically lasting 1–2 minutes, and sensory in nature, although weakness may be experienced. Prolonged neurologic deficits lasting more than a few minutes necessitates MRI of the spine to secure a diagnosis. In the acute scenario, radicular pain is felt and may be accompanied by transient paresis and

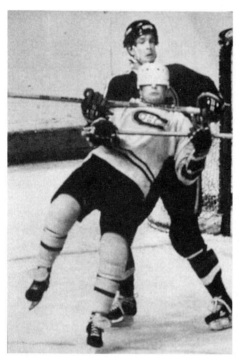

FIG 29-3 Protection against laryngeal fractures is almost impossible. Symptoms are loss of airway, hemoptysis, crepitus, and loss of the Adam's apple prominence. The need for cricothyroidotomy or tracheotomy has to be considered. (Canadian Press Photo.)

tenderness at Erb's point, the most superficial site of the brachial plexus. The radicular symptoms resolve over minutes, but tenderness persists. With C5 and C6 injury, pain and tingling are felt in the lateral arm, thumb, and index finger, with paresis in the biceps, deltoid, supraspinatus, and infraspinatus muscles. If there is any weakness of elbow flexion or shoulder external rotation or abduction, the athlete should not return to competition and should be followed closely.

A player may return to play if symptoms clear after seconds to minutes, they have a painless cervical spine range of motion, negative stretch tests, negative axial compression and resistive hand pressure tests, and normal strength on manual muscle testing (Koffler and Kelly, 2002). One needs to ensure that the patient does not have a transient cervical myelopathy. This will involve two extremities, either both arms, both legs, or ipsilateral arm and leg (Akau et al., 1993).

Transient neurologic deficit symptoms must lead to a thorough workup for ligamentous or bony spinal injury. Plain x-rays with flexion–extension views are completed first, followed by CT, MRI, or somatosensory evoked potentials if required. A finding of significant cervical spine stenosis on MRI is an absolute contraindication to playing contact sports such as hockey (Cantu, 1997).

The best prevention program for neck injuries is an isometric program or isokinetics using the Nautilus hydragym type of equipment prior to the hockey season. The neck and trapezial muscles require strengthening. Holding the neck muscles tightly against the points of compass, north, south, east and west, for periods of 10 seconds, and repeating for three sets of 30, is a good isometric preventative exercise. Flexibility is also the key to protection against neck and back injuries, and a full preseason flexibility program is highly recommended.

SHOULDER INJURIES

Injuries to the shoulder include possible trauma to the neck, shoulder, clavicle, chest, upper ribs, or arm. The greatest proportion of shoulder injuries are classified as minor in nature but can inhibit the ability to play effectively due to the physical nature of the game. The cause of injury is commonly a collision with an opponent or the boards or falling on an outstretched arm. The most common shoulder injuries in ice hockey are

- Acromioclavicular separation
- Glenohumeral joint dislocation/subluxation
- Sternoclavicular fractures

Acromioclavicular Separation

Acromioclavicular (AC) separation may be caused by a projectile force into the boards, a direct blow onto the AC joint with a stick, a direct fall on the shoulder, or a fall on an outstretched arm or point of the elbow. These mechanisms temporarily force the tip of the scapula (acromion) away from the collarbone (clavicle). AC separations can be classified into three main types:

- *First degree:* a stretch of the ligaments with no major break in the continuity between the acromion and the clavicle.
- *Second degree:* a partial tear of the ligaments. On visual examination, the distal end of the clavicle appears to ride somewhat higher.
- *Third degree:* a complete disruption of both the joint capsule and the coracoclavicular ligaments. Physical examination reveals an obvious depression of the scapula with what appears to be an elevation of the clavicle.

Often players with a first-degree AC separation never miss a shift in the game and experience point tenderness over the joint. With a second-degree AC separation, athletes do not need surgical intervention, and immobilization of the joint until the symptoms subside is quite beneficial. Protection over the area is imperative on return to play with well-constructed shoulder pads that emphasize rigid collar protection and possibly a protective doughnut pad over the AC joint. The point tenderness can remain for up to 12 weeks after injury, but if persistent discomfort is felt, suspect a distal clavicular bone irritation, which is positive on bone scan. A few more severe third-degree separations have been documented with complete dislocation of the clavicle at the AC joint, and management of this type of injury is surgical, especially if it occurs on the dominant side. A player also may develop posttraumatic osteolysis of the distal end of the clavicle, and this should be considered if pain is persistent. X-ray shows cyst formation and resorption.

Disability varies with the type of separation, with variable amounts of time off from hockey. Most AC dislocations are treated conservatively because studies comparing nonoperative versus operative treatment have not shown better outcomes with surgery (Weinstein et al., 1995). However, not all patients do well with conservative treatment, and some surgeons recommend surgery for young patients in certain situations.

Glenohumeral Dislocation

Approximately 20% of shoulder injuries in ice hockey are shoulder dislocations.[41] This is caused most commonly by a direct blow to an arm (humerus) that is extended backward with a violent twisting motion that overcomes the shoulder capsular restraints. The player notes a definite pop and/or sensation that the shoulder is out of place. Shoulder dislocations are often classified in the direction of instability. The most common type of instability in hockey is the traumatic anterior dislocation of the shoulder. Player age appears to be a more important factor than length of immobilization, specific rehabilitation program, or degree of initial trauma. Players who sustain an initial dislocation before the age of 20 years as a result of minimal trauma have the highest risk of recurrent dislocation. There has been a reported 92% recurrence rate in individuals aged 20 years or younger at the time of initial dislocation.

The traumatic acute anterior dislocation of the glenohumeral joint should be reduced as quickly as possible following a thorough physical and neurovascular examination and plain radiographs. Early relocation eliminates compression of neurovascular structures and minimizes the amount of muscle spasm that must be overcome to obtain reduction.

Treatment consists of immobilization for comfort, with range of motion and isometric exercises beginning as early as possible. Isokinetic exercises may begin at 3–6 weeks, with biceps strengthening being key (Burra and Andrews, 2002). Treatment concerns with glenohumeral dislocations include the following:

- There may be excessive bleeding internally.
- Weakening of the rotator cuff tendons is more common in patients older than 40 years. This should be suspected especially if persistent pain and weakness do not improve within 2 weeks of reduction. An MRI should be obtained to rule out a rotator cuff pathologic condition.
- After immobilization is discontinued, the patient should gradually progress through a rehabilitation program that emphasizes strengthening of the rotator cuff and scapular musculature.
- Prerequisites for return to hockey are a full range of motion, return of strength to greater than 90% of the opposite side, and absence of pain.
- A harness that limits abduction and outward rotation may be used to avoid recurrent injury.
- Surgical intervention is very successful in hockey players if apprehension compromises the patient's ability to perform despite a conservative trial of treatment.

Arthroscopic surgery is frequently used in the preliminary stages to diagnose rotator cuff tears, Hill-Sach's lesions, glenoid rim fractures, and capsulolabral pathology. In contact sports such as hockey, arthroscopic repair is still controversial and open repair is favored for stability. Open repair does have problems cosmetically with scarring and also with decreased external rotation. However, 80–90% of players in all sports return to their pre-injury level (Burra and Andrews, 2002).

Clavicular Fractures

Clavicle fractures are usually classified into three groups based on which part of the clavicle is fractured:

- 80% occur in the middle third.
- 15% occur in the lateral third.
- 5% occur in the medial third.

Most commonly clavicular fractures are caused by a direct impact to the clavicle. When the middle third of the clavicle is fractured, the shoulder slumps forward and inward as the player attempts to hold the arm against the chest to protect against any shoulder movements. Direct tenderness and palpable deformity are often present at the fracture site. Reduction of a middle-third clavicle fracture is easily accomplished by drawing the shoulders upward and backward as the end fragments are manipulated into alignment. The great majority of clavicle fractures are treated conservatively in a sling for comfort. Indications for operative treatment are

- neurovascular involvement
- open fractures
- fractures that progress to nonunion

Sternoclavicular Dislocation

Sternoclavicular dislocations can occur either anteriorly or posteriorly. A posterior dislocation is usually caused by a direct force and is more significant because of the proximity of important mediastinal structures (e.g., subclavian vein, cardiac vessels, trachea, esophagus, pleura). Emergency medical treatment of this injury may be required on site. This requires pulling the clavicle anteriorly and away from deeper structures either with a towel clip around the clavicle or even with a towel roll between the scapula. With traction on the shoulder joint in a posterior direction, the joint should reduce. Anterior dislocations are more common and not life threatening. Surgical repair of the sternoclavicular joint is difficult, but stability is of great importance.

Overuse Injuries

Overuse injuries of the shoulder are fairly common because players shoot repetitively. Players may develop rotator cuff tendonitis or tuberosity impingement. They exhibit the typical painful arc from 45–110°. Rest, anti-inflammatories, and subsequent strengthening programs are appropriate initial management strategies. Cybex testing and arthrograms are useful for diagnosis in extreme cases. Arthroscopy of the shoulder with subsequent Cybex-based rehabilitation has been quite successful.

UPPER EXTREMITY INJURIES

The most common upper extremity injuries in ice hockey are

- disruption of the ulnar collateral ligament at the metacarpophalangeal joint of the thumb

- fracture of the wrist at the scaphoid bone
- rupture of the flexor digitorum profundus tendon

Disruption of the Ulnar Collateral Ligament at the Metacarpophalangeal Joint of the Thumb

Commonly known as *Gamekeeper's* or *skier's thumb*, the rupture of the ulnar collateral ligament of the first metacarpophalangeal (MCP) joint results from a forced lateral stress with the MCP joint in nearly full extension. A player usually falls with the stick in hand and abducts the MCP joint of the thumb (Cox et al., 1995; Daly et al., 1990). Hockey players are more vulnerable to this injury because of the manner in which the stick is held. It is important to recognize the injury because surgery may be required to re-attach the ulnar collateral ligament. Failure to treat this injury adequately results in a weak pinch and grasp.

A partial tear can be differentiated from a complete tear by obtaining AP stress views of the thumb MCP joint. If angulation of the thumb MCP joint is more than 30° with a radially directed stress compared with the uninjured side, the injury is considered a complete tear.

The physical findings with disruption of the ulnar collateral ligament of the thumb are tenderness over the ulnar aspect of the MCP joint and exquisite pain with abduction stress testing. There is also significant joint laxity when testing the thumb with the MCP and interphalangeal joints both in a flexed position. The *Stenner lesion* is an interposition of the adductor aponeurosis between the torn ulnar collateral ligament ends that can be induced by stress testing the ligament. It is a complication that must be recognized and surgically corrected early if treatment is to be successful. Recommended treatment is summarized as follows.

Grades I and II: Incomplete Lesions

- Immobilize with a hand-based thumb spica cast for 3 weeks.
- Players with grade I–II injuries can often practice and compete in a hand-based spica cast within days of the injury.
- At 3 weeks, reevaluate for stability and discomfort.
- Begin active and gentle passive range of motion exercises and progress to strengthening exercises.
- Removable splint to be worn for protection.
- At 8 weeks, patient should be asymptomatic, and the splint can be discontinued except for sports.
- Continue strengthening exercises.

Grade III: Complete Rupture

- Immobilize with a hand-based thumb spica cast for 3–6 weeks.
- Consider primary surgical repair if a Stenner lesion is suspected. At 3 weeks, remove bulky dressing.
- Fit with wrist and thumb static splint or a hand-based thumb spica cast.
- At 6 weeks, begin dynamic splinting for range of motion.
- Begin active and gentle passive range of motion exercises.
- At 8 weeks, begin active strengthening exercises.
- At 12 weeks, allow patient to return to activity.
- Playing thumb splint should be worn.

Prevention of this type of injury is attempted through lock thumb mechanisms within the hockey glove. Protective measures include the leather tab at the end of the glove thumb, which should not be cut.

Fracture of the Scaphoid Bone

This injury is one of the most dreaded injuries by hockey players because of the time necessary for proper healing and the complications that can occur. The classic symptoms are snuff box tenderness, pain over the volar aspect of the scaphoid bone, and pain with forced compaction of the first metacarpal. Any sign of scaphoid fracture, with or without fracture on the scaphoid radiographs, require the player to be treated with scaphoid immobilization. It is not unusual for radiographs to first show evidence of fracture at 2–5 weeks.

Due to the high nonunion rates for these injuries, early diagnosis and appropriate casting are indicated. The recommended immobilization of this fracture is 8–12 weeks with a complete thumb spica cast and incorporating about two thirds of the forearm. Blood supply is confined to the distal pole in some cases and increases the healing time and the incidence of nonunion, avascular necrosis of the proximal fragment, and osteoarthritis. During immobilization, the player should not play because of the tremendous amount of motion that the scaphoid has in the cast as a result of gripping the hockey stick. Given the amount of contact in hockey, one has to consider earlier open reduction of a scaphoid nonunion in a professional player. Following cast removal, a player is usually able to regain hand function through activity; thus, extensive rehabilitation is not usually warranted.

Jersey Finger

This injury is an avulsion of the flexor digitorum profundus tendon and is a commonly missed injury. The injury occurs when a player grasps an opponent's jersey by flexing the digit, with the distal phalanx forced into hyperextension at the same time. The tendon is avulsed from its insertion and may be associated with an avulsion fracture. The injury commonly involves the fourth digit because it is functionally the longest finger when the hand is in a grasping position. Physical examination reveals swelling and tenderness over the distal interphalangeal (DIP) joint and the distal end of the tendon. The tendon may have retracted to the proximal interphalangeal (PIP) joint level or to the level of the MCP joint. The patient is unable to flex the DIP joint of the affected finger when testing the tendon in isolation. An x-ray should be taken to rule out a fracture. Treatment must be surgical to reattach the tendon to the distal phalanx. The best prognosis is offered with surgery within 2–3 weeks of injury. A missed injury is much more difficult to repair because the tendon has retracted and presents difficulty in being brought back out distally.

LOWER BACK, THORACIC, AND ABDOMINAL INJURIES

Fortunately, injuries to the spine are not among the most common in ice hockey (Daly et al., 1990), but when they do occur, they can be the most devastating and disabling (also refer to the section on the neck). Back pain is often muscular. After conservative management of back pain, unresolving pain should be evaluated with an x-ray and bone scan to rule out more sinister medical problems, such as disrupted posterior spinal elements in acute spondylolysis. The most common lumbar region injuries in hockey are as follows:

- *Lumbar strain:* Most common type of back pain and accounts for at least 70% of all low back pain. Caused by a stretch or microtearing of the muscles of the spine, but it usually responds well to treatment.
- *Facet joint syndrome:* These small joints of the spine can become sprained or inflamed when under extreme force, as with excess twisting or hyperextension of the spine.
- *Herniated lumbar disk:* This is usually the most severe of low back disorders. The motion of skating puts increased pressure on the disk, which can herniate out at a point of weakness or injury. This herniation can place pressure on the spinal nerves, resulting in radiating pain into the buttocks and down the legs.
- *Degenerative disk disease:* Degenerative changes occur after repetitive wear and tear on the spine. As the gelatinous disk becomes thinner, excess pressure is placed on the facet joints and nerves. Eventually, synovitis and osteophyte formation occur.

Although these four conditions are found most commonly in active hockey players, there are still many other potential conditions to consider, such as acute spondylolysis. A thorough history and physical examination are required for all back pains, and radiologic imaging will be required for some. The treatment of each individual back problem varies, but the principles remain the same.

1. *Trunk stabilization.* The *rigid cylinder concept* is one in which the muscles of the trunk are fully strengthened to stabilize the vertebral column. This protects the neural elements and the annular portion of the disk by shifting certain force vectors to the stronger muscles without sacrificing flexibility.
2. *Trunk strength.* The quadriceps and gluteal muscles are very important in the skating motion and must be trained to offer both explosive power and endurance. This improves the resistance to fatigue and protects the spine through improved biomechanical posture.
3. *Trunk flexibility.* Tight hip flexors, hamstrings, and erector spinae muscles increase the compressive forces on the facets and disks when the player assumes the skating position. Therefore, proper stretching of these muscles is imperative.
4. *Overall conditioning.* The player's overall physical conditioning is the single most important factor in the prevention of injuries.

Thoracic and Abdominal Injuries

The most common problems are as follows.

Rib Fractures

Rib fractures are commonly caused by forced compression of the rib cage and can result in significant pain. Displaced rib fractures can cause internal trauma with pneumothorax and/or hemothorax. Splenic trauma has been reported in up to 20% of left lower rib fractures and liver trauma in up to 10% of right lower rib fractures. Never underestimate the severity of rib fractures with regard to medical emergencies. A player may return to play with a minor rib fracture once healing has begun and pain has diminished enough to sustain play in a contact game.

Intra-abdominal Blunt Trauma

In contact sports one must consider blunt trauma with all abdominal complaints. Off-ice examination should include vital signs and a full physical examination. Any point or rebound tenderness, guarding, decreased bowel sounds, back pain in the absence of back trauma, shoulder tip pain, hematuria, hypotension, or tachycardia should alert the examiner to the possibility of significant injury. The spleen and liver are the most likely organs to be injured in blunt abdominal trauma. The spleen may sustain a subcapsular rupture with large hematoma formation. This subcapsular structure may lethally rupture at any time (see Chapter 18).

Slapshot Gut

This injury is a tear in the external oblique muscle that normally occurs in the external oblique aponeurosis of the lower abdomen. Often conventional investigations including ultrasound, x-rays, CT, and MRI do not show any abnormality because they are performed in a static state and the defect is evident only in a dynamic state. Conservative treatment is usually unsuccessful because the opposing portions of the muscle do not approximate close enough to allow for scar formation. Surgical repair of the tear is relatively simple. Some surgeons perform adductor partial or complete releases to decrease the pelvic tension and increase the blood flow to the groin region. Eleven professional NHL players with refractory pain and paresthesia in the lower abdomen with negative investigations were referred for a study (Lacroix et al., 1998). Surgical findings were tears of the external oblique aponeurosis and external oblique muscle with ilioinguinal nerve entrapment. Repair of the external oblique tear, ablation of the ilioinguinal nerve, and 12 weeks of physiotherapy enabled all players to return to professional ice hockey careers. Another study with 22 NHL players undergoing surgical ablation of the ilioinguinal nerve and reinforcement of the external oblique aponeurosis with a Goretex mesh found 82% to be pain free after rehabilitation and 85% able to continue their NHL careers (Irshad et al., 2001).

Women

Breast

The natural support for breasts is minimal, composed mostly of adipose tissue plus skin and some deep fascial structures. Studies of breast motion have been done and have shown considerable breast movement in up-down and spiral motions (Lorentzon and Lawson, 1987). In addition, larger breasts exert more force against the chest wall than smaller breasts. A bra is important to reduce movement and should be made of mostly nonelastic material with good absorbing capabilities, restrict movement in all directions, and have covered clasps and hooks to limit abrasion. It is also extremely important to wear proper chest protectors made of an impenetrable material to decrease trauma to the breast.

Nipple abrasions are common if abrasive material is worn next to the skin. A good bra also will help prevent this. Cold injury can occur in female hockey players; perspiration with evaporation and wind chill if in an outdoor arena make the nipple sore and sensitive. This is best avoided by wearing wind breaking material and proper clothing. There is no specific treatment.

Trauma to the breast consists mainly of mild contusions from elbows, sticks, and pucks. Edema and ecchymosis are the presenting findings and gradually resolve. Treat early with ice. Heavier blows to the breast can cause hematomas. Most resolve spontaneously, but they may need to be evacuated if they are increasing in size or pain or if there is a possible infection. Occasionally, a nodule remains that may need to be excised. There is no evidence that this trauma leads to cancer. Breast augmentation is not recommended in hockey players because trauma can lead to rupture of the prosthesis and bleeding with breast deformity.

LOWER EXTREMITY INJURIES

Groin

The groin is a very common site of muscle strain because skating requires forceful contraction of the hip adductors.[3] Goaltenders are also particularly prone to injure this area. Groin area injuries may include the hip adductor group, the iliopsoas, the rectus femoris, and the internal oblique muscles and peripheral nerve entrapments. Most commonly this injury causes an untimely absence from play with a poor response to treatment using conventional modalities or exercises. The loading of the adductor muscles during high-intensity exercise such as hockey may lead to injury and inflammation along the adductor origin, especially the adductor magnus. Pain may occur along the origin and radiate into the rectus abdomens as well as the symphysis pubis. The differential diagnosis must include inguinal hernia, osteitis pubis, and stress fractures of the hip or pelvis.

Groin Treatment Program

1. Early use of ice packs, compression, and elevation.
2. Second- or third-degree muscle strains require crutches with no weight-bearing for 48–72 hours to allow collagen fibers to scar over the strained area.
3. Soft tissue mobilization is necessary to address the fibrosis and adaptive shortening of the musculature. Fibrosis secondary to injury can predispose the muscle to further injury.
4. Retraining of the injured area once it has healed should progress as follows: Begin with isometrics without external loading, dynamic training without loading (pool workout), isometric training with external loading, dynamic training with loading, stretching, and finally, sport-specific training.

Some athletes with chronic tendonitis benefit from as much as 6 months away from their sport if they can possibly do it. Players need to be discouraged from repetitively traumatizing the region, leading to chronic tendonitis through reaggravation. Injury can be prevented by stretching prior to every game and practice. Prevention can begin in the preseason by measuring hip strength of players to identify those at risk for adductor muscle strains (Tyler et al., 2001). This study showed a player was 17 times more likely to sustain an adductor muscle injury if his adductor strength was less than 80% of his abductor strength.

Knee

Most knee injuries in hockey are of the collateral ligaments, but the anterior cruciate ligament (ACL) and the menisci are also frequently injured. Most injuries occur from contact, mostly with an opponent's knee, but they also may occur with contact with the boards or posts. Although hockey skates allow the feet to move and the foot is not fixed, there are still very severe injuries.

Medial Collateral Ligament Sprain

The hockey player skates with the knee in an almost constantly flexed position. Injury is caused by an overstretching of the ligament by a valgus and internal torsion strain, often when hit by an opposing player on the lateral aspect. This mechanism of injury is also the most common for an ACL injury. In children, it is critical not to miss epiphyseal damage.

Grade I sprains are tearing or stretching of some ligament fibers, with no or minimal loss of function. *Grade II sprains* consist of rupture of some of the fibers resulting in some loss of function. *Grade III sprains* are complete ruptures of the ligament from the bone. There is total loss of stability and function.

Surgery is not advantageous in the treatment of this type of injury. Treatment generally is conservative, and return to play should be accompanied by a custom fit or off-the-shelf brace. In contrast, lateral collateral ligament disruptions are often associated with posterior lateral corner damage and surgery is required for an optimal functional result.

Anterior Cruciate Ligament Sprains

Important historical features are the presence of a pop, crack, or noise at the time of the injury; immediate swelling suggesting hemarthrosis. The physical examination may be quite difficult to perform initially given the large muscle bulk of many players and the spasm existing after injury. In many players with an increased tolerance to pain, a mere lack of pain does not preclude serious injury.

Treatment with reconstructive surgery is a strong possibility, especially for competitive athletes. Joint capsule or cartilage tear increases joint instability, thereby increasing potential complications. If joint instability remains, degenerative changes will develop.

Meniscus

Injury is most commonly from a quick rotational, shearing, or squatting force at the knee joint. Physical findings include a positive McMurray's test, joint line tenderness, and a positive Apley's compression test. Occasionally a player is unable to extend the knee due to a mechanical block of the meniscus into the intra-articular notch. Indications for arthroscopy of meniscal tears include:

- Failure to respond to nonsurgical treatment.
- Positive physical examination and typical symptoms of joint line catching and pain, effusions, locking, and giving way.

Preventative Concepts for Knee Injuries

- Good quadriceps and hamstring strengthening.
- Maintenance of good overall body weight and composition.

- Maintenance of a good overall fitness level.
- Speed and agility training for the lower extremity.

After any injury, strength should be maximized prior to return to play. Players should be able to cut, turn both ways, and pivot with hard forces on their knees without symptoms. A full Cybex examination with 100% return to function is an excellent guide for when to return to play.

Patellar pain and abnormal patellar tracking are common in hockey but less severe than in the jumping sports. The cause in hockey is likely to be drills that involve jumping, squatting, and dropping to the knees on the ice.

Women

In the United States, the NCAA records athletic injuries for certain sports, but only for men's ice hockey, not for women's. In the NCAA's comparable sports (gymnastics, soccer, and basketball), women sustained more knee injuries than men (Hutchinson and Ireland, 1995), including between two and four times as many ACL injuries. Other studies also have supported this finding (Gray et al., 1985; Kelly and Rosenberg, 1997; Murray and Livingston, 1995). Of significance, however, male ice hockey players sustained fewer ACL injuries than men in other sports. Some possible explanations for the increased number of ACL injuries in women include poorer conditioning, increased ligamentous laxity, alignment of the lower extremity (e.g., increased Q angle), and muscle development. The high number of noncontact ACL injuries in women may be related to a smaller ACL and femoral notch space.[46] It is possible that a future study of ACL injuries in ice hockey players will reveal a greater increase in injuries in women versus injuries in men.

Ankle

Ankle injuries do occur in hockey despite the stiff skate, although the skate does offer some prevention against inversion injury. The force to the knee joint when a player is skating hard can be over 600 lb. The force is less in the ankle joint because it is locked in the skate, but there is still an equivalent force of at least two times the player's body weight. An important part of prevention in young players is fitting them with the correct skates. Buying oversized skates for a child to grow into is still common, but should be discouraged.

Rehabilitation of an ankle injury is most important. Fortunately, hockey players are going back into a skate boot, which also provides additional ankle support after an injury. After an ankle injury, it is possible to have weakness of the hip flexors, quadriceps, hamstrings, and calf musculature. After 8 weeks of inactivity, 40% of the strength is lost in the ligaments. Therapy must concentrate on strengthening these groups as well as residual mechanical instability, peroneal weakness, proprioceptive defects, and quick-response fibers of the lower extremity. For the hockey player, therapy should build up to cuts, pivots, tight figure-of-8s, agility exercises, and jumping.

Foot

Problems with the feet are much less common than one would imagine. Hockey players usually fit their skates very tightly, with a thin cotton sock or none at all. With a tight, form-fitting skate there is a tendency to calcaneal bumps, pressure sores on the medial malleolus, or areas of ganglionic-type swelling adjacent to the medial malleolus. Tenosynovitis and tendonitis of the anterior tibial tendons and extensor tendons of the feet can occur. Players usually respond by altering the skate. Sorbothane, moleskin, or low-density foam also can be introduced into the skate. For tenosynovitis of the ankle, excision of the synovial material or removal of the tendon sheath may be required. A metatarsal fracture may occur after a direct blow to the foot, and foot x-rays should be performed with management dependent on the degree of injury.

Morton's neuroma may be excruciatingly uncomfortable in a skate. The player may complain of the sensation of a nail sticking up in the skate. Treatment consists of adequate forefoot room in the skate, corticosteroid injections, ultrasound, and padding. Surgery may be required if conservative therapy is not successful.

Women

Bunions, which are an inflammation of the bursa over the medial first metatarsal, are more common in women in general. This may be due to increased pronation as well as inappropriately narrow and high footwear. When looking for footwear, and importantly, an ice skate, one must remember that a woman's foot is built differently from a man's. The female foot is wider in the forefoot than in the hindfoot (Arendt, 1994). Because most ice skates are built on a man's model, a women's foot may experience problems. To correct movement of the foot in the skate, a tighter fit at the heel may be required, especially because hockey requires many accelerations and decelerations. Surgery eventually can correct the deformity, but the player may be out of play for many months.

Other

Lacerations

Lacerations of the ankle and foot occur, requiring evaluation of underlying tendon function. Boot-top injuries include injury to the anterior tibial tendon, extensor hallucis longus, and extensor communis tendons or the dorsalis artery, vein, or nerve. These injuries are rare in comparison with other injuries in hockey, but several cases have been presented in the literature (Simonet and Sim, 1995). One must suspect this injury when injury has occurred to the anterior aspect of the ankle generally by a skate blade. Severe damage can occur with a seemingly small superficial laceration, and missed injuries can be devastating for athletes. A careful physical examination must be performed, and investigations may include an MRI and wound exploration. Surgery is required to correct any obvious deficits. To prevent such injuries, all players should wear the skate tongue in the upright position and under the shin pad.

Lower Leg Pain

The posterior tibial tendonitis that hockey players develop is treated identically to that in runners. Progression to periostitis and anterior compartment syndrome may occur. The common precipitant in hockey is dry land training such as running and additional exercises in pretraining. In a hockey player who develops shin pain, aerobic training should be conducted in some other sport such as cycling.

Medial Tarsal Tunnel Syndrome

An athlete often incurs entrapment of the posterior tibial nerve as it enters the fiberoseous tarsal tunnel beneath the flexor retinaculum on the medial side of the ankle. At this stage, the nerve divides into the medial and lateral calcaneal or plantar nerves, and the player is left with pain, numbness, burning, and a sensation of impairment on the sole of the foot. The complaint is accentuated by playing for long periods of time. Occasionally an intrinsic muscle weakness is manifested in the distal lateral surface of the foot and along the medial longitudinal arch. Tinel's sign modified by tapping over the area of entrapment is usually positive. If nerve conduction studies are positive, surgical decompression is indicated.

Women

The female anatomy has a wider pelvis, femoral neck anteversion with varus hip, valgus knees, external tibial tubercle rotation, and pronation of the hindfoot combining to increase the Q angle (Pearl, 1993). There is no proof that these anatomic differences result in any decrease in athletic performance. Injuries in female athletes of different sports, which are seen more commonly, are as follows:

1. Iliotibial band (ITB) friction syndrome with pain or snapping over the greater trochanter is common around the hip. Athletes may also suffer lateral knee pain. Treatment is with ITB stretches, ice, anti-inflammatories, and vastus medialis strengthening.
2. Greater trochanteric bursitis is common due to anatomic differences of the hip and a tight ITB. Treat with stretching, anti-inflammatories, and conditioning.
3. Retropatellar pain is very common and may be aggravated in hockey conditioning off ice (hill running, squats, and knee flexion and extension exercises). The patella comes in contact with the femoral trochlea at 30° of flexion. The differential diagnosis is large, but it is important to look for vastus medialis obliquus (VMO) atrophy. In addition, a triad of fat pad hypertrophy, inflammation of the patellar tendon, and medial plica tenderness may exist. Treatment includes strengthening, anti-inflammatories, Cybex, transcutaneous electrical nerve stimulation (TENS), and possible surgery.
4. Lateral knee pain is the second most common problem in the athletic woman, either as a result of ITB friction, synovial interposition, or fat pad interposition. Lateral collateral knee sprains, as well as lateral meniscal injury, must also be ruled out.
5. Medial knee pain is often from VMO atrophy; therefore, treatment is strengthening. Treatment of medial collateral ligament sprains in women is slightly different from that in men and may require medial orthotics and increased VMO strengthening.

THE FEMALE HOCKEY PLAYER

Since the 1970s, female participation in sports has increased tremendously, starting with Title IX legislation in the United States providing equal opportunities in physical education and athletics for women in institutions receiving federal funds (Warren and Shangold, 1997). Several other factors have played a role: research showing the benefits of exercise, increased media attention to these benefits, the physician's role in encouraging exercise, and a change in the societal perception of exercise for women.

Historians will recall the first time women played hockey back in 1889, when Lord Stanley's daughters played the game in the backyard (Webb, 1997). Since then, women's hockey has grown substantially and is still doing so. In Canada, between 1987 and 1997, the number of registered female players increased by 250% (Dryden et al., 2000). In the United States, the number of players increased by 260% between 1990 and 1995 (Dryden et al., 2000). In 1995 the combined total of registered players from both countries was approximately 50,000 (Dryden et al., 2000). The first women's world championships took place in 1990, in Ottawa, Canada, with Team Canada taking the gold. In the 1998 Winter Olympics, women's ice hockey was given full-medal status for the first time. Now as an Olympic event, women's hockey is expected to grow further and make even more noticeable gains with both the public and the press.

Despite greater participation in the sport, the body of literature on women's hockey is small, with very few statistics and case reports. Most research has been conducted on male hockey players at all levels. Female injuries are specific with regard to the reproductive organs, but there is no significant difference in frequency or types of injuries in women when compared with men (all sports) (Pearl, 1993). Injuries to women are sports related not gender related (Rubin, 1991). However, certain injuries are more common in women than in men: patellofemoral disorders (19.6% of all female injuries in sports versus 7.4% of males (Rubin, 1991), recurrent patellar dislocations (4.6% for women, 0.7% for men, in all sports (DeHaven and Lintner, 1996), spondylolysis, stress fractures, shin splints, bunions, and swimmer's shoulder.

The game is different than men's hockey in that muscle and power are less a component and speed, fast passes, and carrying the puck occur more in the women's game. Body checking was banned in 1990, but contact along the boards is allowed. Face shields are mandatory.

One study performed to compare male and female hockey player injuries in recreational leagues found a rate of 7.5 injuries per 1000 player exposures for females and 12.2 injuries per 1000 player exposures for men (Dryden et al., 2000). Injury severity was less in the female league, and anatomic distribution of injury was similar to the male players. The one exception was the high rate of injury to the lower back in females (13.6%), an area uncommonly injured in male players. Differences in overall rate of injury may relate to mandatory facial protection in the female league, body mass, speed, game forces, gender-specific behaviors, and mechanical differences (Dryden et al., 2000). Higher rates of injury would be anticipated if body checking were allowed in either league.

Another study by Schick found no significant differences between male and female rates of injury (Voaklander et al., 1996), although low back injuries were more common in females. This study involved more competitive teams than Dryden's study. The most common injuries in Dryden's study of recreational players were strains, sprains, and contusions, whereas concussion was the most common in the competitive players.

After puberty, a major gender difference is in muscle mass, giving men greater power and speed. Women, however, can gain great strength (up to 44%) without significant increases in muscle mass (Wilmore, 1979). Given the overall increase in muscle mass in men, power is increased, thus subjecting men to increased forces during play. Women, on the other hand, may rely more on speed and agility in their game. If both genders are subjected to the same coaching, training, and conditioning, the actual injury patterns vary mostly from sport to sport and not between the genders (Pearl, 1993).

Reproductive System

Despite the concerns early on in female sports about damaging reproductive organs, the female system is well-protected within the bony pelvis, with few cases of trauma. One anecdotal case (Mueller and Ryan, 1991) reports an IUD perforating the uterus following a pelvic blow in a field hockey game. It is only during pregnancy, when growth has carried on beyond the pelvis after the fourth month, that protection is decreased. It is best to not participate in contact sports beyond this time. The complaint of pelvic pain in the female athlete may be musculoskeletal, gastrointestinal, or genitourinary (Short et al., 1995). Localizing pain is difficult given the close proximity of the viscera and surrounding musculoskeletal elements. An MRI is very useful in clarifying musculoskeletal injuries of the pelvis.

Female athletes have increased irregularities of the menstrual cycle (28% in college varsity athletes) (Pearl, 1993). Delayed puberty also occurs with increased frequency in female athletes, and its long-term effects are not clear. During adolescence, normal bone mass gain occurs, but this is lessened in late-maturing females due to the lack of estrogen (Constantini and Warren, 1994). In addition, amenorrheic women lose bone mass at the rate of 5% per year, similar to the rate seen in menopause. Of greater interest is the bone mass density in female athletes not concerned about thinness, which is often the case in hockey. In a study of female rowers who were oligo/amenorrheic, vertebral bone content was the same as in matched nonathletic women (Constantini and Warren, 1994). However, conflicting data are also available that have shown a decrease in bone mass density in athletes with menstrual irregularities (Fruth and Worrell, 1995). The osteopenia that may result from decreased bone mass density increases players' risk of injury, including stress fractures. If growth is complete, as measured by closed epiphyseal plates, and menarche has not occurred by age 16, hormonal therapy should be started as prevention (Constantini and Warren, 1994).

There are two different types of amenorrhea: one related to low body weight, which is less likely to occur in hockey players, and another hormonal pattern where low weight is not required. The latter pattern may occur in hockey players, because muscle mass is important, and weight and body fat not as much of a concern as in gymnasts, for instance. This *athlete's amenorrhea* has shown increased levels of luteinizing hormone and androgens, but future research is still required (Rubin, 1991). Treatment includes calcium supplement, nutritional counseling, a possible change in training intensity, and hormone replacement. Recommendations for the evaluation and treatment of amenorrhea in adolescent females from the American Academy of Pediatrics' Committee of Sports Medicine are as follows (AAP Committee on Sports Medicine, 1989):

- *All:* Evaluation of menses and diet, counsel on nutrition; monitor menses, diet, growth, weight, and skin fold thickness; calcium supplementation, 1200–1500 mg/d.

- *If amenorrheic:* Physical examination, endocrine evaluation, and exclude pregnancy and anorexia.
- *If less than 3 years after menarche:* Decrease exercise intensity, improve nutrition.
- *If more than 3 years after menarche or after age 16:* Start low-dose OCP.

Steroids

In one study, steroid use among older teens was 5% in males and 1% in females (all sports) (Warren and Shangold, 1997). Given the nature of hockey and its reliance on speed, power, and strength, it is possible for the percentage of women using steroids to be higher if they are hockey players. In women, side effects include hirsutism, increased muscularity, deeper voice, male-pattern baldness, hypertrophy of the clitoris, acne, menstrual disorders, and increased aggressiveness. Oral steroids may cause elevation of liver enzymes, and long-term use may result in peliosis hepatitis. Other effects include increased low- and high-density lipoproteins, hypertension, decreased glucose tolerance, decreased thyroid hormones and immunoglobulins, and possibly early growth plate epiphyseal fusion.

HIGH-PERFORMANCE TRAINING IN HOCKEY

Sport-specific training is important to improve performance. Training programs should be task specific to improve fitness and maximize the energy demands placed on players (Schlerer, 1978). Studies have shown that players involved in hockey-related training programs show greater improvement in skating performance than players only training through games (Greer et al., 1992). Further studies have suggested that players do not receive enough on-ice game and practice challenge to maintain and increase their level of fitness, leading to detraining. With the average NHL on-ice game time being 16 minutes per player and poor exercise intensities during practices, detraining occurs (Schlerer, 1978). Thus, proper training programs must be in place for all levels both to improve playing ability and to decrease injury risk.

Physiologic Characteristics of the Sport

1. Energy requirements of the sport are characterized by fast, explosive skating, and quick and sudden changes in direction.
2. Motor development requiring agility for stick handling, passing, shooting, and playmaking with teammates is necessary.
3. Muscular strength and balance are required for on-ice activities, including body checking, absorbing hits by opponents, and crashing into boards, posts, and ice.

Ice hockey demands a complex interaction of several specific physiologic components, many of which serve to provide a base for advanced high-performance training. Physiologic components are as follows:

1. Aerobic energy system
2. Anaerobic energy system
3. Muscular strength
4. Power
5. Muscular flexibility
6. Agility

Aerobic Energy System

Aerobic training prepares the on-ice energy supply and recovery process and builds the base needed to handle more intense anaerobic training. The aerobic system is vital to the recovery process between bouts of intense exercise. Adjacent slow oxidative muscle fibers also can contribute by reoxidizing lactic acid if they are well conditioned, even if the slow-twitch fibers have not been recruited for the skating action. Players' heart rates during a single shift could exceed 90% of the age-adjusted maximum. During this event, players would have a far greater dependence on the anaerobic energy system.

Anaerobic Energy System

The anaerobic energy system provides the major source of energy for muscle contraction during the exertion phase of hockey. Bursts of maximal effort place explicit demands on the anaerobic system. Fast, explosive movements demand a rapid supply of ATP energy. Anaerobic ATP production peaks at 30–45 seconds and has an upper limit of 120 seconds, depending on the intensity. If the athlete is not trained properly, an inhibitive action on performance results, providing submaximal efforts.

Muscular Strength

Programs are designed to increase lean body mass, improve absolute strength, and provide a base for power training. Absolute strength is necessary for contact. Sport-specific exercises help to lower the center of gravity and increase inertia. Lower body strength contributes to skating, acceleration, agility, and pelvic stability. Upper body strength improves body checking, shooting, and puck-control skills. Muscle balance is important for injury prevention and sport performance. A joint may be more susceptible to injury when there is a strength imbalance between muscle groups.

Power

Power is a fundamental requirement for on-ice activities, particularly when propulsion of the total body is required. The hockey player often executes sharp changes in direction and accelerates quickly. Explosive power is arguably the most important physical parameter in ice hockey.

Muscular Flexibility

Muscular flexibility is very important when a player must execute powerful, explosive movements. Flexibility decreases injuries and improves execution. Players who fail to extend the rear leg during the skating motion seriously hinder their skating speed and power. Flexibility training should target the lumbar region, hip, groin, quadriceps, and hamstrings.

Agility

Agility becomes vital when the athlete must make quick, sudden changes in direction, such as those during one-on-one situations to maneuver around the opposition. Complex agility skills distinguish the elite player.

Ice Hockey Safety

To make ice hockey safer, the most important change must be that of attitude. Players must be educated about the true protective value of safety equipment. Coaches need to teach players the correct way to play and not to tolerate or promote intentional violence. Fans and parents must encourage officials to enforce rules and to prevent high-risk behavior.

Women

In strength training, men develop hypertrophy of muscles because they have much higher levels of androgenic hormones. Women may do the same weight training and also become strong, but they do not develop markedly enlarged muscles. In endurance training, women are found to have a lower maximal oxygen consumption compared with men. This difference is due to larger heart size and thus greater stroke volume and more hemoglobin in men. Thus the training target VO_2 max in women is somewhat lower.

The Canadian National Team and university teams in Canada (University of Toronto) have off-season training manuals for female hockey players. For example, the July national training manual includes the following: strength training 3 days a week, plyometric workouts twice a week, pool work twice a week, a long cardiovascular workout once a week, two shorter anaerobic activities each week such as biking or rollerblading (goal is to perform high-intensity exercise for a short time period and rest for a short time in between), and an abdominal program, with 1 day of rest each week. By August, the on-ice training begins to increase from twice the first week up to four to five times for the last week. The best training drills are high-intensity scrimmage, during which the players are encouraged to do some gamelike drills. The month also continues with pliometrics (such as medicine ball throws, leap frog), anaerobic work, and emphasis on flexibility, especially in the lower back, groin, hamstrings, hip flexors, iliotibial band, quadriceps, and calves. Emphasis is also on abdominals, with a workout 6 days a week.

The University of Toronto training manual for off-season includes a general preparation phase for 2 months, a specific preparation phase for 1 month, and a precompetitive phase for the final month. The first 3 months include strength, flexibility, and aerobic activities. The first 2 months build up muscle strength and general physical conditioning, increasing intensity gradually. Coaches and trainers have noticed a lack of strength in the upper body specifically, predisposing players to injury. Thus greater emphasis is placed on these muscles in this training period. The third month aims activity toward sport-specific exercises to achieve greater speed and power. On-ice intensity also increases gradually. In the last month, more speed, power, and specific skills are worked on and include exhibition games prior to the competitive season.

THE RECREATIONAL PLAYER

In addition to being subject to the same injuries as professional players, the recreational player is also at risk for possible cardiac events (Atwal et al., 2002). A recent article suggests that of the 500,000 male recreational hockey players in Canada, some may be at risk for cardiac events as they exercise at extremes of intensity. In 113 male volunteers, 70% of the Holter monitor data sets showed poor heart rate recovery, 2 data sets showed nonsustained ventricular tachycardia, and 15 sets showed ST depression. Although clinical significance is unknown, it is an important area to be studied and suggests that the game may be dangerous to a player's health.

PROPER FITTING OF PROTECTIVE EQUIPMENT

The following describes what to look for when fitting or buying new equipment. Properly fitted equipment can significantly reduce the chance of injury and improve the athlete's skating performance.

Skates

A hockey skate usually will fit a half size smaller than regular street shoes. Ensure that there are no wrinkles in the sock when tightening the skate up. With foot and toes to the front of the boot, you should be able to place one finger between the boot and the heel of the foot. When lacing up the skate, bang the heel against the floor to ensure support. The first three to four eyelets should be snug, the next three loose, and the final two to four very snug. Do not wrap the lace around the ankle, because this may inhibit circulation and irritate the tendons. The skate tongues should be behind the shin guard to ensure maximum protection for the shins. If the hard shell is cracked, replace immediately because of the increased chance of a serious toe or foot injury. Never buy skates that are too big. This can seriously inhibit skating development.

Shin Guards

The sizes will vary from junior (8–13 inches) to senior (14–16 inches). The cup of the shin guard should be centered directly over the kneecap. The top of the shin guard should overlap roughly 2 inches with the bottom of the hockey pant. With the skates on, the pads should rest 1 inch above the foot when it is fully flexed.

Pants

Hockey pants should be fitted with shin guards in place. The belt should be fitted just above the hip bone and allow for snug adjustment. The pants should have as much padding as possible without restricting movement. The player should be able to fully squat with the pants and shin guards on, with the padding in the pants staying in the same position.

Shoulder Pads

Make sure that the shoulder pads cover the shoulders, upper back, chest, and upper arms to just meet the elbow pads. The protective caps should be placed on top of the shoulders. The back of the shoulder pads should slightly overlap with the pants to ensure maximum protection of the spine. To guarantee full range of motion, the player should be able to lift the arms just above shoulder height without the pads digging into the neck area.

Elbow Pads

Ensure that elbow pads are properly fitted to each arm; some pads vary protection depending on left or right elbow. The donut inside the pad should be placed on the point of the elbow. The elbow pad should fit tightly and lock into the elbow. The pads should extend to the bottom of the shoulder pads and down the forearms to where the tops of the gloves start. The player should be able to fully flex the elbow without constriction from the straps. The straps usually wear out first, so either get new ones or secure them with tape.

Gloves

Hockey gloves should fit like loose winter gloves over the fingers. The top of the glove should extend to the bottom of the elbow pad to ensure full forearm protection. To ensure maximal protection, with your hand in the glove, push the back of the glove with your other fingers. This compression should not be felt inside the glove. Test the glove with a hockey stick and stick handle on the spot for a few minutes to ensure freedom of motion and to locate any spots that might cause blisters.

Helmet

All helmets in Canada must be approved by the Canadian Standards Association (CSA) and will have a sticker indicating this. They are generally measured in junior and senior sizes depending on head sizes from $6\frac{1}{2}$–$7\frac{3}{4}$ inches. The helmet should be snug on the head after adjustments are made. Shake the head from side to side, back and forth, ensuring that the helmet does not move and causes no discomfort. The front of the helmet should be just above the eyebrows. The chin strap should be placed securely under the chin for a snug fit. Occasionally check the inside foam of the helmet. Press the thumb against the padding. If the padding returns to the original position, this is a good sign that the foam is still protective. If the padding breaks or cracks, the helmet should be replaced.

Face Protectors/Masks

All masks must be CSA approved and will have a sticker indicating this. Make sure that the cage is compatible with the helmet. The mask should allow for one finger to fit between the bottom of the chin and the chin cup of the protector.

Throat Protectors

The protector should fit snugly, but not too tight. It should completely cover the throat, and with bib styles, the upper chest area.

Undergarments

Undergarments should be cool and comfortable to avoid irritation of the skin. Always wear a single pair of socks to offer comfort and moisture-absorbing ability.

Athletic Support

Choose an appropriately sized protective cup and strap that is effective for shock absorption. Females should wear a jill. If the cup is cracked or the strap is frayed, replace it immediately.

Women

Some companies have lines of equipment specifically for women:
- Different sizes.
- Pants: Better fitting waist and thinner kidney pads so they fit better with the shoulder pads.
- Gloves: Smaller fit decreases hand motion inside glove.

- Shoulder pads: Two pieces across the breast area enables better arm movement.
- Neck guards: Normal, although most women do not use the neck flap because it does not fit as well with the shoulder pads.

Goalies

Pads

Always fit the pads with your skates on. Kneel down into each pad and make sure the kneecap is in the middle of the knee roll. The pad should extend from the toe of the skate to 4 inches above the knee. The top of the pad should fit approximately 3 inches above the bottom of the pants.

Catcher and Blocker

Lower the blocker and glove to the side, and they should not be able to fall off. The blocker should be comfortable, easy to grip, and able to control the stick for a proper fit. The catcher must have a heavily padded cuff that overlaps the arm pads.

Upper Body Protection

Ensure that all straps are fastened and used properly. The arm padding should extend down past the blocker to the wrist while allowing full range of motion in the wrist and elbow. The body pad should tuck into the pants about 2 inches below the navel.

Throat Protectors

The protector can be either the hanging kind or have a snug fit around the neck (Fig. 29-4). The bib-style protector should be worn beneath the chest protector. *Tip*: Throat protectors protect against skate lacerations and cuts but *not* against spinal injuries. Make sure that all Velcro straps are in good shape, and replace the protector when it is damaged.

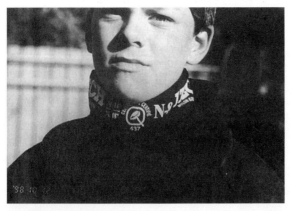

FIG 29-4 Plastic mesh collar for an 8-year-old goalie. They are larger for older players.

Pants and Athletic Supports

Goaltenders should wear a special athletic supporter and cup with extra protection. The pants are specifically designed to absorb and disperse the high impact from pucks. Ensure that the pants are loose enough around the waist to allow for the belly pad to tuck into them. *Tip*: Padding is heavier than regular pants and therefore may require the use of suspenders.

Face Mask Protection

The mask should be CSA approved and specifically designed for goaltenders due to the increased chance of pucks hitting the mask at high speeds.

Sticks

Sticks should be comfortable in the crouch position. The lie of the stick should be flat on the ice when the goaltender is in the crouch position. The length of the paddle also should be comfortable in this position.

REFERENCES

Akau CK, Press JM, Gooch JL. Sports medicine: 4. Spine and Head Injuries. *Arch Phys Med Rehabil.* 1993;74:S443–S446.

American Academy of Pediatrics: Committee on Sports Medicine: Amenorrhea in adolescent athletes. *Pediatrics.* 1989;84:394–395.

Arendt EA. Orthopaedic issues for active and athletic women. *Clin Sports Med.* 1994;13:483–503.

Atwal S, Porter J, MacDonald P. Cardiovascular effects of strenuous exercise in adult recreational hockey: The Hockey Heart Study. *CMAJ.* 2002;166:303–307.

Benoit BG, Russell NA, Richard MT, et al. Epidural hematoma: Report of seven cases with delayed evolution of symptoms. *Can J Neurol Sci.* 1982;9:321–324.

Benson BW, Mohtadi NG, Rose MS. Head and neck injuries among ice hockey players wearing full face shields vs half face shields. *JAMA.* 1999;282:2328–2332.

Benson BW, Rose MS, Meeuwisse WH, Kissick J, Roberts WO. The impact of face shield use on concussions in ice hockey. A Multivariate Analysis/ Commentary. *Br J Sports Med.* 2002;36:27–32.

Burra G, Andrews JR. Acute shoulder and elbow dislocations in the athlete. *Orthop Clinics North Am.* 2002;33:471–495.

Cantu RC. Stingers, transient quadriplegia, and cervical spinal stenosis: return to play criteria. *Med Sci Sports Exerc.* 1997;29:233–235.

Cantu RC, Voy R. Second impact syndrome: A risk in any sport. *Phys Sports Med.* 1995;23:27–36.

Constantini NW, Warren MP. Special problems of the female athlete. *Bailliere's Clin Rheum.* 1994;8:199–219.

Cox MH, Miles DS, Verde TJ, Rhodes EC. Applied physiology of ice hockey. *Sports Med.* 1995;19:184–201.

Daly PJ, Sim FH, Simonet WT. Ice hockey injuries: A review. *Sports Med.* 1990;10:122–131.

DeHaven KE, Lintner DM. Athletic injuries: Comparison by age, sport and gender. *Am J Sports Med.* 1986;14:218–224.

Dick RW. A summary of head and neck injuries in collegiate athletics using the NCAA Injury Surveillance System. In: Hoerner EF, ed. *Head and Neck Injuries in Sports.* Philadelphia: American Society for Testing and Materials; 1994.

Dryden DM, Francescutti LH, Rowe BH, Spence JC, Voaklander DC. Epidemiology of women's recreational ice hockey injuries. *Med Sci Sports Exerc.* 2000;32:1378–1383.

Fekete JF. Severe brain injury and death following minor hockey accidents: The effectiveness of the "safety helmets" of amateur hockey players. *Can Med Assoc J.* 1968;99:1234–1239.

Fruth SJ, Worrell TW. Factors associated with menstrual irregularities and decreased bone mineral density in female athletes. *J Orthop Sports Phys Ther.* 1995;22:26–38.

Gray J, Taunton JE, McKenzie DC, et al. A survey of injuries to the anterior cruciate ligament of the knee in female basketball players. *Int J Sports Med.* 1985;6:314–316.

Greer N, Serfass R, Picanatto W. The effects of a hockey-specific training program on performance of bantam players. *Can J Sports Sci.* 1992;17:65–69.

Hart LE, Walker L. Women's recreational ice hockey injuries. *Clin J Sport Med.* 2001;11:64.

Honey CR. Brain injury in ice hockey. *Clin J Sport Med.* 1998;8:43–46.

Hutchinson MR, Ireland ML. Knee injuries in female athletes. *Sports Med.* 1995;19:288–302.

Ing E, Ing T, Ing S. The effect of a hockey visor and sports goggles on visual function. *Can J Ophthalmol.* 2002;37:161–167.

Irshad K, Feldman LS, Lavoie C, Lacroix VJ, Mulder DS, Brown RA. Operative management of "hockey groin syndrome": 12 years of experience in National Hockey League players. *Surgery.* 2001;130:759–764.

Juhn MS, Brolinson PG, Duffey T, et al. Violence and injury in ice hockey: American Osteopathic Academy of Sports Medicine. *Clin J Sports Med.* 2002;12:46–51.

Kelly JP, Rosenberg JH. Diagnosis and management of concussion in sports. *Neurology.* 1997;48:575–580.

Koffler KM, Kelly JD IV. Neurovascular trauma in athletes. *Orthop Clin North Am.* 2002;33:523–534.

Lacroix VJ, Kinnear DG, Mulder DS, Brown RA. Lower abdominal pain syndrome in national hockey players: a report of 11 cases. *Clin J Sport Med.* 1998;8:5–9.

Lahti H, Sena J, Ylipaavalniemi P. Dental injuries in ice hockey games and training. *Med Sci Sports Exerc.* 2002;34:400–402.

LaPrade RF, Burnett QM, Zarzour R, Moss R. The effect of the mandatory use of face masks on facial lacerations and head and neck injuries in ice hockey. A prospective study. *Am J Sports Med.* 1995;23:773–775.

Leblanc KE. Concussions in sports: Guidelines for return to competition. *Am Family Phys.* 1994;50:801–806.

Lorentzen D, Lawson L. Selected sports bras: A biomechanical analysis of breast motion while jogging. *Phys Sportsmed.* 1987;15:128–139.

Lorentzon R, Wedren H, Pietila T. Incidence, nature and causes of ice hockey injuries. A three-year prospective study of a Swedish elite ice hockey team. *Am J Sports Med.* 1988a;392–396.

Lorentzon R, Wedren H, Pietila T, Gustavsson B. Injuries in international ice hockey. A prospective, comparative study of injury incidence and injury types in international and Swedish elite ice hockey. *Am J Sports Med.* 1988b;16:389–391.

Maron BJ, Poliac LC, Kaplan JA, Mueller FO. Blunt impact to the chest leading to sudden death from cardiac arrest during sports activities. *N Engl J Med.* 1995;333:337–342.

Maroon JC, Bailes JE. Athletes with cervical spine injury. *Spine.* 1996;21:2294–2299.

Molsa J, Kujala U, Nasman O, Lehtipuu TP, Airaksinen O. Injury profile in ice hockey from the 1970's through the 1990s in Finland. *Am J Sports Med.* 2000;28:322–327.

Molsa JJ, Tegner Y, Alaranta H, Myllynen P, Kujala UM. Spinal cord injuries in ice hockey in Finland and Sweden from 1980 to 1996. *Int J Sports Med.* 1999;20:64–67.

Mueller FO, Ryan AJ. *Prevention of Athletic Injuries: The Role of the Sports Medicine Team.* Philadelphia: F.A. Davis; 1991.

Murray TM, Livingston LA. Hockey helmets, face masks, and injurious behaviour. *Pediatrics.* 1995;95:419–421.

Pashby TJ. Eye injuries in Canadian Hockey. Phase III: Older players now most at risk. *Can Med Assoc J.* 1979;121:643–644.

Pashby TJ. Eye injuries in Canadian amateur hockey, still a concern. *Can J Ophthalmol.* 1987;22:293–295.

Pearl AJ, ed: *The athletic female. American Orthopaedic Society for Sports Medicine.* Champaign, Ill:, Human Kinetics; 1993.

Pelletier RL, Montelpare WJ, Stark RM. Intercollegiate ice hockey injuries. A case for uniform definitions and reports. *Am J Sports Med.* 1993;21:78–81.

Rubin CJ. Sports injuries in the female athlete. *N J Med.* 1991;88:643–645.

Schlerer KA. *The seventy year history of the International Ice Hockey Federation, 1908–1978.* Munich: Prospect Presse Service; 1978.

Short JW, Pedowitz RA, Strong JA, Speer KP. The evaluation of pelvic injury in the female athlete. *Sports Med.* 1995;20:422–428.

Sim FH, Chao EY. Injury potential in modern ice hockey. *Am J Sports Med.* 1978;6:378–384.

Simonet WT, Sim L. Boot-top tendon lacerations in ice hockey. *J Trauma.* 1995;38:30–31.

Stuart MJ, Smith A. Injuries in Junior A Ice Hockey. A three-year prospective study. *Am J Sports Med.* 1995;23:458–461.

Stuart MJ, Smith AM, Malo-Ortiguera SA, Fischer TL, Larson DR. A comparison of facial protection and the incidence of head, neck and facial injuries in Junior A hockey players. *Am J Sports Med.* 2002;30:39–44.

Stuart MJ, Smith AM, Nieva JJ. Injuries in youth ice hockey: A pilot surveillance strategy. *Mayo Clin Proc.* 1995;70:350–356.

Summary and Agreement Statement on the 1st International Symposium on Concussion in Sport. *Clin J Sport Med.* 2002;12:6–11.

Tator CH. Neck injuries in ice hockey: A recent, unsolved problem with many contributing factors. *Clin Sports Med.* 1987;6:101–114.

Tator CH, Carson JD, Cushman R. Hockey injuries of the spine in Canada, 1966–1996. *CMAJ.* 2000;162:787–788.

Tyler TF, Nicholas SJ, Campbell RJ, McHugh MP. The association of hip strength and flexibility with the incidence of adductor muscle strains in professional ice hockey players. *Am J Sports Med.* 2001;29:124–128.

Voaklander DC, Saunders LD, Quinnery HA. Correlates of facial protection use by adult recreational ice hockey players. *Can J Public Health.* 1996;87:381–382.

Voaklander DC, Saunders LD, Quinney HA, et al. Epidemiology of recreational and old-timer ice hockey injuries. *Clin J Sport Med.* 1996;6:15–21.

Warren MP, Shangold MM. *Sports gynecology: Problems and care of the athletic female.* Cambridge, Mass: Blackwell Science; 1997.

Webb M. Hockey Moments with Marg. *Univ Toronto Magazine.* 1997;XXV:10–13.

Weinstein DM, McCann PD, McIlveen SJ, Flatow EL, Bigliani LU. Surgical treatment of complete acromioclavicular dislocations. *Am J Sports Med.* 1995;23:324–331.

Wilmore J. Alteration in strength, body composition, and anthropometric measurements to a ten week training program. *Med Sci Sports.* 1979;6:133.

30 | Basketball Injuries

Douglas W. Richards, Paul H. Marks, Ato Sekyi-Out,
and Gilbert Yee

QUICK REFERENCE

Factors Affecting Basketball Injuries

- Gender—ACL injuries more common in women than men
- Playing surfaces—synthetic surfaces higher incidence
- Games versus practice—injuries more frequent in games
- Position played—no difference in incidence of injuries
- Shoes and ankle stabilization—athletes preference but recommend tape/brace/high cut shoes
- Proper training and conditioning—most important factor in injury prevention

Specific Common Injuries in Basketball

Ankle and Foot

- Ankle ligament injuries—most common
- Tendon injuries—Achilles, posterior tibialis, flexor hallucis, peronei
- Fractures—anterior avulsion calcaneus, navicular tuberosity, os trigonum, fifth metatarsal
- Heel pain and fasciitis
- Anterior ankle impingement
- Osteochondritis dissecans
- Hallux rigidus

Knee Injuries

- Ligamentous—ACL most common
- Meniscus
- Jumper's knee
- Patellofemoral pain/arthrosis

Upper Extremity Injuries

- Jammed fingers
- Fractures/dislocations/ligamentous
- Mallet finger
- Gamekeeper's thumb

Eye Injuries

- Encourage use of protective eyewear
- Corneal abrasions
- Lid lacerations
- Orbital blowout fractures
- Scleral lacerations

Oral and Dental Injuries

- Encourage use of mouth guard
- Lacerations
- Maxillary and mandibular fractures

441

- Temporomandibular sprains and contusions
- Dental fractures, luxations, and avulsions

Adolescent Basketball Player

- Physeal injuries
- Apophysitis

Specific Injuries

- Ankle and foot: Tillaux/Triplane fracture, Sever disease, accessory navicular
- Knee injuries—Osgood-Schlatter, Sinden-Larsen-Johanssen, tibial eminence/tibial tubercle fracture
- Hand injuries—fracture epiphysis at base of proximal phalanx

Basketball is a sport that enjoys wide popularity among people of many ages and both sexes in most parts of the world. In this chapter, we examine the epidemiology, prevention, and management of basketball injuries.

INCIDENCE OF INJURY IN BASKETBALL

Information about injury rates in basketball may be derived from several different types of studies. Prospective longitudinal examinations of all injuries occurring within a given team or league (Gomez et al., 1996; Henry et al., 1982; NBTA, 1998; NCAA, 1990), provide the best estimates. Other studies, based on retrospective questionnaires (Rocca, 1997; Leanderson et al., 1993; Weir and Watson, 1996), or analysis of emergency room or other medical encounters (Brison et al., 1992; Chandy and Grana, 1985; de Loes, 1995; Hickey et al., 1997; Kujala et al., 1995), suffer from sample bias and underreporting of injuries, but add some additional information. In all of these paradigms, the estimates vary widely, at least in part because of different definitions or detection thresholds for injury (the protocols requiring an athlete to miss time from participation fail to report the mildest injuries). Various authors report injury rates per athlete-year, per athlete-hour, or per athlete-exposure (where an exposure is one game or practice, regardless of actual minutes of participation). Table 30-1 combines and summarizes the range of available estimates of the overall incidence of injury in basketball, expressed as injuries per 1000 athlete-exposures.

Many authors have reported a breakdown of injury incidence by timecourse and/or anatomic region of injury (Gomez et al., 1995; Henry et al., 1982; Hickey et al., 1997; McKay et al., 1996; NBTA, 1998; NCAA, 1990; Rocca, 1997; Yde and Buhl-Nielsen, 1988; Zvifac and Thompson, 1996). Not surprisingly, the reported relative incidence of different injuries in basketball varies somewhat among them, likely due to the variation in tracking methods, thresholds of injury detection, and injury definition used in these studies. Nonetheless, certain trends emerge clearly, and are approximated in

TABLE 30-1 Incidence of Injury per 1000 Athlete-Exposures

Gender	Level of play	Incidence of injury
Female	Elite	4–18
	Recreational	0.5–4.0
Male	Elite	5–12
	Recreational	0.3–6.0

TABLE 30-2 Relative Incidence of Injuries by Anatomic Region

Anatomic Region	Acute injuries (%)	Chronic/Overuse injuries (%)
Ankle and foot	30	10
Knee	20	40
Other lower extremity (calf, shin, thigh, groin, hip)	15	15
Hand/wrist	10	5
Face/eyes/mouth	10	—
Low back	5	15
Other	15	15

Table 30-2. Acute injuries most commonly affect the ankle, knee, hand, or face, and chronic or overuse syndromes are most common in the knee, low back, foot, and ankle. Our discussion of specific injuries later in this chapter focuses on these problems with significant incidence in basketball.

FACTORS AFFECTING BASKETBALL INJURIES

A number of factors can be seen in the literature to correlate with, perhaps cause, or contribute to the variance in the incidence of basketball injuries. Although some of these are obviously inherent to the nature of the game, many of them can be affected through timely appropriate intervention by trainers, coaches, officials, and physicians. Such interventions are the cornerstone of injury prevention.

Gender

Some disagreement exists in the literature as to whether overall injury rates differ between men and women. Some studies have reported higher rates for female participants (Chandy and Grana, 1985; Zelisko et al., 1982), but many others have found no difference or even slightly higher rates for men (Brison et al., 1992; DeHaven and Lintner, 1986; de Loes, 1995; Kujala et al., 1995; NCAA, 1990; Payne et al., 1997; Yde and Buhl-Nielsen, 1988, 1990; Weir and Watson, 1996). Considering all of these data, we can say that overall injury rates reported for women's and men's basketball at comparable levels of play have not consistently been shown to be significantly different statistically. However, certain specific injuries are more common in women (and presumably others among men, although these have not been focused on in studies).

Among acute injuries, disruption of the anterior cruciate ligament (ACL) while playing basketball is more common in women by a ratio of perhaps 4:1 (Arendt and Dick, 1995; Arendt and Teitz, 1997; Ireland and Wall, 1990). Among women, noncontact mechanisms of ACL injury are more common (Arendt and Dick, 1995). Speculation on why this may be includes theories on less favorable muscle balance, coordination, or proprioception (Ball et al., 1996; Hewett et al., 1996; Huston and Wojtys, 1996; Marks et al., 1998), intercondylar notch width (LaPrade and Burnett, 1994; Souryal and Freeman, 1993), and the effect of female hormones on tissue strength. Further research is required to assert the cause of this problem with any confidence. In the meantime, all players, but especially women, would perhaps be well advised to pay particular attention to muscle balance and neuromuscular coordination during training (see the section on training and conditioning).

Playing Surfaces

Basketball is played on a variety of surfaces, from the asphalt and concrete of urban playgrounds to double-sprung maple hardwood gym floors. Personal experience providing medical coverage for 3-on-3 tournaments on asphalt reveals what would be expected in terms of acute injuries—more abrasions and contusions from falling down than occur on a wooden floor. With respect to overuse syndromes from accumulation of microtrauma, many of us suspect that tendinopathies, enthesopathies, and stress fractures are all more common when the game is played on harder surfaces. One of us (D.W.R.), who has traveled with a Canadian national team to many tournaments, has seen the number of athletes on the team suffering from patellar enthesitis (*jumper's knee*) go from 4 to 12 after 1 week of tournament play on a rubberized concrete floor (the team had practiced only on hardwood before the tournament). Interestingly, the host team (Brazil), which trained regularly on this surface, did not experience any higher an incidence of enthesitis than is normal in elite basketball. Perhaps gradual conditioning to playing on harder surfaces may actually strengthen entheses, tendons, or other tissues.

Minkoff et al. (1994) cite a study performed by an independent research company for a flooring manufacturer (Maple Flooring Manufacturers Association, 1988), which showed almost twice the incidence of injuries on synthetic surfaces as on maple hardwood floors in high schools. They point out that a lesser difference (10% higher incidence on synthetic floors) has been observed in college basketball (NCAA, 1990).

Games Versus Practices

The intensity of practices varies with the time of season, level of play, particular team and coach, and other circumstances. Nonetheless, it comes as no surprise that injuries are relatively more frequent in games. The relative incidence of injury in games has been reported to be between two (NBTA, 1998) and seven (Gomez et al., 1996) times as high in games as in practices. Most teams need some amount of game-like drills or intra-squad scrimmaging to be ready for competition, but coaches are well advised to remember that their athletes' risk of injury is significantly higher in these situations.

Position Played

Insufficient data and/or insufficient analysis thereof, do not allow any confident assertion about the vulnerability of certain positions to general or particular injuries. No positional trends have been observed in the NBA (NBTA, 1998), and trends not shown to be statistically significant have been observed in other leagues (Henry et al., 1982; Hickey et al., 1997; McKay et al., 1996; NCAA, 1990; Rocca, 1997; Yde and Buhl-Nielsen, 1998; Zelisko et al., 1982; Zvifac and Thompson, 1996).

Shoes and Ankle Stabilizers

Most basketball players wear high-top or medium-cut sneakers designed specifically for basketball. Many also wear ankle stabilizers (braces) or have their ankles strapped with zinc oxide trainer's tape. There are two issues to consider in choosing both sneakers and whether or not to use additional ankle support: their effects on injury and performance.

In the laboratory, ankle stabilizers, ankle taping, and high-cut shoes have all been shown to reduce the range of motion of rearfoot inversion, with no reliable differences across studies (Beynnon and Renström, 1991; Bunch et al., 1985; Garrick and Requa, 1973; Greene and Hillman, 1990; Greene and Wight, 1990; Gross et al., 1994; Karlsson et al., 1993; Ottaviani et al., 1995; Shapiro et al., 1994; Stacoff et al., 1996; Wilkerson, 1991). Several of these studies showed that the restricting effect of tape was reduced after exercise (Beynnon and Renström, 1991; Bunch et al., 1985; Furnich et al., 1981; Greene and Hillman, 1990; Greene and Wight, 1990; Shapiro et al., 1994), leading the authors to question whether re-usable stabilizers (braces) are not a better choice. However, all of these laboratory studies suffer from questionable extrapolation from restricted range of motion to prevention of ankle sprains.

More important, some clinical studies have analyzed the effect of stabilizers or tape on the actual incidence of ankle sprains. In a retrospective multisport study, it was found that the combination of lace-up braces and low-cut shoes was most effective (Rovere et al., 1988). The authors suspect the low-cut shoes encouraged brace wearers to retighten their braces during competitions. The only published randomized prospective clinical trial of ankle braces in basketball was associated with a statistically significant reduction in the frequency of ankle sprains (Sitler et al., 1994). Another prospective, randomized trial examined the effect of high-cut versus low-cut shoes on ankle sprains in basketball, and found no significant differences in injury rates (Barrett et al., 1993).

Braces or tape may reduce ankle injury, but many athletes are concerned, or have a perception, that they inhibit athletic performance. Several studies have provided some evidence of this (Brizuela et al., 1997; Burks et al., 1990; MacKean et al., 1995). However, several others disagree, finding no significant effect on performance (Gross et al., 1994; Locke et al., 1997; Pienkowski et al., 1995; Robinson et al., 1986). These latter studies include several prospective, randomized, longer-term trials, lending more credence to their findings. It may be that wearing braces or taping requires some habituation to negate a temporary inhibition of performance found when they are first used.

In the end, it is (or should be) an athlete's choice whether or not to wear protective stabilizers or tape, and what type of shoes to wear. In our opinion, athletes would be well advised to use either professionally applied tape or a reputable ankle stabilizer (brace), and perhaps wear high-cut shoes. Lace-up shoes and/or braces should be retightened during a game if they loosen perceptibly. We feel the evidence warrants assurance to athletes that these preventive measures will not significantly alter their performance, but will prevent some ankle sprains.

Training and Conditioning

We believe that proper training and conditioning is the single most important intervention in preventing injuries in basketball, or sports in general. There is some literature to bolster that contention (Anonymous, 1993); however, that is based to some extent on conventional wisdom and common sense. Aside from injury prevention, physical conditioning also has the important goal of improving athletic performance. Although it is not the focus of this chapter, we examine several aspects of training and conditioning for basketball from a combined injury preventive and performance enhancing perspective.

Adaptation to Specific Overload

Commonly accepted wisdom in sports medicine includes the principles of *overload* and *specific adaptation to imposed demand*, which collectively assert that gradually progressive training and conditioning prevents injuries through strengthening of tissues in response to overloads that stimulate hypertrophy without significantly exceeding those tissues' envelope of load acceptance. There are many laboratory studies that corroborate that connective tissues respond to physical activity with hypertrophy (Chandler and Kibler, 1993). In spite of the obvious inference that stronger tissues should lead to less trauma, there are few clinical studies that convincingly demonstrate this. Nonetheless, it remains conventional wisdom. Coupled with the demonstrated improvements in performance flowing from specific overload, it forms the cornerstone of athletic training and conditioning.

Training Variables and Training Errors

Many variables in the design of a training program can affect the desired outcomes. The frequency and duration of training sessions are the two most apparent; taken together, these are sometimes said to represent the volume of training. Equally important is the intensity of training in each session, which includes the strength, work, and power involved in executing prescribed movements or activities. Attempts to increase any of the variables that determine volume or intensity of training by too much in one increment, or too quickly, are commonly called training errors. These errors of commission have been shown to cause injury (Taunton, 1993).

It is common practice in basketball, as in many other sports, to start the preseason training camp with two per day workouts. This volume and intensity is often more than the athletes are accustomed to (despite warnings "report to camp in shape"). Our experience at the university, national team, and professional levels in basketball reveals an unfortunately high injury rate during this preseason training camp (unpublished data). Dialogue with coaches and trainers is an important mechanism to induce change in this aspect of the culture of sport, including basketball. Having said that, it is equally or perhaps more important for basketball players in elite leagues to train during their off-season so that training camp does not represent a training error.

Periodization

Training regimens in basketball should be periodized across a 1-year cycle, so that attempts to alter an athlete's anatomic (e.g., hypertrophy) or physiologic (e.g., power) substrate significantly occur during the competitive off season. At other times, training can focus on technical skill development and so on (Stone and Steingard, 1993).

Flexibility

That flexibility prevents injury and/or improves performance is another item of conventional wisdom with less scientific corroboration than one might expect. There are no studies that specifically show injury reduction through flexibility in basketball. The literature on flexibility and injury prevention in sports in general is controversial (Stanish and McVicar, 1993); nonetheless, stretching is widely practiced and recommended.

It is increasingly common to avoid static stretching as part of the warm-up routine. Many believe that warming up tissues through gradual active movements is better. Attempts to improve flexibility through static stretching or proprioceptive neuromuscular facilitation may best be reserved for sessions between games or practices.

Strength, Power, and Endurance

Basketball is demanding of most aspects of locomotion. It requires strength, speed, and power over a wide range of time intervals. Hence, the basketball athlete requires truly balanced or broad development of muscular strength, speed, strength endurance; and well-developed energy provision by all three systems for the production or resynthesis of intramuscular ATP (phosphocreatine, anaerobic glycolysis, and aerobic glycolysis). Basketball athletes training programs must, therefore, incorporate regimens of activity of sufficient specificity as to develop all of the necessary physiologic substrate for the game.

Balance, Coordination, Stability, and Proprioception

It is important to balance the strength and flexibility of agonists and antagonists across each motion segment (e.g., strengthen flexion and extension of the knee, and stretch both quadriceps and hamstrings). Although this is true in general, it has received most attention with respect to the contribution of muscle imbalance to the rupture of ACLs (Ball et al., 1996; Hewett et al., 1996; Huston and Wojtys, 1995; Johnson et al., 1992; Marks et al., 1998). It is also important to strengthen the short, stabilizing muscles across each motion segment as much as the stronger, prime movers of that segment (e.g., the rotator cuff muscles must be strengthened as well as pectoralis major).

Accumulated Exposure

Data from the National Basketball Association indicates that more experienced players are injured more frequently (NBTA, 1990). One obvious reason explaining this might be that virtually all overuse injuries have some component of accumulated microtrauma in their etiology. Accumulated exposures would be expected to generate such accumulated microtrauma. However, other confounding factors exist (such as more playing time for some more experienced players).

Fatigue

Data from the most detailed prospective observations of basketball injuries reveal that injuries are perhaps twice as common in the second half of games, and much less common in the first quarter (NCAA, 1990; NBTA, 1990). Whether this is due to fatigue as the game goes on or confounding factors such as increased participation of less-experienced or skilled players (nonstarters), or increased intensity of play in the late parts of the game, is not clear.

Level of Competition

As seen in Table 30-1, injury rates are higher among elite competitors than their recreational counterparts. No good statistical analyses exist to tell us what amount of this variance is due to the increased intensity or skill level of play per se, but we suspect that some of it is. Confounding variables correlated with elite play that might contribute to the increased injury rate independent of the intensity or skill level of play include length of games, frequency of exposure (less rest time between exposures), accumulated exposures (see above), different officiating or interpretation of rules (see below), and so on.

Rules and Their Interpretation

Basketball is, in the rulebooks, a noncontact sport. One would expect then that traumatic injuries due to collisions (other than with the floor) would be minimal. However, all that have played or watched it at a competitive level know that certain amounts of contact are explicitly or implicitly tolerated. At the highest competitive levels, collisions with considerable transfer of momentum occur routinely, and collisions with other players are responsible for a significant percentage of injuries (NBTA, 1990). It follows that proper enforcement of the rules of the game, and some control over the level of collisions tolerated, might contribute to the prevention of basketball injuries, as it does in other sports (Jørgensen, 1993). Certainly, the extent to which elbows to heads, or hands on faces, are tolerated has such an effect.

Preexisting Disease or Injury

As in any sport, a basketball player with a past history of injury or illness may face increased risk of recurrence or other new injuries. Three situations warrant comment. History of significant musculoskeletal injury or disease may pre-dispose to a higher risk of further injury. For example, basketball players with a history of ankle injuries are up to five times more likely to sustain an additional ankle injury compared to previously uninjured players (McKay et al., 2001). Appropriate screening for, and advice about, such predisposing conditions should be provided to participants in organized basketball programs.

Cardiovascular problems may predispose a basketball player to further illness or even sudden death with intense activity. Recommendations for screening and guidelines for participation are discussed in the section on Sudden Death.

Past history of concussion has been shown to increase risk of future concussions. Previous loss of consciousness (Grade 3 concussion using the American Academy of Neurology (AAN) classification (Kelly and Rosenburg, 1997) increases relative risk of concussion by a factor of four in high school football (Gerberich et al., 1983). Although this may not be exactly the case in basketball, it would seem reasonable to suspect that prior history of significant concussion in a basketball player may have increased risk of a recurrence with further competition. Athletes with prior history of head injury should be advised of these risks before competing.

General Medical Considerations

Athletes playing basketball are subject to the same wide spectrum of general health disorders as those in most other sports. A physician caring for a basketball team or athlete needs to consider, and attempt to prevent or be prepared to deal with, all these issues; such as, exercise-induced bronchospasm, diabetes, exercise in pregnancy, dermatologic conditions, respiratory infections, and so on. We do not consider these further, as their prevention, diagnosis, and management are not specific to basketball. There is one general medical problem that stands out as having a significant incidence in basketball, which warrants closer consideration.

Sudden Death Syndrome

The American College of Cardiology and the American College of Sports Medicine have sponsored two conferences to formulate recommendations or guidelines for participation in sports for people with known cardiovascular disease or risks (Maron and Mitchell, 1994; Mitchell, Maron et al., 1985). One of the task forces in each of these conferences has classified sports according to their static and dynamic cardiovascular requirements. Basketball is classified as a high-intensity sport with moderate static and high dynamic demands (Mitchell, Blomqvist, et al., 1985, 1994).

Approximately 35% of the sudden deaths occurring in sports in the United States occur in basketball (Maron et al., 1996). However, it is not clear how disproportionate that may or may not be when compared to sports of similar intensity and normalized for participation rates in the United States. Nonetheless, publicity associated with the deaths of several well-known basketball players has generated a perception that playing basketball confers disproportionate risk of sudden death (Maron, 1993; Thomas and Cantwell, 1990; Van Camp, 1993), which may or may not be true.

Of sudden deaths among young people playing sports in the United States, 85% are of cardiovascular cause. Most of these are due to hypertrophic cardiomyopathies, with fewer due to anomalous or otherwise deficient coronary circulation (Epstein et al., 1985; Maron et al., 1985, 1996; Thompson et al., 1994; Maron et al., 1996). Hypertrophic cardiomyopathy is more common in African Americans than in Caucasian Americans. The high participation rate in basketball among African Americans may explain the apparent high incidence of sudden death in basketball to some extent. Even fewer of these sudden deaths are caused by cardiovascular anomalies such as aortic root dilatation and aortic dissection associated with Marfan syndrome (Lazar, 1997); however, the high prevalence of Marfan among tall people, and the prevalence of tall people in basketball, has led to obvious concern for possible risks to marfanoid hoopsters.

The two Bethesda conferences have generated detailed and specific recommendations for participation among people with identified disease, including coronary artery disease, congenital malformations, acquired valvular disease, cardiomyopathies, systemic hypertension, and arrhythmias. The reader is referred to these sources for details. These recommendations have led to scrutiny of the efficiency and effectiveness of screening for abnormalities that would predict risk and/or preclude or limit participation based on the Bethesda guidelines. Routine history taking and physical examination appears to be of limited value (Maron et al., 1996; Fuller et al., 1997), but 12-lead resting electrocardiography may yield as much as 1 potentially high-risk individual per 255 tests (Fuller et al., 1997). Stress electrocardiography is even more effective, but inefficient such that it is only useful as a routing screening test at the elite levels of the game.

SPECIFIC COMMON INJURIES IN BASKETBALL

Ankle and Foot

As noted in Table 30-2, foot and ankle injuries represent the most commonly seen acute and chronic problems arising from basketball.

Ankle Ligament Injuries

By far the most common acute injury in basketball (other than minor contusions, which go unreported) is a sprain of the lateral ankle ligaments, especially the anterior talofibular ligament (DeHaven and Lintner, 1986; Garrick, 1977, 1987; Leanderson et al., 1993). The bony architecture of the ankle is the primary stabilizer of the mortise in the weight-bearing position. The lateral ligament complex includes the anterior talofibular ligament, calcaneofibular ligament, and posterior talofibular ligament. The anterior talofibular ligament becomes the significant static stabilizer when the ankle is plantarflexed or rotated. The basketball court provides an ideal situation for the usual mechanism of first-time injury to the lateral ligamentous complex, as the player lands on the plantarflexed foot after a jump. In crowded situations under the boards, this plantarflexed foot too often lands on another player's foot resulting in an inversion injury of the ankle.

The calcaneofibular ligament becomes more important with the ankle in dorsiflexion. However, the calcaneofibular ligament is rarely injured in isolation but is usually injured in association with the anterior talofibular ligament during massive inversion injuries.

The medial, deltoid ligament consists of strong superficial and deep fibers that originate from the medial malleolus and fan out to the navicular, sustentaculum, and the talus. The deltoid contributes to resistance of internal rotation along with the anterior talofibular ligament. The dorsiflexion and eversion or external rotation forces necessary to rupture the deltoid ligament are not commonly seen on the basketball court.

In addition to the mechanism of injury, the physician should determine whether the patient was able to bear weight following the injury, because this is often an indicator of severity of injury. The presence of an audible snap or crack, the degree of swelling, and the presence of bruising following injury should be noted, although they have no bearing on the degree of injury. In adolescent patients, it is important to determine whether the patient is skeletally mature, because physeal injuries to the distal tibia and fibula are more common than ligamentous injuries in children; these areas should be palpated. The areas of maximum tenderness should be determined by examination. Palpation should also include the proximal fibula and the remainder of the foot to rule out associated injuries. Range of motion should be compared to the uninjured limb and is often limited by both pain and swelling. In the acutely injured ankle, stability testing can be difficult and is best performed early, while swelling is minimal. The anterior drawer test is positive when the talus subluxes forward on the ankle. A clunk may or may not be heard. The test signifies disruption of the anterior talofibular ligament. Positive inversion stress at neutral dorsiflexion signifies injury to the calcaneofibular ligament.

The need for roentgenographic evaluation of the ankle following injury is now more clearly defined by the Ottawa rules (Leddy et al., 1998; Steill et al., 1992, 1993). When pain and tenderness are more directly over the malleoli (rather than their anterior aspects where commonly injured ligaments originate), or when there is an inability to bear weight, AP, lateral, and mortise views are recommended. Foot x-rays are required if the tenderness is localized on either the base of the fifth metatarsal or the navicular. MRI evaluation of the acutely injured ankle may reveal subchondral bone contusions or other lesions not easily detected by either clinical examination or x-rays (Fig. 30-1).

Management of ankle sprains has been well reviewed elsewhere (Ogilvie-Harris and Gilbart, 1995; Shrier, 1995). Immediate management of the injured ankle includes protection from re-injury through modified activity (non-weightbearing if this causes significant pain) and taping or bracing, compression, and elevation to prevent swelling, ice or other cryotherapy,

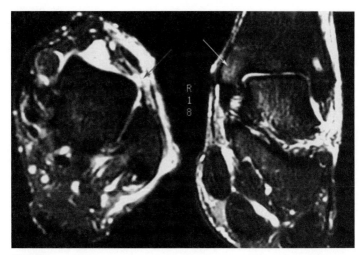

FIG 30-1 MRI of an acutely sprained ankle in an NBA athlete. Arrows indicate a disrupted anterior talofibular ligament and an area of bone contusion medially.

early mobilization, and perhaps NSAIDs. Immobilization and surgery have not been shown to yield better results and are not indicated except perhaps in the most severe injuries, such as complete dislocations. Muscle and tendon strengthening and postural stability exercises follow early mobilization. Gradually incorporate functional activities that are part of basketball, such as sudden stops and starts, lateral cuts, and landing on toes, into the rehabilitation protocol. The ankle should be protected by taping and/or a stabilizer for at least 12 weeks after the return to basketball, if this was not already being done prior to injury.

Tendon Injuries

The Achilles, posterior tibialis, flexor hallucis, and peronei tendons are susceptible to both acute and chronic overuse injuries that can lead to disabling dysfunction. The Achilles tendon must support forces about the ankle during normal gait that are up to five times body mass. The repetitive jumping activity in basketball subjects the tendon to even higher forces. Furthermore, the region of the Achilles tendon 2–6 cm proximal to its bony insertion has a precarious blood supply that makes it most prone to injury (Carr and Norris, 1989).

Insertional Achilles tendinitis is seen within the last 2 cm over the distal tendon. Tendinitis in this area can be associated with a calcaneal posterosuperior prominence that contributes to the symptoms of local tenderness and impingement pain. Retrocalcaneal bursitis may be a resulting or exacerbating factor. Intratendonous calcification and fibrous degeneration have been observed in surgical specimens.

Noninsertional Achilles tendinitis is classified by stage and histology (Puddu et al., 1976). Isolated peritendinitis (stage 1) involves acute, chronic, or recurring inflammation of the peritenon with localized symptoms of pain, warmth, swelling, tenderness, and difficulty bearing weight. In stage 2 peri-tendinitis with tendonosis, there are fibrovascular degenerative changes with the tendon substance. Symptoms are similar to stage 1; however, a mass may be palpated. Pure tendonosis is seen in stage 3 with areas of atrophy, fibrovascular degeneration, or calcification without inflammatory changes. Swelling is minimal in this stage, and the palpable nodule is nontender. The latter stages may lead to rupture in the watershed region.

Initial treatment of Achilles tendinitis is nonsurgical. Basketball activities are modified, or in severe cases discontinued, until sufficient progress allows for nondestructive return to previous levels of functional activity. Gradually progressive strengthening, with careful attention to the magnitude and speed of eccentric loads, is often successful (Curwin and Stanish, 1985). Adjuvant therapy such as NSAIDs and ice can be used. A heel wedge of 1–2 cm in height can significantly reduce pain (Lowdon et al., 1984). Cortisone injections are not recommended, even for stage 1 disease, because they can weaken the tendon and predispose it to spontaneous rupture. Insertional Achilles tendinitis may be difficult to treat in the basketball player. Modifications of the heel counter in the shoe may be necessary to alleviate direct pressure here. There may be a role for extracorporeal shock wave therapy in the treatment of refractory Achilles tendinosis prior to surgical intervention. Only when all conservative therapy fails should debridement of degenerative and calcified tissue and excision of any posterosuperior bony prominence be considered.

Complete ruptures of the Achilles tendon typically occur in the middle-aged males involved in activities that produce eccentric elongation of the tendon. Rupture of the tendon in the young adult or adolescent is unusual. A history of sudden onset of pain and swelling following minor trauma is common. Patients describe a sudden pop or a sensation of being hit from behind. There is a palpable defect in the tendon, although significant swelling and ecchymosis may mask this sign. The patient is unable to perform a single heel rise. The Thompson test, performed by having the patient kneel over a chair and squeezing the calf, is used to confirm the diagnosis. The absence of a passive plantarflexion of the foot during this maneuver is diagnostic.

Ultrasonography and MRI have both been used to evaluate both acute and chronic Achilles tendonopathy. Ultrasound can distinguish inflammation of the peritenon from either complete or partial rupture (Kainberger et al., 1990). MRI also distinguishes rupture from inflammation or degeneration of tendon or peritenon (Quinn et al., 1987). The optimum treatment for the acute ruptures of the Achilles tendon remains controversial. In a prospective randomized study comparing operative and nonoperative management of acute ruptures of the Achilles tendon, the rate of re-rupture was 8% in the nonoperative group compared with 4% in the surgical group (Nistor, 1981). However, no significant difference in the strength of plantarflexion was demonstrated. In general, the management of an acute Achilles tendon rupture in a basketball player needs to be individualized following a detailed discussion of the risks and benefits with the patient. At the elite level, the normal practice would lean toward surgical repair.

Basketball players can present with dysfunction of the tibialis posterior tendon. Biomechanical factors expose this tendon to stresses of repeated trauma in the region of the medial malleolus. In this same area, the mesotenon is scarce and a consistent area of hypovascularity is produced just distal to the medial malleolus (Frey et al., 1990). Johnson and Strom (1989) have classified this entity into three stages. The young basketball athlete is most likely to present with stage 1 disease, which is characterized by pain, swelling, and mild weakness of the posterior tibial tendon, but no secondary foot deformity (Woods and Leach, 1991). The pain may not be confined to the region between the navicular and the medial malleolus, but may extend to behind the malleolus proximally for some distance. Local tenderness and swelling are consistent with the tenosynovitis. Although the patient is able to perform a single limb stance, the task is often painful. Rupture of the tibialis posterior tendon without foot deformity, stage 2, is even more uncommon in young athletes. The diagnosis of tibialis posterior tendon dysfunction is the basketball player is made clinically. MRI has been found to be useful in evaluating the status of the tendon preoperatively when conservative measures fail (Conti et al., 1992). Early diagnosis is crucial to prevent the onset of progressive foot deformity. The basketball player who presents with stage 1 tendinopathy can be managed initially with a non-weightbearing cast to help resolve the acute symptoms, followed by fitting in a UCBL (University of California Biomechanics Laboratory) orthosis, which provides support to the longitudinal arch, limiting heel valgus. Acute rupture, when seen in the young athlete, should be treated surgically utilizing flexor digitorum longus or flexor hallucis longus to augmentation the posterior tibialis tendon (Mann and Thompson, 1985).

The flexor hallucis tendon is also prone to repetitive trauma in the basketball player. At the level of the talus, the FHL tendon passes through a restrictive fibrous osseous tunnel. Functionally the long flexor of the great toe is important for push-off. This explains why the highest incidence of FHL tendinitis occurs in ballet dancers and jumpers. Overuse activities can lead to a stenosing tenosynovitis and secondary posterior ankle impingement if the cycle is not halted. In addition to the usual site of impingement at the entrance of the fibro-osseous tunnel, stenosis may occur proximally behind the medial malleolus or distally, between the hallux sesamoids. Pain is localized deep to the medial side of the Achilles tendon. This can be exacerbated by resisted plantarflexion or passive dorsiflexion of the great toe with the ankle and first metatarsal supported in a neutral position (Gould, 1981). MRI is useful when the diagnosis is unclear. Nonsurgical treatment with rest, ice, and NSAIDs is usually successful. In the early phase of treatment, taping the great toe in a position of plantarflexion may also help. When conservative measures fail, tenosynovectomy and debridement are indicated.

The peronei both play a role as dynamic lateral stabilizers of the ankle joint. The peroneus longus tendon is necessary for normal lateral push-off. Despite its long course from behind the fibular malleolus to its insertion on the first metatarsal, acute rupture and tenosynovitis of peroneus longus is rare. The peroneus brevis is closer to the fibula and the lateral malleolus, and although acute rupture of the peroneus brevis tendon is rare, degenerative tears of this tendon are common (Sammarco and DiRaimondo, 1989). The severity of the pathology can range from mild fraying to extensive longitudinal tears (Sobel et al., 1991). Pain and swelling are located behind the lateral malleolus and can be exacerbated by passive inversion of the ankle or eversion against resistance. The ankle should also be assessed for associated recurrent instability. MRI can localize abnormal pathology. Temporary modification of activity, orthotic support for the medial longitudinal arch, and strengthening exercises for TP and FHL are cornerstones of treatment. NSAIDs may be adjuvant therapy. Intratendonous debridement is indicated only if nonsurgical measures are unsuccessful.

Subluxation of the peroneal tendons occurs when the superior peroneal retinaculum avulses from its fibular attachment during acute dorsiflexion of the ankle coupled with a forced contraction of the peronei (Eckert et al., 1976). These injuries are often mistaken for ligamentous injuries; however, the pain and tenderness of the acute peroneal subluxation is retromalleolor. Radiographs may demonstrate small fragments of bone at the site where the retinaculum avulsed form the distal fibula. Recurrent instability of the peroneal tendons is unusual and presents with a history of recurrent and often painful snapping over the distal fibula. This can sometimes be managed adequately with taping that includes a pad over the peroneal tendons. When symptomatic recurrent subluxation of the peronei is unmanageable and sufficiently bothersome, soft tissue reconstruction may be considered (Zoellner and Clancy, 1979).

Fractures

Anterior avulsion fractures of the calcaneus can occur in basketball players. The bifurcate ligament, originating from the anterior calcaneal process and attaching to both the cuboid and the navicular, avulses off its proximal attachment during an inversion-plantarflexion mechanism. These fractures may initially be diagnosed as severe ligament sprains and recovery may be prolonged. Pain is localized to the region of the sinus tarsi. The oblique radiograph of the foot may identify an avulsed fragment of bone. Nonoperative treatment with cast immobilization usually yields good results. Surgery is reserved for fractures with large avulsion fragments or for symptomatic nonunions (Degan et al., 1982).

Fractures of the navicular tuberosity occur with forced eversion of the foot and subsequent avulsion of the posterior tibial tendon as it forcefully contracts. The fracture is usually held in an undisplaced position by the multiple slips of the tibialis posterior tendon to other bones, and the insertion of the deltoid to the navicular. Tenderness is localized and x-rays are helpful in distinguishing the lesion from an accessory os naviculare. Cast immobilization is usually all that is required of the acute injury. Although they usually heal with fibrous union, this is often asymptomatic. Excision of the avulsed fragment is indicated for symptomatic nonunions. Stress fractures of the navicular can also be seen in basketball players and the diagnosis should always be considered in any athlete with chronic vague midfoot pain from repeated jumping and running (Torg et al., 1982). Undisplaced fractures are treated in non-weightbearing casts for 6–8 weeks. Displaced fractures require stabilization.

The os trigonum is a posterolateral accessory ossicle seen in only 10% of the population. Fractures of the os trigonum are most commonly seen in dancers or soccer players, but can be seen in basketball players when the plantarflexed foot takes the weight of another player's body (Ihle and Cochran, 1982). Stress fractures of the os trigonum can also occur in the absence of any specific history of trauma. Pain is posterior, although symptoms may be vague. Swelling and bruising may be present. Because of the proximity to the flexor hallucis longus tendon, motion of the great toe may exacerbate the pain. The lateral x-ray is used to identify the irregular borders suggestive of an acute fracture of the os trigonum. Bone scan is also used to distinguish the normal os trigonum for fracture or fibrous detachment. Early immobilization is usually successful. When pain is persistent in the presence of increased uptake on bone scan, excision is advocated.

The Jones fracture of the proximal diaphysis of the fifth metatarsal, and the avulsion fracture of the same bone are two distinct entities with varying locations, injury mechanism, and prognoses (DeLee et al., 1983). Either can occur in isolation in the basketball player, and they must be distinguished to implement adequate treatment. The region of the proximal diaphysis of the fifth metatarsal is relatively hypovascular and this contributes to the significant risk of delayed or nonunion of the Jones fracture (Smith et al., 1998). Historically, the avulsion fracture is felt to arise from force contraction of the peroneus brevis tendon at the tuberosity. In contrast, the acute Jones fracture occurs when the forefoot is loaded laterally while pivoting. The chronic form is a fatigue fracture, typically occurring in the young athlete. Fractures at the base of the fifth metatarsal present with local tenderness. Radiographs may initially be normal in the fatigue fracture, and bone scan may be needed to confirm the suspicion. The current standard care for the elite basketball athlete with an acute Jones fracture is percutaneous screw fixation (Fig. 30-2); however, the acute Jones fracture and the more benign tuberosity avulsion fracture may be treated in a below knee nonweightbearing cast for 6 weeks. Longer periods of casting are needed for delayed unions of Jones fractures, but operative treatment is again advised for the young or high-level athlete with this problem. Established nonunions require internal fixation.

Heel Pain and Fasciitis

Heels pain is extremely common among all athletes. The differential for this complaint is large and includes plantar fasciitis, bursitis, tendinitis and apophysitis, fracture, nerve entrapment, tumor, foreign body, and infection (Graham, 1983). History and physical examination usually help to differentiate the pathology. Radiographs, bone scan, MRI, and electrophysiology are ordered as needed when the diagnosis remains unclear. The pain of plantar fasciitis is accentuated by running or jumping activities. Pain can be intense in the morning following a prolonged sleep with the foot in the plantarflexed position. Tenderness is typically plantar and medially where the fascia originates from the medial calcaneal tuberosity. The mainstay of treatment of plantar fasciitis is nonsurgical with a strict regimen of NSAIDs, heels pads, foot orthotics, and stretching of the plantar fascia and Achilles tendon. Cortisone injections in the region of pathology may be useful. A night dorsiflexion splint can be used for both acute flare ups and as a preventive measure. Extracorporeal shock wave therapy is an option in recalcitrant cases. Plantar fascia release should only be performed after a prolong period of unsuccessful conservative therapy (Leach et al., 1986).

Anterior Ankle Impingement

The pathogenesis of anterior ankle impingement in the basketball player probably begins with a traumatic injury to the lateral ankle ligaments. Subsequent laxity and synovial and capsular soft tissue scarring contribute to the pathology. Osteophytes then develop specifically between the distal tibia and the neck of the talus. Pain is with dorsiflexion activities and as osteophytes enlarge, range of motion can be restricted. Lateral x-rays reveal the site of disease. Conservative therapy begins with either a heel rise or a negative heel. When this fails or if ankle motion continues to be restricted, excision

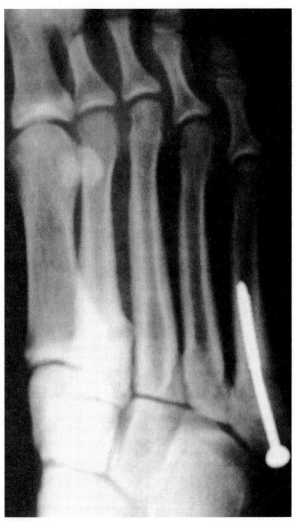

FIG 30-2 Postoperative x-ray after percutaneous screw fixation of an acute Jones fracture in an NBA athlete.

of the osteophyte is performed either openly or arthroscopically (Ferkel et al., 1991).

Osteochondritis Dissecans

Osteochondral defects of the talar dome can occur insidiously. Traumatic lesions are more commonly posteromedial; atraumatic lesions are usually anterolateral. Symptoms are related not only to the size and the location of the lesion, but also to its stability. Pain, locking, or a feeling of giving way can all be presenting symptoms. When plain radiographs do not show the defect, computed tomography or MRI is indicated (De Smet et al., 1990). In the skeletally immature basketball player, the prognosis with conservative therapy is good, and a brief period in a patella tendon bearing cast will usually suffice. Operative treatment after unsuccessful conservative management in adults depends on the size, location, and stability of the fragment (Alexander and Lichtman, 1980).

Hallux Rigidus

Defined as arthritis of the first metatarsophalangeal joint of the great toe, this is seen in sports that involve sudden starts, stops, and jumping. Continued repetitive activity can lead to synovitis and arthrosis. Osteophyte formation occurs on the dorsal portion of the metatarsal head, which causes impingement with dorsiflexion and resultant pain. Plantarflexion is reduced and painful secondary to the stretching of the dorsal capsule as well as the extensor hallucis longus tendon over the osteophyte. Examination notably reveals a palpable ridge over the dorsum of the metatarsal with reduced range of motion. The athlete favors push-off on the lateral border of the foot as opposed to the front due to pain with dorsiflexion (McDermott, 1993). Instead of a transverse crease over the toe box of the shoe, an oblique crease can be seen. Radiographs reveal a dorsal osteophyte on the metatarsal head and joint space narrowing. Initial treatment should involve modification of athletic shoe wear, consisting of a more rigid and rocker bottom sole to minimize the dorsiflexion required. Failing this, surgical intervention involves a chielectomy of the dorsal third of the metatarsal head. This alleviates the dorsal impingement and improves pain and motion. Arthrodesis is generally reserved for individuals with severe degenerative changes throughout the joint. However, this may limit further involvement in competitive basketball.

Knee Injuries

Basketball players are prone to a variety of acute and overuse injuries about the knee. The great majority of these injuries arise from noncontact mechanisms.

Acute Knee Injuries

With frequent episodes of acceleration and deceleration, internal and external tibial rotation, and continuous pivoting, the opportunity to injure the ACL during basketball activity is high. The player with an acutely injured ACL is almost always unable to return to the basketball court following the traumatic event. A pop or tear heard on the court is sensitive for an ACL injury. Early swelling is suggestive of an acute hemarthrosis. Weightbearing is difficult but may not correlate with injury severity. Injury-specific tests such as the Lachman, anterior drawer, and the pivot shift usually confirm the diagnosis, but may be difficult to perform in the acutely swollen knee. The Lachman test appears to be the most reliable in the acutely injured knee, so the court side examination may be most telling following game injuries (Torg et al., 1976). MRI demonstrates the acute or chronic tear as well as associated bone bruises and meniscal injuries (Marks and Fowler, 1993) (Fig. 30-3). The definitive management of the ACL-deficient knee is individualized to the patient's activities and level of participation. Although initial management involves physical therapy to restore range of motion and

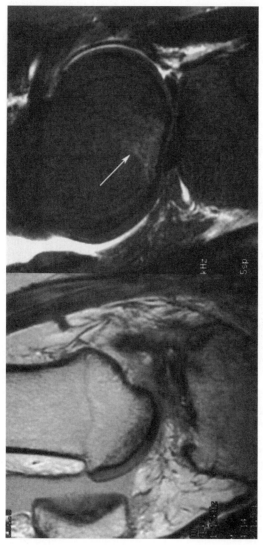

FIG 30-3 MRI of an acute ACL rupture in an NBA athlete. Images reveal areas of subchondral bone contusion in addition to the disruption of the ligament.

muscle strengthening, the young basketball athlete who wishes to continue playing competitively is unlikely to tolerate the cutting and pivoting that the game demands without reconstruction. Returning to basketball without ACL reconstruction most often results in tearing of the remaining menisci. The role of functional or rehabilitative braces following ACL injuries remains controversial. Braces are generally used to supplement the nonoperative rehabilitation regimen or the surgical ACL reconstruction; the player who returns to basketball should not be under the impression that the brace will prevent further injury (Mishra et al., 1989; Ott and Clancy, 1993).

Meniscal injuries can occur in isolation or in association with ACL or medial collateral ligament (MCL) tears. Pain is localized over the joint line, and the painful arc of motion depends on the location of the pathology. Mechanical symptoms such as locking, giving way, and swelling may also be evident. McMurray's test helpful when present but is not specific for meniscal disease. MRI is the investigation of choice when physical examination remains unclear. When symptoms are significantly disabling, therapeutic arthroscopy is required for repair or partial meniscectomy, followed by rehabilitation and gradual return to sport. The reparable meniscus lesion requires protected weightbearing for 4–6 weeks. The basketball player with a reparable meniscus tear and a torn ACL warrants more aggressive treatment of the ligament injury to increase the chance of a successful cartilage repair (Johnson et al., 1992).

Overuse Injuries of the Knee Extensor Mechanism

Derangement of the patellar mechanism is extremely common in basketball players particularly at the competitive levels (King et al., 1990; NBTA, 1990; NCAA, 1990). Microscopic tissue failure and/or inflammation along the patellar or quadriceps tendons or their insertional entheses at the patella or tibia are collectively known as *jumper's knee*. Eccentric contractions during repeated jumping predisposes the basketball player to this sometimes disabling problem (Curwin and Stanish, 1985). Patients can present with activity-related anterior knee pain and tenderness over the patellar tendon at its bony insertion. Pathologic changes in this area include acute or chronic inflammation and mucoid degeneration. MRI is valuable in demonstrating the extent of disease (El-Khoury et al., 1992) (Fig. 30-4). A strict training program with eccentric strengthening is critical in avoiding or treating jumper's knee (Curwin and Stanish, 1985). Early diagnosis is the key to implementing prompt treatment and halting the cycle of inflammation. NSAIDs, ice, ultrasound therapy, and a period of avoidance of jumping is the initial treatment. Eventually, eccentric contractions can be attempted but isometric and concentric activity must be mastered first.

The requirement to temporarily curtail jumping is usually the biggest barrier to successful treatment in basketball players. It is often difficult to obtain a suitable interval free of further damaging eccentric exercise (jumping) during which the extensor mechanism can be gradually strengthened. Noncompliance in this regard explains the high prevalence of chronic patellar enthesopathy in basketball.

Cortisone injections in the region of the patellar tendon should be completely avoided; steroids weaken the tendon and may lead to spontaneous rupture (Kennedy and Willes, 1991). Ruptures of the patella tendon or the quadriceps tendon may also occur after weakening by chronic inflammation or following an acute eccentric contraction. Disruptions of the extensor

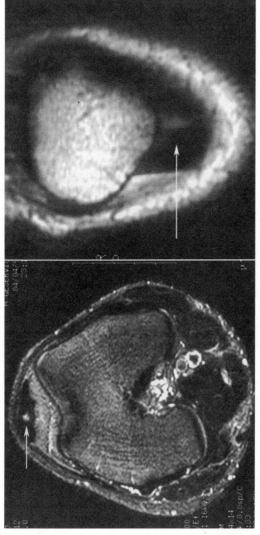

FIG 30-4 MRI of acute "jumper's knee" in an NBA athlete. The typical findings of patellar tendon enthesopathy are seen as an area of increased signal in the central third of the tendon just distal to the interior pole of the patella (arrows).

mechanisms warrant surgical management, and when treated early, good results are achieved (Kelly et al., 1984). Rarely, a chronic case of jumper's knee is refractory to all nonoperative measures when they are given adequate trials. Only then is surgical debridement indicated.

Patellofemoral pain and eventually arthrosis often occurs with repeated running and jumping. It comes as no surprise that basketball is fertile ground for this problem. Maltracking of the patella caused by dynamic forces (imbalance of quadriceps strength between vasti medialis and lateralis, or rotation of the knee with hyperpronation of the foot) or rotational abnormalities of the femur or tibia are often implicated in this syndrome (van Kampen and Huiskes, 1990).

Patellofemoral pain is best prevented and treated with proper training, conditioning, and equipment. The basketball player regardless of caliber should avoid open-chain kinetic exercises that tend to place excessive stress on the patellofemoral joint. Increasing endurance and strengthening gradually avoids sudden stresses of the patellar mechanism. Careful attention to alignment of the foot and knee, awareness of muscle tone in vastus medialis, and core strengthening of the pelvis and trunk are critical to achieve strengthening of the quadriceps mechanism. Motion control features in the shoe can be helpful in preventing contributory hyperpronation. Unfortunately, basketball shoes do not come in as wide a spectrum of stabilizing features as shoes for running per se. It is, therefore, often necessary to replace the manufacturer's insole with one custom fitted to the athlete's foot, with built-in corrections or support to prevent hyperpronation.

Conservative therapy is usually successful, and surgery is rarely indicated for the patient with a documented structural abnormality whose symptoms do not resolve with therapy. Such surgery is usually limited to minimal debridement.

Upper Extremity Injuries

As noted, injuries to the hand and wrist are very common in basketball (Choyce et al., 1998; Henry et al., 1982; Hickey et al., 1997; Kujala et al., 1995; NBTA, 1990; NCAA, 1990; Rocca, 1997; Weir and Watson, 1996; Yde and Buhl-Nielsen, 1988; Zelisko et al., 1982; Zvifac and Thompson, 1996). Before commenting on specific hand and wrist injuries, we note that the treatment of these injuries in basketball is very aggressive. Early consultation with a hand specialist is critical. Early mobilization and functional splinting often allow a return to activity much quicker than is suggested by the hand surgery literature. Early compression of injured digits, usually with COBAN wrap is critical to prevent excessive swelling. Where hand specialists often use volar splints, we fashion a dorsal splint to allow volar contact with a basketball. Although the ideal angle of flexion for splinting of some injuries varies, we usually splint a finger with the hand placed on a basketball, such that the flexion of the digits matches the curve of the ball. This allows as early as possible return to partial basketball activities, and minimizes the loss of ball skills during rehabilitation from hand injuries. This is most critical for injuries to the primary shooting hand.

Injuries to the Fingers

Injuries to digits two to five are most common. Commonly referred to by players as a *jammed finger*, there are several variations on this theme. The proximal interphalangeal joints (PIPJs) are most often injured, followed by the distal interphalangeal (DIP) joints, phalanges, metacarpals, metacarpophalangeal (MCP) joints, and the carpal metacarpal joints (CMCJs).

Injuries to the PIPs include fractures and dislocations as well as sprains and ruptures of the collateral ligaments. Collateral sprain or tears occur with hyperabduction or hyperadduction at the PIP. The radial collateral ligament is injured most frequently compared to the ulnar collateral ligament (Wilson, McGinty, 1993). Treatment is conservative with buddy taping and early range of motion. Usually the athlete is able to return to basketball quickly with functional splinting or taping.

Volar plate rupture occurs with hyperextension of the PIPs and leads to dorsal PIPs dislocation. Tenderness is over the volar plate of the joint and lateral x-rays confirm the direction of the distal fragment (Fig. 30-5). These isolated dislocations are usually stable following closed reduction, and can be treated with 4–5 days of immobilization followed by early range of motion (Kahler and McCue, 1992). Dorsal PIPs fracture dislocations may be more difficult to treat. The fracture is an avulsion of the volar base of the middle phalanx that can vary in size and when the collateral ligaments are attached to this fragment, the fracture is unstable. Stable fracture-dislocations can be treated with early mobilization, similar to the isolated dislocations. Unstable fracture-dislocations require extension block splinting or open reduction with fixation if the fragment involves more than 50% of the articular surface, or excision and volar plate advancement, if the fragment is irreparable. The principle of any treatment option should be to obtain and maintain joint congruity and to initiate early range of motion and maximize joint function.

Volar dislocations at the PIP are less common. They occur after forced varus or valgus load with a volar impact. The pathology includes injury to one of the collateral, an incomplete volar plate tear, and a disruption of the central slip. The acute finger is swollen over the PIP. The injury may be missed because the patient may use the lateral bands to extend the PIP. However, weakness is demonstrated with resisted extension and pain is dorsal. It is the central slip injury, which if left unrecognized, will lead to a posttraumatic boutonniere deformity. For this reason, these injuries are best treated early with extension splinting and close observation (Incavo et al., 1989).

Soft tissue injuries of the MCP joints are common in basketball players. Dorsal dislocations occur with forced hyperextension of the joint. Simple dislocations are easy to reduce and should temporarily be splinted in 70° of flexion to avoid contracture of the collateral ligaments and subsequent stiffness. Complex dislocations are irreducible due to soft tissue interposition of the volar plate. The metacarpal head is trapped between the lumbrical radially and the flexor digitorum profundus tendon ulnarly. Open reduction is necessary.

Intra-articular fractures at the MCP joint can usually be treated nonoperatively with brief immobilization and buddy taping, and then early mobilization. Surgery is reserved for fractures with large fragments that can be reduced and surgically stabilized.

Avulsion of the extensor mechanism at the DIP joint may result in a mallet finger if left unrecognized (Culver, 1990). This injury is common in basketball with axial loading of the finger against the ball. It may be associated with an avulsion fracture of the distal phalanx. In the skeletally immature patient, this is a Salter-Harris type I or III fracture. Dorsal extension splinting is used to prevent late a mallet deformity and recurrent subluxation. This is worn full time for 3 weeks followed by another 3 weeks

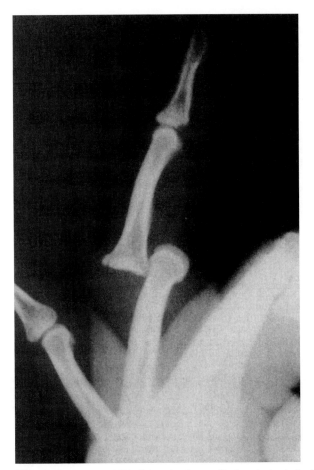

FIG 30-5 A dorsal PIPJ dislocation in an elite female basketball player.

of wear as the player returns back to activities (Crawford, 1984). Surgery is recommended for joint subluxation associated with large fragments.

Fractures or dislocations of any of the CMC joints of the other digits may occur after direct trauma or crush, from the weight of an opponents body. Dorsal dislocations are more common at this joint and it is often the lateral or oblique x-rays that demonstrate the pathology. These are usually stable following reduction. Dislocation of multiple CMC joints should be treated surgically. The reverse Bennett's fracture is an intra-articular fracture at the base of the fifth metacarpal that mirrors the thumb fracture. The deforming force is the extensor carpi ulnaris tendon. This fracture must be reduced and held reduced by casting or preferably pin fixation.

Thumb Injuries

The human thumb by nature of its mobility and ability to oppose in space is prone to a number of very common injuries. Bony stability is imperative in controlling and handling the basketball. The thumb is commonly injured in falls on the floor, when jammed on the rim during a dunk or when struck by an opponent.

Gamekeeper's thumb, or injury to the ulnar collateral ligament (UCL) at the metacarpophalangeal joint of the thumb is the most common of these injuries, and occurs with hyperextension and hyperabduction of the joint. The UCL usually avulses distally, and the adductor pollicis aponeurosis may come to interpose and prevent proper reduction and healing of the ligament to bone, a complication known as the *Stener lesion* (Abrahamsson et al., 1990). Acute injuries present with pain and tenderness directly over the site of the UCL at the thumb MCP. Plain radiographs are taken to demonstrate any avulsion fractures from the proximal phalanx. Only after plain radiographs are assessed should stress views be taken. Angulation of greater than 35°, or 15° compared to the uninjured side confirms a complete tear of the UCL and surgery is recommended to prevent chronic instability and joint incongruity. Surgery is also indicated if the joint is irreducible, or if intra-articular bony fragments are seen on plain radiographs. Incomplete tears can be treated with immobilization in a thumb spica for a period of days to a few weeks (depending on severity) with the MCP at 30° of flexion, followed by functional taping or splinting.

Dislocation of the thumb MCP occurs from forced hyperextension. Closed reduction should be attempted by first adducting and flexing the thumb metacarpal, which relaxes the intrinsic musculature. Following this, the proximal phalanx should be hyperextended followed by traction. Isolated longitudinal traction may lead to interposition of the volar plate, flexor pollicus longus, and sesamoids resulting in a complex often irreducible dislocation and should be avoided (Rettig, W., personal communication, 1994). A hand specialist should be consulted to determine stability postreduction. Complete collateral ligament injury and distal volar plate ruptures may require operative management (Rettig, W., personal communication, 1994).

A Bennett fracture involves the intra-articular surface of the base of the first metacarpal. It is caused by a fall or direct load on the thumb. The smaller metatarsal base fragment is held in its proper position by the strong volar oblique ligament. The pull of the abductor pollicus longus then displaces the metacarpal proximally. Operative intervention is generally required for this fracture dislocation.

The Rolando fracture is a comminuted intra-articular fracture of the base of the first metacarpal. Operative management is typically required for this fracture.

Wrist Injuries

Injuries to the carpus can be bony, ligamentous, or cartilaginous. History usually reveals a fall on the outstretched hand. The exact site of pain and tenderness must be determined on physical examination and radiographs including anterioposterior, lateral, and oblique should always be taken. MRI or ultrasonography may be used to assist diagnosis of triangular fibrocartilage injury. The management of wrist injuries in basketball does not differ significantly from what is done for athletes in other sports (or nonathletes).

Orofacial Injuries

The aspect of the game of basketball played in the paint, or in the key under the basket, generates many injuries to the face. Players jostling for position under the net, holding their opponents at bay (*boxing out*) with arms and elbows, and fighting for possession of a ball rebounding from a missed shot attempt all make for many elbows and fingers in faces.

Eye Injuries

The frequency and types of eye injuries in elite basketball have been well documented (Zagelbaum et al., 1995). Corneal abrasions, lid lacerations, orbital blowout fractures, and scleral lacerations all occur with significant frequency. Symptoms that contraindicate a return to play without ophthalmologic (slit lamp) examination and/or treatment are significant loss of vision, photophobia, diplopia, sudden onset of visual flashes, or floaters.

Initial examination must include visual acuity, visual fields, close inspection of the eyelid margins and canthi, ophthalmoscopic examination of iris detail and the fundus, extra-ocular movements, pupil shape and responsiveness, corneal/scleral integrity (using fluorescein stain and cobalt blue light), and palpation of the orbital margins and peri-orbital tissues. Return to play without further examination or treatment is contraindicated by loss of visual acuity (this makes a baseline assessment important); loss of visual fields (suspected detached retina); unclear iris details (suspected hyphema); loss of extra-ocular movements or diplopia with extremes of range (suspected blow-out fracture); subcutaneous emphysema or palpable tender deformity of orbital margins (suspected blow-out fracture); laceration of lid margins, canthi, cornea, or sclera; or swelling that prevents adequate opening of the palpebral fissure.

Many of these injuries, certainly the ones caused by fingers poking eyes, could be prevented by the use of polycarbonate lens protective eyewear. Although frames and lenses of sufficient strength to merit CSA approval for racquet sports would probably also help prevent some blow-out fractures, thinner polycarbonate lenses (inadequate for racquet sports), such as Oakley eye guards, perform admirably in basketball. The ball is large enough that impact with such thinner polycarbonate lenses does not cause them to crack into the eye (Easterbrook, 1998). An increasing number of players in the NBA are starting to see the light and protect their vision.

Oral and Dental Injuries

Injuries to the lips, cheeks, jaw, and teeth are common in basketball. These are also caused mostly by contact with opponent's elbows. Lip and cheek lacerations, maxillary and mandibular fractures, temporomandibular sprains and contusions, and dental fractures, luxations, and avulsions all occur too frequently (Flanders and Bhat, 1995). Some tooth avulsions have been reported from entanglement with the net (Kumamoto et al., 1997).

Prevention is most desirable. Aside from issues surrounding officiating and interpretation of the rules of the game, the most obvious preventive measure is the use of custom-fitted mouthguards. Also important is to have elective dental work taken care of in a timely fashion, to prevent in-season dental emergencies, as well as to reduce the risk of mandibular fracture after extractions (elective extractions should occur as soon as possible after the end of a season, to allow maximum time for bone healing before the next season).

When covering basketball games without the luxury of an attending dentist, the physician's kit should include a few dental supplies: eugenol (oil of clove) for the relief of dental pain, a stock or boil and bite mouthguard for emergency use in the absence of a custom-fitted guard, a container of Hank's balanced salt solution (available from 3M Company as the Save-a-Tooth kit) for the preservation of avulsed teeth, and temporary filling material (such as zinc oxide paste). Luxated teeth should be reduced immediately. Avulsed teeth should be replaced in the socket from whence they came, if that can be identified. If multiple teeth have been avulsed, it may be better to place them in Hank's solution (milk, saline, or water are better than nothing) and let a dentist sort them out. Avulsed teeth should not be debrided of any loose tissue remaining attached to them (see Chapter 14).

THE ADOLESCENT BASKETBALL PLAYER

Over the past several years there has been a growth in organized adolescent sport programs, particularly basketball. With such structured programs, children are seeing more repetitive training and increased playing time on the court. The former potentially predisposes to more overuse type injuries, and the latter increases the risk for acute traumatic injuries. There are different injury patterns found between children and adults that merit discussion.

In adolescents, growing bone has increased plasticity and porosity. In acute traumatic episodes, a substantial degree of deformation occurs prior to fracture. Physeal injuries should always be considered and suspected in this population. Trauma that results in injury to the musculotendinous junctions may lead to apophyseal avulsions. In overuse injuries, repetitive microtrauma to the apophysis leads to repetitive small avulsions with subsequent healing at the weaker bone–cartilage interface. This is classically referred to as *apophysitis*. The physeal plate can also be affected by repetitive trauma. Microtrauma to the physis can result in arrest and loss in longitudinal growth (Caine et al., 1997). This has been recognized to occur in the wrist with high-impact activities such as gymnastics; however, it has not been shown to occur in the lower extremities.

Specific Injuries

Foot and Ankle

Inversion injuries to the ankle can commonly lead to sprain or injury to the lateral ligament complex. However, close attention should be paid to the distal physis of the fibula and tibia. Physeal injuries of the distal fibula can occur with the same mechanism of injury as lateral ankle sprains and can be easily be overlooked. A careful physical examination is necessary to determine whether there is tenderness to palpation over these regions. In cases of physeal injury, a short period of immobilization may be required.

A tillaux and triplane fracture is an ankle fracture unique to the adolescent. The distal tibia physis first closes in the medial and central regions with the anterolateral aspect closing last (Dailiana et al., 1999). During this phase, forced external rotation, as often seen in cutting and contact sports, may result in a fracture involving the lateral aspect of distal tibial physis. Any displacement necessitates operative intervention (Kling 1990). Growth arrest, however, is less of a concern as the physis is nearing complete closure.

Sever's disease or calcaneal apophysitis is an overuse injury caused by repetitive microfracture and inflammation to the calcaneal apophysis secondary to the pull of the triceps surae musculature. It presents as activity-related pain with tenderness over the Achilles tendon insertion into the calcaneus. Although this is generally seen in sports requiring running (Micheli and Fehlandt, 1992), it is particularly prevalent during the growth phases when adolescents are often relegated to the less forgiving gymnasium floor surfaces. Pain occurs with resisted plantarflexion as well as the extremes of dorsiflexion. Treatment is conservative with heel cord stretching, heelpads, and modifications to activity dictated by pain. This condition is usually self-limiting. Other apophysites, such as accessory navicular syndrome, may be seen in adolescent athletes (Conti, 1994). An accessory navicular is a normal variant found in up to 12% of the population. It may be associated with flatfeet. Symptoms are related to the repetitive pull of the tibialis posterior tendon insertion into the navicular. Cases can usually be managed conservatively; however, refractory cases may require surgical excision.

Knee Injuries

Adolescent jumper's knee presents as a traction apophysitis of the tibial tubercle called *Osgood-Schlatter's disease. Sinden-Larsen-Johanssen syndrome* refers to the inflammation of the patellar tendon at the inferior pole of the patella. Signs and symptoms of these entities are similar to the adult forms and treatment is nonoperative.

ACL injuries are commonly seen in adolescents; however, controversy exists regarding definitive management of this injury. Traditionally, authors have advocated rehabilitation and protection of the knee with bracing until skeletal maturity before reconstruction. Recent studies of intra-articular surgical reconstruction, however, have demonstrated that the risks to the growth plate are low (Aichroth et al., 2002; Lo et al., 1998) and the risks of not reconstructing the ligament are high.

Tibial eminence fractures occur as a result of an avulsion injury from an axial force directed along the ACL. Undisplaced fractures can be treated in a long leg cast; however, displaced fractures usually require operative intervention. Malunited fractures not only result in ACL laxity but can also block full extension as it impinges in the intercondylar notch. Residual objective ACL instability has been demonstrated in some series and correlated to the amount of initial displacement (Wiley and Baxter, 1990; Willis et al., 1993). However, most athletes do not have subjective instability with, 84% being able to return to their pre-injury sports level (Schoenecker, Luhmann, 2002).

Tibial tubercle fractures occur in the adolescents during maximum contraction of the quadriceps during jumping or landing. These injuries usually occur close to skeletal maturity at about fifteen years of age (Schoenecker and Luhmann, 2002). Displaced fractures require operative intervention.

Hand Injuries

Due to its anatomic position, adolescents are more predisposed to fractures of the epiphysis at the base of the proximal phalanx at the MCP joint compared to the IP joints (Barton, 1979; Fischer et al., 1994; Garcia-Moral, 1990). Bogumill (1983) showed that the collateral ligaments of the MCP joints attach directly on to the epiphysis at the base of the proximal phalanx. In contrast, the collateral ligaments of the IP joints span the epiphyseal plate, thereby protecting it. As a result, Salter-Harris type III injuries occur as the epiphyseal plate fails before the collateral ligaments. Similar injuries also occur in the distal phalanx and represent an avulsion injury from the extensor mechanism. This may lead to a Salter-Harris I or III injury. Anatomic reduction is required and prompt referral to a hand specialist is recommended.

REFERENCES

Abrahamsson SO, Solerman C, Lundborg G, et al. Diagnosis of displaced ulnar collateral ligament of the metacarpophalangeal joint of the thumb. *J Hand Surg.* 1990;15A:457–460.

Aichroth P, Patel D, Zorrila P. The natural history and treatment of rupture of the anterior cruciate ligament in children and adolescents. A prospective review. *J Bone Joint Surg Br.* 2002;84:38–41.

Alexander AH, Lichtman DM. Surgical treatment of transchondral talar-dome fractures (osteochondritis dissecans): Long term follow up. *J Bone Joint Surg Am.* 1980;62A:646–652.

Arendt EA, Dick R. Knee injury patterns among men and women in collegiate basketball and soccer - NCAA data and review of literature. *Am J Sports Med.* 1995;23:694–701.

Arendt EA, Teitz CC. The lower extremities. In: Teitz CC, ed. *The female athlete.* Rosemont, Ill: American Academy of Orthopaedic Surgeons; 1997;45–62.

Ball KA, Evans RE, Marks PH, Richards DW. *The effect of hip and knee angle on force generation in quadriceps/hamstring knee strength: Implications for ACL injury.* Québec, QC: Canadian Orthopaedic Association; 1996.

Barrett JR, Tanji JL, Drake C, Fuller D, Kawasaki RI, Fenton RM. High-top versus low-top shoes for the prevention of ankle sprains in basketball players— A prospective randomized study. *Am J Sports Med.* 1993;21:582–585.

Barton NJ. Fractures of the phalanges of the hand in children. *Hand.* 1979;11:134–143.

Beynnon BD, Renström PAFH. The effect of bracing and taping in sports. *Annales Chirurgiae et Gynaecologiae.* 1991;80:230–238.

Bogumill GP. A morphologic study of the relationship of collateral ligaments to growth plates in the digits. *J Hand Surg.* 1983;8:74–79.

Brison RJ, Macnab RBJ, Arthur-Quinney H, Voaklander DC. *The epidemiology of contact sport injuries treated in an emergency department.* Gloucester, ON: Canadian Fitness and Lifestyle Research Institute; 1992.

Brizuela G, Llana S, Ferrandis R, Garcia-Belenguer AC. The influence of basketball shoes with increased ankle support on shock attenuation and performance in running and jumping. *J Sports Sci.* 1997;15:505–515.

Bunch RP, Bednarski K, Holland D, Macinanti R. Ankle joint support: A comparison of reusable lace-on braces with taping and wrapping. *Phys Sportsmed.* 1985;13:59–63.

Burks RT, Bean BG, Marcus R, Barker HB. Analysis of athletic performance with prophylactic ankle devices. *Am J Sports Med.* 1990;19:104–106.

Caine D, Howe W, Ross W, Bergman G. Does repetitive physical loading inhibit radial growth in female gymnasts? *Clin J Sports Med.* 1997;7:302–308.

Carr AJ, Norris SH. The blood supply of the calcaneal tendon. *J Bone Joint Surg Br.* 1989;71B:100–101.

Chandler TJ, Kibler WB. Muscle training in injury prevention. In: Renström PAFH, ed. *Sports injuries: Basic principles of prevention and care.* Oxford: Blackwell Scientific Publications; 1993;252–261.

Chandy TA, Grana WA. Secondary school athletic injuries in boys and girls. A three year comparison. *Phys Sportsmed.* 1985;13:106–111.

Choyce MQ, Potts M, Maitra AK. A profile of sports hand injuries in an accident and emergency department. *J Accident Emerg Med.* 1998;15:35–38.

Conti S, Michelson J, Jahss MM. Clinical significance of magnetic resonance imaging in preoperative planning for reconstruction of posterior tibial tendon ruptures. *Foot Ankle.* 1992;13:208–214.

Conti S. Posterior tibial tendon problems in athletes. *Orthop Clin North Am.* 1994;25:109–121.

Crawford GP. The moulded polythene splint for mallet finger deformities. *J Hand Surg.* 1984;9A:231–237.

Culver JE. Sport-related fractures of the hand and wrist. *Clin Sports Med.* 1990;9:85–109.

Curwin S, Stanish W. *Tendinitis: Its etiology and treatment.* London: Churchill, Livingstone; 1985.

Dailiana Z, Malizos K, Zacharis K, et al. Distal tibial epiphyseal fractures in adolescents. *Am J Orthop.* 1999;28:309–312.

de Loes M. Epidemiology of sports injuries in the Swiss organization "Youth and Sports" 1987–1989. Injuries, exposure and risks of main diagnoses. *Int J Sports Med.* 1995;16:134–138.

De Smet AA, Fisher R, Burnstein MI, et al. Value of MR imaging in staging osteochondral lesions of the talus (osteochondritis dissecans): Results in 14 patients. *Am J Roentgenol.* 1990;154:555–558.

Degan T, Morrey B, Braun D. Surgical excision for anterior process fracture of the calcaneus. *J Bone Joint Surg.* 1982;64A:519.

DeHaven KE, Lintner DM. Athletic injuries: Comparison by age, sports and gender. *Am J Sports Med.* 1986;14:218.

DeLee JC, Evans JP, Julian J. Stress fracture of the fifth metatarsal. *Am J Sports Med.* 1983;11:349–353.

Easterbrook M. Eye protection for basketball. Personal communication; 1998.

Eckert WR, Lakes M, Davis E. Acute rupture of the peroneal retinaculum. *J Bone Joint Surg Am.* 1976;58A:670.

El-Khoury GY, Wira RL, Berbaum KS, et al. MR imaging of patellar tendonitis. *Radiology.* 1992;184:849–854.

Epstein SE, Blomqvist CG, Buja LM, Haskell WL, Ryan TJ, Thompson PD. Task Force V: Ischemic Heart Disease. *J Am Coll Cardiol.* 1985;6:1222–1224.

Ferkel R, Karsel R, Del Pizzo W, et al. Arthroscopic treatment of anterolateral impingement of the ankle. *Am J Sports Med.* 1991;19:440.

Fischer M, McElfresh E. Physeal and periphyseal injuries of the hand. *Hand Clin.* 1994;10:287–301.

Flanders RA, Bhat M. The incidence of orofacial injuries in sports: A study in Illinois. *J Am Dent Assoc.* 1995;126:491–496.

Frey C, Shereff M, Greenidge N. Vascularity of the posterior tibial tendon. *J Bone Joint Surg Am.* 1990;72A:884–888.

Fuller CM, McNulty CM, Spring DA, et al. Prospective screening of 5,615 high school athletes for risk of sudden cardiac death. *Med Sci Sports Exerc.* 1997;29:1131–1138.

Furnich RM, Ellison AE, Guerin GJ. The measured effect of taping on combined foot and ankle motion before and after exercise. *Am J Sports Med.* 1981;9:165–170.

Garcia-Moral C. Injuries to the hand and wrist. In: Sullivan G, Grana W, eds. *The Pediatric Athlete.* Baltimore: Port City Press, AAOS; 1990;155–165.

Garrick JG. The frequency of injury, mechanism of injury: The frequency of injury, mechanism of injury and epidemiology of ankle sprains and epidemiology of ankle sprains. *Am J Sports Med.* 1977;5:241–242.

Garrick JG. Epidemiology of foot and ankle injuries. *Med Sport Sci.* 1987;23:991–997.

Garrick JG, Requa RK. Role of external support in the prevention of ankle sprains. *Med Sci Sports Exerc.* 1973;5:200–203.

Gerberich S, Priest JD, Boen JR, Straub CP, Maxwell RE. Concussion incidences and severity in secondary school varsity football players. *Am J Public Health.* 1983;73:1370–1375.

Gomez E, DeLee JC, Farney WC. Incidence of injury in Texas girls' high school basketball. *Am J Sports Med.* 1996;24:684–687.

Gould N. Stenosing tenosynovitis of the flexor hallucis longus tendon at the great toe. *Foot Ankle.* 1981;2:46–48.

Graham CE. Painful heel syndrome: Rationale of diagnosis and treatment. *Foot Ankle.* 1983;3:261–267.

Greene TA, Hillman SK. Comparison of support provided by a semirigid orthosis and adhesive ankle taping before, during, and after exercise. *Am J Sports Med.* 1990;18:498–506.

Greene TA, Wight CR. A comparative support evaluation of three ankle orthoses before, during, and after exercise. *J Orthop Sports Phys Ther.* 1990;11:453–466.

Gross MT, Batten AM, Lamm AL, et al. Comparison of DonJoy ankle ligament protector and subtalar sling ankle taping in restricting foot and ankle motion before, during, and after exercise. *J Orthop Sports Phys Ther.* 1994;19:33–41.

Gross MT, Everts JR, Robertson SJ, Roskin DS, Young KD. Effect of DonJoy ankle ligament protector and Aircast sport-stirrup orthoses on functional performance. *J Orthop Sports Phys Ther.* 1994;22:77–81.

Henry JH, Lareau B, Neigut D. The injury rate in professional basketball. *Am J Sports Med.* 1982;10:16–18.

Hewett TE, Stroupe AL, Nance TA, Noyes FR. Plyometric training in female athletes - Decreased impact forces and increased hamstring torques. *Am J Sports Med.* 1996;24:765–773.

Hickey GJ, Fricker PA, McDonald WA. Injuries to young elite female basketball players of a six-year period. *Clin J Sports Med.* 1997;7:252–256.

Huston LJ, Wojtys EM. Neuromuscular performance characteristics in elite female athletes. *Am J Sports Med.* 1996;24:427–436.

Ihle CI, Cochran RM. Fracture of the fused os trigonum. *Am J Sports Med.* 1982;10:47–50.

Incavo SJ, Morgan JV, Hilfrank BC. Extension splinting of palmar plate avulsion injuries of the proximal interphalangeal joint. *J Hand Surg.* 1989;14a:659–661.

Ireland ML, Wall C. Epidemiology and comparison of knee injuries in elite male and female United States basketball athletes. *Med Sci Sports Exerc.* 1990;22:592.

Johnson KA, Strom DE. Tibialis posterior tendon dysfunction. *Clin Orthop.* 1989;239:196.

Johnson RJ, Beynnon BD, Nichols CE, et al. Current concepts review: The treatment of injuries of the anterior cruciate ligament. *J Bone Joint Surg Am.* 1992;74A:140–151.

Jørgensen U. Regulations and officiating in injury prevention. In: Renström PAFH, ed. *Sports injuries: Basic principles of prevention and care.* Oxford: Blackwell Scientific; 1993;213–219.

Kahler DM, McCue FC III. Metacarpophalangeal and proximal interphalangeal joint injuries of the hand, including the thumb. *Clin Sports Med.* 1992;11:57–76.

Kainberger FM, Engel A, Barton P, et al. Injury of the Achilles tendon: Diagnosis with sonography. *Am J Roentgenol.* 1990;155:1031–1036.

Karlsson J, Sward L, Andreasson GO. The effect of taping on ankle stability; practical implications. *Sports Med.* 1993;16:210–215.

Kelly DW, Carter VS, Jobe FW, et al. Patellar and quadriceps tendon ruptures-jumper's knee. *Am J Sports Med.* 1984;12:375.

Kelly JP, Rosenburg JH. Diagnosis and management of concussion in sports. *Neurology.* 1997;48:575–580.

Kennedy JC, Willes RB. The effects of local steroid injections on tendons. *Am J Sports Med.* 1991;4:11.

King JB, Perry DJ, Mourad K, et al. Lesions of the patellar ligament. *J Bone Joint Surg Br.* 1990;72B:46–48.

Kling T. Operative treatment of ankle fractures in children. *Orthop Clin North Am.* 1990;21:381–392.

Kujala UM, Taimela S, Antti-Poika I, Orava S, Tuominen R, Myllynen P. Acute injuries in soccer, ice hockey, volleyball, basketball, judo, and karate - Analysis of National Registry data. *Br Med J.* 1995;311:1465–1468.

Kumamoto DP, Winters J, Novickas D, Mesa K. Tooth avulsions resulting from basketball net entanglement. *J Am Dent Assoc.* 1997;128:1273–1275.

LaPrade RF, Burnett QM II. Femoral intercondylar notch stenosis and correlation to anterior cruciate ligament injuries: A prospective study. *Am J Sports Med.* 1994;22:198–203.

Lazar JM. Marfan syndrome: Cardiovascular manifestations and exercise implications. *Phys Sportsmed.* 1997;25:34–39.

Leach RE, Seavey MS, Salter DK. Results of surgery in athletes with plantar fasciitis. *Foot Ankle.* 1986;7:156–161.

Leanderson J, Nemeth G, Eriksson E. Ankle injuries in basketball players. *Knee Surg Sport Traumatol Arthrosc.* 1993;1:200–202.

Leddy JJ, Smolinski RJ, Lawrence J, Snyder JL, Priore RL. Prospective evaluation of the Ottawa Ankle Rules in a university sports medicine center, with a modification to increase specificity for identifying malleolar fractures. *Am J Sports Med.* 1998;26:158–165.

Lo I, Bell D, Fowler P. Anterior cruciate ligament injuries in the skeletally immature patient. *Instructional Course Lectures.* 1998;47:351–359.

Locke A, Sitler M, Aland C, Kimura I. Long-term use of a softshell prophylactic ankle stabilizer on speed, agility, and vertical jump performance. *J Sport Rehabil.* 1997;6:235–245.

Lowdon A, Bader DL, Mowet AG. The effect of heel pads on the treatment of Achilles tendinitis: A double blind trial. *Am J Sports Med.* 1984;12:431.

MacKean LC, Bell G, Burnham RS. Prophylactic ankle bracing vs. taping: Effects on functional performance in female basketball players. *J Orthop Sports Phys Ther.* 1995;22:77–81.

Mann RA, Thompson FM. Rupture of the posterior tibial tendon causing flat foot. Surgical treatment. *J Bone Joint Surg Am.* 1985;67A:556–561.

Maple Flooring Manufacturers Association (MFMA). *Incidence of injury study: Maple flooring vs. synthetic.* Northbrook, Ill: Maple Flooring Manufacturers Association; 1998.

Marks PH, Ball KA, Evans RE, Richards DW, Brooks-Hill AL. *Effect of hip and knee angle on hamstring/quadriceps knee strength: Implications for ACL injury.* Beaver Creek, Col: ACL Study Group; 1998.

Marks PH, Fowler PJ. Imaging modalities for assessing the anterior cruciate ligament deficient knee. *Orthopaedics.* 1993;16:417–424.

Maron BJ. Sudden death in young athletes—Lessons from the Hank Gathers affair. *N Engl J Med.* 1993;329:55–57.

Maron BJ, Gaffney FA, Jeresaty RM, McKenna WJ, Miller WW. Task Force III: Hypertrophic cardiomyopathy, other myopericardial diseases and mitral valve prolapse. *J Am Coll Cardiol.* 1985;6:1215–1217.

Maron BJ, Mitchell JH. 26th Bethesda Conference: Recommendations for determining eligibility for competition in athletes with cardiovascular abnormalities. *J Am Coll Cardiol.* 1994;24:845–899.

Maron BJ, Shirani J, Poliac LC, Mathenge R, Roberts WC, Mueller FO. Sudden death in young competitive athletes—Clinical, demographic, and pathological profiles. *JAMA.* 1996;276:199–204.

McKay G, Payne W, Goldie P, Oakes B, Stanley J. A comparison of the injuries sustained by female basketball and netball players. *Aust J Sci Med Sport.* 1996;28:12–17.

McKay G, Goldie P, Payne W, Oakes B. Ankle injuries in basketball: Injury rate and risk factors. *Br J Sports Med.* 2001;35:103–108.

Micheli L, Fehlandt A. Overuse injuries to tendons and apophyses in children and adolescents. *Clin Sports Med.* 1992;11:713–724.

Minkoff J, Simonson BG, Sherman OH, Cavaliere G. Injuries in basketball. In Renström PAFH, ed. *Clinical practice of sports injury prevention and care.* Oxford: Blackwell Scientific Publications; 1994;303–353.

Mishra DK, Daniel DM, Stone ML. The use of functional knee braces in the control of pathological anterior knee laxity. *Clin Orthop.* 1989;241:213–220.

Mitchell JH, Blomqvist CG, Haskell WL, et al. Classification of sports. *J Am Coll Cardiol.* 1985;6:1198–1199.

Mitchell JH, Haskell WL, Raven PB. Classification of sports. *J Am Coll Cardiol.* 1994;24:864–866.

Mitchell JH, Maron BJ, Epstein SE. 16th Bethesda Conference—Cardiovascular abnormalities in the athlete: Recommendations regarding eligibility for competition. *J Am Coll Cardiol.* 1985;6:1185–1232.

National Basketball Trainers Association (NBTA). *Injury report, 1989–90.* National Basketball Trainers Association; 1990.

National Collegiate Athletics Association (NCAA). *1989-90, Basketball. National Collegiate Athletics Association injury surveillance statistics.* Indianapolis: NCAA; 1990.

Nistor L. Surgical and non-surgical treatment of Achilles tendon rupture: A prospective randomized study. *J Bone Joint Surg Am.* 1981;63A:394–399.

Ogilvie-Harris DJ, Gilbart M. Treatment modalities for soft tissue injuries of the ankle: A critical review. *Clin J Sport Med.* 1995;5:175–186.

Ott JW, Clancy WG. Functional knee braces: Review. *Orthopaedics.* 1993;16:171–176.

Ottaviani RA, Ashton-Miller JA, Kothari SU, Wojtys EM. Basketball shoe height and the maximal muscular resistance to applied ankle inversion and eversion moments. *Am J Sports Med.* 1995;23:418–423.

Payne KA, Berg K, Latin RW. Ankle injuries and ankle strength, flexibility, and proprioception in college basketball players. *J Athletic Training.* 1997;32:221–225.

Pienkowski D, McMorrow M, Shapiro R, Caborn DNM, Stayton J. The effect of ankle stabilizers on athletic performance—A randomized prospective study. *Am J Sports Med.* 1995;23:757–762.

Puddu G, Ippolito E, Postacchini F. A classification of Achilles tendon disease. *Am J Sports Med.* 1976;6:731–734.

Quinn SF, Murray WT, Clark RA, et al. Achilles tendon: MR imaging at 1.5 T. *Radiology.* 1987;164:767–770.

Renström PAH, ed. *Sports injuries: Basic principles of prevention and care.* Oxford: Blackwell Scientific Publications; 1993.

Rettig A, Adsit W. Athletic injuries of the hand and wrist. In Griffin L, ed. *Orthopaedic knowledge update: Sports medicine.* Rosemont, Ill: AAOS; 1994;205–224.

Robinson JR, Frederick EC, Cooper LB. Systematic ankle stabilization and the effect on performance. *Med Sci Sports Exerc.* 1986;18:625–628.

Rocca G. Basketball traumatology. Epidemiologic study. *Medicina dello Sport.* 1997;50:317–324.

Rovere GD, Clarke TJ, Yates SC, Burley K. Retrospective comparison of taping and ankle stabilizers in preventing ankle injuries. *Am J Sports Med.* 1988;16:228–233.

Sammarco GJ, DiRaimondo CV. Chronic peroneus brevis tendon lesion. *Foot Ankle.* 1989;9:163–170.

Schoenecker P, Luhmann S. Knee and leg: Pediatric aspects. In: Koval K, ed. *Orthopaedic knowledge update 7.* Rosemont, Ill: AAOS; 2002;465–478.

Shapiro MS, Kabo JM, Mitchell PW, Loren G, Tsenter M. Ankle sprain prophylaxis: An analysis of the stabilizing effects of braces and tape. *Am J Sports Med.* 1994;22:78–82.

Shrier I. Treatment of lateral collateral ligament sprains of the ankle: A critical appraisal of the literature. *Clin J Sport Med.* 1995;5:187–195.

Sitler M, Ryan J, Wheeler B, et al. The efficacy of a semirigid ankle stabilizer to reduce acute ankle injuries in basketball—A randomized clinical study at West Point. *Am J Sports Med.* 1994;22:454–461.

Smith JW, Arnoczky SP, Hersh A. The intraosseous blood supply of the fifth metatarsal: Implications for proximal fracture healing. *Foot Ankle.* 1998;13:143–152.

Sobel M, DiCarlo EF, Bohne WH, Collins L. Longitudinal splitting of the peroneus brevis tendon: An anatomical and histological study of cadaveric material. *Foot Ankle.* 1991;12:165

Souryal TO, Freeman TR. Intercondylar notch size and anterior cruciate ligament injuries in athletes: A prospective study. *Am J Sports Med.* 1993;21:535–539.

Stacoff A, Steger J, Stussi E, Reinschmidt C. Lateral stability in sideward cutting movements. *Med Sci Sports Exerc.* 1996;28:350–358.

Stanish WD, McVicar SF. Flexibility in injury prevention. In: Renström PAFH, ed. *Sports injuries: Basic principles of prevention and care.* Oxford: Blackwell Scientific; 1993;262–276.

Steill IG, Greenberg GH, McKnight RD, et al. A study to develop clinical decision rules for the use of radiography in acute ankle injuries. *Ann Emerg Med.* 1992;21:384–390.

Steill IG, Greenberg GH, McKnight RD, et al. Decision rules for the use of radiography in acute ankle injuries: Refinement and prospective validation. *JAMA.* 1993;269:1127–1132.

Stone WJ, Steingard PM. Year-Round Conditioning for Basketball. In Steingard PM, ed. *Basketball injuries.* Philadelphia: Saunders; 1993;173–191.

Taunton JE. Training errors. In Renström PAFH, ed. *Sports injuries: Basic principles of prevention and care.* Oxford: Blackwell Scientific; 1993;205–212.

Thomas RJ, Cantwell JD. Sudden death during basketball games. *Phys Sportsmed.* 1990;18:75–78.

Thompson PD, Klocke FJ, Levine BD, Van Camp SP. Task force 5: Coronary artery disease. *J Am Coll Cardiol.* 1994;24:888–892.

Torg JS, Conrad W, Kalen V. Clinical diagnosis of anterior cruciate ligament instability in the athlete. *Am J Sports Med.* 1976;4:84.

Torg JS, Pavlov H, Cooley LH, et al. Stress fractures of the tarsal navicular: A retrospective review of twenty-one cases. *J Bone Joint Surg Am.* 1982;64A:700–712.

Van Camp SP. What can we learn from Reggie Lewis' death? *Phys Sportsmed.* 1993;21:73–74.

van Kampen A, Huiskes R. The three-dimensional tracking pattern of the human patella. *J Orthop Res.* 1990;8:372–382.

Weir MA, Watson AWS. A twelve month study of sports injuries in one Irish school. *Irish J Med Sci.* 1996;165:165–169.

Wiley J, Baxter M. Tibial spine fractures in children. *Clin Orthop.* 1990;225:54–60.

Willis R, Blokker C, Stoll T, et al. Long-term follow-up of anterior tibial eminence fractures. *J Pediatr Orthop.* 1993;13:361–364.

Wilkerson GB. Comparative biomechanical effects of the standard method of ankle taping and a taping method designed to enhance subtalar stability. *Am J Sports Med.* 1991;19:588–595.

Wilson RL, McGinty LD. Common hand and wrist injuries in basketball players. *Clin Sports Med.* 1993;12:265–291.

Woods W, Leach R. Posterior tibial tendon in athletic people. *Am J Sports Med.* 1991;19:495

Yde JR, Buhl-Nielsen A. An epidemiological and traumatological analysis of injuries in a Danish basketball club. *Ugeskrift for Laeger.* 1988;150:142–144.

Yde JR, Buhl-Nielsen A. Sports injuries in adolescent's ball games: soccer, handball and basketball. *Br J Sports Med.* 1990;24:51–54.

Zagelbaum BM, Starkey C, Hersh PS, Donnenfeld ED, Perry HD, Jeffers JB. The National Basketball Association eye injury study. *Arch Ophthalmol.* 1995;113:749–752.

Zelisko JA, Noble HB, Porter M. A comparison of men's and women's professional basketball injuries. *Am J Sports Med.* 1982;10:297–299.

Zoellner G, Clancy W Jr. Recurrent dislocation of the peroneal tendon. *J Bone Joint Surg Am.* 1979;61A:292–294.

Zvifac J, Thompson W. Basketball. In: Caine DJ, ed. *Epidemiology of sports injuries.* Champaign, Ill: Human Kinetics; 1996;86–97.

31 | Football Injuries

Don Johnson and Paul Johnson

QUICK LOOK

- Injury prevention is improved with cardiovascular training, strength training, and flexibility.
- Shoulder injuries common to football include anterior shoulder dislocation, acromioclavicular sprains, clavicle fractures, and tendon ruptures.
- Wrist and hand injuries common to football include scaphoid fracture, phalangeal dislocations, metacarpal and phalangeal fracture, and Bennett's fracture.
- Spine injuries common to football include burners and stingers, musculoligamentous sprain of the spine, intervertebral disk injury, fractures and stress fractures of the pars intra-articularis, and fracture dislocation of the cervical spine.
- Thigh injuries common to football include contusion to the quadriceps, exertional muscle cramps, adductor strain, and hamstring strain.
- Knee injuries common to football include medial, anterior, and posterior cruciate ligament sprains, and meniscus cartilage tear.
- Lower leg injuries common to football include stress fracture, shin splints, compartment syndrome, and calf muscle strains.
- Ankle injuries common to football include lateral and deltoid ligament sprains, osteochondral talus fracture, Achilles tendonitis and tears, and posterior tibial tendon rupture.
- Foot injuries common to football include plantar fascial injury, metatarsal fracture, Jones fracture, and first metatarsal–phalangeal joint injury (turf toe).
- Return to play decisions are difficult on the sidelines and there are specific injuries not to miss.

Football (Fig. 31-1) is a collision-contact sport and injuries are inevitable. It is the responsibility of the team physician and athletic trainer to provide a high standard of care for the athletes. Immediate attention to proper assessment of game and practice injury and illness with a coordinated treatment effort may prevent long-term disability or even death. Prevention strategies and rehearsed emergency protocols are critical to care of the severe problems that can occur in football.

PREVENTION

The best prevention of an injury is proper conditioning. *Conditioning* consists of three elements: cardiovascular training, strength training, and flexibility exercises. The coaches, athletic trainers, and strength coaches will design individual programs consisting of both endurance and interval training. The most specific and efficient exercise for football is running. For the lineman, the exercise bike or Stairmaster will work better. The cardiovascular training program should be specific for a player's position. Most football players are advocates of weight lifting for strength training. The key is developing a training program that targets their weak muscle groups based on preseason testing. Hamstring tears are one of the most common injuries for receivers and defensive backs. If there is a detectable weakness, then the training program should address this area for strengthening. Not

475

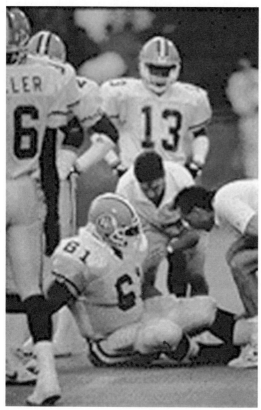

FIG 31-1   Injuries are an inevitable part of the game of football.

only are free-weight exercises important, but also sport-specific plyometric exercises should be instituted. The other essential area to emphasize is the flexibility of commonly injured muscle groups. The wide receivers and deep backs, who are sprinters, should emphasize both strength and stretching of the hamstrings to avoid tearing. Most of the anterior cruciate ligament (ACL) injuries occur with a noncontact twisting injury. This is often a maneuver that the athlete has done many times in the past and it is hard to believe that a specific exercise can prevent this injury. The best prevention is by running the same pattern repeatedly to condition the specific muscles involved.

Heat and cold injury protocols should be reviewed before each season and preseason conditioning should emphasize acclimatization to the heat. Heat stress is amplified by the occlusive nature of the uniform and pads. The onsite team should rehearse the protocols for spine injury and airway management on a regular basis. The helmet should be left on unless there is airway compromise.

COMMON INJURIES

Shoulder

Most upper extremity injuries are caused by a fall on the outstretched arm. The shoulder pads protect the shoulder structures from the trauma of direct impact on the shoulder.

Anterior Shoulder Dislocations

The mechanism of injury is by forced abduction and external rotation of the shoulder. The underlying pathology is tearing of the capsulolabral complex from the anterior glenoid rim. The symptoms of pain, limited motion, and a square shoulder deformity make the diagnosis. The treatment of the dislocation should be early reduction. The author does not think it is appropriate to reduce the dislocation on the field, although it is often done. On occasion, it is possible to reduce it on the bench with the athlete prone and the arm hanging over the side of the bench. It is more prudent to take the athlete into the dressing room to perform the reduction.

The easiest method is to have the athlete lie prone on the bench, letting the arm hang over the edge of the bench. Many times, with gentle traction downward on the elbow, the shoulder reduces. If it does not reduce easily, the tip of the scapula may be rotated medially with the other hand. If the shoulder still does not reduce easily, whatever method of reduction is used, the athlete should be transported to the hospital. The reduction of the dislocation is confirmed by asking the athlete to touch the opposite shoulder with the involved hand. If they can perform this maneuver, the shoulder is reduced.

The question of whether to attempt a reduction without an x-ray is controversial. A physician experienced at the diagnosis and manipulation of the dislocated shoulder who does not believe that this is a fracture of the surgical neck of the humerus can attempt reduction. A postreduction radiograph should always be obtained.

Acromioclavicular Joint Sprains

Injuries to the acromioclavicular (AC) joint can still occur in spite of shoulder pads. The diagnosis is made by pain, tenderness, and deformity at the AC joint (Fig. 31-2). The injuries are classified into six grades:
- *Grade 1:* Pain and tenderness, with no deformity.
- *Grade 2:* Pain, tenderness, and slight separation with a prominent end of the clavicle.
- *Grade 3:* Pain, tenderness, and marked separation of the joint with a prominent end of the clavicle.
- *Grades 4–6:* These three more severe grades of injury are very rare.

Treatment is based on the grading of the injury:

- *Grade 1:* Symptomatic treatment only. May return to play when the pain is tolerable and the range of motion is adequate to perform the needed skills; for some players that can be the next game.
- *Grade 2:* Requires a sling, analgesics, physiotherapy, and may be out of play for 2–4 weeks, depending on the severity of the symptoms.
- *Grade 3:* Requires protection and reduction in a brace. There is considerable controversy concerning this degree of injury, and in some instances,

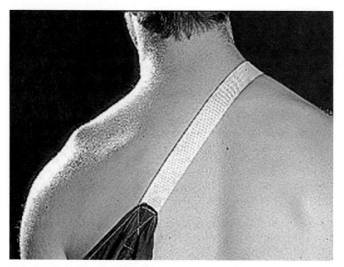

FIG 31-2 The appearance of the superior subluxation of the outer end of the clavicle in a grade 3 AC joint injury.

open reduction and internal fixation is the best treatment. This depends on the athlete's position. For example, a quarterback with a grade 3 AC joint dislocation on his throwing arm should have an operative reduction and will be out of practice and play for 6–8 weeks. The hardware will need to be removed before returning to play.

Clavicle Fractures

Clavicle fractures result from a fall on the outstretched arm. The diagnosis can be made on the sidelines by palpating the clavicle. This injury should be confirmed by x-ray and immobilized in a figure-of-8 bandage if displaced and a sling if undisplaced. Clavicle fractures take 6–8 weeks to heal. There is very little physiotherapy that can be done in the early fracture healing stages. Riding an exercise bike will maintain some cardiovascular fitness during the healing stages. Most clavicle fractures heal with conservative treatment. The only indication for operative fixation is if there is marked displacement of the fragments or neurovascular compromise.

Tendon Ruptures

Tendon ruptures of the upper extremity are common but sometimes overlooked. The rupture of the long head of the biceps is caused by a violent flexion of the elbow and shoulder. Pain, swelling, and deformity of the biceps are quite evident and make the diagnosis evident. When the biceps is flexed it looks like a "Popeye" muscle. Treatment is generally conservative.

The distal rupture of the biceps at the elbow is more difficult to diagnose, but careful palpation in the antecubital fossa reveals the absence of the tendon on elbow flexion. The torn tendon is usually surgically reattached to the radius.

Wrist and Hand

Scaphoid Fracture

The scaphoid is often injured by a fall on the outstretched arm. Pain, swelling, and tenderness in the anatomic snuff box of the wrist make the diagnosis of a scaphoid fracture. The fracture may be confirmed by an x-ray, although it is common that the fracture not show up on initial plain x-rays. In the early phase, the wrist should be immobilized and a bone scan performed. If the plain x-rays and bone scan are negative, then the possibility of a scaphoid fracture is remote. A clenched fist view of the wrist may reveal a scapholunate instability that may mimic a scaphoid fracture. The treatment of a scaphoid fracture is cast immobilization for 6–12 weeks until good calcium bridging of the fracture is demonstrated on x-ray and the site is nontender. A significantly displaced scaphoid fracture or a scapholunate dislocation may require surgical open reduction and internal fixation.

Phalangeal Dislocation

Dislocation of the fingers is extremely common and used to be called *coach's finger*, because the coach often reduced them. Pain, swelling, and deformity make the diagnosis of a joint dislocation. Management is gentle longitudinal traction to reduce the joint. It is acceptable to attempt a gentle closed reduction without an x-ray. The association of fracture is fairly common, and a postreduction x-ray is mandatory to confirm the reduction and to rule out an associated fracture. Immobilization of the dislocated finger by taping to the next finger and allowing the athlete to play is acceptable.

Metacarpal and Phalangeal Fractures

These fractures are produced by direct blows or crush injury. The diagnosis is by pain, swelling, and bony tenderness. X-ray is essential to confirm any suspicious injury. Treatment of undisplaced fractures is cast immobilization. Displaced fractures may require closed reduction; some require surgical open reduction and fixation. Undisplaced fractures of the 2nd and 3rd metacarpals may have adequate support from the surrounding tissue to play with a soft cast or padded splint.

Bennett's Fracture

The Bennett's fracture is a displaced fracture at the base of the thumb. The mechanism occurs by jamming the thumb. Pain, swelling, and tenderness at the base of the thumb with a positive x-ray make the diagnosis. Closed reduction of the fracture may be adequate, but an open surgical reduction is usually necessary to ensure adequate alignment and future function.

Tendon Injuries

Tendon injuries also occur in the hand. The long flexor of the finger may be ruptured distally when the player grabs another player's shirt (*jersey finger*). The violent flexion ruptures the tendon from the distal phalanx. Diagnosis is made by examining for lack of flexion of the distal phalanx. Treatment is by surgical reattachment.

Spine

Burners and Stingers

Burners and stingers are traction injuries to the brachial plexus. When the athlete falls on his head and the neck is flexed to the opposite side, traction on the nerves produces a sensation like hitting the funny bone in the elbow. These injuries may be a mild nuisance or quite severe and prevent the athlete from playing for most of the season. Many times, the first injury is mild, and reinjury causes prolonged disability.

The diagnosis of stingers is made by the history of injury and examination of the neck by flexing to the side of the injury and reproducing the symptoms. Treatment is to protect the neck with a horse collar attached to the shoulder pads to reduce excessive lateral flexion of the neck. If the symptoms persist, then the athlete must be taken out of play until the symptoms subside. Gentle mobilization exercises and therapeutic heat applications provide symptomatic relief.

Musculoligamentous Sprain of the Spine

There are many injuries that occur to the spine in football that are categorized as *back sprain*. The diagnosis is by history of back pain, local spinal tenderness, and restricted range of motion but a normal neurologic examination. Back sprains are usually minor, and the athlete may miss a few practices but is ready to play the next game. If the symptoms persist or worsen, then further investigation is indicated.

Intervertebral Disk Injury

Many back sprains are injuries to the disk, but may be difficult to diagnose early in the course of the injury. If a lumbar or cervical injury does not improve quickly, reexamination and further investigation is necessary. If the athlete has radiating pain with or without neurologic symptoms, then a CT scan or MRI should be ordered to assess for disk protrusion or fragmentation. Most disk injuries may be treated conservatively. Disk herniation with a neurologic deficit may require early surgical intervention. Conservative treatment may keep the athlete out of play for 6–12 weeks or longer.

Fracture and Stress Fracture of the Pars Intra-articularis

Persistent back pain that does not settle in a lineman is often a *pars intra-articularis fracture*, which is produced by repeated extension of the spine. Routine x-rays of the spine may reveal a fracture or even spondylolysis. A bone scan will help to determine whether this is of recent origin and may demonstrate a stress fracture. The CT scan is the best method to evaluate this injury. Initial treatment is conservative with rest and back exercises. Surgical intervention may be required if spondylolysis progresses.

Fracture Dislocation of the Cervical Spine

This injury is rare, but for sports physicians and athletic trainers on the sidelines, it is the most feared injury. Every time an athlete goes down on the field of play and does not get up quickly the first thought is, "Please move your arms or legs." Because serious neck injury is uncommon, it is important to review the evacuation protocol regularly. In the Canadian Football League there is always an ambulance on the sidelines. If a serious neck injury occurs, the ambulance crew with the backboard should be called on to evacuate the player. If a fracture is suspected, it is more prudent to move the athlete to the hospital than to try to evaluate this injury in the training room. The neck is immobilized in a collar with the helmet left on, and the athlete is transferred to the hospital for x-ray and evaluation. After the initial screening x-rays, the helmet can be removed without moving the neck, and follow up x-rays or CT scanning can be done. It is critical to remember that the shoulder pads elevate the neck off the table about 4 inches and the head has to be supported when the helmet is removed.

Thigh

Contusion to Quadriceps

A deep bruise to the quadriceps muscle due to a direct blow can cause extensive short-term disability. Pain, swelling, local tenderness, and limited range of motion of the knee make the diagnosis of a quadriceps contusion.

Immediate treatment is ice, compression, elevation, and full knee flexion splinting to put the quadriceps at full length to minimize bleeding into the muscle. The injury may be evaluated by the degree of loss of knee flexion in 1–2 days. If there is only 45° of knee flexion, this injury will take several weeks to improve. Physiotherapy modalities, such as ultrasound, contrast baths, and local stretching of the muscle, will improve comfort and may speed healing. Once the injury has settled, strength training is important to regain muscle power lost to disuse.

Adductor Strain

A strain of the adductors may be diagnosed by pain, swelling, local tenderness in the adductor muscle or at the tendon–bone junction, and limited abduction range of motion at the hip. The adductor group is essential for sprinting and cutting. With a severe injury to the tendon–bone transition or avulsion fracture, the athlete may be disabled for 6 months. The treatment should be initially ice, compression, and analgesics for pain control. Ultrasound and stretching will also aid in the healing of the injury. For some chronic tendon–bone junction pain syndromes, a cortisone injection may help with pain relief and allow more intensive rehabilitation programs. The muscle must also be strengthened after the initial inflammation has settled.

Hamstring Strain and Tear

The hamstring strain is one of the most common injuries in players who sprint, such as running backs, receivers, and defensive backs. The hamstring strain is diagnosed by examining for local tenderness of the muscle, pain with resisted hamstring curls or stretches, and limited straight-leg raising. If the straight leg raise is limited to 45°, this injury will probably keep the athlete out of play for 4–6 weeks. Treatment is with ice, compression, ultrasound, and gentle stretching. Strength training is resumed when the athlete is able to jog. In spite of a palpable defect in the muscle, the usual treatment for hamstring muscle injuries is nonsurgical.

Knee

Medial Ligament Sprain

The medial collateral ligament (MCL) is injured by a valgus or lateral force against the outside of the knee when another player falls or tackles against

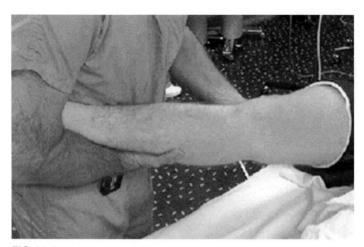

FIG 31-3 The grading of the medial ligament injury is done by applying a valgus force against the knee and observing the degree of ligament laxity in both the full extension and 30° of knee flexion positions.

the lateral side of the knee. The diagnosis is made by pain, swelling, local tenderness over the ligament on the medial side, limited range of motion of the knee, and a feeling of instability when weight bearing. To aid in planning the treatment, the injury severity is categorized into three grades by the examination (Fig. 31-3).

- *Grade 1:* local pain and tenderness without instability on examination.
- *Grade 2:* local pain, swelling, tenderness, and laxity of the ligament on valgus stress, but an endpoint can be felt on stressing the ligament.
- *Grade 3:* often very little pain, moderate swelling, and marked instability on valgus stress with no endpoint to the examination. With laxity at full extension, injury to the cruciate ligaments must be considered.

Management depends on the grade or severity of the sprain to the ligament.

- *Grade 1:* ice, compression, and hinged knee sleeve for comfort, ligament protection, and stability; return to sport in 2–3 weeks with medial and lateral hinged brace protection only.
- *Grade 2:* ice, compression, and protection for 4–6 weeks in a double upright brace that allows range of motion but prevents valgus stress on the knee. An extension block at 15–30° may be used, but is not necessary for a stable knee. Strengthening exercises including the bike and Stairmaster may be instituted early.
- *Grade 3:* ice, compression, and protection with a knee brace as used for grade 2 injuries. Strengthening exercises can be started when comfort allows. It usually takes 10–12 weeks to return to sport. It is extremely rare to have an isolated grade 3 MCL strain, so be certain that an associated ACL injury is not present by performing a Lachman test. It has been shown that initial conservative treatment of the MCL injury followed by late reconstruction of the ACL provides the best results if there is no associated meniscus cartilage injury. A ruptured lateral collateral ligament is

usually associated with damage to the posterior corner support structures and these injuries require immediate surgical repair.

Anterior Cruciate Ligament Tear

The most common mechanism of injury of the ACL is a noncontact pivot injury. The athlete hears a pop and experiences immediate pain and instability with swelling ensuing over the next several hours. Sideline examination reveals a positive Lachman test. The athlete will often walk around and feel better in 10–15 minutes and will want to go back in the game. The seriousness of the injury must be impressed on the athlete; at this stage the injury can progress to the meniscus or articular cartilage and have a poor long-term outcome. Approximately half of cruciate ligament injuries are isolated and have no associated meniscal injury. With proper management, these have a good long-term outlook.

The diagnosis of an anterior cruciate ligament injury is made by pain, swelling, limited range of motion, and a positive Lachman test (Fig. 31-4). The Lachman test is an important diagnostic tool to master. You are examining to feel the endpoint of anterior excursion of the tibia in relation to the femur; if it is soft and different from the uninjured knee, an injury to the ACL should be suspected. The Lachman and pivot shift tests should be documented in the preseason physical examination. This information can be referred to later in the season when the athlete has a knee injury. It is unusual to be able to do a pivot shift on the acutely injured knee, especially more than one time, so you have to rely on the Lachman test to make the clinical diagnosis. Because many football players have large legs, and it is difficult to get them to relax, the drop leg Lachman test (Fig. 31-5) is much easier to perform. The leg is dropped over the edge of the examining bed, the foot held between the examiners knees, and the tibia is pulled forward.

If the Lachman test is positive and the athlete is going to have surgery, you do not have to order an MRI to confirm the ACL tear. The only

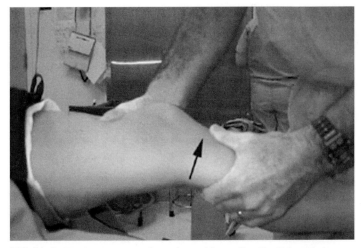

FIG 31-4 The Lachman test is performed by pulling the tibia anterior with the knee flexed at 30°.

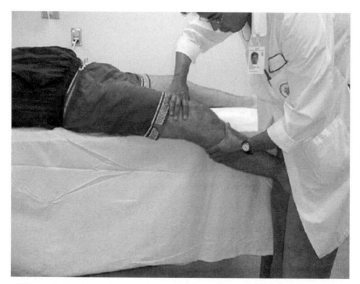

FIG 31-5 The drop leg Lachman is performed by flexing the leg over the edge of the bed and pulling the tibia forward.

indication for an MRI is to rule out a meniscal injury if considering delaying surgery until the end of the season, or if clinical suspicion for ACL disruption is high but the Lachman test is negative. If the MRI was positive for both an ACL and meniscal tear, then surgery should be scheduled during the season. In this situation, the MRI could change the course of treatment. A routine preoperative MRI does not change the treatment plan. The treatment for an ACL tear in a pivoting athlete is surgery. The timing of the surgery may be controversial. If a lineman has an isolated ACL tear, they may be rehabilitated and return to play in 1 month in a brace. Surgery may then be performed at the end of the season because the risk of reinjury is low. The presence of a meniscal tear is generally an indication to repair the meniscus and reconstruct the ACL. If the MRI is negative for meniscal injury, then you can feel safe in allowing the athlete to return to play in a brace. This program will usually not be successful in a running back or receiver, and these athletes should have surgery when the swelling subsides and range of motion is nearly normal. The criteria to return to play are no pain, full range of motion, no effusion, and equal strength measured on Cybex testing.

Meniscal Tear

The meniscus is usually torn by a compression and rotation mechanism. The duck walk (or baseball catcher's squat position) is a good example of the mechanism that tears the posterior horn of the medial meniscus. The duck walk is also a good provocative test for the chronic meniscal tear. The history of flexion and rotation of the knee followed by pain and swelling make the diagnosis of meniscal injury. The swelling often does not occur until the next day. The clinical signs of meniscal tear are effusion, tenderness, and pain with flexion and rotation, the McMurray test (Fig. 31-6).

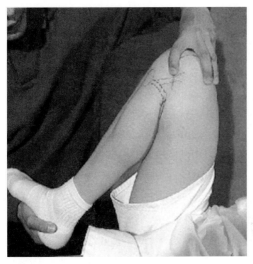

FIG 31-6 The McMurray test is performed by flexing the knee and rotating the tibia to pinch an unstable fragment of meniscus between the tibia and femur.

The Apley compression test may also be useful. It is performed in the prone position by flexing the knee to 90° and compressing the tibia against the femur. A positive test is pain and snapping of the meniscus between the femur and the tibia. Placing the knee in full flexion often provokes pain from a meniscus tear. If the knee can obtain full extension (it is not locked), then conservative treatment should be instituted (ice, compression, and elevation). Contrast baths in the whirlpool and gentle range of motion exercises should be started early. If the knee lacks full extension, x-rays should be done to rule out avulsion fractures and loose bodies. The MRI confirms the bucket handle tear of the meniscus. This should be treated surgically as quickly as possible.

Posterior Cruciate Ligament Injury

The mechanism of injury to the posterior cruciate ligament (PCL) is a direct blow to the anterior aspect of the tibia. This may occur by falling on the front of the knee with the foot plantar flexed. The blow occurs directly to the tibial tubercle and drives the tibia posteriorly tearing the PCL. Pain, swelling, limited motion, and a positive posterior drawer test (Fig. 31-7) make the diagnosis. Once you determine the neutral tibial step-off by comparing the tibial plateau position on both knees, you can grade the posterior drawer test. The quadriceps-neutral position may also be determined by having the patient contract their quadriceps with the knee at 70°. This pulls the tibia forward to the neutral position. There are three grades of PCL injury:

- *Grade 1:* Tibial plateau palpated and forward of the femur, 0–5 mm posterior displacement.
- *Grade 2:* Tibial plateau slightly palpable or equal with the femur, 5–10 mm of posterior displacement.
- *Grade 3:* Tibial plateau posterior to the femur, 10–15 mm of posterior displacement.

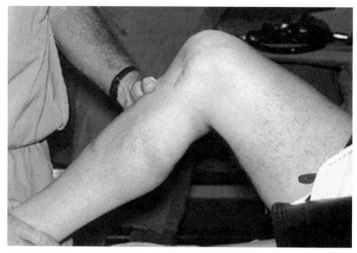

FIG 31-7   The posterior drawer test is performed by pushing the tibia posteriorly with the knee flexed to 90°.

Most of the isolated PCL injuries are grade 1 or 2. The grade 3 injuries are usually associated with other ligament injuries such as the posterolateral corner. It is important to determine if there is any associated injury. The isolated injury may be treated conservatively, but combined injuries generally require surgery. The common posterolateral corner injury may be detected by examining for external rotation of the tibia at 30° and 90° of knee flexion.

Quadriceps Tendon Rupture

The patellar tendon and quadriceps both can be ruptured by sudden quick stops while running. These injuries are massive and require urgent surgical treatment. Cortisone injections weaken the tendon and should not be used on weight-bearing tendons such as the patellar tendon, quadriceps tendon, or Achilles tendon. Pain, swelling, local tenderness, and lack of active knee extension make the diagnosis. The defect in the tendon is palpable. The treatment is surgical repair and the athlete may need 6 months to recover.

Lower Leg

Stress Fracture

Stress fractures are less common in football than other running and jumping sports. The mechanism is overuse in an unconditioned player. They are more likely to occur at the end of training camp after twice daily workouts. The common sites are the proximal tibia, the distal fibula, and the metatarsal shafts. Uncommon sites are the tarsal navicular and the calcaneous. Pain, swelling, and local bony tenderness make the diagnosis. The stress fracture may not show clinical signs on the x-ray for 3–4 weeks. The bone scan will be positive within a few days of injury. Treatment is relative rest of the bone with alternate activities for conditioning. No immobilization is required. A bone stimulator may speed healing.

Shin Splints and Compartment Syndrome

Shin splints are a pain syndrome along the front of the tibia caused by running in the unconditioned state. The shin splint is a stress syndrome of the muscle attachment to bone. It is important to differentiate shin splints from *compartment syndrome*, which is characterized by pain and swelling in the anterior or lateral muscle compartments of the lower leg. The muscle swells up to 30% with exercise. If there has been a bruise to the compartment or the fascial sheath is tight, the muscle may swell enough to obstruct venous outflow, increasing the volume within the compartment. This may become a surgical emergency if the swelling is sufficient to cut off the arterial blood supply. The severity of the pain will alert the medical staff to the more urgent compartment syndrome. The diagnosis of compartment syndrome is pain increased by plantar flexion of the ankle. More severe signs are pallor, pulselessness, and peripheral neuropathy. The treatment for compartment syndrome is to release the fascia around the involved muscle. Compartment syndromes may occur from acute trauma or from chronic exertional mechanisms.

Pain, swelling, and local tenderness along the anterolateral border of the tibia make the diagnosis of shin splints. Pain along the posterior medial border the tibia is usually due to posterior tibialis strain. Treatment consists of ice, compression, elevation, stretching, and rest; in some cases, foot orthotics can be helpful.

Calf Muscle Pull, Strains, and Tears

Muscle pulls and tears are extremely common in football owing to the explosive nature of the activity. Muscle tears are graded into three levels—mild strain, partial tear, and complete tears. Pain, swelling, local muscle tenderness, and deformity make the diagnosis. Treatment is ice, compression, and elevation. Ultrasound and interferential current treatments help to reduce pain and swelling. The degree of tear is an estimate for the length of time to return to sport. The criteria for return to sport are no pain, no swelling, full range of joint motion, and equal strength on Cybex muscle testing.

Ankle

Lateral Ligament Sprain

Rolling over on the ankle or an inversion sprain injures the lateral ligaments. Pain, swelling, local tenderness, and instability of the ankle joint make the diagnosis. The anterior drawer test of the ankle and the inversion stress test determine the lateral ankle stability. The degree of instability can be measured by performing these tests and taking an x-ray at the maximum degree of laxity. Ankle sprains are graded like all ligament sprains into three levels. However, all grades are treated conservatively. The grade 3 sprain may be treated in a clam shell–type splint (such as an Aircast) that is removable for physiotherapy exercises. All sprains benefit from a protective lace-up ankle brace for the first 3 months after injury.

Chronic persistent ankle pain 3 months after injury may prevent the player from returning to sport. An MRI or CT scan of the ankle joint should be considered to rule out an occult fracture. The ankle joint may have to be injected with steroids to help reduce synovitis. If the pain persists in spite of the injection, then arthroscopy of the ankle may be necessary to diagnose the soft tissue impingement.

Deltoid Ligament Ankle Injury

Injury of the medial deltoid ligament is less common than lateral ligament injury. The mechanism of injury is an eversion stress to the ankle. Pain, swelling, and local tenderness suggest the diagnosis. Initial treatment is ice, compression, elevation, and protective splinting. Ultrasound and range of motion exercises are necessary to regain full motion.

Osteochondral Fracture of the Talus

The inversion injury may be severe enough to produce a shear force to the dome of the talus and detach a fragment of bone and articular surface. The osteochondral fracture may heal if undisplaced. If displaced, arthroscopy and removal of the loose fragment may be required. Pain, swelling, and loss of range of motion are the clinical signs that make the diagnosis. Plain x-rays will usually demonstrate the lesion. Occasionally, a CT scan of the talus may be required to evaluate the osteochondral lesion.

Achilles Tendonitis and Tendon Tears

Achilles tendonitis occurs with running overuse. Prevention is to stretch and gradually warm up. Treatment consists of stretching, icing, ultrasound, and a heel raise in the shoe.

The Achilles tendon is torn by a violent contraction of the gastrocnemius muscle in sprinting. A loud pop followed by pain and swelling make the diagnosis. A palpable defect in the tendon and a positive Thompson test are the clinical signs of a complete rupture of the tendon. Squeezing the gastrocnemius muscle when the patient is supine comprises the Thompson test (Fig. 31-8) (calf compression test). A positive test is the failure of the ankle to plantar flex when the muscle is squeezed. The opposite side is used for comparison.

Achilles tendon tears can be treated with casting in the equines position or by surgically suturing the torn ends of the tendon together. Most athletes chose surgical repair and are usually out of competition for 6 months.

Posterior Tibial Tendon Rupture

This is an uncommon tendon rupture. It produces a flat foot appearance. The athlete is unable to toe raise without the foot remaining in a pronated position. The treatment is to surgically suture the tendon or to augment the repair with another tendon.

Foot

Plantar Fascia Injury

The plantar fascia may be injured by a sprinting action or a forced dorsiflexion of the foot. Pain, swelling, and local tenderness of the fascia along its course and at the insertion on the os calcis make the diagnosis. Treatment consists of ice, compression, and taping of the arch to protect it while the soft tissues heal. An arch support and night splint may speed the healing process.

Metatarsal Fracture

Metatarsal fractures are caused by a direct blow, such as another player stepping on the foot. Pain, swelling, and local bony tenderness make the diag-

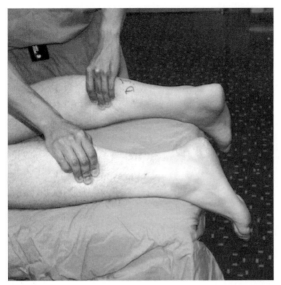

FIG 31-8   The Thompson test is performed by squeezing the calf. The injured right leg does not plantar flex when squeezed due to the loss of continuity of Achilles tendon.

nosis. The x-ray confirms the fracture. The treatment is by cast immobilization for 4–6 weeks. Physiotherapy after cast removal regains range of motion and strength of the foot.

Jones Fracture of the Fifth Metatarsal

The Jones fracture is a fracture of the base of the fifth metatarsal caused by an inversion motion of the ankle. Pain, swelling, and local bony tenderness of the fifth metatarsal base make the diagnosis. The x-ray confirms that the fracture is through the metaphyseal region of the bone. The avulsion fracture of the base of the fifth metatarsal has a different outcome. The avulsion can be treated conservatively with a stiff shoe; the Jones fracture may require surgical reduction and pinning to return the athlete to sport.

Metatarsophalangeal Joint Injury: Turf Toe

Turf toe is caused by hyperextension of the great toe. Pain, swelling, and limited motion of the metatarsophalangeal joint make the diagnosis. The x-ray is negative for fracture. Treatment is conservative with ice, compression, and elevation. Anti-inflammatory medications help to reduce swelling. Other physiotherapy modalities such as interferential current will also help to reduce pain and swelling. An intra-articular steroid injection may reduce the inflammation and speed recovery. This injury may persist throughout the season and only gets better when the athlete has time to rest in the off season. An orthosis with an extension to the tip of the toe to stiffen the shoe may allow the athlete to complete the season.

RETURN TO SPORT: DIFFICULT DECISIONS ON THE SIDELINES

Knee Ligament Sprain

A careful sideline examination must determine if there is any laxity of the joint. If laxity is detected, then the athlete must be sidelined. Type 1 injuries, or those with no laxity, may return to play, based on the severity of pain.

Assessment of the ACL is the most difficult, due to muscle guarding that protects the joint. You may have to do the Lachman test several times to catch the athlete relaxed. The initial examination before the swelling has started to accumulate is the most accurate and gives the best opportunity to make the diagnosis early. The drop leg Lachman test is an effective method to relax the hamstrings after acute injury.

Acromioclavicular Joint Injury

If there is no significant prominence of the outer end of the clavicle, type 1 injury, the athlete may return to play. Make sure that you stress the joint by adduction of the shoulder or by longitudinal traction to examine for mobility of the outer end of the clavicle.

Shoulder Dislocation

If this is a first-time dislocation that reduces, the athlete should be protected and kept out of play. If this is a recurrent dislocation that reduces easily, and the athlete has minimal pain and a good range of motion, he or she may return to play as pain dictates.

Hamstring Injury

Return to play after a hamstring injury is a difficult assessment. After a period of rest and icing, have the athlete run on the sidelines to assess the degree of functional impairment. If the strain is grade 1, and they are able to run, cut, and stop, then they may return to sport. Often this call is made by the athlete, who feels that they are unable to perform satisfactorily.

Quadriceps Contusion

Quadriceps contusions are similar to hamstrings strains. Minor injuries may be iced, wrapped, and the athlete returned to play. An athlete with a serious quadriceps hematoma with less than 90° of knee flexion should be removed from the game. This injury may take up to 6–8 weeks to return to play.

SPECIFIC INJURIES NOT TO MISS

Be overcautious and have a high index of suspicion for these injuries. Always think the worst-case scenario. If you always have these injuries in mind, you will not overlook them.

- Cervical spine injuries
- Anterior cruciate ligament injuries
- Occult fractures—scaphoid
- Compartment syndrome
- Cerebral concussion
- Exertional heat stroke

32 | Baseball Injuries

Borna Meisami, Richard G. Clarnette, Chris Hand, and Anthony Miniaci

QUICK LOOK

- The focus is the chronic and overuse injuries specifically related to baseball.
- Emphasis on those areas where diagnosis and treatment may be difficult.
- The mechanics of throwing is discussed in detail to understanding how most chronic injuries occur.
- Review specific injuries of the shoulder and elbow in adults and in the skeletally immature.

In the assessment of an injured baseball player of any age at any level, the physician must have a thorough and systematic approach to arrive at the correct diagnosis. In the acute setting on must rule out fractures, dislocations, ligament injuries, and musculotendinous injuries. In those with chronic symptoms, the differential diagnosis may include the following: stress fractures, osteochondral lesions, arthritic conditions, joint instability and subluxation, neuropathies, and tendonitis or tendinopathy.

THROWING

Throwing is a very important aspect of baseball for all players involved, not exclusively for the pitcher. Most chronic and overuse injuries in baseball are caused by throwing; it is an activity that has been extensively researched by many authors using electromyographic (EMG) analysis (Andrews et al., 1995; Hancock and Hawkins, 1996; Jobe et al., 1984). Studies have been performed on both professional and amateur pitchers, allowing interesting comparisons between the two groups. The pitch motion is a continuous flowing motion, but for the purpose of description and analysis it can be divided into five stages (Figs 32-1, 32-2, and 32-3) (Hancock and Hawkins, 1996).

Stage 1: Windup

The *windup* occurs from the initial movement until the ball leaves the gloved hand. This is a very important phase whereby the leading leg is lifted and the pitcher's center of gravity is placed over the pitching rubber. From here the pitcher is well balanced to move into the cocking phase. There is little strain on any particular muscle group during this phase.

Stage 2: Early Cocking

This phase begins when the ball leaves the gloved hand and ends as the front foot strikes the ground. During this phase the arm is elevated and abducted to 90° together with early external rotation of the shoulder. EMG studies show the deltoid is the dominant upper limb muscle during this phase and mainly acts to hold the shoulder in abduction (Jobe et al., 1983). During this phase there is also a lot of lower limb and trunk activity. The pelvis rotates toward the target, causing a coiling effect on the trunk. The leading leg is powerfully extended toward the home plate, which increases the coiling effect.

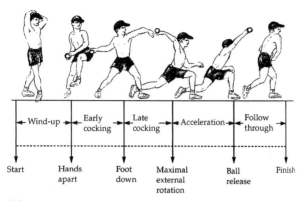

FIG 32-1 The five phases of pitching.

Stage 3: Late Cocking

This phase begins as the front foot contacts the ground and ends with the first forward motion of the ball. During this phase the enormous amount of energy that has been built up in coiling of the trunk is now transferred to the arm. As the trunk and lower body unwind and begin to translate toward the home plate, the hand and ball remain relatively motionless. To allow this to occur, the shoulder moves into a position of extreme external rotation. At the beginning of this phase the shoulder is usually in a position of approximately 90° of abduction and 90–120° of external rotation and by the end of the late cocking maximal external rotation will be reached that may be up to 180°. In nonathletes, 90° of shoulder external rotation is considered normal; therefore, one can begin to appreciate the enormous stress being placed on the pitcher's shoulder as it is rotated externally to almost 180°.

It is during this phase, as the shoulder and trunk move ahead of the hand and forearm, that the elbow, which is flexed to approximately 90°, is put under an extreme valgus load that stretches the medical structures and compresses the lateral structures. EMG studies show an enormous amount of rotator cuff activity during this phase. Infraspinatus and teres minor work concentrically during stage 2, acting as external rotators of the shoulder. During late cocking their activity peaks as these muscles function to stabilize the humeral head and draw it posteriorly, thus protecting against anterior subluxation. Supraspinatus contracts isometrically to help with humeral head stabilization. Subscapularis is inactive initially but then undergoes its peak activity late in stage 3 as it contracts eccentrically to decelerate the external rotation and protect the anterior of the joint from ligament damage and subluxation. Latissimus dorsi and pectoralis major also act eccentrically during late cocking to decelerate the external rotation of the humerus (Jobe et al., 1984).

Stage 4: Acceleration

This phase begins with the first forward motion of the ball, which corresponds to the beginning of internal rotation of the humerus. The angular velocity achieved here is up to 7000° per second, and the ball velocity goes from 0–90 miles per hour in about 50 milliseconds. The large amount of

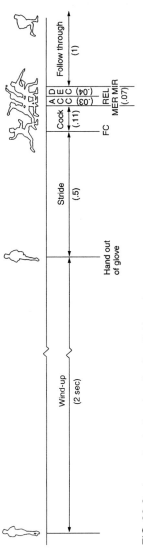

FIG 32-2 Approximate time lengths for pitching phases.

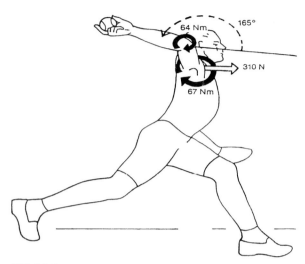

FIG 32-3   Rotation of shoulder in throwing motion.

energy stored in the previous stages is transferred to the ball during this phase with surprisingly little muscle activity required.

Strong contraction of triceps muscle forces the elbow into rapid extension, at velocities averaging over 4000° per second. During this phase the triceps muscle, its tendon, and the olecranon are all exposed to injury.

EMG studies show that the rotator cuff muscles of professional pitchers are relatively inactive during this phase, although in injured and amateur pitchers this is often not the case. It has been shown that amateurs have high levels of activity in both the rotator cuff and the biceps during the acceleration phase, and this may predispose them to an increased likelihood of overuse injuries and possibly to superior labral injuries (Fleisig et al., 1995).

The major activity in professional athletes is in the pectoralis major and latissimus dorsi, which act concentrically to accelerate the humerus into internal rotation. Triceps activity is also maximal during this phase, acting to extend the elbow, but it begins to fire in late cocking and may have some role in helping to stabilize the shoulder by its long head attachment (Jobe et al., 1984).

Stage 5: Follow Through

This phase begins with ball release and ends when motion ceases. It is a very violent phase as the muscles of the upper limb attempt to resist the 200-lb outward force on the arm, mostly by the use of powerful eccentric contraction. Despite the strong contraction of the biceps, the elbow still reaches full extension, and at this point, the olecranon strikes the olecranon fossa of the humerus.

EMG studies show activity particularly in the rotator cuff muscles, which act to stabilize and decelerate the glenohumeral joint, and also in the trapezius, serratus anterior, and the rhomboid muscles, which control and decelerate the scapula. Teres minor is particularly active in this phase as it contracts eccentrically to decelerate the humerus, which is forcefully rotating internally at this point (Hancock and Hawkins, 1996).

Biceps and brachialis have been shown to fire synchronously through this stage and are thought to act mainly to decelerate the elbow, which is undergoing quite violent extension (Basmajian and Latif, 1957; Jobe et al., 1983). The strong pull of the biceps may be important in the development of labral and superior labrum from anterior to posterior (SLAP) lesions in the shoulder (Fleisig et al., 1995; Snyder et al, 1990).

Understanding the mechanics of throwing helps the clinician to appreciate the extreme forces placed on the bones, ligaments, and muscles of the body. It is known that eccentric loading of muscles places them at most risk of injury and that is partly why the act of throwing is so stressful, particularly on the rotator cuff. If the rotator cuff is weakened or injured, then more stress is placed on the static stabilizers, especially the glenoid labrum and the anterior glenohumeral ligaments (Fleisig et al., 1995). The untrained or injured athlete often places even more stress on the rotator cuff and biceps as they attempt to compensate for a deficiency in technique or shield an injury (Glousman, 1993). This may lead to an overuse injury and tendonitis of the rotator cuff that weakens the rotator cuff and thereby predisposes the individual to further damage to the ligaments of the shoulder. Instability, through physiologic laxity or pathologic ligament damage, can then allow secondary rotator cuff damage owing to impingement, and thus a vicious cycle is entered (Jobe, 1996).

In the elbow, pathology occurs owing to tension on the medial side of the joint, compression on the lateral side of the joint, and impaction posteriorly. The region of the joint most affected is partly determined by the age of the individual and their skeletal maturity, as these factors determine which anatomic structures are most vulnerable.

EPIDEMIOLOGY

Baseball is one of the most popular sports in North America. In 1981 there were estimated to be approximately 13,000,000 children playing baseball. Approximately half of the amateur players are aged between 6 and 12. The number of amateurs playing some form of organized baseball had risen to estimated 16 million in the United States by 2000 (Yen and Metzl, 2000). A survey of over 2800 Little League baseball players in 1994 concluded that baseball was a safe activity with low rate of injury (Pasternack et al., 1996.). Severe injuries occurred in only 11 cases, giving a rate of only 0.08 severe injuries per 1000 player-hours. Impacts by the ball caused more than half of the severe injuries and were usually facial. There have been several cases of fatal comotio cordis associated with youth baseball, but it is a rare injury. Overuse injuries were generally not severe but accounted for 19% of the injuries incurred.

SHOULDER INJURIES IN ADULTS

Throwing places very high demands on the shoulder, and in the pursuit of speed the anatomic structures of the shoulder are put under loads that may be greater than can be tolerated. The shoulder enjoys the greatest freedom of motion of any joint, and this is owing largely to the lack of bony congruity between the humeral head and glenoid. The shoulder is mainly reliant on the ligaments and muscles to give it stability, and in particular the superior, middle, and inferior glenohumeral ligaments and the rotator cuff muscles play a key role. Athletes and especially throwing athletes tend to have relatively lax ligaments, allowing them the advantage of an increased range of motion, but putting them at increased risk of instability. Throwing injuries in skeletally mature athletes can be grouped into two main categories: macrotrauma and microtrauma (Jobe, 1996).

Macrotraumatic injuries, such as acute rotator cuff tears, acute shoulder dislocations, and fractures, are generally specific events that are relatively simple to diagnose. A large rotator cuff tear in a throwing athlete is likely to require investigation and surgical repair to optimize the final result. Dislocations require reduction and a short period of immobilization, but the risk of subsequent instability in young athletes is very high and surgical intervention will probably be required.

Microtraumatic or *overuse injuries* are more common; they tend to be insidious in their onset and may be difficult to diagnose. In understanding the biomechanics of throwing, one can appreciate those structures most at risk of failure. The rotator cuff is placed under extreme loads and often contracts eccentrically, which puts it under even greater stress. Subscapularis is loaded maximally in late cocking and teres minor in the follow-through stage. Tendonitis, fatigue, or failure of the rotator cuff leads to further stress on the glenohumeral ligaments, particularly in the anterior quadrants. Excessive external rotation with reduced internal rotation of the shoulder is a common finding in pitchers and is presumably an adaptive phenomenon that allows greater velocity to be achieved. This, however, results in posterior capsular tightness that forces the center of rotation anteriorly, and this places further stress on the anterior ligaments and predisposes to impingement.

IMPINGEMENT AND INSTABILITY

These entities are discussed together, because they are interrelated and interdependent. *Subacromial impingement* was described by Neer (1973, 1983) and refers to the impingement of the superior portion of the rotator cuff against the anterior acromion and coracoacromial ligament. Bigliani's work (1986) showed that hooked acromions were more commonly associated with rotator cuff tears, and this added support to the concept of a mechanical injury occurring as the rotator cuff was impinging against the anterior acromion.

Associated with the mechanical impingement are subacromial and acromioclavicular spurs, subacromial adhesions, fibrosis, and bursal-sided partial-thickness tears. This type of impingement syndrome is usually seen patients over the age of 40 unless there is an anatomic variant, such as an os acromiale. Based on this, Neer (1972, 1983) described the anterior acromioplasty, and given the appropriate pathology good results have been achieved with this operative technique.

Unfortunately, shoulder pain became synonymous with *impingement*, and this led to some patients being treated inappropriately. In young, overhead throwing athletes treated with anterior acromioplasty, whether open or arthroscopic, fewer than 50% of cases were achieving good results and returning to their sports, leading to the conclusion that the pathology was different in this group of patients (Glousman, 1993; Tibone et al., 1985).

Pathophysiology

It is now clear that there are different types of impingement requiring different treatment regimes as discussed in the following sections (Jobe, 1996).

Classic Anterior Impingement

This is impingement syndrome as described by Neer (1972). It is rare under the age of 40 years and in throwing athletes, and therefore the clinician should consider other types of impingement syndrome. Anatomic variations, such as an unstable os acromiale or a type III (hooked) acromion, need to be excluded, because they will predispose an individual to this type of impingement.

Anterior Impingement Secondary to Tight Posterior Capsule or Instability

Posterior capsular tightness is a common finding in throwing athletes and can be recognized by an excess range of external rotation with a limited range of internal rotation. Its effect is to shift the center of rotation anteriorly and predispose the individual to anterior impingement. Ligamentous laxity particularly in an anterior direction can also result in secondary anterior impingement. Acromioplasty and coracoacromial ligament resection are contraindicated in these instances, because it further destabilizes the shoulder.

Internal Impingement (Superior Glenoid Impingement)

More recently, the concept of internal impingement has been recognized, and this is especially important in throwing athletes (Jobe, 1997; Walch et al., 1992). Arthroscopic examination in many of these individuals did not show subacromial bursitis or bursal-sided rotator cuff pathology, but instead revealed incomplete articular-sided tears of the posterosuperior cuff, injury, and reaction of the posterosuperior labrum. This is owing to internal impingement of the cuff against the glenoid and occurs with the arm in abduction and external rotation. (This can be visualized arthroscopically.) Bony changes on the greater tuberosity and posterosuperior glenoid were also occasionally seen.

The relationship that this type of impingement has with instability is not yet fully established. Jobe (1996) believes weakness of subscapular or incompetence of the inferior glenohumeral ligament results in hyperangulation and inferior subluxation of the shoulder during abduction and external rotation and that this allows impingement of the rotator cuff against the glenoid.

Pure instability can also occur without impingement and can be classified according to direction (anterior, posterior, inferior, or multidirectional), etiology (traumatic or atraumatic), frequency (acute, recurrent, or chronic), degree (subluxation or dislocation), and volition (Cofield and Irving, 1987). Typically, the throwing athlete has anteroinferior or multidirectional instability that is atraumatic (owing to overuse).

Having recognized that there is a spectrum of pathology from pure impingement to pure instability, Jobe and colleagues have classified throwing athletes with shoulder pain into four groups (Glousman, 1993; Jobe et al., 1990).

- *Group 1:* pain secondary to pure impingement
- *Group 2:* pain secondary to instability owing to anterior ligament and labral injury with secondary impingement
- *Group 3:* pain secondary to instability owing to hyperelastic capsular ligaments with secondary impingement
- *Group 4:* pain secondary to pure instability without secondary impingement

Evaluation

Anterior impingement with rotator cuff tendonitis is suggested by shoulder pain related to overhead activities and often by night pain. There is tenderness along the subacromial bursa, a painful abduction arc, and positive impingement test as described by Neer and Hawkins (Hawkins and Kennedy, 1980; Neer, 1983; Neer and Welsh, 1997).

Superior glenoid impingement gives a slightly different clinical picture, with chronic dorsal shoulder pain that is characteristically worse in the acceleration phase of the pitch when the impingement is maximal (Jobe 1996). Examination reveals tenderness along the posterior joint line with impingement in a position of 90° of abduction together with full external rotation and horizontal extension. This is the same arm position used to test for anterior instability in the apprehension test, although with superior impingement the athlete experiences pain rather than apprehension. Applying a posterior force to the proximal humerus while repeating the test often reduces the pain in much the same way as apprehension can be reduced using the relocation test in a patient with anterior instability (Kvitne and Jobe, 1993).

Rotator cuff tears are unusual in young athletes, but can occur and are suggested by atrophy and weakness of the rotator cuff. Subscapularis is best assessed using the liftoff test, as described by Gerber and Krushell (1991). This is performed with the arm internally rotated so that the dorsal surface of the hand rests on the lower back. Actively lifting the hand away from the back and resisting force suggests integrity of the subscapularis. The external rotators, teres minor, and infraspinatus can be tested with the arm by the side and elbow flexed to 90°. In this position impingement should not be present so that painful inhibition of muscle activity is eliminated. Supraspinatus can be most effectively isolated and tested with arms in 90° of scapular elevation and full internal rotation.

Instability usually takes the form of repeated transient subluxations that may be symptomatic to the athlete as a feeling of instability with the shoulder feeling loose, or it may cause pain that is usually felt over the posterior aspect of the shoulder in the late cocking or early acceleration phase. Occasionally, the subluxation may cause momentary traction on the brachial plexus giving rise to *dead arm syndrome* (Leffert and Gumley, 1987). On examination, shoulder instability may be anterior, posterior, or inferior. It may be very obvious and easy to demonstrate, or it may be very subtle and difficult to diagnose. In all cases one needs a relaxed, cooperative patient and a gentle technique.

In the shoulder it is difficult to know if the translation felt is subluxation to an abnormal position or relocation to a normal position. It is also important to remember that a normal shoulder has a degree of physiologic laxity and can translate significantly, and this can be particularly evident under anesthesia (Harryman et al., 1995). Comparison to the opposite side is vital, as is very careful palpation to feel when the joint is properly located (Miniaci et al., 1995). Subluxation, apprehension, and the reproduction of the patient's pain may all be positive examination findings. The following examination, tests are used to determine the degree and direction of instability.

Load-and-Shift Test

With the patient comfortably seated and with hands in the lap, one can perform the anteroposterior translation or load-and-shift test. To perform this test the right humeral head is grasped with the right hand, while the left hand is positioned over the top of the shoulder girdle so that the scapula can be stabilized. Simultaneously, the posterior joint line is palpated with the thumb while the anterior shoulder is palpated with the index and middle fingers. The right hand then loads the joint to ensure concentric reduction and then applies anterior and posterior shearing forces. The direction and amount of translation can then be determined and graded using a scale of 0–3 (grade 0 for no instability; grade 1 for mild translation of less than 1 cm; grade 2 for moderate translation of 1–2 cm, or to the glenoid rim; and grade 3 for severe translation of greater than 2 cm, or over the glenoid rim). The fingers of the left hand should be positioned with the middle finger on the coracoid and index finger on the humeral head. In this way abnormal anterior translation can be appreciated, as the index finger moves forward relative to the middle finger. To perform the apprehension test, move the right hand to the patient's right wrist and keep the left hand on the shoulder. With the arm in adduction and internal rotation the shoulder will not be anteriorly subluxated. From this position bring the arm into abduction and external rotation while using the left hand to palpate any anterior subluxation (Leffert and Gumley, 1987). Using the left thumb to push the humeral head forward can augment the test.

Apprehension (Crank) Test and Relocation Test

The remaining tests are best performed with the patient supine with the shoulder brought just beyond the edge of the examination table beginning with the apprehension or crank test. The test is performed by external rotation of the abducted arm. Classically, it is performed with the arm at 90° of abduction, but this can be varied to stress different portions of the glenohumeral ligament complex. While one hand rotates and abducts the arm, the other should be used to palpate the anterior and posterior shoulder to reference the direction of any movement. The test can be augmented by pushing the humeral head anteriorly from behind. Finally, the relocation test can be performed by pushing posteriorly on the upper part of the humerus. This part of the test is positive if the apprehension of pain is relieved, thereby allowing further external rotation before reemergence of the patient's symptoms. Patients with classical anterior impingement often experience pain without apprehension during the apprehension test, with the pain being relieved by the relocation maneuver.

Sulcus Sign

Applying inferior traction to the arm assesses inferior instability. Gross instability is demonstrated by visible widening of the subacromial space with a sulcus appearing in the adjacent area just distal to the lateral acromion (*sulcus sign*). It is important to remember that normal shoulders can translate significantly (Harryman et al., 1990). It is also important to appreciate the significance of generalized ligamentous laxity, particularly in patients with multidirectional instability. The examiner should test for this by looking for elbow, finger, and thumb hyperextension together with knee recurvatum and increased ankle dorsiflexion.

Posterior Apprehension

Posterior apprehension is elicited by maximally internally rotating the humerus with the shoulder in 90° of abduction and then applying a posteriorly directed force on the humeral head. In a positive test the patient feels as if the shoulder is about to dislocate. O'Driscoll (1991) found this test to be highly sensitive and specific for posterior shoulder instability. It can be differentiated from impingement by the absence of relief after injecting local anesthetic into the subacromial space. Often, however, posterior instability is not associated with pain or apprehension, and so most clinical tests rely on the detection of the subluxation that occurs in certain arm positions.

Posterior Subluxation Testing

Posterior subluxation usually occurs with the arm in adduction and internal rotation combined with some degree of flexion. Abduction and external rotation relocate the subluxated shoulder. This test, devised by the senior author, utilizes these observations in a clinical test similar to Ortolani's test for hip subluxation. To assess the right shoulder, the examiner stands in the axillary region of the patient who is supine with the right shoulder off the edge of the bed. The examiner's left hand takes the elbow and positions the arm in a position of adduction, internal rotation, and 70–90° of flexion. The examiner's right hand is positioned over the top of the shoulder with the thumb on the anterior shoulder and fingers on the posterior joint line. With the arm in this position, the thumb of the right hand is used to apply a posterior force on the humeral head to achieve posterior subluxation. With the shoulder subluxated the humeral head fills the normal hollow that is present below the acromion. From this position the arm is brought out slowly into abduction and external rotation and will, at some point, relocate with a clunk, which is palpable with the right hand.

Investigation

Routine radiographic evaluations are an essential component of the assessment and should include an anteroposterior, axillary, and lateral view of the shoulder in the plane of the scapula. These can be supplemented with the caudal-tilt view (a 10° tilt of the x-ray beam) for assessing the supraspinatus outlet (Neer and Welsh, 1977). Pathologic findings predisposing to impingement include subacromial spurs, acromioclavicular spurs, a hooked acromion, or an os acromiale. Evidence of instability may include a bony Bankart lesion, glenoid erosion, a Hill-Sachs lesion, or subluxation of the glenohumeral joint. Supplementary radiologic tests such as arthrography, CT, and MRI are usually not necessary. CT is the best modality to assess any bony defects if required. MRI is very sensitive and shows signal changes in the rotator cuff in asymptomatic individuals. It is the modality of choice in the evaluation of suspected rotator cuff tears.

Management

Group 1: Pain Secondary to Pure Impingement

This is an uncommon group of athletes, usually over the age of 35, with impingement and no instability. Treatment is initially conservative with avoidance of throwing, stretching, and rotator cuff strengthening. Only after 6–12 months of conservative treatment should surgical treatment be considered. Arthroscopic acromioplasty may then be indicated if there are acromial spurs or an acromial hook together with bursal inflammation or bursal-sided rotator cuff pathology. If the athlete has a rotator cuff tear and no instability then operative repair may be indicated if conservative measures fail or if the tear is large. The prognosis for return to the athlete's former level of performance is, however, very poor (Tibone et al., 1986).

Group 2: Pain Secondary to Instability Owing to Anterior Ligament and Labral Injury with Secondary Impingement

This group has superior or anterior impingement owing to a definite anteroinferior ligamentous or labral injury. They do not have multidirectional laxity and therefore do not have posterior subluxation. Initial treatment is conservative with rest from throwing activities and anti-inflammatory medication to resolve the rotator cuff tendonitis. This is followed by therapy with particular emphasis on rotator cuff strengthening, scapular stabilization, and posterior stretching. This leads to an improvement in some; however, others fail, especially if they have significant structural pathology, such as a large Bankart or Hill-Sachs lesion. Surgery may then be indicated in the form of a capsulolabral repair (unless there are very large bony defects requiring more complex reconstructive surgery).

Group 3: Pain Secondary to Instability Owing to Hyperelastic Capsular Ligaments with Secondary Impingement

This group is similar to group 2 except they tend to have multidirectional laxity that affects both shoulders and often have generalized ligamentous laxity. They also have features of rotator cuff tendonitis and impingement. For this group, nonoperative treatment is the mainstay of therapy with emphasis on rotator cuff strengthening and scapular stabilization. Surgery may be indicated if there is failure of nonoperative management, but without a discrete pathologic entity and in the face of laxity in all the ligaments, success cannot be guaranteed. Surgery usually takes the form of a capsulolabral reconstruction together with a capsular shift to effectively tighten the ligaments. In this case the balance between obtaining stability and not over-tightening the shoulder is difficult to achieve. The other concern is that tightening the anterior structures alone may accentuate a previous and subtle posterior instability. It is partly owing to these technical difficulties that nonoperative treatment is pursued so vigorously in these cases.

Group 4: Pain Secondary to Pure Instability without Secondary Impingement

These athletes have instability without impingement. If the instability is multidirectional and associated with generalized ligamentous laxity as in group 3, then they are managed along similar guidelines with emphasis on nonoperative management. If they have a more discrete pathologic lesion such as a Bankart lesion, they are more likely to fail nonoperative management and have a better prognosis with surgery.

SUPERIOR LABRAL AND BICEPS LESIONS

The long head of biceps tendon runs up the bicipital groove under the transverse ligament and then runs through the shoulder joint to attach to the superior glenoid via the superior labrum. The biceps tendon and superior labrum can be involved in various pathologic processes, including bicipital tendonitis, biceps rupture, biceps tendon subluxation or dislocation, and tears of the superior labrum. Since the advent of arthroscopy, lesions of the superior labrum and biceps anchor have been more clearly defined and classified (Snyder et al., 1990).

Pathophysiology

Throwing is associated with high activity in biceps, and this is thought to predispose the athlete to superior labral tears, including SLAP lesions (Fig. 32-4).

Evaluation

Superior labral lesions are often associated with instability, and the symptoms may be nonspecific. Anterior shoulder pain, clicking, and popping may, however, be due to labral or biceps lesion (Snyder et al., 1990). The following tests may help to isolate biceps or labral pathology.

Yergason's Test

In this test the elbow is flexed to 90° and the forearm is pronated (Yergason, 1931). At this point the examiner holds the patient's wrist to resist active supination by the patient. Pain in the bicipital groove is a positive test and indicates possible wear or tendonitis of the biceps tendon.

Speed's Test

This involves having the patient forward flex the shoulder against resistance while maintaining the elbow in extension and the forearm in supination. Pain or tenderness in the bicipital groove indicates bicipital tendonitis. Field and Savoie (1993) found this test to cause nonspecific shoulder pain in all of their series of patients with superior labral lesions, suggesting that it does test for the competence of the biceps anchor.

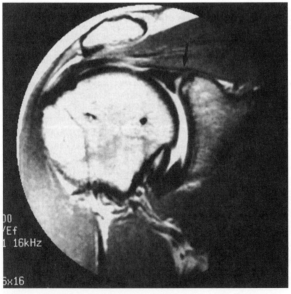

FIG 32-4 Slap lesion (superior labral tears from anterior to posterior).

Clunk Test

The clunk test has been described, whereby the arm is rotated and loaded from a position of extension to one of forward flexion. A clunk-like sensation may be felt if a free labral fragment is caught in the joint. This test is similar to the McMurray's test of the knee. Studies have shown that a click on manipulation of the glenohumeral joint is a common finding in patients with labral tears even in the absence of joint instability (Glascow et al., 1992; Liu et al., 1996).

Investigation

These lesions are difficult to diagnose and certain investigations may be very valuable. Usually contrast is required to show the pathology with any degree of sensitivity. CT arthrography and MR arthrography have both been shown to be effective.

Management

Treatment depends on the degree of damage to the labrum and the stability of the biceps. In many cases involving young athletes there is superior labral damage and associated mechanical instability of the biceps anchor requiring fixation (Rames and Karzel, 1993). In most cases repairs of this type can be achieved arthroscopically.

BENNET LESION

Posterior ossification of the shoulder is a lesion first described by Bennett in 1947 (Fig. 32-5). He described a deposit of bone on the posterior inferior border of glenoid fossa that he thought was owing to traction by the origin of the long head of triceps and was an exostosis. He believed the

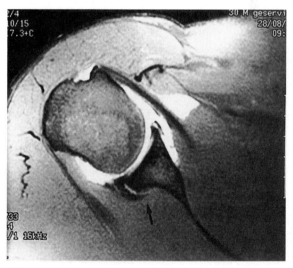

FIG 32-5   Bennett lesion.

lesion caused symptoms by local irritation of the capsule, synovium, and axillary nerve. Further studies using arthrography, CT, MRI, arthroscopy, and histologic evidence have provided further knowledge. The lesion is extra-articular, in the region of the posterior band of the inferior gleno-humeral ligament complex (IGHLC) and is not related to the long head of the biceps (Ferrari et al., 1994; O'Brien et al., 1990). The lesion is commonly associated with intra-articular pathology, most commonly tears of the posterosuperior labrum, but also posteroinferior labral tears, posterior instability, and posterior undersurface rotator cuff tears (Ferrari et al., 1994). Histologic and MRI studies have not demonstrated any cancelous bone or bone marrow, and this suggests that the lesion is neither an exostosis nor an osteophyte. It has been shown to be reactive new bone formation at capsular insertion to the posterior glenoid.

Pathophysiology

The cause of the lesion remains unclear, but it seems most likely to be owing to traction on the posterior band of the IGHLC, either during late cocking when subscapularis contraction may cause posterior subluxation of the glenohumeral joint, or during follow-through when there are large distractive forces on these ligaments.

Evaluation

Symptoms may be gradual in onset or develop suddenly (Bennett, 1947). Pain is felt posteriorly with occasional radiation to the deltoid region. Pitchers can throw hard only for a limited time, and as pain increases performance declines. Often the shoulder is asymptomatic and functions normally unless the athlete attempts to throw hard. In a series of seven pitchers with Bennett lesions, all had posterior shoulder pain, mostly in the follow-through phase of the pitch; some experienced it only during cocking. All had posterior glenoid tenderness, two had evidence of posterior instability, and none exhibited any anterior instability (Ferrari et al., 1994).

Investigation

The lesion cannot usually be seen on standard shoulder radiographs. A modified anteroposterior radiograph with the arm in 90° of abduction and in maximal external rotation and the beam tilted 5° cephalad brings the abnormal area of the glenoid into relief (Bennett, 1947). CT is the investigation of choice to demonstrate the bony abnormality and shows extra-articular curvilinear calcification originating from the posterior inferior glenoid extending toward the humeral head. MRI shows the lesion, although it is not as good as CT in demonstrating cortical bone. It is, however, more sensitive in defining the commonly associated intra-articular pathology, particularly if combined with arthrographic techniques.

Management

Bennett (1959) described how the lesion could be approached and removed using a posterior approach to the shoulder but stated that operative treatment was not advisable. There is no agreement as to the cause or treatment of the lesion. Most agree that a trial of nonoperative management involving rest, nonsteroidal anti-inflammatory drugs (NSAIDs), and rehabilitation should be undertaken before anything more aggressive is considered. Lombardo et al. (1977) reported on a series of four pitchers who failed nonoperative treatment and underwent open posterior excision of the lesion with "encouraging" results. It is not clearly stated if they returned to their former level of competition. In Ferrari et al.'s (1994) series of seven pitchers (six professional) all but one returned to their former level of performance after surgery, which involved arthroscopy and treatment of the intra-articular pathology without visualization or treatment of the lesion itself.

SHOULDER INJURIES IN CHILDREN

Even though the elbow is more commonly affected in skeletally immature baseball players than the shoulder, significant lesions can occur at this site owing to the unique stresses encountered as a result of pitching. The pathology seen in children is different from adults owing to the presence of growth plates, which are weaker than the surrounding ligaments and joint capsule. The proximal humerus has three centers of ossification involving the head and the greater and lesser tuberosities, which coalesce at age 7 and fuse to the shaft at approximately 20 years. Acute injuries to the shoulder girdle can occur in baseball owing to falls and collisions, and these may result in variety of fractures and growth plate injuries.

The chronic overuse injury that occurs due to repetitive trauma associated with pitching is *Little Leaguer's shoulder*. This was first described by Dotter in 1953, who believed that the injury was owing to fracture through the proximal physeal plate. Adams (1966) reported a similar injury in five adolescent pitchers. He believed the injury was owing to a repetitive traction injury of the proximal humeral physis. All boys in his series were between 13 and 15 years of age and presented with vague shoulder pain at the end of hard throwing motions. All had over-development of the affected shoulder but there was little else to find on examination, except for occasional local tenderness and pain on jerking the outstretched arm. Comparative x-ray studies are the key to making the correct diagnosis, revealing widening of the proximal humeral epiphysis and demineralization of the proximal epiphysis, without evidence of avascular necrosis.

The condition usually responds rapidly to rest, and there is unlikely to be any long-term sequelae. Some authors have recommended that pitching be ceased until the physis has closed, although others suggest that one season of rest is usually adequate (Adams, 1966; Tibone, 1983).

ELBOW INJURIES IN ADULTS

Acute and chronic valgus and hyperextension stress produce a different set of pathologic entities in the adult than in the child. The weakest link in the growing immature elbow is the growing epiphysis and the intervening physeal plates. In the young adult it is the ligaments that tend to fail initially (Pincivero et al., 1994). The medial collateral ligament complex consists of three parts: an anterior oblique bundle, a posterior oblique bundle, and a transverse band, which is of little functional significance. The anterior oblique band arises from the medial epicondyle and inserts into the medial border of the coronoid process, and it is the primary stabilizer against valgus stress with the elbow in extension. The posterior bundle is a fan-shaped ligament that arises from the medial epicondyle and inserts into the olecranon; it is taut with the elbow in flexion (Morrey and An, 1985; Regan et al., 1991).

Repetitive forceful valgus stress is associated with the development of the medial stress syndrome that can involve a number of different pathological entities, including the valgus-extension overload syndrome, medial collateral ligament injuries, and ulnar neuritis.

Andrews and Timmerman (1995) found that in professional baseball pitchers undergoing surgery for elbow injuries, the most common types of pathology were posteromedial olecranon osteophyte, ulnar collateral ligament injury, and ulnar neuritis.

Valgus-Extension Overload

Pathophysiology

Pitching results in very high valgus and extension forces on the elbow, and this can lead to a specific impingement syndrome in the posterior compartment of the elbow. Wilson et al. (1983) drew attention to this syndrome and the importance of recognizing the medial as well as posterior osteophyte formation that occurs on the olecranon owing to attenuation of the medial ligament. Hypertrophy of the distal humerus adds to the impingement by narrowing the olecranon fossa.

Evaluation

Pain is felt posteromedially and often increases during the game. Pain is often associated with poor pitching control that the pitcher may attempt to compensate for by snapping the elbow, which may further reduce control. Localized tenderness with pain or valgus stressing in extension is the classic examination finding. There may be associated ulnar neuritis owing to impingement of the ulnar nerve on the osteophyte.

Investigation

Plain x-rays with axial images will usually demonstrate the posteromedial osteophyte formation on olecranon. Occasionally the lesion is cartilaginous and recognized only at arthroscopy.

Management

Rest and NSAIDs should be used initially to reduce any associated synovitis. An attempt should be made to improve the range of motion without producing pain using a careful stretching program. If this fails to resolve the symptoms, surgical excision is highly successful.

Medial Collateral Ligament Injuries

Pathophysiology

The anterior bundle is the most important stabilizer against valgus stress. Injury is usually a chronic overuse syndrome but may be an acute event.

Evaluation

Often there is a history of chronic medial-sided elbow pain related to throwing. Acutely there is tenderness and swelling that is maximal toward the ulnar attachment of the ligament, as this is where the ligament avulsion occurs. Stability testing of the medial collateral ligament can be performed by applying a valgus stress to the elbow held in approximately 25° of flexion, which unlocks the olecranon from its fossa. The clinician must look carefully for evidence of ulnar neuritis, which is often associated.

Investigation

Stress views comparing both elbows often aid in confirmation of the diagnosis. X-rays may show spur formation in the region of the coronoid process of the ulna and calcification in the region of the medial ligament. A quite distinctive change seen in baseball pitchers is single or multiple ossicles of bone seen along the course of the medial ligament (Bennett, 1959).

Treatment

Most athletes are managed conservatively with a period of rest, ice, and NSAIDs, followed by therapy to regain motion and strength. Chronic instability with pain and inability to throw after 6 months of conservative therapy may be an indication for ligament repair or reconstruction. Jobe et al. (1986) reported that 10 out of 16 throwing athletes returned to their former level of sport after a ligament reconstruction using autologous tendon grafts.

Ulnar Neuritis

Pathophysiology

Ulnar neuritis is common in throwing and pitching athletes and is usually owing to mechanical irritation, which can be from repetitive tension, compression, or friction. In the arm the nerve passes from the extensor compartment to the flexor compartment about 8–10 cm above the elbow joint. Here it passes through the fibrous arcade of Struthers where it may be compressed. It passes distally to course posterior to the medial epicondyle and enters the cubital tunnel. Within this tunnel the nerve lies adjacent to the medial epicondyle and medial edge of trochlea and is roofed by the triangular arcuate ligament, which extends from the medial border of the olecranon to the medial epicondyle. After exiting the tunnel the nerve then passes between the two heads of flexor carpi ulnaris. Compression of the nerve can occur at any point along its course but in the case of throwing athletes one of several pathologic entities tends to occur:

1. Traction neuritis may exist due to valgus deformity of valgus instability.
2. Compression of the nerve against posteromedial osteophytes that is seen as part of the valgus extension overload (Wadsworth, 1977).
3. Subluxation of the nerve with friction of the ulnar nerve (Wadsworth, 1977).

Evaluation

Usually there is insidious onset of ulnar-sided elbow pain with associated paresthesia in the ulnar nerve distribution. Examination may reveal tenderness or instability of the nerve at the elbow together with a positive Tinel's sign. Neurologic abnormalities may be present, but are often subtle or absent.

Investigation

Radiographs of the elbow may reveal spur formation or calcification in the region of the ulnar nerve or medial collateral ligament. EMG studies should be done but may be negative in up to half of the cases.

Management

Initial treatment involves rest, activity modification, and NSAIDs followed by therapy, particularly aimed at strengthening of the flexor and pronator groups. The likelihood of resolution if symptoms are chronic is relatively poor, and surgery may be indicated. This usually involves anterior transposition of the nerve.

ELBOW INJURIES IN CHILDREN AND ADOLESCENTS

Chronic conditions affecting the elbow are rare in the general population but are relatively common among baseball players owing to the stress of throwing. The elbow is the most frequent area of complaint in children and adolescent baseball players (Gugenheim et al., 1976). As previously outlined, the main forces are tensile on the medial side of the elbow and compressive on the lateral and posterior aspects of the elbow.

Little Leaguer's elbow describes the abnormal changes that occur in the pitching elbows of the skeletally immature. It may refer to medial epicondylar abnormalities (accelerated growth and separation or fragmentation of the epiphysis), osteochondritis of the capitellum, or osteochondritis of the radial head in any combination (Adams, 1965).

It is important to have some understanding of the way the elbow ossifies and the order in which the epiphyses appear and fuse. At birth the entire elbow is a radiolucent cartilaginous anlage. During childhood the different regions of the elbow undergo ossification in a predictable sequence starting with the capitellum, which begins to ossify at approximately 2 years of age. This is followed by ossification in the radial head epiphysis at about 4–5 years, the medial epicondylar epiphysis at about 5–7 years, the trochlear epiphysis at 8–9 years, and the lateral epicondyle and olecranon that appear between 9 and 11 years of age. There is quite a significant amount of variation, depending on the physiologic maturity of the individual; for this reason the epiphyses tend to appear earlier in girls. Fusion of the ossified epiphyses to the shaft of the bone occurs at between the ages of 13 and 16 in boys and 11 and 14 in girls, with the trochlea being the first to fuse (Pappas, 1982). Pappas uses skeletal maturity to define three stages of development that render the elbow susceptible to different pathologic processes.

1. *Childhood*—This includes children up to the age of about 11–12, when the secondary ossification centers are appearing but have not yet fused to the shaft. During this time the cartilage anlage is being vascularized and ossified, and is highly vulnerable to excess physical forces. Injury at this time is likely to cause degeneration and necrosis of the epiphysis followed later by regeneration. This is an osteochondrosis and it may affect the medial epicondyle, olecranon, trochlea, or capitellum. Osteochondrosis of the capitellum is known as *Panner's disease*.

2. *Adolescence*—This is the period that begins when all secondary centers have appeared and ends when all long bones physes have fused (up to the age of approximately 14 in girls and 17 in boys). In this time period, the secondary center has been formed and is now most vulnerable at its periphery, which is at its junction with the physis (growth plate) and at its articular surface. Injury at this time results in subchondral avascular necrosis (osteochondritis dissecans), which usually affects the capitellum, and physeal separations and nonunions, which usually affect the medial epicondyle or olecranon.

3. *Young adult*—This period encompasses the first 3–5 years after closure of the physes. During this period we begin to see the emergence of adult

types of pathology, but one can still see late presentations and sequelae of the adolescent problems.

Osteochondritis Dissecans of the Capitellum

Pathophysiology

In this condition there is fragmentation and possible separation of a portion of the articular surface (Pappas, 1982). Repetitive compressive and shearing forces are thought to be important etiologic factors (Clanton and DeLee, 1982; Pappas, 1982). In adolescents it is commonly seen in conjunction with abnormalities of the medial epicondyle together with enlargement and deformity of the radial head, and it is then often called *Little Leaguer's elbow* (Adams, 1965).

Evaluation

The first symptom may be pain after a season of pitching, which later becomes more severe and activity related, and may be associated with intermittent swelling. As the disease progresses there is often a loss of full extension followed by the loss of pronation and supination. Catching, locking, and intermittent severe pain suggest the presence of loose intra-articular fragments. Examination may reveal a joint effusion, local tenderness over the capitellum, loss of range particularly in extension, and crepitus on movement.

Investigation

Sequential changes can be seen on plain x-ray, although CT scanning may be more sensitive in evaluating the more subtle changes. Evaluation of the overlying articular cartilage requires the use of either arthrography or MRI. The earliest changes on plain radiographs are an area of subchondral rarefaction surrounded by a sclerotic rim. Later there is flattening of the capitellum seen particularly on the lateral view, followed by fragmentation and possibly the development of loose bodies (Clanton and DeLee, 1982).

Treatment

The mainstay of treatment is conservative, with rest and avoidance of throwing. This needs to continue until healing of the capitellum, which can be followed by serial x-rays taken at 6-month intervals. Arthroscopic surgery is reserved for those cases where there is evidence of loose or unstable fragments causing mechanical symptoms (Morrey, 1994).

Osteochondrosis of the Capitellum: Panner's Disease

Pathophysiology

This is abnormal growth or ossification of the capitellar epiphysis and occurs at a younger age than osteochondritis dissecans. It was first described by Panner in 1927 and was likened to Legg-Perthe's disease of the hip. It is seen most commonly in children between the ages of 5 and 10 and is more common in baseball players and gymnasts than in the general population. It is thought to occur as a result of vascular insufficiency during the critical stages of ossification.

Evaluation

Pain, local tenderness, and loss of motion are the most common features. The development of unstable or loose osteochondral fragments causing mechanical symptoms such as locking is unusual in this condition.

Investigation

The radiologic changes are similar in sequence to those occurring in Legge-Perthe's disease, with sclerosis and fragmentation followed by lucency and later by re-ossification. MRI can also be used and shows the typical sequence seen when there is avascular necrosis of bone with loss of the high signal normally seen in healthy bone marrow on T1-weighted images. These changes occur much earlier than radiographic changes.

Management

Rest and cessation of throwing activities usually result in the resolution of symptoms. Radiologic follow up until there is re-ossification and healing should occur before consideration is given to resumption of activities.

Osteochondritis of the Olecranon

Pathophysiology

The development of the condition is similar to what has already been outlined in case of capitellum.

Evaluation

These adolescents present with pain, swelling, and tenderness.

Investigation

Radiologic investigation reveals fragmentation and irregularity of the epiphysis, and in these cases comparison to the opposite side is often helpful.

Management

Treatment is symptomatic with rest and activity modification until resolution, which may take several months.

Olecranon Epiphyseal Nonunion or Stress Fracture

Pathophysiology

This is owing to failure of fusion of the olecranon physeal plate, which normally occurs at about 16 years of age in boys. It has been reported in baseball players and may be related to the repetitive stress of pitching.

Evaluation

There is pain, swelling, weakness, and tenderness present. Radiographs may show widening of the physeal line or simply failure of the epiphysis to fuse. There is considerable variation in the appearance and position of the physeal line so comparison with the opposite side is vital.

Management

Treatment initially involves a period of immobilization in an attempt to achieve union, but it may require operative fixation if this fails.

Disorders of the Medial Epicondyle

Pathophysiology

The medial epicondyle is the site of origin of the medial collateral ligament and the powerful forearm flexors. Throwing and in particular pitching place enormous stresses through this region, and in those who are skeletally immature, it is the medial epicondylar epiphysis and the intervening growth plate that are most susceptible to injury. It is also important to consider ulnar nerve pathology, which may be coexistent. The ulnar nerve may be unstable in the ulnar groove, allowing irritation and an ulnar nerve palsy to occur.

Evaluation

The overuse syndrome is characterized by insidious onset of medial-sided elbow pain with localized tenderness and pain on valgus stressing of the joint. Occasionally, an acute separation of the epiphysis can occur with sudden onset of severe pain.

Investigation

Adams (965) showed radiographic changes in 100% of Little League pitchers between the ages of 9 and 14. These changes included accelerated growth, separation, or fragmentation of the epiphysis as compared to the nonthrowing side. At least 45% of the pitchers were symptomatic but only on direct questioning, and the study concluded by recommending guidelines for young pitchers that limit the amount of pitching and abolish the throwing of curve balls, which places even more stress on the elbow.

Management

Separation of the epiphysis by 1 cm or more together with valgus instability is an indication for surgery, with open reduction and fixation of the fragment being the goal. Most cases are less severe without instability and can be managed by rest and activity modification.

CONFOUNDING CONDITIONS

Overuse of the arm, especially in the pitchers, and performing activities that unduly stress the arm are significant factors in development of chronic injuries of the upper limb. Disregard for proper fundamentals of pitching and throwing is an example of this. Introduction of off-speed pitches too early in the career of a young pitcher, which mechanically stress the elbow and shoulder, along with increased ligamentous laxity of younger players, can lead to serious and chronic injuries (Clark, 2002).

PREVENTION

Baseball is generally considered to be a safe sport. Nevertheless almost 500,000 baseball-related injuries are treated yearly in the United States. There are important preventative measures that can be utilized by parents and coaches to reduce the risk of both acute and chronic injuries. Equipment should be fitted and worn properly. This includes cleated baseball shoes and batting helmet, which should be worn while waiting to bat, at the plate, and while running the bases. Additionally, catchers should always wear a helmet, facemask, throat guard, long-molded chest protector, protective supporter, catcher's mitt, and shin guards. Position players need the appropriate baseball glove for their specific position. Facial protective devices that attach to batting helmets are available and can reduce the risk of serious facial injuries.

Stretching the muscles and taking time to perform the appropriate warm up are very important. Warm up should start with a 3- to 5-minute duration of jumping jacks, stationary cycling, or running, followed by slow and gentle stretching. Pitchers should concentrate on the shoulder, arm, and back muscles. Catchers should focus on the muscles of the legs and back.

Overuse is to be avoided, especially in pitchers. Different leagues have specific guidelines for number of pitches allowed per week. The usual number of innings allowed is between 4 and 10. The number of pitches thrown should be carefully followed. It is reasonable to aim for maximum of 80–100 pitches in a game and 30–40 pitches in a practice. Finally, one must be able to recognize the signs and symptoms of injuries such as pain, swelling, and limitation of motion. One should not attempt to "play through the pain" (American Academy of Orthopaedic Surgeons, 2003).

SIDELINE TIPS

Knowledge of first aid is important and one must be able to treat facial cuts, bruises, minor tendonitis, strains, and sprains. Ice is the universal first aid treatment and should always be available. One must remember that in children injuries that resemble sprains in adults could indeed be physeal fractures. One must have a plan for transferring the player safely to medical personnel in case of more serious injuries such as concussions, dislocations, or fractures (American Academy of Orthopaedic Surgeons).

SUMMARY

Baseball continues to be a popular sport with increasing numbers of participants over a wide age range. Falls, collisions, and direct impact injuries occur, but these are relatively easy to diagnose with appropriate diligence. Injuries that are relatively unique to baseball occur owing to repetitive chronic stress overload, most commonly owing to pitching. An understanding of the mechanics of throwing gives the clinician important insight into how these injuries occur and which anatomic structures are most at risk. The clinician also needs to appreciate how the age of the individual significantly alters the likely spectrum of pathology encountered in a given joint or region. This is because the anatomic structures that are most susceptible to injury change as the individual matures.

Appropriate injury prevention strategies are also important and can be logically developed with knowledge of the pathology that occurs with overuse, particularly in the skeletally immature, who are most susceptible to long-term complications, especially in the elbow joint.

REFERENCES

Adams JE. Injury to the throwing arm: A study of traumatic changes in the elbow joint of boy baseball players. *Cal Med*. 1965;102:127–132.

Adams JE. Little league shoulder: Osteochondrosis of the proximal humeral epiphysis in boy baseball pitchers. *Calif Med*. 1966;105:22–25.

American Academy of Orthopaedic Surgeons. Tips to prevent baseball injuries. *Prevent Injuries America*. 2003. Accessed April 2, 2003 from URL: orthoinfo.aaos.org/category.cfm

Andrews JR, Timmerman LA. Outcome of elbow surgery in professional baseball players. *Am J Sports Med.* 1995;23:407–413.

Andrews JR, Timmerman LA, Wilk KE. Baseball. In: Petrone FA, ed. *Athletic injuries of the shoulder.* New York, McGraw-Hill; 1995.

Basmajian JV, Latif A. Integrated actions and functions of the chief flexors of the elbow: A detailed electromyographic analysis. *J Bone Joint Surg Am.* 1957;39:1106–1118.

Bennett GE. Elbow and shoulder lesions of baseball players. *Am J Surg.* 1959;98:484–492.

Bennett GE. Shoulder and elbow lesions distinctive of baseball players. *Ann Surg.* 1947;126:107–110.

Bigliani LU, Morrison DS, April EW. Morphology of the acromion and its relationship to rotator cuff tears. *Orthop Trans.* 1986;10:459–460.

Clanton TO, DeLee JC. Osteochondritis dissecans. History, pathophysiology and current treatment concepts. *Clin Orthop.* 1982;(167):50–64.

Clark B. Care and prevention of Little League arm injuries. *HSES 802 course: Injury Prevention in Exercise and Sport.* Kansas City: University of Kansas; 2002.

Cofield RH, Irving JF. Evaluation and classification of shoulder instability. With special reference to examination under anesthesia. *Clin Orthop.* 1987;(223):32–43.

Dotter WE. Little Leaguer's shoulder. Fracture of the proximal humeral epiphyseal cartilage due to baseball pitching. *Guthrie Clin Bull.* 1953;23:68–72.

Ferrari JD, Ferrari DA, Coumas J, Pappas AM. Posterior ossification of the shoulder: The Bennett lesion. Etiology, diagnosis, and treatment. *Am J Sports Med.* 1994;22:171–155; discussion 175–176.

Field LD, Savoie FH 3rd. Arthroscopic suture repair of superior labral detachment lesions of the shoulder. *Am J Sports Med.* 1993;21:783–790.

Fleisig GS, Andrews JR, Dillman CJ, Escamilla RF. Kinetics of baseball pitching with implications about injury mechanisms. *Am J Sports Med.* 1995;23:233–239.

Gerber C, Krushell RJ. Isolated rupture of the tendon of the subscapularis muscle. Clinical features in 16 cases. *J Bone Joint Surg Br.* 1991;73:389–394.

Glascow S, Bruce RA, Yacobucci GN, et al. Arthroscopic resection of glenoid labral tears in the athlete. *Arthroscopy.* 1992;8:48–54.

Glousman RE. Instability versus impingement syndrome in the throwing athlete. *Orthop Clin North Am.* 1993;24:89–99.

Gugenheim JJ, Stanley RF, Woods GW, Tullos HS. Little League survey: The Houston study. *Am J Sports Med.* 1976;4:189–200.

Hancock RE, Hawkins RJ. Applications of electromyography in the throwing shoulder. *Clin Orthop.* 1996;(330):84–97.

Harryman DT 2nd, Sidles JA, Clark JM, McQuade KL, Gibb TD, Matsen FA 3d. Translation of the humeral head on the glenoid with passive glenohumeral motion. *J Bone Joint Surg Am.* 1990;72:1334–1343.

Hawkins RJ, Kennedy JC. Impingement syndrome in athletes. *Am J Sports Med.* 1980;8:151–158.

Jobe CM. Superior glenoid impingement. Current concepts. *Clin Orthop.* 1996;(330):98–107.

Jobe CM. Superior glenoid impingement. *Orthop Clin North Am.* 1997;28:137–143.

Jobe FW, Kao JT. Throwing sports. In: Hawkins RJ, Misamore GW, eds. *Shoulder injuries in the athlete.* New York: Churchill Livingstone; 1996;389–401.

Jobe FW, Moynes DR, Tibone JE, Perry J. An EMG analysis of the shoulder in pitching. A second report. *Am J Sports Med.* 1984;12:218–220.

Jobe FW, Pink M. Classification and treatment of shoulder dysfunction in the overhead athlete. *J Orthop Sports Phys Ther.* 1993;18:427–432.

Jobe FW, Stark H, Lombardo SJ. Reconstruction of the ulnar collateral ligament in athletes. *J Bone Joint Surg Am.* 1986;68:1158–1163.

Jobe FW, Tibone JE, Jobe CM, et al. The shoulder in sports. In: Rockwood CA, Matsen FA, eds, *The Shoulder.* Philadelphia: Saunders; 1990;961–990.

Jobe FW, Tibone JE, Perry J, Moynes D. An EMG analysis of the shoulder in throwing and pitching. A preliminary report. *Am J Sports Med.* 1983;11:3–5.

Kvitne RS, Jobe FW. The diagnosis and treatment of anterior instability in the throwing athlete. *Clin Orthop.* 1993;(291):107–123.

Leffert RD, Gumley G. The relationship between dead arm syndrome and thoracic outlet syndrome. *Clin Orthop.* 1987;(223):20–31.

Liu SH, Henry MH, Nuccion S, Shapiro MS, Dorey F. Diagnosis of glenoid labral tears. A comparison between magnetic resonance imaging and clinical examinations. *Am J Sports Med.* 1996;24:149–154.

Lombardo SJ, Jobe FW, Kerlan RK, Carter VS, Shields CL. Posterior shoulder lesions in throwing athletes. *Am J Sports Med.* 1977;5:106–110.

Miniaci A, Dowdy PA, Fowler PJ Clinical assessment of shoulder injuries. In: Chan KM, ed. *Sports injuries of the hand and upper limb.* New York: Churchill Livingstone; 1995.

Morrey BF. Osteochondritis dissecans. In DeLee JC, Drez D, eds. *Orthopaedic sports medicine: Principles and practice.* Philadelphia: Saunders; 1994;908–912.

Morrey BF, An KN. Functional anatomy of the ligaments of the elbow. *Clin Orthop.* 1985;(201):84–90.

Neer CS 2nd. Anterior acromioplasty for the chronic impingement syndrome in the shoulder: A preliminary report. *J Bone Joint Surg Am.* 1972;54:41–50.

Neer CS 2nd. Impingement lesions. *Clin Orthop.* 1983;(173):70–77.

Neer CS 2nd, Welsh RP. The shoulder in sports. *Orthop Clin North Am.* 1977;8:583–591.

Neer CS 2nd, Welsh RP. The shoulder in sports. *Orthop Clin North Am.* 1977;8:583–591.

O'Brien SJ, Neves MC, Arnoczky SP, et al. The anatomy and histology of the inferior glenohumeral ligament complex of the shoulder. *Am J Sports Med.* 1990;18:449–456.

O'Driscoll SW. A reliable and simple test for posterior instability of the shoulder. *J Bone Joint Surg Br.* 1991;73:50.

Panner HJ. An affection of the capitulum humeri resembling Calve-Perthes' disease of the hip. *Acta Radiologica.* 1927;8:617.

Pappas AM. Elbow problems associated with baseball during childhood and adolescence. *Clin Orthop.* 1982;(164):30–41.

Pasternack JS, Veenema KR, Callahan CM. Baseball injuries: A Little League survey. *Pediatrics.* 1996;98:445–448.

Pincivero DM, Heinrichs K, Perrin DH. Medial elbow stability. Clinical implications. *Sports Med.* 1994;18:141–148.

Rames RD, Karzel RP. Injuries to the glenoid labrum, including slap lesions. *Orthop Clin North Am.* 1993;24:45–53.

Regan WD, Korinek SL, Morrey BF, An KN. Biomechanical study of ligaments around the elbow joint. *Clin Orthop.* 1991;(271):170–179.

Snyder SJ, Karzel RP, Del Pizzo W, Ferkel RD, Friedman MJ. SLAP lesions of the shoulder. *Arthroscopy.* 1990;6:274–279.

Tibone JE. Shoulder problems of adolescents. How they differ from those of adults. *Clin Sports Med.* 1983;2:423–427.

Tibone JE, Elrod B, Jobe FW, et al. Surgical treatment of tears of the rotator cuff in athletes. *J Bone Joint Surg Am.* 1986;68:887–891.

Tibone JE, Jobe FW, Kerlan RK, et al. Shoulder impingement syndrome in athletes treated by an anterior acromioplasty. *Clin Orthop* 1985;(198):134–140.

Wadsworth TG. The external compression syndrome of the ulnar nerve at the cubital tunnel. *Clin Orthop.* 1977;(124):189–204.

Walch G, Liotard JP, Boileau P, Noel E. Postero-superior glenoid impingement. Another impingement of the shoulder. *J Radiol.* 1993;74:47–50.

Wilson FD, Andrews JR, Blackburn TA, McClusky G. Valgus extension overload in the pitching elbow. *Am J Sports Med.* 1983;11:83–88.

Yen K, Metzl J. Sports-specific concerns in the young athlete: Baseball. *Pediatric Emergency Care.* 2000;16:215–220.

Yergason RM. Supination sign. *J Bone Joint Surg Am.* 1931;13:160.

33 | Soccer Injuries

Steven R. Elias

THE IMPORTANCE OF SOCCER IN THE WORLD OF SPORTS

As a team sport, soccer is played most regularly in the greatest number of countries around the world; in most countries—other than the United States—it is known as *football*. There are an estimated 200 million participants worldwide (Patel et al., 2002). Because of the dynamic involvement of national federations and state and regional sport authorities, youth league, high school, college, and professional levels have flourished, making soccer the fastest growing team sport in North America (Darley and Barsan, 1992). The Soccer Industry Council of America (1997) reported 18.1 million participants greater than 6 years of age with 10.9 million men and 7.2 million women. Approximately 13.4 million (74%) were under 18 years of age and 4.7 million (26%) 18 and over. In the United States, the growth of youth soccer is estimated to range from 11–22% annually. Soccer has emerged as the sport with the greatest number of youth players participating in scheduled league competition. It ranks second to basketball in the number of participants from ages 6–11 and third after basketball and volleyball in the 12–17 age group (Table 33-1).

One reason for soccer's popularity is the perception that soccer is a safe sport (Sullivan and Gross, 1980; Tegner et al., 1990; Ward, 1987). Compared with American football, which is a more contact-oriented sport, soccer appears to be relatively safe for younger players who, under 12 years of age (starting at age 5 years), sustained half as many injuries as their counterparts playing American football. In the teenage group, the number of injuries is five times higher in American football than in soccer (Lindenfeld et al., 1994; Schmidt-Olsen and Bunemann, 1985). The most common causes of soccer injuries are related to physical conditioning and training, equipment, playing field, and skills.

HISTORY OF SOCCER

Earlier forms of *soccer* were played in ancient Greece and Rome, although the origins of soccer in its current form can be traced back to England in the mid-19th century. A peoples game played by apprentices and farm boys since the 4th century yielded *Mob football*—a rowdy and dangerous street game. "The football field was the length of the town, the players might be as many as five hundred, the conflict continued all day long; vast numbers of windows and legs were broken, and there were even some deaths" (Association of Football Statisticians, 2002). This turmoil illustrated the need to establish a more orderly game.

TABLE 33-1 Youth Team Sports Rankings

	12–17 Years	6–11 Years
Basketball	12,702	9520 [1]
Volleyball	8706	3825 [5]
Soccer	6034	7376 [2]
Football (tackle)	5435	2603 [6]
Softball	5418	4690 [4]
Baseball	4444	5047 [3]
Hockey	785	431 [7]

The Football Association, formed in 1863, was a union of local football clubs, all of which had been playing under their own sets of rules. The goal of the Football Association was to adopt a unified set of rules defining the field and procedures of play. Consensus was reached only after advocates of the Rugby School withdrew from the negotiations, leading to the independent evolution of the Rugby Union game and soccer association.

Among the rules established by the Football Association were the following:

No player shall run with the ball. Neither tripping nor hacking shall be allowed, and no player shall use his hands to hold or push his adversary. A player shall not be allowed to throw the ball or pass it to another with his hands. No player shall be allowed to take the ball from the ground with his hands under any pretext whatever while it is in play. No player shall be allowed to wear projecting nails, iron plates, or gutta percha on the soles or heels of his boots.

The initial rules did not specify the number of players or length of play; these decisions were left to the discretion of local team captains. Association rules were not, by any means, widely accepted and many local teams continued to play by the set of rules established through local custom.

In the United States, soccer emerged as a collegiate sport on the east coast. The Oneida Soccer Club was formed in Boston in 1862 with subsequent development of teams at other colleges. The first intercollegiate game resembling the current game of soccer occurred in 1869 in New Brunswick, New Jersey, between Princeton and Rutgers with an adaptation of the 1863 English Football Association rules. The ball could be moved with all parts of the body, including the hands, but not carried or thrown. The English custom of 11 players per side was more widely adopted by 1870.

However, as in England, there continued to be a competing interest in Rugby with the first intercollegiate game of Rugby played between Harvard and McGill University of Montreal in 1874. This trend eventually led to the temporary demise of college soccer when Harvard, Princeton, and Columbia formed the Intercollegiate Football Association and adopted Rugby-style rules.

The saying in England, "Soccer is a game for gentlemen played by hooligans; rugby is a game for hooligans played by gentlemen," characterizes the evolution of the two games in the United States. The upper class schools continued to play rugby while working class industrial communities in the northeastern United States played soccer, influenced by the influx of new immigrants from Europe who brought with them the homeland traditions of soccer.

In the 20th century, the popularity of soccer as a professional sport waxed and waned. Throughout the mainstream United States, the game still does not generate the widespread passion and commercial appeal of American-rules football or baseball. Nevertheless, the popularity of soccer as a sport for youth and the emergence of female teams as credible competitors suggests that soccer is on its way to achieving parity in the American sporting landscape.

FACTORS OF INJURY

Characteristics of the Game

Unlike other contact sports, such as American football and rugby, serious injuries in soccer are uncommon. To understand the nature of soccer injuries as compared with rugby and American football, it is necessary to review some basic movements of the game. In soccer, the goalkeeper is the only one among the 11 team members who can touch the ball with the hands (and only within certain areas of the field). The soccer player may kick the ball, but also hit with the head or any other part of his or her body except the upper extremities. The use of the head to advance the ball is unique to soccer and contributes to the risk of head trauma.

Soccer is a hybrid aerobic-anaerobic game (played on a field 105 × 70 m) in which players must rapidly run short distances at various speeds and also cover substantial distances over the course of a 90-minute game. The demands of rapid deceleration, pivoting, lateral and backward displacement, jumping combined with the kicking motion, and contact with other players all contribute to the risk of injury.

Furthermore, the duration and intensity of sustained play over two 45-minutes halves (30- to 40-minute halves for younger players) makes fatigue a major factor in injury. A soccer player spends 70–80% of the time running and jogging with the remaining time engaged in high-intensity sprinting (Patel et al., 2002).

Position of Play

Offensive forwards, defensive fullbacks, and the goalkeeper suffer the most injuries. The goalkeeper is the only player on the field who can legally use his or her hands on the ball, provided it is done inside the penalty zone. So, even if soccer is not a contact-oriented sport, it is in fact a body contact game played with little or no equipment. Because it puts great demands on stamina, numerous injuries do occur. In indoor soccer, the injury rates are similar for goalkeepers and other players. Goalkeepers more often injure fingers, heads, elbows, or hands; other players more commonly incur ankle, knee, or thigh injuries (Lindenfeld et al., 1994).

Intrinsic Factors

Factors related to players, such as joint instability, muscle tightness, inadequate rehabilitation after injury, or lack of training, account for 42% of injuries (Ekstrand and Gillquist, 1983a). In this report, 24% of injuries were owing to unsatisfactory playing surfaces; 17% to equipment, inadequate shoes, or nonuse of shin guards; 12% to rule infractions and foul play; and 29% to chance. A combination of these factors is also fairly common.

EPIDEMIOLOGY

Many injuries occur in soccer players, but this may more reflect the popularity of the game than its dangers. Soccer is generally considered to be a safe sport with a high proportion of minor injuries. Serious injuries are the exception, not the rule.

Classification of Injury

Injuries are classified as either traumatic or overuse (Table 33-2). *Traumatic injury* is caused by either a direct blow or an indirect mechanism and accounts for about 70% of injuries. Trauma accounts for about 70% of injuries. A total of 45% of all injuries result from contact, and affect more often the lower and youth divisions (45%), whereas players at the senior level are reported to have only a 30% incidence of tackling injuries. Tackling causes more than 50% of knee injuries (Nielsen and Yde, 1989). *Overuse*

TABLE 33-2 Classification of Injuries

Trauma: 70%
        Direct contusion: 20%
            Bone
            Soft tissues
        Indirect
            Sprain
            Strain
Overuse injuries: 30%
        Tendinitis or bursitis: 23%
        Shin pain

injuries account for remaining 30%. In traumatic injuries, sprains account for 29%, bursitis or tendinitis for 23%, contusions for 20%, and strains for 28% (Ekstrand and Gillquist, 1983b).

Anatomic Distribution of Injury

More than 80% of soccer injuries in adults involve the lower extremities, with ankle sprain being the most common (35%) (Nielsen and Yde, 1989). A Spanish soccer study by Naves showed the lower extremities sustained 70% of all injuries (Table 33-3) (Pardon, 1977). In youth soccer, only 60% of the injuries occur in the lower extremities, with about 20% involving ankle sprains and strains. Twenty percent are contusions and 6% are knee sprains and strains (Keller, 1987). Youth players sustain a relative increase in upper extremity and head/face injuries (Metzl and Micheli, 1998). Head and neck injuries comprise 4.9–22.0% of the total (American Academy of Pediatrics, 2000) and includes concussions, which account for 1–3% of injuries. Rare injuries in youth players include acute neck sprains, disk herniations, fracture/dislocations, and central cord compression. Maxillofacial injuries include nasal, mandibular and zygomatic fractures, dental injuries (tooth avulsions and fractures), orbital blow-out fractures, and eye injuries (hyphemas, corneal abrasions, and retinal injuries) (Patel et al., 2002). Soccer is secondary only to basketball in the incidence of orofacial and dental injuries (American Academy of Pediatrics, 2000).

Upper extremity injuries comprise 15% of youth soccer injuries (range 3–30%) (Patel et al., 2002) with involvement of the shoulder in 1.8–2.6% and hand in 6.3% of the total injuries. Fractures are more frequent in the upper extremity than in the lower extremity (American Academy of Pediatrics, 2000). Lower extremity injuries range from 60–90% of all injuries in youth players. Groin injuries represent 5–8% of injuries. Hip and pelvis injuries are less common and include osteitis pubis, iliac apophysitis/hip

TABLE 33-3 Injuries in Soccer

Area of body	%	Injuries of extremities	%
Lower extremity	70	Ankle	22
Upper extremity	19	Knee	20
Trunk	6	Thigh	15
Head and neck	5	Elbow	9
		Foot	8
		Wrist	8
		Hand	7
		Shoulder	6
		Others	5

pointers, avulsion fractures, and femoral neck stress fractures. Thigh contusions occur in 10–45% of players (Patel et al., 2002). Knee injuries constitute 10–26% of total injuries (Patel et al., 2002) and are the most common soccer injury. Knee injuries are responsible for nearly 50% of major injuries in soccer (Metzl and Micheli, 1998). Anterior cruciate ligament (ACL) disruptions are the most common cause of major injury with a rate twice greater in women compared to men. The medial collateral ligament (MCL) is the most common site of all knee injuries (Patel et al., 2002). Ankle injuries (13.0–23.1% of total) (American Academy of Pediatrics, 2000) are the second most common injury and generally occur with an inversion mechanism (Patel et al., 2002). Foot (0.3–28.0%) (American Academy of Pediatrics, 2000) injuries include plantar fasciitis, foot sprains, and turf toe. Stress fractures involving the second through fifth metatarsals represent the most common stress fractures in soccer players. Subluxation of the peroneus brevis and tibialis posterior also occurs in youth soccer players (Patel et al., 2002). There is an increased incidence of calcaneal apophysitis or Sever disease in skeletally immature soccer players attributed to the impact demands of running in cleated shoes without adequate heel cushion or arch support, especially when playing fields are dry and hard (American Academy of Pediatrics, 2000).

Severity of Injury

There are a variety of systems describing severity of soccer injuries. One useful scheme categorizes injury based on a retrospective assessment of time away from play. Injuries are classified as *minor* if the injuries cause little or no loss of activity. *Major injuries* require ongoing medical care and result in absence from play for more than 1 month, and *moderate injuries* are in between. About 60% of all injuries are considered to be minor, 27% moderate, and 11% severe (Ekstrand and Gillquist, 1983a).

Youth soccer players sustain a greater proportion of minor soccer injuries than adults. In adults, 60–75% of injuries are considered minor and include strains, sprains, and contusions. In youth players, over 85% of the injuries are considered minor (Metzl and Micheli, 1998).

Mortality over a period of 20 years, between 1938 and 1959, was 0.6–1.2 per 100,000 players per year, 33% secondary to head injuries (Fields, 1989). The National Center for Catastrophic Sport Injury tracked catastrophic injuries sustained by direct contact from 1982 through 2001. The fatality rate for male high school participants was 0.13 (per 100,000 participants) for soccer and 0.30 for football (Mueller and Cantu, 2002). It is estimated that the rate for soccer is lower now than in the mid-20th century, because of improved safety measures, such as better conditioning, training, and environment precautions. Collision with goal posts is the primary mechanism for fatalities in soccer. The United States Consumer Product Safety Commission documented 18 fatalities from 27 injuries related to falling goalposts between 1979 and 1993, and most were not game play related. The mean age of the subjects in this series was 10 years (American Academy of Pediatrics, 2000).

Context of Injury

The injury incidence during games is highest among players participating at higher levels. Soccer injuries occur more frequently during games than during practice (Nielsen and Yde, 1989). In 1991, Ekstrand studied amateur Swedish male players with an average age of 25 showing rates of 7.6 injuries per 1000 player-hours during practice and 16.9 per 1000 player-hours during games (Metzl and Micheli, 1998).

The rate of soccer injury for indoor play is 6.1 times higher than for outdoor play. The significant difference in injury rates may be explained by differences between artificial turf and natural grass playing surfaces and by wall collisions (American Academy of Pediatrics, 2000). In indoor soccer, male players aged 25 years old or older have the highest injury rate. The most common cause of injury is collision with another player, which accounts for about 30% of all injuries; about 16% occur when a player is kicked by an opponent. There does not seem to be a significant difference in the rate of ligament injury for male and female players in indoor settings. However, male players sustain more ankle injuries than female players do; women have a higher rate of knee ligament injuries (Lindenfeld et al., 1994).

Mechanism of Injury

A total of 45% of all injuries result from contact, and affect more often the lower adult age groups and the youth divisions (45%), whereas players at the senior level are reported to have only a 30% incidence of tackling injuries. On the other hand, overuse syndromes represent about 37% of all the injuries. Tackling causes more than 50% of knee injuries (Nielsen and Yde, 1989).

Age and Gender

In the United States, the National Electronic Injury Surveillance System tracked soccer-related injuries between 1992 and 1994 and estimated between 146,00 and 160,000 soccer injuries annually. Approximately 45% of the injuries occurred in players under age 15 with 85% occurring in players through 23 years of age (American Academy of Pediatrics, 2000).

Youth epidemiologic studies reveal tournament-related injury rates ranging from a low of 2.38 injuries per 1000 player-hours in Kentucky to rates of 14 injuries per 1000 player-hours for boys and 32 injuries per 1000 player-hours for girls at the Norway Cup Soccer Tournament. Rates at the Norway Cup subsequently decreased to 6.9 (boys) and 8.3 (girls) per 1000 player-hours when the studies were repeated in 1997. Elias showed similar injury trends at the USA Cup tournament in Minnesota. Highest injury rates occurred in the Under-16 and Under-18 female groups and lowest rates in Under-19 female and Under-12 male groups (Elias, 2001).

The development of girls' and women's soccer has provided an increasing opportunity for women to experience popular team and contact sport activities (Brynhildsen et al., 1990; Engstrom et al., 1991). Soccer has become more popular among girls and women, and it is now played in more than 50 countries. Lack of proper conditioning was cited as being responsible for many of the injuries in female athletes by early reports that demonstrated that more injuries occur in female than in male athletes (Arendt, 1994; Engstrom et al., 1991). Soccer data showed an increase in serious injuries to women and girls during the 1970s. Later studies showed more equal distribution in injury rates, probably owing to the improvement in the level of play (Nilsson and Rooas, 1978; Sullivan and Gross, 1980).

This trend was demonstrated in the USA Cup study of youth tournament play with female rates (per 1000 player-hours) ranging from a high of 20 in 1988 to a low of 10 in 1996; male rates ranged from a high of 20 in 1988 to a low of 8 in 1996. The USA Cup study also showed that women sustained injury at rates slightly greater than men with a trend toward less significant differences in rates. Women did show a relative increased susceptibility to heat illness, knee injuries, and ankle sprains compared to men (Elias, 2001).

A review of an National Collegiate Athletic Association Injury Surveillance System supports the notion that there are similar injury rates in men's and women's sports with comparable rules. In the same study, female soccer players experienced a higher percentage of severe knee injuries than their counterparts, especially with respect to the ACL (Arendt, 1994). On the other hand, comparing with all injuries for men and women, there was an equal percentage of occurrences, but exposure was twice for men. In other words, the distribution of injury is the same but the nature differs, with women being more susceptible to injuries. Knee injury rate is similar in men (16%) and women (18%). Men generally sustain more knee injuries to all structures of the knee except for ACL. Women sustain twice as many ACL injuries as men, and more than half of all ACL injuries are noncontact in nature (Arendt, 1994).

The most common injuries in female soccer players are sprains to the lower extremity. Overuse injuries are responsible for more than 40% of persistent symptoms. Women are more prone to sustain patellar dislocations than men, whereas men incur more dislocations to the upper extremity (Brynhildsen et al., 1990).

SPECIFIC INJURIES

The Ankle

The ankle is the part most often injured in soccer. The most common injury is sprain produced by a forceful inversion of the plantar-flexed foot. The severity of the sprain may vary from a single elongation to complete disruption of multiple ligaments, mainly the anterior talofibular and calcaneofibular ligaments. The ultimate injury, dislocation of the joint, may be associated with a fracture of one or many components of the ankle and foot (Fig. 33-1). Another mechanism of injury of ankle sprain is a forceful eversion when a player boots the ground instead of the ball, resulting in a deltoid ligament injury that may also be associated with a fibular fracture. Sometimes rupture of the syndesmotic inferior talofibular ligament may result in a sprain injury requiring a long period of recovery.

Ankle sprains are usually treated conservatively with compressive taping or bracing for ligament protection. It is recommended that a player wear an ankle orthosis to minimize the high risk of recurrence. Definitive treatment of complete dislocation is controversial in the elite athlete, and the orthopedic surgeon may recommend operative treatment to repair all the ligaments to promote optimal healing and early rehabilitation. The evaluation and management of foot and ankle injuries is presented in detail in Chapter 26.

One complication of ankle sprain in soccer players has been described as a meniscoid lesion of the ankle (McCarrol et al., 1987). This lesion is rare and characterized by pain, persistent swelling, and trapping. If the same complaints persist after a minimum of 6 months of conservative treatment that includes rehabilitation protective devices, anti-inflammatory medication, and occasional periods of rest, surgery may be indicated. The pathology of

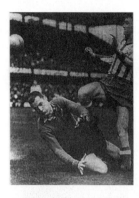
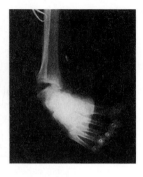
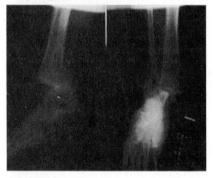

FIG 33-1 Fracture dislocation of left ankle. This patient required an open reduction. He would be out of action for 6 months or more. Soccer players have to be among the fittest of all athletes to tolerate this demanding sport. Fracture dislocations of the ankle require immediate relocation if possible and early operation.

the internal derangement of the ankle is a band of white, fibrotic, meniscus-like tissue from an old torn ligament lying between the fibula and the talus. The removal of this lesion appears to be an effective treatment and can be done arthroscopically.

Contusions of the foot and fractures of the metatarsals, especially the fifth, are common. They are produced by kicking or when a player's foot is stepped on. Fracture of the base of the fifth metatarsal is usually caused by a strong pull on the peroneus brevis tendon. Treatment is surgical when there is displacement. The subtalar and other tarsal joints may be sprained or fractured and an MR or CT imaging may be required to elucidate the cause of chronic pain.

Footballer's Ankle

This condition is a chronic periostitis or peritendinitis with calcification that occurs on the anterior margin of the lower end of the tibia and over the talus.

It is owing to the way a player ordinarily kicks the ball with the foot in plantar flexion and slight inversion with the ball making contact with the dorsal and medial aspects of the foot.

Thigh Injuries

A history of thigh muscle strains is found in 60% of players (Ekstrand and Gillquist, 1983b). Soft tissue injuries of the thigh can result in an inter- or intramuscular hematoma. The very serious ones are intramuscular, where the muscle sheath remains intact, entrapping the hematoma and increasing the risk for traumatic compartment syndrome and myositis ossificans. Treatment includes a compression dressing with the muscle at full length, ice, elevation, and crutch walking; massage is contraindicated. For a quadriceps contusion, the leg needs to be splinted in a fully flexed position, and a hinged post-operative brace works well to maintain a comfortable flexed position. Measure the limb circumference to track the swelling and if necessary monitor the extent of the clot with x-ray or repeat Doppler ultrasound studies. Give analgesics for pain, but do not use nonsteroidal anti-inflammatories. If active bleeding with or without compartment syndrome, surgical intervention may be warranted. If the patient is worse after 72 hours with unremitting severe pain and increasing immobility, take the patient to the operating room. Well-trained experts have used the plastic surgery technique of high-vacuum liposuction to remove the hematoma. Open reduction and direct release of the hematoma, which lies right on top of the bone, is an alternate treatment that is occasionally used in some centers. Once the clot has been evacuated, treatment is the same as for other first-degree injuries.

The Knee

Injuries to the knee include sprains of the collateral and cruciate ligaments (mainly MCL and ACL) and tears of the menisci. The incidence of meniscus injuries in soccer is as high as 35% of knee injuries in some series (Brynhildsen et al., 1990). Because the leg may be fixed to the ground by cleats on the soccer shoe, sudden uncontrolled rotation and flexion changes of the body position during passing, running, or collision with another player (Fig. 33-2) may produce sudden rotation of the femur relative to the fixed lower leg causing injuries to the meniscus and knee joint. Even though soccer is a sport with great demands on the knee, the incidence of knee injuries in soccer players is one-fifth that of the comparable American football player populations (Pritchett, 1981). Tackling causes more than 50% of knee injuries and ligament sprains often occur when a player is tackled with the loaded leg fixed on the ground (Nielsen and Yde, 1989). High friction between the shoe and surface may produce excessive force on the knee or ankle, but too little traction can contribute to slipping injury. Thus, the use of a properly cleated shoe balances the risk of high- and low-traction joint injuries (Ekstrand and Gillquist, 1983).

The incidence of chondral injuries in soccer players has been reported and may result from high velocities, and repetitive pivoting, deceleration that the knee experiences, placing extreme stress on the articular cartilage (Levy et al., 1996). Chondral injuries are believed to occur through two distinct mechanisms: abrasive wear with superficial fibrillation and large shear forces disrupting the deep cartilage ultrastructure. The pathology found on arthroscopy is a full-thickness chondral delamination exposing subchondral

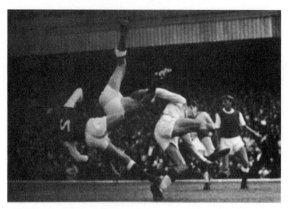

FIG 33-2 All the players shown were injured in this collision. Evidence of great speed, and impact of play.

bone at the base of the lesion. These lesions are more often seen on the femoral condoyle, but the patella facet or the trochlea may also be involved in the knee. It is possible that the same type of lesion occurs in other joints such as the ankle. The treatment of chondral lesions is controversial, but at the present time, debridement to bleeding bone and stimulation of fibrocartilage is the most common surgical treatment. Partial-thickness lesions may be treated by an open vertical lesion and drilling or microfracturing of the subchondral bone. Autogenous core osteochondral (mosaic) graft and allografts have been tried with varying success. Attempts to fill isolated chondral lesions with laboratory-grown cartilage cells and to stimulate chondrogenesis with reversed periosteum are experimental techniques with an unknown long-term outcome (Leach and Corbett, 1996).

The Groin

Because soccer players manipulate the ball with their legs, groin injuries are fairly common. They are caused by sudden, powerful overstretching of the leg and thigh in abduction and external rotation, especially if there is an opposing force such as an opponent's foot at full speed and in full swing or the ground. These forces may overstretch the fibers of the muscles or tendons, the bony tissue of the pelvic ring, the sacroiliac joint, and the pubic symphysis.

Adolescent soccer players may sustain avulsion fractures of pelvic apophysis, such as the anteroinferior iliac spine where the rectus femoris originates, the anterosuperior iliac spine where the sartorius is inserted, or the ischial tuberosity where the hamstring originates (Fig. 33-3). Avulsion of the lesser trochanter site of insertion of the psoas iliac muscle also occurs. Those avulsions are generally treated nonoperatively with excellent functional outcomes. If the avulsion gap is too great to allow bone bridging, the apophysis may have to be surgically fixed.

Groin pain also occurs as a rare overuse syndrome that begins with an adductor strain, leading first to tendinitis followed by chondritis, osteitis, and formation of necrotic foci in the pubis or ossification along the pubis or in

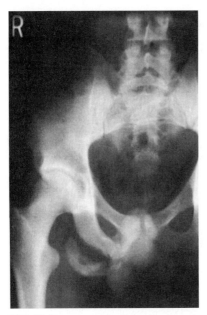

FIG 33-3 Pictured is a 17-year-old male sprinter who lunged at the finish line and sustained avulsion of ischium, hamstring origin. This heals with 2–3 months judicious rest.

the attached muscles appearing as a calcifying tendinitis. This may cause a temporary or even permanent disability. Other pathologies in the area should be looked at, such as abdominal wall strain, sportsman's and inguinal hernia, hip, sacrum, pelvic rotation, or lower back afflictions. Groin pain is treated by rest, physical therapy, anti-inflammatory drugs, and rehabilitation. Steroid injection is not generally recommended, but if it is necessary, one infiltration of the painful area with a local anesthetic along with a water-soluble corticosteroid solution may be cautiously used (Smodlaka, 1980). Sacroiliac joint, symphysis pubis, and lower lumbar joint mobilization may improve pain and function. In rare cases, surgical intervention where the abductor origin is partially detached from the pubic tubercle and pectineal line is necessary to relieve the pain.

Shin Pain and Anterior Tibial Compartment Syndrome

Pain along the medial half distal border of the tibia often represents a medial periostitis. A stress fracture of the tibia or the fibula should be considered as a cause of the pain. Pain, swelling, and limping are the main symptoms. X-rays may be normal initially, but bone scintigraphy confirms the diagnosis. Treatment consists of restriction from sport activities until complete bone healing has occurred.

Anterior tibial compartment syndrome has been reported in soccer players (Kurosawa et al., 1991). It may be produced acutely by a kick from another player or chronically from running. Acute compartment syndrome may also be associated with a leg fracture. Pain, swelling, and tenderness are the

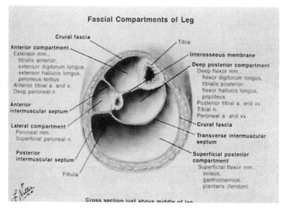

FIG 33-4 Acute compartment syndrome is a true surgical emergency. Chronic compartment syndrome can be operated on electively. The medial tibia and posterior and lateral (anterior) compartments are released.

precursors of the onset, followed by weakness of the foot dorsiflexors and numbness in the sural nerve distribution. The trauma patient must be followed closely and monitored for sensation and muscle activity. Development of acute compartment syndrome occurs in a matter of hours, and unremitting pain and progressive loss of dorsiflexion and motor function of the foot after trauma is a much clearer indication of compartment syndrome than the symptoms and signs that develop with chronic exertional compartment syndrome. Peroneal nerve injury and medial periostitis must be considered in the differential diagnosis. In the case of acute compartment syndrome (Fig. 33-4), a surgical fasciotomy must be performed. In chronic recurrent cases, surgical treatment is often the only alternative to giving up the sport (see Chapter 24).

The Upper Extremity

Injuries to upper extremities in soccer players account for nearly 20% of all injuries (Pardon, 1977). Acromioclavicular or sternoclavicular shoulder joint sprains and rotator cuff strains occur with falls. A forceful backward motion while throwing the ball from the sideline with the arm highly extended or in abduction and external rotation may dislocate the shoulder joint.

The elbow is the most frequently affected joint in the upper extremity, and contusion is the most frequent cause. Radial head fractures and medial collateral ligament sprains occur, but frank dislocations are rare. Because only goalies handle the ball with the hands, they sustain most of the hand injuries. Falls on an outstretched hand cause most of the upper extremity injuries and the wrist is often sprained or fractured in soccer. Colles' and related wrist fractures occur most commonly with falls. Soft tissue contusions, sprains, and dislocation of the fingers are the most frequent hand fractures.

The Trunk

Injuries to the trunk represent about 6% of all injuries (Pardon, 1977). Contusions, muscle strains, or rib fractures caused by kicks and blows from the elbows are the usual mechanisms. Injuries can also occur from falls on the ball and to the ground. There are occasional injuries to the organs of the trunk and abdomen.

The Head and Neck

Injuries to the head and neck represent about 5% of all injuries (Pardon, 1977). Injuries ranging from sprains to muscle strains are frequent in all players, especially the goalkeeper. Fatal head injuries are rare, but concussions are common (Fields, 1989). The mechanism of injury varies. Incorrectly heading the ball with the neck flexed or extended may cause increased head motion and a change in momentum of the head may contribute to concussion. Goalies and field players sustain concussions from head-to-head, head-to-ground, head-to-elbow or foot contact and occasionally from a forcefully kicked ball strike to the head. Goalkeepers also strike their heads against goalposts.

Concussions, skull fractures, and epidural or subdural hematomas have all been reported following collision injury (Darley and Barsan, 1992). Improvement in ball construction, particularly the addition of a plastic coating to prevent water logging of the ball, seems to cause less severe head injuries and is considered the most important change in the prevention of head injuries. In fact, the older leather balls could absorb water, increasing its weight by 20% or more. However, we have to remember that even heading the ball correctly produces forcible impact and can cause headaches that may last for several days. Proper techniques coaching may help prevent soccer-related head-to-head injuries. Many minor head injuries that soccer players sustain in collisions are probably underdiagnosed or overlooked. Heading the ball or a blow to the head may also result in neck injuries, and soccer players may develop premature degenerative changes in the cervical spine (Kurosawa et al., 1991). Understanding the etiology of head and neck injuries can initiate preventive measures. Controlled head contact with the ball or heading is as valuable a skill as shooting on goal, but it places the player at risk of injury from ball as well as from other players simultaneously trying to head the ball. Core and neck strengthening are critical elements in neck and head injury.

The Eye

Blunt trauma to the eye occurs in soccer. Hyphema is the most common traumatic disorder and may lead to secondary glaucoma. Corneal abrasion, lens trauma, pupillary defects, orbital fracture, retinal hemorrhage, and retinal detachment also occur (Orlando, 1988). Eye injuries are usually unilateral and caused by a kicked ball striking the eye and periorbital region at close range, a kicking foot of another player, or a hit by the skull of an opponent attempting a header. Athletes who need vision correction should wear contact lenses or sports glasses with polycarbonate lenses and frames. It is estimated that serious complications occur in 25% of sports-related eye injuries. Protective devices should be mandatory for one-eyed athletes to minimize any risk of eye injury (Orlando, 1988).

MANAGEMENT OF SOCCER INJURIES ON THE SIDELINES

The responsibility of the physician, trainer, coach, and organization authorities should be defined in advance within accepted principles of injury management. A logical approach to on-the-field evaluation and management is essential for proper on-the-field decisions and necessary first aid measures. Decisions regarding playability of the injured athlete during a game situation are the sole responsibility of the team physician. In the absence of a physician, the decision becomes the responsibility of the athlete trainer or coach, if an athletic trainer is not available. A parent should be involved in the final decision when a minor player is involved. As a matter of course the most qualified individual on the field, be it the physician, athletic trainer, or coach, should determine the nature and extent of acute soccer injury. Understanding the mechanisms of injury along with a careful history and examination is critical to ascertaining the correct diagnosis.

Basic principles of management following an injury must be respected and an injured player should be removed from the contest. One must restrict play of the injured athlete to observe, listen, examine, and initiate treatment when indicated. Before return to play, a functional evaluation is necessary. The best time for accurate assessment of the degree of damage is immediately following the injury when muscle spasm is absent, pain is not severe, and swelling has not yet developed. The priority is the evaluation of the ABCs, state of consciousness, the general appearance of the athlete, the color of the skin, the ability to move, the respiratory rate, and the presence of abrasions, lacerations, pain, deformity, or bleeding. A conscious athlete can relate the injury experience, indicate the injury site, and describe the injury mechanism. It is important to know if the athlete felt something popping, breaking, or going out, and if the disability was immediate, all of which reflect on injury severity. Rapid swelling after injury is an important guide to assessing the severity and type of injury sustained. Swelling that develops immediately after injury indicates bleeding within the joint, resulting in a hemarthrosis. If the swelling appears the day after injury, usually it is owing to synovial fluid as a result of a reactive synovitis. During the examination, the physician must search for tenderness, crepitus, stability, weakness, dysfunction, sensory defects, and range of motion. A careful evaluation prior to moving an injured player is critical and severe injuries should be appropriately splinted on the field of play.

Initial treatment is based on the acronym RICE (rest, ice, compression, evaluation), the key steps in the initial management of acute injuries. Application of ice is used for controlling pain and hemorrhage; compression to increase the pressure on the tissue, decreasing the extravasation of fluid, and minimizing the hemorrhage and swelling. Elevation increases venous return and decreases swelling; immobilization decreases pain and minimizes swelling of the injured part.

Playability

If after careful examination, the injury appears to be insignificant and a functional evaluation is satisfactory, the athlete can safely be allowed to return to play. If abnormal function is observed, then further participation should be delayed until a more thorough evaluation can be completed. There are several findings that suggest significant injury and mitigate against a return to play.

1. A pop at the time of injury
2. Inability to bear full weight on the leg while walking
3. The inability to run or change direction

4. Loss of motion
5. Instability or false motion
6. Pain or immediate swelling

The presence of any of these findings demands the removal of the athlete from the game and a more thorough evaluation of the injured part. The return to play decision cascade is presented in Chapter 7.

Injury Reduction

Muscle tightness predisposes to strain, and the question has been raised whether soccer training itself can lead to muscle shortness. It has been observed that most ranges of motion would be reduced after training without stretching and that all motion is reduced at 24 hours. The situation can be corrected with a stretching exercise program (Moller et al., 1985). A session of stretching exercises seems to be effective in countering the decrease in range of joint motion normally caused by a standard soccer work-out. Stretching consists of isometric contractions followed by relaxation and then passive lengthening or elongation of the muscle.

Playing in Hot Weather

Soccer players playing in hot humid weather who are not acclimated to heat are at increased risk of exercise heat exhaustion or heat stroke. In hot environments, the athletic trainer, team physician, or sport authorities must initiate modifications in play to reduce heat injury risk, including shorter playing periods, more water and rest breaks, and unlimited substitutions. Modifications are critical in tournament situations where athletes are away from home and from parental supervision.

A big part of the coaching plan on a humid day should be regularly scheduling substitutions. At the end of the game, the players will not be exhausted from the heat and more likely to perform well in subsequent tournament games. In addition, replacing sweat losses helps to prevent heat stroke and exercise exhaustion. Athletes practicing or playing on hot, humid days should learn to replace sweat losses without taking in too much water. A simple guideline is to keep the urine color pale yellow, like lemonade, not dark like apple juice.

Players, coaches, officials, and parents should be informed of the potential for heat injury. Guidelines used at the USA Soccer Cup Tournament based on wet bulb globe temperature (WBGT), with quarterly fluid breaks at WBGT over 65°F, shortened game times or unlimited substitution at WBGT over 73°F, and moving midday games to earlier or later times at WBGT over 82°F have been effective in reducing the incidence of heat-related illness (Elias et al., 1991). Additional effective interventions include canceling all nongame-related activities that are not in air conditioned areas, setting up wading pools for postgame cool downs, and encouraging participants to return to air conditioned homes and hotels during nongame times. An event should not be scheduled at the hottest time of the day or year and the insidious nature of dehydration should be recognized. Heat stroke and exercise exhaustion presenting symptoms usually include dizziness, light-headedness, weakness, headache, hyperventilation, mild disorientation, nausea, and syncope. Affected players with any central nervous system changes should have a rectal temperature measured to rule out heat stroke, and be allowed to rest in an air conditioned area with ice packs applied to the groin, neck, and axillae with oral hydration. Intravenous hydration is occasionally required.

Playing Surface

Another aspect of player safety and injury prevention is the playing surface, either outdoors or indoors. Soccer is played outdoors on grass or artificial turf and indoors on the various floor and artificial turf surfaces. Artificial turf is not always a stable static surface, and with use and exposure irreversible changes occur in its physical makeup. The diminished impact absorption capacity clearly seems detrimental to player safety, although some players prefer to play on artificial turf because grass surfaces provide a less uniform playing surface in wet and dry conditions. There are more soccer injuries on artificial surfaces than on grass.

Protective Gear

The general use of shin pads by the players has decreased injury rates in soccer. The use of a mouthguard would decrease dental injuries and might decrease the severity of concussions. There is no evidence for other protective equipment in soccer, although helmets, especially for goalkeepers, and padded goalposts have been discussed.

CONCLUSION

Soccer is a dynamic game and the most popular team sport in the world. It is considered safe for both genders in youth soccer, even at the highly competitive levels. It is a sport with few and generally minor injuries, but unfortunately permanent disability and even fatalities may result from soccer injuries. Relative to safety, according to international rules, there are no game stoppages and few substitutions; thus, fluid replenishment is a problem that may be minimized simple by rule modifications that provide for fluid intake during play.

ACKNOWLEDGMENT

The author acknowledges the contribution of Rejean Grenier, who wrote this chapter for the first edition of the book.

REFERENCES

American Academy of Pediatrics Committee on Sports Medicine and Fitness. Injuries in youth soccer: A subject review. *Pediatrics.* 2000;105:659–661.

Arendt EA: Orthopaedic issues for active and athletic women. *Clin Sport Med.* 1994;13:483–503.

Association of Football Statisticians. *The History of Football.* Accessed from URL: http://11v11.co.uk/linkpage.php3?linkpageid=3, 2002.

Brynhildsen J, Ekstrand J, Jeppsson A, Tropp H. Previous injuries and persisting symptoms in female soccer players. *Int J Sports Med.* 1990;11:489–492.

Darley SW, Barsan WG. Head injuries in soccer. *Phys Sports Med.* 1992;20:79–85.

Ekstrand J, Gillquist J. Incidence of soccer injuries and their relation to training and team success. *Am J Sports Med.* 1983a;11:63–67.

Ekstrand J, Gillquist J. Avoidability of soccer injuries. *Int J Sports Med.* 1983;4:124–128.

Elias SR. 10-year trend in USA Cup soccer injuries: 1988–1997. *Med Sci Sports Exerc.* 2001;33:359–367.

Elias SR, Roberts WO, et al. Team sports in hot weather: Guidelines for modifying youth soccer. *Phys Sports Med.* 1991;19:67–80.

Engstrom B, Johansson C, Tornkvist H. Soccer injuries among elite female players. *Am J Sports Med.* 1991;19:372–375.

Fields KB. Head injuries in soccer. *Phys Sports Med.* 1989;17:69–73.

Keller CS. The medical aspects of soccer injuries: Epidemiology. *Am J Sports Med.* 1987;15:230–237.

Kurosawa H, Yamanoi T, Yamakoshi K. Radiographic findings of degeneration in cervical spines of middle-aged soccer players. *Skeletal Radiol.* 1991;20:437–440.

Leach R, Corbett M. Anterior tibial compartment syndrome in soccer players. *Am J Sports Med.* 1996;24:634–639.

Levy AS, Lohnes J, Sculley S, LeCroy M, Garrett W. Chondral delamination of the knee in soccer players. *Am J Sports Med.* 1996;24:634–639.

Lindenfeld TN, Schmitt DJ, Hendy MP, Mangine RE, Noyes FR. Incidence of injury in indoor soccer. *Am J Sports Med.* 1994;22:364–371.

McCarrol JR, Schrader JW, Shelbourne KD, Rettig AC, Bisesi MA. Meniscoid lesions of the ankle in soccer players. *Am J Sports Med.* 1987;15:255–257.

Metzl JD, Micheli LJ. Youth Soccer: An epidemiologic perspective. *Clin Sports Med.* 1998;17:663–673.

Moller MH, Oberg BE, Gillquist J. Stretching exercises and soccer: Effect of stretching on range of motion in the lower extremity in connection with soccer training. *Int J Sports Med.* 1985;6:50–52.

Mueller FO, Cantu RC. National Center for Catastrophic Sport Injury Research. Accessed http://www.unc.edu/depts/nccsi, 2002.

Nielsen AB, Yde J. Epidemiology and traumatology of injuries in soccer. *Am J Sports Med.* 1989;17:803–807.

Nilsson S, Rooas A. Soccer injuries in adolescents. *Am J Sports Med.* 1978;6:358–361.

Orlando RG. Soccer-related eye injuries in children and adolescents. *Phys Sports Med.* 1988;18:103–106.

Pardon ET. Lower extremities are site of most soccer injuries. *Phys Sports Med.* 1977;43–48.

Patel DR, Stier B, Luckstead EF. Major international sport profiles. *Pediatr Clin North Am.* 2002;49:769–792.

Pritchett JW. Cost of high school soccer injuries. *Am J Sports Med.* 1981;9:64–66.

Schmidt-Olsen S, Bunemann LKH. Soccer injuries in youth. *Br J Sports Med.* 1985;19:161–164.

Smodlaka VN. Groin pain in soccer players. *Phys Sports Med.* 1980;8:57–61.

Soccer Industry Council of America. 1997. North Palm Beach, FL. 33408.

Sullivan JA, Gross WA. Evaluation of injuries in youth soccer. *Am J Sports Med.* 1980;8:325–327.

Tegner Y, Henriksson A, et al: Avulsion of the anterior-inferior iliac spine in young soccer players. *Clin Sports Med.* 1990;2:143–148.

Ward A. Soccer: Safe kicks for kids. *Phys Sports Med.* 1987;15:151–158.

SUGGESTED READINGS

Chantrane A. Knee joint in soccer players: Osteoarthritis and axis deviation. *Med Sci Sports Exerc.* 1985;17:434–439.

Ekstrand J, Nigg BM. Surface-related injuries in soccer. *Sports Med.* 1989;8:56–62.

Ekstrand J. Soccer injuries and their mechanism: A prospective study. *Med Sci Sport Exerc.* 1993;15:267–270.

Engstrom B. Does a major knee injury definitely sideline an elite soccer player? *Am J Sports Med.* 1990;18:101–105.

Hanson PG, Angevine M, et al. Osteitis pubis in sports activities. *Phys Sports Med.* 111–114, 1978.

Kirkendall DT. The applied sport science of soccer. *Phys Sports Med.* 1985;13:53–59.

Maehlum S, Dahl E. Frequency of injuries in a youth soccer tournament. *Phys Sports Med.* 1986;14:73–79.

McMaster WC, Maarten W. Injuries in soccer. *Am J Sports Med.* 1978;6:354–357.

Neyret P, Donedll ST. Partial meniscectomy and anterior cruciate ligament rupture in soccer players: A study with a minimum of 20 years follow-up. *Am J Sports Med.* 1993;21:455–460.

34 | Cross-Country Ski Injuries

Janus D. Butcher

Cross-country skiing is an ancient sport that originated several thousand years ago in Scandinavia. Skiing probably evolved as a convenient form of transportation in these snow-covered northern climates. Most of the early written references to skiing describe its use by the Norwegian military (Levinson and Christensen, 1999). It has since evolved into an integral part of Scandinavian and Finnish culture that has been imported into countries throughout the northern and southern extremes of the planet. Although cross-country skiing was relatively unchanged from its remote beginnings, in the past 25 years dramatic equipment and technique innovations have revolutionized the sport.

The history of competitive skiing can be traced back to the Norwegian military in the late 18th century. Subsequently, civilian ski clubs formed to promote the sport and competition. The most famous ski race, the Holmenkollen, takes place each March in Oslo, Norway, and traces its roots back to these club competitions in 1879 (Vaage and Kristensen, 1992). In recent years, marathon-distance races have been organized in all countries of northern, central, and Eastern Europe as well as Japan, North America, and Australia. China initiated its first *Loppet* race in 2003.

In the United States, a full calendar of local, regional, and national marathon races are scheduled throughout the winter months. The largest of these, the American Birkebeiner, is 52 km long with over 7000 participants. High school and college cross-country ski teams are common in the northeast, upper Midwest, and western states. These competitions include races 5–15 km in length with both classic stride and skating formats.

The International Ski Federation (FIS) governs international competition. The FIS establishes race rules, schedules, doping control systems, athlete injury surveillance and, most other aspects of World Cup and World Championship racing. The specific events held at elite competitions are varied in both distance and technique. Formats include sprint (1 km), sprint relay, middle distance (5, 10, and 15 km), team relay (4 × 5 and 4 × 10 km), long distance (30 and 50 km), classic/skate pursuit, and others. One unique aspect of elite cross-country skiing is that the athletes frequently compete as both sprinters (1 km) and marathon skiers (30 or 50 km) within the same race schedule. Most competitors train and race in both the classical and skating techniques, which are described in greater detail below.

The sport of cross-country skiing has undergone dramatic changes over the past 25 years. Currently, two very distinct techniques are used: the diagonal stride (classic) and ski-skating (freestyle). The diagonal stride technique has been used for centuries and remains a popular style for ski touring and back country skiing. In the diagonal stride forward, propulsion is accomplished through alternating kick and glide actions of the skis (Fig. 34-1). This requires a full stop of the kick ski to propel the skier forward. Backward slip of the planted ski is limited by the application of high-friction kick wax on the cambered portion of the ski surface. The requirement to plant the ski to generate thrust limits the maximum speeds

Janus D. Butcher is solely responsible for this material; the views expressed herein are his alone and in no way reflect those of his employer.

533

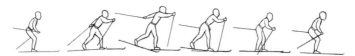

FIG 34-1   Diagram of classic or diagonal stride technique.

obtainable (Renstrom and Johnson, 1989). In the diagonal stride, the poles are used primarily for balance but can contribute up to 30% of forward thrust in higher-level skiers (Renstrom and Johnson, 1989). Double poling is utilized because increasing the tempo limits the effectiveness of the kick and glide action.

Since Bill Koch introduced the ski-skating technique to US skiers with his dramatic victory in the 1982 World Cup, the very nature of the sport has changed. This new technique rapidly evolved and has become the method of choice for most recreational prepared track skiers. Skating is the only technique used in biathlon and Nordic combined (ski jumping and cross-country skiing) competitions. The skating technique generates forward momentum by driving the skis at an angle to the direction of travel in a motion analogous to speed skating (Fig. 34-2). There is no kick phase and thus no stopping of the ski during the cycle. Several different strides (V1 skate, V2 skate, Marathon skate) are utilized depending on terrain and skier tempo. Double poling is used in most skating strides to transfer upper body energy to the skiing surface and can provide up to 60% of the forward propulsive force (Smith, 1992).

In studies evaluating the biomechanics of these techniques, skating has been shown to be much more energy efficient than the diagonal stride technique (Hoffman and Clifford, 1990). In addition, there is no need for high-friction kick wax, so low-friction glide waxes can be used along the entire surface of the ski. These factors combined with the use of extremely light-weight construction materials such as carbon fiber and Kevlar as well as improvements in skiing surface preparation have resulted in a 10–30% increase in average speed since the 1950s (Hoffman and Clifford, 1990; Street, 1992).

INJURY EPIDEMIOLOGY AND PATHOPHYSIOLOGY

Previous studies conducted when only the classic technique was used reported injury rates of between 0.1 and 5.63 injuries per 1000 skiers (Boyle et al., 1981; Sherry and Asquith, 1987). This low injury rate has long been questioned but has been difficult to measure accurately (Lyons and Porter, 1978). Unfortunately the study of the true incidence of injuries in cross-country skiing is complicated by the very nature of the sport. Cross-country skiing is not confined to specific slopes or areas, but rather, is possible wherever there is snow. In the limited data available from more confined

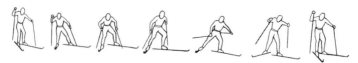

FIG 34-2   Diagram of V₁ skating technique.

circumstances, such as endurance races, the incidence was found to be substantially higher at 10–35 per 1000 skiers (Butcher and Brannen, 1998; Renstrom and Johnson, 1989).

As the sport has changed with new techniques and equipment, so too have the reported injuries among a growing population of skiers (Bovard, 1994; Dorsen, 1986; Lawson et al., 1992; Lindsay et al., 1993; Schelkun, 1992). Equipment–injury relationships that have been suggested include increased pole length, which accentuates demands on the shoulder and elbow and stiffer bindings and rigid boot construction with heel–ski fixation devices, which may increase the risk of ankle and knee injuries. The equipment–injury relationships are largely anecdotal at this point; few studies have compared injury patterns between the two techniques. The biomechanics of the new technique are also suggested in the changing injury patterns. The skating stride places significantly greater demands on the hip adductors and external rotators, muscle groups that may not be worked by traditional dry land training techniques such as running or cycling (Renstrom and Johnson, 1989). In addition, the greater emphasis on upper body strength in the double-poling action has been implicated in increasing upper extremity overuse injuries (Dorsen, 1986).

A great deal of research has been done to delineate the biomechanics and biokinetics of this new technique (Hoffman and Clifford, 1990; Renstrom and Johnson, 1989; Smith, 1992; Street, 1992). However, until recently little work had been done to support the reports of changing injury patterns associated with ski-skating. A questionnaire was used to evaluate back pain in the two skiing techniques (Eriksson et al., 1996). This study found that over 90% of skiers reported low back pain while using the classical technique but none complained of these symptoms while skating. Another study reported increased lower extremity complaints in skiers using the skating technique and a greater incidence of trunk complaints with the classical technique (Beate-Claudia, 1995). In a recent report of injuries occurring during a long-distance event where the skating technique was the dominant style used, the injury rate was found to be higher than reported for similar races in the preskating period (Butcher and Brannen, 1998). This report, however, did not specifically compare injuries between the two techniques.

Studies describing the distribution of musculoskeletal injuries in mass participation events demonstrated that lower extremity injuries are somewhat more common than upper extremity injuries (55% vs. 35%). The distribution of injuries is sprains/twists 40.4%, fractures 27.4%, contusions 16.4%, lacerations 9.3%, dislocations 5.8%, other 0.7%. The most frequently encountered acute orthopedic complaints include thumb ulnar collateral ligament strain, knee medial collateral ligament sprain, and plantar fascia strain. The most common overuse injuries include sacroilliitis, first metatarsophalngeal degenerative joint disease/synovitis, lateral ankle pain, and wrist tendinitis. Common medical illnesses reported include exhaustion/dehydration, cold injury, gastrointestinal symptoms, photokeratitis, and bronchospasm.

SPECIFIC INJURIES

Acute Injuries

Severe acute injuries are uncommon in cross-country skiing. Although major knee ligament injuries, shoulder dislocations, and fractures do occur, none are specifically associated with cross-country skiing (Morris and Hoffman, 1999). Most fractures are associated with a fall on the outstretched hand, collisions with trees during falls, loss of control on the track. These injuries are well-covered elsewhere in this text. One relatively common acute injury, skiers thumb, will be discussed below. By and large, most cross-country ski injuries are related to acute or chronic overuse.

Low Back

Sacroiliitis

The sacroiliac (SI) joint is a biconcave articulation of the hemipelvis to the sacrum. It has relatively small rotational motion but functions primarily to transmit force from the lower extremity to the spine. Sacroiliac dysfunction is the most common cause of low back pain in the skier. Injury can result from direct trauma associated with a fall, but more commonly arises from repetitive loading. Symptoms stem from inflammation in the SI joint. Contributing factors in this injury include SI joint hypermobility, excessive shear forces, and relative core strength deficits.

Typically, the athlete experiences tenderness at the SI joint and relative hypomobility on the affected side with a standing knee to chest test. The FABER test (flexion, abduction, and external rotation) usually elicits symptoms. This test is performed with the athlete supine; the hip is abducted with the knee in flexion and the leg externally rotated, producing pain in the ipsilateral SI joint. Neurologic examination is normal. Radiographs may demonstrate arthrosis or degenerative disease of the lower spine. MRI is useful if disk disease is suspected.

Treatment is aimed first at pain relief and may include oral analgesics/anti-inflammatory medications, joint mobilization treatments, ice packing, and stretching. Long-term management aims at improving SI function through core stabilization and muscle balance training (Thera-ball program, Pilates, or similar). Technique and equipment issues should also be reviewed.

Piriformis Syndrome

The piriformis muscle originates at the sacrum and inserts on the greater trochanter. It functions primarily in external rotation of the lower extremity. The sciatic nerve lies deep to the muscle and may pass through the muscle belly in up to 15% of athletes. Symptoms arise from piriformis muscle spasm, insertional inflammation, or irritation of the sciatic nerve.

Typically, the athlete complains of an aching pain in the buttocks often associated with sciatica. Symptoms may subside with skiing but will be worse at rest or with prolonged sitting. Examination reveals marked tenderness over the gluteal prominence. Pain can be reproduced with resisted abduction and external rotation of the hip, as well as with passive internal rotation of the hip (examined with the patient lying supine and the knee in full extension). The neurologic examination is usually normal, but the straight-leg raise may be positive.

Treatment should first address pain control. The principles of PRICEMM (protection, rest, ice, compression, elevation, medications, and modalities) may be useful to alleviate muscle spasm and inflammation. Deep tissue massage such as Rolfing may be helpful. Chiropractic, osteopathic, or physical therapy mobilization treatments are also frequently beneficial. Definitive treatment involves physical therapy directed at improving flexibility and correcting any associated underlying SI dysfunction.

Lower Extremity Injuries

Greater Trochanter Bursitis

Trochanteric bursitis results from irritation of any of three bursa overlying the superior margin of the greater trochanter. This arises from either direct trauma or chronic overuse in the setting of SI joint dysfunction. Associated etiologic factors include tightness in the tensor fascialata/iliotibial band, leg length discrepancy, gait anomalies, shortened hip abductors or external rotators, increased varus angulation of the hip, or a broad pelvic structure.

Skiers typically complain of a deep, aching, lateral hip pain that may extend into the buttocks or down into the lateral knee. The pain is aggravated by activity, local pressure, or stretching, and is often worse at night. Palpation over the bony prominence of the greater trochanter and slightly inferiorly or posteriorly elicits tenderness. Pain is often reproduced with resisted hip abduction and external rotation. A functional or anatomic leg length discrepancy is common. Findings of SI dysfunction including tenderness and restricted motion are almost universal. Ober's test is often helpful. To perform this test, the patient lies on their unaffected side with both hips and knees initially flexed. The affected hip and knee are then extended stressing the soft tissues over the greater trochanter. This test demonstrates poor flexibility in the iliotibial band and allows focal palpation of the effected bursa.

Treatment involves pain management, usually with anti-inflammatory medications, and activity modification to limit symptoms. Local corticosteroid injection is often effective in relieving symptoms. Because of the relatively large volume of this bursa, 10 cc of lidocaine with 80 mg of triamcinolone should be injected at the point of maximal tenderness. Definitive treatment usually involves rehabilitative exercises aimed at improving flexibility of the iliotibial band, SI function, and hip rotator strength. A comprehensive core stabilization program designed to improve strength and function of the low back, pelvis, and bilateral lower extremities should accompany this. Weight loss, conditioning, and proper lifting technique can aid in preventing recurrent or chronic injury.

Retropatellar Knee Pain (Patellofemoral Dysfunction)

Patellofemoral dysfunction (PFD) is the most common cause of chronic knee pain in the skier. PFD usually develops as an overuse injury in the setting of knee malalignment. Etiologic factors in PFD are described as both intrinsic (those related to anatomy, strength, and function) and extrinsic (external factors). Intrinsic factors include patellar malalignment (increased Q angle, patella alta or baja, lateral patellar tilt), quadriceps muscle imbalance, poor hamstring and quadriceps tendon flexibility, iliotibial band tightness, vastus medialis oblique (VMO) hypoplasia, and foot biomechanics. Contributing extrinsic factors include inappropriate ski equipment, precipitous changes in training volume, and poor training technique, to name a few.

Symptoms may arise from patellar chondral injury (chondomalacia patellae), synovial pinch, synovitis, or an irritated medial plica. Symptoms typically begin days to weeks after beginning a new routine or changing training intensity or volume. Pain is retro- or peripatellar without associated joint line symptoms. In addition to pain with skiing, symptoms may be exacerbated with running, climbing stars, or sitting with the knee flexed for extended periods of time. A retropatellar grinding sensation and snapping or popping with activity is common; however, swelling is usually minimal.

Clinical signs of malalignment are common. These include a lateral J shift of the patella (lateral tracking with active extension), an increased Q angle, positive Ober's test (see trochanteric bursitis), and over-pronated gait. The patellar grind test is usually positive. To perform this the patient lies supine with the knee flexed 10° and pressure is applied to the proximal patella or quadriceps tendon as the patient actively extends the knee. The test is considered positive if it produces pain. Other frequent physical findings include peripatellar tenderness, mild swelling, and a small joint effusion.

Radiographs are usually normal; however, subtle findings of malalignment may be seen. These include a lateral shift of the patella on the anterior-posterior weight-bearing view and a lateral tilt of the patella on sunrise view. MRI is usually not helpful.

Treatment is aimed at relieving symptoms and improving functional patellar alignment. PRICEMM provides a useful guide for symptom modifying measures. Oral anti-inflammatory medications or injected corticosteroids (80 mg of triamcinolone in 8 cc of lidocaine) are often helpful in alleviating pain. The use of an open patella knee sleeve and arch supports may also be helpful for symptom relief.

An aggressive physical therapy program should include quadriceps, iliotibial band, and hamstring stretching, balanced quadriceps strengthening (with particular attention to VMO function), and kinetic chain strengthening of the pelvis and trunk. These symptoms tend to be chronic and episodic even with adequate therapy. It is helpful to educate the athlete regarding the nature of this condition.

Occasionally, surgery may be useful in individuals with the more severe form (chondromalacia patellae). Patients with these severe symptoms and clinical evidence of chondromalacia may benefit from arthroscopic evaluation and lateral patellar release.

Patellar or Quadriceps Tendinitis

Extensor tendinitis is more common in classic technique. It is associated with similar underlying intrinsic and extrinsic factors as found in PFD (malalignment, inappropriate equipment, and technical deficiencies).

Symptoms are due to inflammation of the tendon, usually at the insertion on the inferior pole of the patella. These symptoms are typically precipitated by eccentric overload. Tenderness is localized to the patellar or quadriceps tendon and may be associated with mild swelling, erythema, and warmth. Stiffness is common after rest. Malalignment is typically seen with an increased Q angle, lateral patellar tracking, and weak ankle dorsiflexors. The posterior muscle–tendon chain and the quadriceps tendon are generally tight.

Treatment is directed toward symptom relief initially with activity modification, nonsteroidal anti-inflammatory drugs (NSAIDs), ice, and elevation. Definitive therapy aims at correcting the functional malalignment and tightness through structured physical therapy. The patient should be advised to continue in alternative, nonpainful, activities while in rehabilitation. The infrapatellar strap has been advocated for symptom relief and may be useful in some individuals. Extracorporeal shock wave therapy has been effective in relieving the discomfort, but this is an off-label indication.

Iliotibial Band Friction Syndrome

The iliotibial band arises from the tensor fascialata muscle in the lateral buttocks and runs along the lateral leg to its insertion at Gerdes tubercle on the anterolateral tibia. Tightness in the iliotibial band leads to friction irritation at the lateral femoral condoyle resulting in inflammation and pain. Predisposing factors include genu varum, leg length discrepancy, and excessive foot pronation. It is more commonly symptomatic with the skating technique.

Patients complain of lateral knee pain that is usually worse with skating or running. The character of the pain is frequently described as aching over the lateral femoral condoyle. Examination reveals marked tenderness and mild swelling along the distal course of the iliotibial band as it crosses the femoral condoyle. Ober's test usually demonstrates tightness in the iliotibial band. To perform this test, the patient is placed on the uninvolved side and both hips flexed 90° with the knees flexed to 90°. The free leg is then maximally extended. Tightness in the iliotibial band is demonstrated if the knee does not fall to the table. This position also provides an ideal position to palpate the iliotibial band.

Pain relief and anti-inflammatory measures follow the general guidelines of PRICEMM. Corticosteroid injection (triamcinolone 40 mg or betamethasone 6 mg) is useful for symptom relief. The tender area is identified (usually at the lateral femoral condoyle the steroid is injected beneath the iliotibial band under sterile technique. Typically 2–3cc of lidocaine is mixed with the steroid to provide immediate relief. Physical therapy is directed at improving iliotibial band flexibility through stretching exercise. Treatment should also address any foot biomechanical issues and underlying SI dysfunction.

Exertional Anterior Compartment Syndrome

In cross-country skiers, exertional compartment syndrome (ECS) typically affects the anterior or lateral compartments representing injury to the tibialis anterior or peroneus brevis muscles, respectively. This is precipitated by exercise-induced swelling of the soft tissue in the confined compartment, leading to ischemic pain in the effected muscle.

This is most common in skating technique where the foot is dorsiflexed and everted during ski recovery (Fig. 34-2). This injury was very prevalent when the technique was first introduced due to the excessive length of the ski and relatively soft binding used with the classic stride. As equipment has been developed specifically for the skating technique, this has become less common. It is now most commonly seen with the use of combination equipment (designed for both skating and classic technique) and with poorly fitted equipment.

Typical symptoms include pain in the anterior or lateral leg with skiing. As the condition progresses, symptoms may persist after skiing. Athletes may complain of dorsal foot or toe numbness or foot drop due to compressive neuropathy. As the condition progresses, the athlete may complain of pain with walking or in the most severe cases, at rest.

Physical examination often demonstrates tenderness and a diffusely swollen feel in the appropriate compartment. Resisted contraction of the tibialis anterior or peroneus brevis may produce pain. Pre- and postexercise compartment pressure testing may be helpful, although it is difficult to reproduce the specific conditions of skiing in the laboratory. The testing is considered positive if pressures at rest are over 15–20 mm Hg and after exertion are over 25–30 mm Hg.

Treatment consists of decreasing compartment inflammation using anti-inflammatory medications and improving function through a balanced stretching and strengthening program. Equipment modifications should be made to utilize a skating-specific boot–binding–ski system. A stiffer binding and shorter ski may also help. In many cases, surgical fasciotomy may be necessary to allow continued participation in skiing.

Peroneus Tendon Injury

Injury to the peroneus tendon can occur with an acute inversion dorsiflexion injury or develop through repetitive overload that leads to tendinitis. With an acute injury, the peroneus tendon can be torn or may be subluxed from the fibular groove with disruption of the overlying retinaculum. Acute injuries occur with both classic and skating techniques, whereas chronic tendinitis is usually seen in the skating technique.

Acute injuries present with pain, swelling, and bruising along the posterior and inferior fibula. The athlete often reports a pop in association with an appropriate mechanism. Following the acute phase, a chronic clicking sensation may be present representing subluxation of the peroneal tendon. Examination may demonstrate subluxation of the effected peroneus tendon when compared to the contralateral ankle. The athlete complains of pain with active or resisted eversion of the ankle. Peroneal tendinitis usually presents with pain and swelling along the posterior and inferior fibula. Pain is worse after skiing and interferes with other activities such as running and walking. Resisted eversion of the foot reproduces pain.

In most of these injuries, an ankle x-ray is useful to rule out associated fracture. In an acute peroneal tear or subluxation, MRI evaluation may be helpful to evaluate the extent of injury.

Acute strain injuries without a complete tear can be treated with immobilization (either casting or Rocker bottom walker boot, depending on extent of injury). This is typically continued for 4–6 weeks. Complete tear of the tendon or avulsion of the retinaculum is best managed surgically. Tendinitis is managed with temporary immobilization in a walker boot followed by active rehabilitation incorporating passive stretching and eccentric overload exercise. Anti-inflammatory medications may be helpful for pain management. Corticosteroid injection may also address discomfort. This is accomplished by injecting a solution of 60 mg of triamcinolone in 2–3 cc of 1% lidocaine into the peroneus sheath. An ankle brace or taping may allow the athlete to continue active training during the rehabilitation process.

Skier's Toe

Skiers toe is frequently used to describe pain in the first metatarsophalangeal (MTP) joint. This may represent either an acute injury (turf toe or acute sesamoid injury) or chronic problem (hallux rigidus, MTP synovitis, or sesamoiditis). In skiers, the chronic form stemming from degenerate joint disease and synovitis is most common and is associated almost exclusively with the classical technique. The mechanism of injury is repetitive extreme extension of the MPT joint.

Pain, swelling, and limited motion are the hallmarks of skiers toe. Symptoms are exacerbated with classical skiing, running, and other activities involving repetitive forced extension of the toe. Radiographs typically demonstrate first MTP degenerative disease. If a stress fracture or sesamoiditis is suspected, a three phase bone scan or limited MRI study may be useful.

Treatment is problematic; the nature of the classic technique mandates a flexible toe in the ski boot. Temporary exclusion of this technique helps to alleviate symptoms. Fortunately, the skating technique involves a rigid soled boot that allows very little flexion; thus, most skiers can skate-ski symptom free. Modifying nonskiing footwear to eliminate flexion with a spring steel insert or rigid orthotic is also beneficial. Severe cases may require temporary use of a rocker bottom boot. NSAIDS are often helpful. In cases with substantial degeneration, the athlete may benefit from surgical intervention.

Upper Extremity

Rotator Cuff Tendinitis and Impingement

Although shoulder problems are uncommon in cross-country skiers, the most common shoulder injury seen is rotator cuff tendinitis. These problems typically arise secondary to functional instability with the forces applied on the glenohumeral joint exceeding the intrinsic strength of the rotator cuff. This is most often seen in skiers using excessively long poles, usually with the skating technique.

Athletes complain of an insidious onset of pain as they transition into the ski season. Pain is localized to the anterior or lateral shoulder and is exacerbated with abduction or forward flexion of the arm. Pain at night is common. Examination usually reveals typical findings of impingement with Hawkins and/or Neer's test reproducing pain. Manual motor testing of the specific rotator cuff component exacerbates the athlete's pain and usually defines the specific muscle/tendon involved.

Plain radiographs may demonstrate subacromial spurring or acromioclavicular (AC) joint arthrosis. An MRI arthrogram should be considered if symptoms persist after treatment. This test is ideal for evaluating for cuff tears or labral injuries.

Treatment is aimed at both pain management and correction of the underlying pathoetiologic factors. Pain management strategies include the use of oral anti-inflammatory medications. Corticosteroid injection may also be effective. Subacromial injection is accomplished by instilling 80 mg of triamcinolone in 8 cc of lidocaine using a lateral approach. The needle is inserted at the junction of the middle and posterior deltoid muscle along the inferior margin of the acromion. A $1\frac{1}{2}$-inch 25-g needle is directed toward the AC joint and the solution infiltrated in a broad pattern. If symptoms persist following injection, a second, intra-articular glenohumeral injection should be considered.

Definitive treatment involves increasing functional stability of the shoulder complex. A gradual rotator cuff strengthening program both encourages healing of the injured tendon and improves intrinsic strength of the rotator cuff. Care must be taken to address associated scapulothoracic dysfunction through aggressive upper thoracic strengthening. Off-season conditioning should be encouraged to maintain rotator cuff strength and allow a problem-free transition to skiing.

Lateral Epicondylitis

Lateral epicondylitis typically refers to tendinitis of the origin of the extensor carpi radialis brevis. The mechanism of injury usually involves repetitive strain with eccentric overload due to resisted wrist extension. It may also arise with a direct blow to the lateral epicondoyle or a single macrotraumatic wrist flexion injury (against active wrist extension).

The skier complains of lateral elbow pain exacerbated with active extension of the wrist. This is seen with pole recovery as the athlete lifts the pole forward. This problem was common for a brief time when horizontal pole grips were marketed. These poles are now rarely used. Examination demonstrates tenderness at the lateral elbow. Elbow range of motion is usually preserved; however, the athlete frequently complains of discomfort with passive flexion of the wrist with the elbow fully extended. Pain with resisted wrist extension is nearly universal. Radiographs are generally not indicated.

Treatment includes analgesia with oral anti-inflammatories, ice massage, and physical modalities (ultrasound and electrical stimulation). Corticosteroid injection is also useful to address pain. In this, 80 mg of triamcinolone in 3 cc of lidocaine is injected into the tendon origin in a fanned pattern. The point of maximal tenderness serves as a useful landmark for this injection. Extracorporeal shock wave therapy has been effective in relieving the discomfort.

Physical therapy with stretching and an eccentric strengthening program is most effective. The athlete should be educated on the gradual improvement to be expected with this problem. Wrist bracing or the use of a counterforce forearm brace may be useful adjuncts to allow the athlete to continue skiing. Instruction on proper technique to avoid pole gripping and excessive wrist extension is also important.

DeQuervein's Tenosynovitis

The repetitive gripping and ulnar/radial deviation motion associated with double poling can lead to tendinitis of the extensor pollicis brevis or abductor pollicis longus. Both tendons occupy the first dorsal wrist compartment and are generally both involved. Symptoms can be insidious in onset or may arise acutely with a traumatic event. Chronic pain is common if untreated.

Typical symptoms include pain and swelling along the radial wrist. The athlete complains of pain with gripping and rotational motions (removing the lid from a jar or turning a doorknob and opening a door). Examination reveals tenderness along extensor thumb, radial wrist, and forearm and pain with resisted thumb abduction or extension. Finklestein's test is performed by placing the thumb in a flexed position beneath the flexed fingers. The wrist is passively flexed to the ulnar side. A positive test produces pain in the first dorsal wrist compartment. Radiographs are not helpful in the diagnosis of DeQuervein's tenosynovitis, but may rule out wrist arthritis or bony injury as a cause of pain.

The principles of PRICEMM are useful for pain relief. Corticosteroid injection may also be beneficial. In this, 60–80 mg of triamcinolone in 3 cc of lidocaine are injected into the tendon sheath within the first dorsal wrist compartment. Protective bracing with a thumb spica splint is helpful and may allow the athlete to continue to ski while being treated. Physical or occupational therapy is often useful to address strength and flexibility issues. Surgical treatment involving a synovectomy may be necessary in persistent cases.

Intersection Syndrome

Intersection syndrome describes a tendinitis/tenosynovitis involving the intersection comprised of extensor pollicis brevis, abductor policis longus, and the wrist extensors. The injury typically arises from repetitive overuse with gripping and wrist extension. The athlete complains of pain along the dorsoradial wrist several centimeters proximal to the carpus. Symptoms are worse with gripping, or twisting motion in wrist.

Examination reveals tenderness and swelling along dorsoradial forearm at the junction of the distal and middle thirds. Pain localized to this area is reproduced with resisted extension of wrist or abduction/extension of the thumb. Crepitance at the intersection is common. Plain radiographs are usually not helpful in this condition but may reveal underlying wrist degenerative joint disease or congenital abnormalities such as Madelungs deformity. MRI usually demonstrates the tendinopathy but is usually not helpful in management.

Treatment for pain includes the tenets of PRICEMM. Protective bracing using a thumb spica brace with the wrist in neutral or slight dorsiflexion may allow the athlete to continue skiing. Physical therapy may be helpful to address strength and flexibility issues. Anti-inflammatory medications may be useful for analgesia and swelling. Corticosteroid injections may also speed the athlete's return to activity. After sterile preparation, 60 mg of triamcinolone with 3–5 cc of lidocaine are injected into the tendon sheaths at the point of tenderness. Surgical treatment is rarely indicated.

Extensor Carpi Ulnaris Tendinitis

Injury arises either from acute strain or repetitive eccentric overload of the extensor carpi ulnaris (ECU) tendon. The ECU is contained in the sixth dorsal wrist compartment and travels just volar to the ulnar styloid and inserts on the dorsal proximal fifth metacarpal. Injury can arise from an acute strain or subluxation resulting from eccentric radial deviation or hypersupination of the wrist, respectively. This injury most commonly occurs with a fall forward with the pole planted. ECU tendinitis may also develop as a result of overuse due to poor poling technique (tight gripping of the pole) or with using poles with an inferior pole extension that applies pressure to the ulnar aspect of the wrist.

The athlete complains of pain at the ulnar wrist exacerbated by wrist extension or resisted ulnar deviation. They may have swelling along the ulnar wrist and hand. The pain often extends into the ulnar forearm. Examination reveals tenderness at the ulnar wrist that extends into the distal forearm. The pain is reproduced with resisted ulnar deviation, passive radial deviation, and resisted wrist extension.

Plain radiographs are useful in acute injuries to rule out fracture. Because ECU tendinopathy is often confused with a triangular fibrocartilage complex (TFCC) injury, an MRI arthrogram is often necessary if symptoms persist after treatment.

Treatment begins with PRICEMM. In acute injuries, a brief period of casting (2–3 weeks) may be helpful. Protective bracing with the wrist in neutral or slight dorsiflexion is usually indicated. Physical therapy addresses inflammation and early mobilization. Anti-inflammatory medications may be useful for analgesia and swelling. Corticosteroid injections are useful in the subacute phase to speed the athlete's return to activity. After sterile preparation 60 mg of triamcinolone with 3–5 cc of lidocaine are injected into the ECU tendon sheath at the ulnar wrist. Surgical treatment is rarely indicated for ECU tendinitis but is frequently required with a TFCC tear.

Skiers Thumb (Ulnar Collateral Ligament)

Injury to the UCL results from valgus stress to the thumb metacarpophalangeal (MCP) joint. This usually results from a fall on an outstretched hand with the ski pole acting as a brake on the thumb proximal phalanx as the hand hits the snow. This results in a hyperabduction injury at the MCP and a partial or complete tear of the ulnar collateral ligaments.

Following trauma, the athlete complains of pain, swelling, and bruising at the ulnar aspect of the thumb MCP. Strain testing (valgus stress) produces pain at the UCL and may demonstrate laxity.

Plain radiograph may show an avulsion fracture. MRI is useful in ruling out a Stener's lesion (UCL ligament entrapment) if significant instability is found on examination.

Immediately following the injury the athlete should be treated with PRICEMM, splinting, and analgesics as needed. Unless a complete disruption is suspected, these injuries are best treated by casting. A thumb spica cast is applied for 3–6 weeks. A complete disruption of the UCL is frequently associated with a Stener's lesion. In general, these should be evaluated by a hand specialist for surgical management. Injuries associated with a small avulsion can be managed with casting. With a large fragment or obvious joint instability, surgical referral is indicated. After immobilization, aggressive physical therapy should be undertaken to regain strength and range of motion.

Common Medical Conditions

For the most part, common medical conditions and illnesses occur with no greater incidence in cross-country skiers than in the general population. The single notable exception is exercise-induced asthma. The competitive Nordic ski season is also the flu season, and influenza immunization may be advisable for all skiers.

Exercise-Induced Asthma

Exercise-induced asthma is a common condition affecting athletes of all ages and levels of participation. Early studies suggested an incidence ranging from 2.8–11.2% (Pierson and Voy, 1988; Rice et al., 1985) with the highest frequency found in track athletes. Exercise-induced asthma effects up to 35% of winter sports athletes with the highest incidence found in cross-country skiers (Larsson et al., 1993; Rundell et al., 2000; Sue-Chu et al., 1996).

Although exercise is a common precipitator of bronchial spasm in individuals with classic asthma, the majority of athletes effected by exercise-induced asthma do not have the classic asthma history. *Exercise-induced asthma* refers to an inflammatory-mediated bronchial response precipitated by exercise. Although the exact mechanism is not established, the commonly cited etiologic factors are low humidity and temperature of inspired air. It is common for athletes to exhibit symptoms intermittently. Typically, the athlete with true exercise-induced asthma develops symptoms only in relatively extreme circumstances. The likelihood of developing symptoms increases with exercise involving a higher minute volume and cold, dry conditions.

The usual symptoms include shortness of breath with exercise that is out of proportion to effort, burning chest pain, postexercise cough, and wheezing. Other red flags include a history of childhood asthma, frequent upper respiratory illnesses, and a chronic cough.

Many testing protocols exist for exercise-induced asthma, from passive chemical challenge to graded treadmill testing (Eggleston, 1984; Garcia de la Rubia, 1998; Mannix et al., 1999). Unfortunately, these tests typically require specialized laboratory settings that may not be readily available to all affected athletes. More recently, nonlaboratory testing protocols have been described and validated. The majority of these protocols use running as the exercise challenge with pre- and postexercise pulmonary function test change as the measured variable (Garcia de la Rubia et al., 1988; Randolph et al., 1997). One study describes a cross-country skiing–specific protocol similar to the free-running test (Ogston and Butcher, 2002). Submaximal tests have also been described. In previous studies, three major factors have been identified that may significantly effect testing sensitivity: exercise load (Carlsen et al., 2000; Rundell et al., 2000), absolute humidity (Rundell et al., 2000), and temperature (Anderson and Daviskas, 2000). Exercise duration is less important (Rundell et al., 2000). Pre-exercise warm-up may also affect test results (de Bisschop et al., 1999).

Exercise-induced asthma is easily managed with medical therapy. Typically a stepped approach is undertaken (Fig. 34-3). If the athlete is felt to have classic asthma, the mainstay of therapy is inhaled corticosteroid with inhaled bronchodilator used for symptom management. These athletes should be identified and treated appropriately. With exercise-induced asthma, the main goal is prevention of airway irritation and bronchospasm through pre-exercise administration of medications.

Preventive medications include short-acting beta-agonists (albuterol, pirbuterol), long-acting beta-agonists (salmeterol), leukotriene inhibitors (montelukast sodium), and chromolyn sodium. The short-acting beta-agonists are usually effective and have the advantage of low cost, ease of use, and high compliance. Aerosolized preparations should be used with a chamber or spacer. Leukotriene inhibitors should be reserved as a second line and should always be used with a beta-agonist as a rescue medication. Chromolyn sodium is rarely effective when used alone and tends to be quite expensive in the required dosages.

If the athlete has more severe symptoms, the longer-acting beta-agonists are useful. Athletes who require second-line medications should be further evaluated and considered for treatment with inhaled corticosteroids (budesonide, fluticasone). Several preparations are available including long-acting beta-agonist/corticosteroid combinations (Advair Diskus, GlaxoWellcome). Inhaled corticosteroid is effective in alleviating the post exercise cough brought on by late phase inflammatory effects of exercise-induced asthma.

Care must be taken to ensure compliance with doping control measures in elite-level skiers. Most asthma medications are restricted and appropriate procedures for documenting their use is required. Recently, the IOC and FIS have begun requiring documented testing of these athletes prior to the use of asthma medications. The USADA hotline is a useful resource for any questions

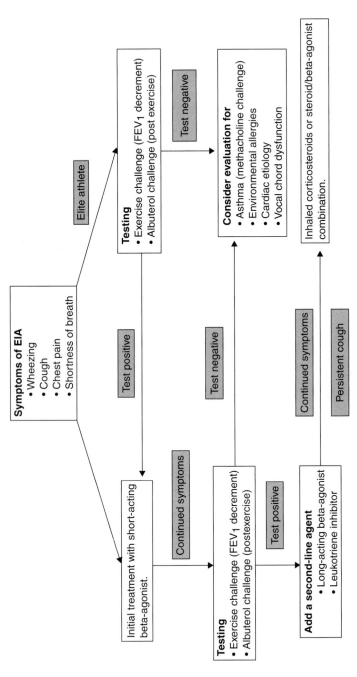

FIG 34-3 Evaluation and management of exercise-induced asthma.

Symptoms of EIA
• Wheezing
• Cough
• Chest pain
• Shortness of breath

Elite athlete

Testing
• Exercise challenge (FEV$_1$ decrement (post exercise)
• Albuterol challenge

Test negative

Test positive

Test negative

Consider evaluation for
• Asthma (methacholine challenge)
• Environmental allergies
• Cardiac etiology
• Vocal chord dysfunction

Inhaled corticosteroids or steroid/beta-agonist combination.

Continued symptoms

Persistent cough

Initial treatment with short-acting beta-agonist.

Continued symptoms

Testing
• Exercise challenge (FEV$_1$ decrement (postexercise)
• Albuterol challenge

Test positive

Add a second-line agent
• Long-acting beta-agonist
• Leukotriene inhibitor

546

regarding the use of these medications (1-800-223-0393). The World Anti-doping Agency also lists prohibited substances (http://www. wada-ama.org).

REFERENCES

Anderson SD, Daviskas E. The mechanism of exercise-induced asthma is ... *J Allergy Clin Immunol.* 2000;106:453–459.

Beate-Claudia F. Verletzungsrisiko, uberlastungsbeschwerden und prophylaktische Moglichkeiten beim skilanglauf. *Sportverl Sportschad.* 1995;9:103–108.

Bovard R. The new ski-skating poles: A role in fracture risk? *Phys Sport Med.* 1994;22:41–47.

Boyle JJ, Johnson RJ, Pope MH. Cross country ski injuries: A prospective study. *Iowa Orthop J.* 1981;1:41–48.

Butcher J, Brannen S. Comparison of injuries in classic and skating Nordic ski techniques. *Clin J Sport Med.* 1998;8:88–91.

Carlsen KH, Engh G, Mork M. Exercise-induced bronchoconstriction depends on exercise load. *Respir Med.* 2000;94:750–755.

de Bisschop C, Guenard H, Desnot P, Vergeret J. Reduction of exercise-induced asthma in children by short, repeated warm ups. *Br J Sports Med.* 1999;33:100–104.

Dorsen P. Overuse injuries from Nordic ski skating. *Phys Sport Med.* 1986;14:34.

Eggleston PA. Methods of exercise challenge. *J Allergy Clin Immunol.* 1984;73:666–669.

Eriksson K, Nemeth G, Eriksson E. Low back pain in elite cross-country skiers: A retrospective epidemiological study. *Scan J Med Sci Sports.* 1996;6:31–35.

Garcia de la Rubia S, Pajaron-Fernandez MJ, Sanchez-Solis M, et al. Exercise-induced asthma in children: a comparative study of free and treadmill running. *Ann Allergy Asthma Immunol.* 1998;80:232–236.

Hoffman MD, Clifford PS. Physiological responses to different cross country skiing techniques on level terrain. *Med Sci Sports Excer.* 1990;22:841–848.

Larsson K, Ohlsen P, Larsson L, Malmberg P, Rydstrom PO, Ulriksen H. High prevalence of asthma in cross country skiers. *BMJ.* 1993 20;307:1326–1329.

Lawson SK, Reid DC, Wiley JP. Anterior compartment pressures in cross-country skiers. *Am J Sports Med.* 1992;20:750–753.

Levinson J, Christensen A, eds. *Encyclopedia of World Sport.* New York: Oxford University Press; 1999.

Lindsay DM, Meeuwisse WH, Vyse A, Mooney ME, Summersides J. Lumbosacral dysfunction in elite cross country skiers. *J Orthop Sports Phys Ther.* 1993;18:580–585.

Lyons JW, Porter RE. Cross country skiing: A benign sport? *JAMA.* 1978;239:334–335.

Mannix ET, Manfredi F, Farber MO. A comparison of two challenge tests for identifying exercise-induced bronchospasm in figure skaters. *Chest.* 1999;115:649–653.

Morris PJ, Hoffman DF. Injuries in cross country skiing. Trail markers for diagnosis and treatment. *Postgrad Med.* 1999;105:89–91, 95–98, 101.

Ogston J, Butcher J. A sport-specific protocol for diagnosing exercise-induced asthma. *Clin J Sport Med.* 2002;12:291–295.

Pierson WE, Voy RO. Exercise-induced bronchospasm in the XXIII summer Olympic games. *N Engl Reg Allergy Proc.* 1988;9:209–213.

Randolph S, Fraser B, Matasavage C. The free running athletic screening test as a screening test for exercise induced asthma in high school. *Allergy Asthma Proc.* 1997;18:311–312.

Renstrom P, Johnson RJ. Cross country skiing injuries and biomechanics. *Sports Med.* 1989;8:346–370.

Rice SG, Bierman CW, Shapiro GG, Furukawa CT, Pierson WE. Identification of exercise-induced asthma among intercollegiate athletes. *Ann Allergy.* 1985;55:790–793.

Rundell KW, Wilber RL, Szmedra L, et al. Exercise induced asthma screening of elite athletes: Field versus laboratory exercise challenge. *Med Sci Sports Exerc.* 2000;32:309–316.

Schelkun PH. Cross country skiing: Ski skating brings speed and new injuries. *Phys Sports Med.* 1992;20:168–174.

Sherry E, Asquith J. Nordic Skiing injuries in Australia. *Med J Australia.* 1987;146:245–246.

Smith GA. Biomechanical analysis of cross country skiing techniques. *Med Sci Sports Excer.* 1992;24:1015–1022.

Street GM. Technological advances in cross country ski equipment. *Med Sci Sports Excer.* 1992;24:1048–1054.

Sue-Chu M, Larsson L, Bjermer L. Prevalence of asthma in young cross-country skiers in central Scandinavia: Differences between Norway and Sweden. *Respir Med.* 1996;90:99–105.

Vaage J, Kristensen T, eds. Hollmenkollen. In: *History and Results.* Oslo: De Norske Bokklubbene; 1992.

35 | Alpine Skiing and Snowboard Injuries

David Thorson

Skiing has been a means of transportation and survival with descriptions of equipment dating to the years before Christ. Skiing was initially a means of getting across snow-covered terrain. To control speed and direction on slopes skiers developed the telemark turn as a method of turning while descending hills. It was well-suited to the skis at the time, which had a fixed toe but free heel. The idea of alpine ski racing seems to have started in the Scandinavian countries in the late 1700s. It did not become popular in the North America until the early 1900s. The excitement of skiing downhill led to the development of bindings and skis that would allow for greater speeds and control. As downhill skiing changed so did injury patterns. In the early 1960s, *snurfing* (snow surfing) was developed but it was not until the early 1970s, when Burton and Sim's snowboards were built and marketed that the huge interest in snowboarding began. The number of alpine skiers plateaued in the late 1980s, but at that same time the sport of snowboarding was taking off and now makes up 25% of people participating in downhill sliding. The technology of the carved snowboard turn led to the development of *shaped skis*, which allow for easier turning and more efficient downhill skiing. These shaped skis have generated significant excitement and new participants in skiing as well as new injury patterns. This chapter reviews injury patterns in snowboarding and alpine skiing as well as giving a few pearls to help raise suspicion for certain unique injuries in these sports.

INJURY RATES

Injury rates for alpine skiing and snowboarding are most often reported as injuries per 1000 skier-days. The rates are inaccurate due to underreporting of less severe injuries, which are often not reported to the ski patrol or do not present to the local emergency room and to the definition of a *skier-day*. Some experts feel that accurate reporting may increase injury rates by 25%. Most injury data are acquired from ski area ski patrol data and emergency room data. It is likely that the rate of underreporting is similar for both alpine skiing and snowboarding. The other area of concern when reviewing the data is the inaccuracy of skier-days. These rates are collected by lift ticket sales and many skiers only ski part days or skip days altogether. As computerization occurs more frequently at ski resorts and each lift ride is associated with a scanned ticket, it will be easier to accurately report exposure to injury based on vertical distances skied or runs made. There has been an attempt to do this in Norway with snowboard injuries.

Multiple review articles agree on injury rates for these two sports. (Bindner and Geiger, 1999; Dunn, 2001; Fukuda et al., 2001; Hunter, 1999; Koehle et al., 2002; O'Neill and McGlone, 1999; Rønning et al., 2001; Sasaki et al., 1999; Young and Niedfeldt, 1999). Alpine skiing injury rates have been tracked for several decades. Prior to 1972 injury rates were reported at 7.8 per 1000 skier-days. After 1972, the injury rates dropped dramatically and now appeared to have plateaued in the range of 2–3 injuries per 1000 skier-days. The likely cause for this reduction is the introduction of the releasable heel binding. The two-mode binding provides release at the toe for twisting falls and release at the heel for forward falls. There are multi-mode bindings available, which provide release at the toe to upward movement and release at the heel to lateral movement. The properly adjusted binding is designed to protect leg below the knee. Proper binding adjustment and daily self-testing are associated with a decrease in lower leg injuries. A reduction of lower leg and ankle injuries by 90% has resulted directly from the introduction of the modern binding. As a result of stiffer boots, two-mode bindings protecting the lower leg, and new ski design (shaped skis) increasing the forces transferred to the knee, the knee is now the vulnerable area; knee injuries and injury rates will be discussed in detail later.

Injury rates for snowboarding are estimated to be double that of alpine skiing at 4–6 per 1000 skier days. Although any body part is vulnerable to injury in contact and collision sports such as skiing and snowboarding, there are patterns that are unique to each. Injury distribution in snowboarders involves the lower extremity only about 33% of the time; in alpine skiing, the lower extremity is involved 66% of the time. Injuries to the upper extremity in snowboarding tend to be more severe than those from skiing; injuries of the lower extremity tend to be more severe in skiers. The introduction of *twin tip skis*, skis designed for the half pipe and terrain park (special areas of the ski area where terrain is built and maintained allowing for various aerial tricks) may change the upper extremity patterns seen in alpine skiing. Injuries can be reduced in both sports by using protective gear and maintaining equipment properly.

Alpine skiing and snowboarding often occur at high altitude and the risk of dehydration and high-altitude pulmonary edema is present. Athletes at altitude experience declines in performance if they do not maintain hydration. Acclimatizing to altitude before competing at altitude, following the rule of "play high, sleep low," and minimizing caffeine and alcohol intake help to prevent problems at altitude.

Even ski waxing places athletes and coaches at risk, with reports of respiratory distress linked to frequent exposure to the fumes of overheated fluorinated waxes and base cleaners. During competition, these waxes improve glide and maintain higher speeds. Anyone waxing skis with fluorocarbon waxes containing should be aware of this problem and use a filtering respirator mask. Wax companies have warnings in their waxing charts regarding this (Appendix).

ALPINE SKI INJURIES

Alpine ski injuries occur at a frequency of 2–3 per 1000 skier-days. Over the past 20 years, there has been a dramatic change in injury patterns. Injuries to the lower leg below the knee have noted a 43% reduction. Lower extremity equipment-related injuries still occur and are often related to poor binding adjustment, causing either pre-release or delayed release. Delay in release allows increasing torque or pressure to the lower leg, resulting in fractures of the lower leg or ankle. Prior to the development of bi- and multimode release bindings, spiral fracture of the lower tibia was the skiers fracture. Prior to the more rigid modern plastic boots, the boot was a single-laced and eventually a double-laced (inner and outer) boot. This less-than-ideal coupling of the boot to the ski was related to the increased occurrence of ankle fractures.

The modern ski boot in combination with advanced binding design has reduced the rates of ankle fractures as well as the frequency of Achilles tendon injuries. Failure of the heelpiece to release transfers forces to the boot top and can cause a transverse boot top fracture, which requires surgery. Skiers who present with symptoms of lateral ankle pain after an internal rotation injury should be evaluated for subluxation of the peroneal tendon from its notch behind the lateral malleolus. High-level skiers will require surgical repair of this injury. Prevention of these injuries is associated with proper binding adjustment for weight, boot sole length and ability. Adjustment in conjunction with torque testing (Appendix 2 and 3) has been associated with a decrease in lower extremity injuries. The increase in lower extremity injuries in children is associated with older, poorly adjusted hand-me-down equipment.

The knee is now the most vulnerable area of the leg and there has been an astronomical rise in knee injuries from the increased stresses placed on the knee with the new equipment and techniques. The tighter coupling of the boot to the ski allows the skier to apply more pressure to the ski edge, which allows the ski to carve a turn. The advance of shaped skis allows skiers to ride an edge like snowboarders. When the skier is off balance, the carving ski can transfer the forces back up the leg to the knee. Knee injuries associated with skiing include medial and lateral collateral ligament injuries as well as meniscus injuries. A fairly unique injury to skiing is the isolated anterior cruciate ligament (ACL) injury. ACL injuries have increased 280 times during the same time period that lower leg injuries decreased. There have been three common patterns of injury associated with ACL injuries.

1. The big bump flat landing (Figure 35-1)
   a. Skier becomes airborne off balance and lands on the flat with the weight on the tails of the skis.
   b. Landing on the tail of the ski applies forces through the boots forward angle (forward lean built into the boot) to the knee.
   c. The skier tries to prevent a fall and while in the back seat position (hips over the tails) fires the quadriceps muscles.

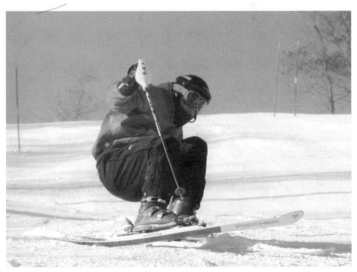

FIG 35-1 Hips behind and lower than the knees places the ACL at risk.

    d. The flexed knee position isolates the ACL, and in combination with the boot levering the lower leg forward at the knee and the quads pulling the lower leg forward from the attachment at the tibial tubercle, the ACL is torn.
2. Forward twisting fall
    a. Commonly associated with MCL but in 20% of cases ACL also
    b. The knee is extended, the skier falls forward between his skis
    c. The inside edge of the ski catches in the snow and the ski rotates the toe of the boot outward placing an external rotation and valgus force on the knee
    d. This places a stress on the MCL and ACL
3. Phantom foot (Figure 35-2)
    a. The skier falls backward between his skis.
    b. The knee is flexed and the hips are below the knee.
    c. The weighted down-hill edged ski begins to turn uphill and places a internal rotational stress on the knee.
    d. This isolates the ACL and causes the tear; *or*
    e. The skier has fallen and is sliding on his hip with the skis across the hill. The skier attempts to recover from the slide and get back up on his skis.
    f. The downhill edge is engaged into the snow to help the skier stop sliding and enable him to get up.
    g. The hips are hyperflexed and the ski begins to turn uphill, placing an internal rotational force on the knee.
    h. The ACL is torn.

Educational videos that teach beginners how to fall have been associated with decreasing ACL injuries. Skiers who fall on their uphill hip should slide until they stop, thus preventing a phantom foot ACL injury. Eventually, as binding technology improves, the ACL may gain protection. This is going

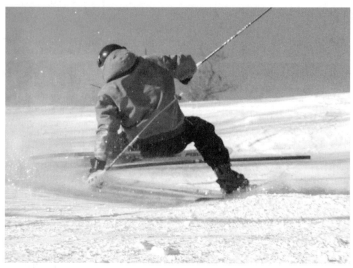

FIG 35-2 Phantom foot.

to be difficult because surrounding muscle strength enhances the strength of the ACL. How a binding will protect an ACL when there is no support from surrounding muscle, and not prematurely release when the surrounding muscles are firing will require a significant advance in technology. There has been talk and prototype boots that have a breakaway upper (the upper shell can collapse rearward) that in theory should protect the knee in a big bump flat landing situation. Whether this can be designed to work for high-level skiers without sacrificing performance is debatable. Bindings that have a mechanism for lateral release at the heel may help prevent MCL and ACL injuries in forward twisting falls. However, this has not been the case so far.

The twisting fall during a carved turn at high speed on groomed runs with smooth snow has been associated with tibial plateau fractures. This is one of the few injuries not showing a bimodal pattern of beginner and expert skiers, but rather seems to affect intermediate skiers on intermediate terrain. These injuries have severe complications if misdiagnosed. Physicians must have a higher level of suspicion when examining an injured skier with an acutely swollen knee. These injuries are also associated with collisions with trees and other objects.

Upper Extremity Injuries

Skier's Thumb

The thumb is the most frequently injured upper extremity body part followed closely by the wrist. *Skier's thumb* is associated with a fall onto the hand while holding a pole. The pole grip isolates the thumb and if it catches in the snow an ulnar collateral ligament (UCL) injury occurs. Some studies indicate that with skier's thumb there is an increased risk of a Stener lesion (the torn UCL edges are separated by fascia) when compared to other UCL injuries. If this is true, ulnar collateral thumb injuries incurred in skiing should be surgically explored and repaired. Special pole grips have been designed to prevent this injury, but have not gained widespread acceptance due to the awkward feeling they have when compared to traditional pole grips. Many authors suggest skiing without pole straps and releasing the pole when you fall as a way of preventing skier's thumb.

Wrist Injuries

Any athlete who falls on an outstretched hand and develops wrist pain requires evaluation for a scaphoid fracture. These fractures are often not visible on plain radiographs. If there is a high clinical suspicion, snuffbox tenderness, or pain at the base of the wrist over the pole of the navicular, a short arm–thumb spica cast should be applied. The cast can be removed after 2 weeks with radiographs repeated. If there is no radiographic evidence of fracture and no pain over the navicular the cast can be left off. If pain persists and x-ray films are still negative, further diagnostic testing is needed or the cast should be reapplied. A navicular fracture requires 6–8 weeks of casting and is at risk for nonunion or avascular necrosis.

Arm and Shoulder Injuries

Forearm fractures rarely occur and are usually associated with collisions with other skiers/snowboarders or stationary objects. Fractures of the humerus are also usually related to collisions, not falls. Shoulder dislocations can occur during a fall or if a ski pole gets caught on something. If a pole wrist strap is used to help hold onto the pole the pole cannot be easily released. The arm is caught and pulled behind the body and the shoulder is dislocated as the skier is twisted and decelerated by the fixed arm. Ski pole manufacturers have developed releasable pole straps to help prevent this injury. Pole baskets are designed to be less likely to become caught in trees or other places. Skiers who ski off trail or in tree areas are encouraged to remove the straps from their wrists.

Head Injuries

Head injuries are occurring with increasing frequency. There have been a number of high-profile deaths recently (Sonny Bono, Michael Kennedy) attributed to head and neck injuries in skiing. The concern is that advances in ski technology (shorter, more shaped skis) have changed skier behavior. There is no question that these skis have made it easier for the beginning and intermediate skier to carve a turn. A carved turn is more efficient and higher speeds are obtained. The better grooming at most ski areas allows less-skilled skiers to ski more advanced terrain. The combination of steeper terrain with higher speed turns increases the risk of falling. Falling at speed on shorter skis is often a backward fall, which can cause the head to hit the snow, or worse yet the skier will slide uncontrollably (slide for life) and impact stationary objects. It is apparent that ski helmets will not prevent death where there is a catastrophic neck injury due to high-speed impacts. Experts seem to disagree on the benefit of helmets for recreational skiing. There does not seem to be disagreement in the reduction in severity of concussion that could be obtained by wearing helmets. The anti-helmet group feels that helmets will increase daredevil behavior and therefore increases injuries. Helmets are being seen on recreational skiers with greater frequency and injury data are currently being gathered. It seems to be reasonable to require helmets for children who rent equipment or even for all children (as is done in some Scandinavian countries). Adults should be encouraged to wear helmets for skiing as they do for bicycling.

Pearls for Alpine Ski Injuries

1. Evaluate lateral ankle pain for peroneal tendon subluxation or disruption.
2. Acute knee pain and swelling may be a tibial plateau fracture not just an ACL injury.
3. ACL injuries in skiing can occur without collateral ligament damage.
4. Teaching skiers how to fall may decrease ACL injuries.
5. Remind skiers of the importance of yearly binding adjustment and daily release self-testing.
6. Skier's thumb carries an increased risk for a Stener lesion, which requires surgery.
7. Recommend helmets for all skiers, especially children and racers.
8. Performance drops off in the face of dehydration and fatigue.
9. Children are at increased risk for injuries partly due to older equipment and poor binding adjustment.

SNOWBOARD INJURIES

Snowboarding is the fastest growing winter sport. Snowboard injury rates are approximately double those encountered in alpine skiing. Two thirds of snowboard injuries involve the upper extremity and these injuries tend to be more severe than those associated with skiing. Snowboarders stand with both feet firmly attached to a single board. Both feet are angled forward for a carving board and outward for a freeride board. The boots are either soft, rigid (like an alpine boot), or a hybrid design. Only rarely is the binding releasable. There are unique injuries to the lower extremity of boarders; however, ACL, collateral ligaments, and lower leg fractures are rare. Most injuries to lower extremities involve the foot and ankle. Because the feet are firmly attached to the board, falling boarders attempt to catch themselves with outstretched arms and hands. These self-preservation attempts are responsible for the high upper extremity injury rate. Injuries to the wrist account for almost 40% of all snowboard injuries; over 60% are fractures. Upper extremity injury rates are different from the leading to the trailing arm, the lead arm being most frequently injured. Heel side falls (falling backward) are often associated with the back of the head striking the snow. Concussions are more frequent in snowboarding than skiing. Snowboarders participate in carving, freeriding, or halfpipes. Aerial maneuvers (impressive height obtained in jumping is called *hospital air*) in freeriding, terrain parks, or the halfpipe are associated with more frequent and severe injuries. Under-reporting is likely, but injury rates for snowboarding are reported at 4–6 per 1000 boarding days. Beginners who do not take lessons are more likely to be injured. Twenty-five percent of injuries were to first time snowboarders and 50% occurred in the first year. Experts, although injured less, tended to have more severe foot and ankle injuries.

Injuries to the Foot and Ankle

Injuries to the foot and ankle account for 15–20% of all snowboard injuries. Foot injuries (distal to the talus) make up less than 2%; about 60% of these injuries are fractures. Fractures of the metatarsal make up over three fourths of all foot fractures and are most common in boarders who wear soft boots. The lead foot is injured twice as often as the trailing foot. Calcaneal and tarsal fractures make up the remaining foot fractures.

Ankle injuries account for about 15% of all snowboard injuries and these ankle injuries are evenly divided between sprains and fractures. Roughly two thirds of ankle fractures involve the lateral or medial malleolus and one third involve the talus. These talar fractures, although rare in other sports, make up almost 2% of all snowboarding injuries and one third of all ankle fractures as well as 15% of all ankle injuries. The lateral process talus fracture has been called the *snowboarders ankle*. This injury is difficult to see on plain radiographs and any persistent lateral ankle pain after snowboarding injury should be evaluated for a lateral process talus fracture with special views or CT scan. This injury may be the result of dorsi flexion and external rotation of the hind foot (there is some disagreement as to the exact biomechanical cause). These injuries can be misdiagnosed as lateral sprains and if not treated appropriately, significant long-term ankle morbidity results.

Injury to the Knee

The knee is injured about 15% of the time. The fixed position of the foot and ankle minimize severe knee injuries and fewer than 13% of knee injuries involve the ACL, compared to 45% in skiers. Most knee injuries are sprains of the medial or lateral collateral ligaments. Fractures of the tibial plateau are rare. Use of hybrid or hard shell boots seems to increase the risk of more severe knee injuries. The lead leg again appears to be more vulnerable. There are not enough data on injury rates associated with releasable snowboard bindings to make any conclusions about improved safety or injury pattern changes.

Upper Extremity Injuries

The upper extremities are the most common area injured in snowboarding. Two thirds of all snowboard injuries involve an upper extremity. The wrist is the most frequently injured area for all snowboarding, accounting for nearly one quarter of all injuries and one half of upper extremity injuries. Upper extremity injuries tend to be more severe than those found in skiing and are most commonly caused by a fall, often after attempting a jump. The lead arm is injured most frequently and the shoulder seems to be injured most often in a forward fall and the wrist most often in a backward fall. The shoulder and clavicle account for about one third of all upper extremity injuries. Fractures account for 50% of all upper extremity injuries, dislocations less than 10%; sprains occur about 25% of the time.

Wrist and Hand Injuries

Injuries to the hand are most likely fractures (almost 50%), but make up less than 10% of all upper extremity injuries. The ulnar collateral ligament of the thumb is rarely injured (less than 2% of all injuries involving the upper extremity). The wrist is the most frequently injured area and it is most often a fracture. Wrist fractures occur most frequently to the leading hand and most often in beginners. Almost three quarters of all wrist injuries are fractures. Intermediate and above snowboarders are more likely sustain scaphoid fractures and wrist dislocations. These injuries usually occur after falling while attempting a jump. Wrist dislocations, lunate fractures, or perilunate fracture/dislocations are rare and almost always associated with aerial attempts ending in a backward fall. There is a gender difference in injuries to upper level snowboarders, but it may be due to numbers of participants more than anything else. The high rate of fractures associated with wrist and hand injuries in snowboarding requires a heightened suspicion and the use of diagnostic imaging (x-ray, CT, etc.). Snowboarders with navicular pain should be treated for a fracture until proven otherwise; plain films may take up to 5 weeks to show the fracture. The use of protective wrist guards can reduce wrist injuries by over 50% and their use needs to be reinforced to all snowboarders, especially beginners who have the highest rate of wrist injuries. Instruction has also been associated with a decrease in injuries in beginning snowboarders. Beginners frequently use rental snowboard equipment and have an increased injury rate. Snowboard rental shops should provide wrist protectors for all snowboard rentals.

Elbow Injuries

Injuries to the elbow comprise less than 10% of all snowboard injuries and severe elbow injuries are eight times more likely in those with intermediate or above abilities. Snowboarders are four times more likely to injure their elbows than alpine skiers. Fractures and dislocations of the elbow are rare in beginner snowboarders. Of all elbow injuries, almost 50% are fractures and nearly 25% are dislocations. Forearm injuries, when reported, are likely to be fractures.

Shoulder Injuries

One third of upper extremity injuries involve the shoulder (only 10% in alpine skiers). Shoulder injuries are most often the result of a forward fall. Almost one third of the injuries are fractures and most fractures involve the clavicle. Dislocations account for 20% of all shoulder injuries. As expected, more severe injuries are associated with higher abilities and aerial attempts. Most often the lead shoulder is injured. The high incidence of fractures and dislocations to the shoulder should raise the index of suspicion and indicates the need for diagnostic studies.

Head and Neck Injuries

The risk of head injury to boarders is two to six times that for skiers and the injuries are more severe. Spinal cord injuries occur four times as often and in younger snowboarders. Head injuries are more common in beginners, but are less severe. Snowboarders, especially beginners, often fall backward and therefore have an increase in occipital head injuries.

Helmets do not prevent serious, catastrophic head and neck injuries. However, helmets are very good at decreasing the severity of occipital injuries. There is considerable discussion in sports medicine circles regarding helmet use. Do they increase at-risk behavior, encourage daredevil activity, and therefore increase risks for injury? Do they protect the head sufficiently to decrease severity and frequency of concussions? Head injuries happen more frequently in beginners. It is doubtful that a helmet would enable these inexperienced boarders to attempt more difficult hills or aerial tricks. A helmet would likely minimize the degree and rate of head injury in this group. It is this author's opinion that snowboarders should be encouraged to wear helmets at all ability levels. All rental shops should provide helmets to renters and children should be required to wear helmets at ski areas.

Snowboard Pearls

1. Encourage snowboarders to wear helmets and wrist protection.
2. Lessons for beginners may decrease injury rates in this group.
3. Lateral ankle pain in a snowboarder may be a lateral talus fracture and this fracture does not show up well on routine x-rays; consider CT imaging.
4. Wrist injuries are frequently associated with fractures; suspect navicular fractures.
5. ACL injuries are less common in boarders.
6. Snowboard injuries are frequently associated with aerial maneuvers and the current trend at ski areas to provide a safer area for aerials (snowboard parks, terrain parks, and halfpipes) may increase safety.
7. Leading side is most frequently injured.

Waxing Precautions

1. Have adequate ventilation.
2. When ironing in waxes they should not be allowed to smoke.
3. Do not expose waxes to open flames.
4. Do not allow fluorocarbon waxes to overheat because they may release toxic fumes.
5. When brushing waxes, use a particle mask and protective eyewear to avoid inhaling or getting wax particles in eyes.

6. When doing base repair or ironing fluorocarbon waxes, a cartridge mask should be worn.
7. Avoid inhaling fumes from base cleaners and use only in well-ventilated areas.

REFERENCES

Bindner SR, Geiger KM. The downside of snowboarding. *Postgraduate Med.* 1999;105:83–88.

Boon AJ, Smith J, Zobitz ME, Amrami KM. Snowboarder's talus fracture. *Am J Sports Med.* 2001;29:333–338.

Bracco D, Favre JB. Pulmonary injury after ski wax inhalation exposure. *Annal Emerg Med.* 1998;32:616–619.

Deibert MC, Aronsson DD, Johnson RJ, Ettlinger CF, Shealy JE. Skiing injuries in children, adolescents, and adults. *J Bone and Joint Surg.* 1998;80:25–32.

Dunn KA. Curbside consult: What are the health hazards of snowboarding? *West J Med.* 2001;174:128–130.

Ferrera PC, McKenna DP, Gilman EA. Injury patterns with snowboarding. *Am J Emerg Med.* 1999;17:575–577.

Finch CF, Kelsall HL. The effectiveness of ski bindings and their professional adjustment for preventing alpine skiing injuries. *Sports Med.* 1998;25:407–416.

Fukuda O, Michiyasu T, Saito T, Endo S. Head injuries in snowboarders compared with head injuries in skiers. *Am J Sports Med.* 2001;29:437–440.

Goulet C, Régnier G, Grimard G, Valois P, Villeneuve P. Risk factors associated with alpine skiing injuries in children. *Am J Sports Med.* 1000;27:644–650.

Hagel BE, Pless IB, Hanley JA. Letters to the editor (re: wrist injuries in snowboarding). *Am J Sports Med.* 2001;29:676–678.

Hame SL, Oakes DA, Markolf KL. Injury to the anterior cruciate ligament during alpine skiing. *Am J Sports Med.* 2002;30:537–540.

Hunter, RE. Skiing injuries. *Am J Sports Med.* 1999;27:381–389.

Idzikowski JR, Janes PC, Abbott PJ. Upper extremity snowboarding injuries. *Am J Sports Med.* 2000;28:825–832.

Kirkpatrick DP, Hunter RE, Janes PC, Mastrangelo J, Nicholas RA. The snowboarder's foot and ankle. *Am J Sports Med.* 1998;26:271–277.

Koehle MS, Lloyd-Smith R, Taunton JE. Alpine ski injuries and their prevention. *Sports Med.* 2002;32:785–793.

Levy AS, Hawkes AP, Hemminger LM, Knight S. An analysis of head injuries among skiers and snowboarders. *J Trauma.* 2002;53:695–704.

Machida T, Hanazaki K, Ishizaka K, et al. Snowboarding injuries of the chest: Comparison with skiing injuries. *J Trauma.* 1999;46:1062–1065.

Matsumoto K, Miyamoto K, Sumi H, SumiY, Shimizu K. Upper extremity injuries in snowboarding and skiing: a comparative study. *Clin J Sports Med.* 2002;12:354–359.

Natri A, Beynnon BD, Ettlinger CF, Johnson RJ, Shealy JE. Alpine ski bindings and injuries. *Sports Med.* 1999;28:35–48.

Oates KM, Van Eenenaam P, Briggs K, Homa K, Sterett WI. Comparative injury rates of uninjured, anterior cruciate ligament-deficient, and reconstructed knees in a skiing population. *Am J Sports Med.* 1999;27:606–610.

O'Neill DF, McGlone MR. Injury risk in first-time snowboarders versus first-time skiers. *Am J Sports Med.* 1999;27:94–97.

Rønning R, Gerner T, Engebretsen L. Risk of injury during alpine and telemark skiing and snowboarding. *Am J Sports Med.* 2000;28:506–508.

Rønning R, Rønning I, Gerner T, Engebretsen L. The efficacy of wrist protectors in preventing snowboarding injuries. *Am J Sports Med.* 2001;29:581–585.

Sacco D, Sartorelli DH, Vane DW. Evaluation of alpine skiing and snowboarding injury in a northeastern state. *J Trauma.* 1998;44:654–659.

Sasaki K, Takagi M, Ida H, Yamakawa M, Ogino T. Severity of upper limb injuries in snowboarding. *Arch Orthop Trauma Surg.* 1999;119:292–295.

Sasaki K, Takagi M, Kiyoshige Y, Ogino T. Snowboarder's wrist: Its severity compared with alpine skiing. *J Trauma.* 1999;46:1059–1061.

Shorter NA, Mooney DP, Harmon BJ. Snowboarding injuries in children and adolescents. *Am J Emerg Med.* 1999;17:261–263.

Smekal V, Kadletz R, Rangger C, Gföller P. A new type of triplane fracture in a 19-year-old snowboarder. *J Trauma.* 2001;50:155–157.

Weir E. Snowboarding injuries: Hitting the slopes. *Can Med Assoc J.* 2001;164:88.

Young CC, Niedfeldt MW. Snowboarding injuries. *Am Fam Phys.* 1999;59:131–136, 141.

36 | Figure Skating

Sami F. Rifat and James L. Moeller

QUICK LOOK

Anorexia Nervosa

- Altered body image
- Fear of gaining weight
- Refusal to maintain weight
- Amenorrhea
- Complete nutritional assessment
- Multidisciplinary treatment approach

Bulimia Nervosa

- Binge eating
- Inappropriate purging behavior
- Behavior occurs at least twice weekly for 3 months
- Complete nutritional assessment
- Multidisciplinary treatment approach

Concussion

- Traumatic brain injury
- Often associated with headache, dizziness, cognitive deficit, nausea, vomiting, and memory loss
- No universally agreed upon grading system or management protocol

Exercise-Induced Bronchospasm

- Distinct from asthma
- Increased risk in those with allergic rhinitis
- Diagnosed with exercise challenge test
- Treated with beta-2 agonist, mast cell stabilizer, leukotreine inhibitor

Ischial Bursitis

- Usually due to repeated falls
- Ice and analgesics first-line treatment
- Stretching exercises and sometimes physical therapy
- Injection as last resort

Fibular Stress Fracture

- Boot top injury
- Often not diagnosed on x-ray
- Bone scan confirms the diagnosis
- Modify or pad the boot to prevent further irritation

Malleolar Bursitis

- Adventitial bursa
- Pad or modify boot
- Iontophoresis sometimes beneficial

- Consider injection
- Surgical removal as last resort

Spondylolysis

- Pars interarticularis stress fracture
- Pain with extension, positive Stork test
- Rest, physical therapy consisting of trunk stabilization
- Bracing or surgery in refractory cases
- The great majority return to normal activity

Spondylolisthesis

- Anterior slippage of vertebral body as a result of spondylolysis
- Mild spondylolisthesis treated with physical therapy
- Mild forms often able to maintain full activity
- More severe forms require surgery and activity modification

Figure skating is an increasingly popular sport with participants of all ages. Originally skating grew from necessity as a mode of transportation across the frozen ponds, lakes, rivers, and streams of northern Europe. Eventually figure skating developed as participants traced preestablished curves or figures on the ice. Figure skating as we know it today traces its origins to an American named Jackson Haines who lived from 1840 to 1875. Haines introduced artistic and expressive dance movements to the sport. Haines' way was not immediately embraced and it was not until the turn of the century that others began to adopt the style of figure skating that we recognize today.

COMMON FIGURE SKATING TERMINOLOGY

- *Connecting steps/footwork:* a series of connected skating movements.
- *Edges:* each skate blade has two edges, an inside and an outside.
- *Figures:* a footwork skill in which patterns are traced on the ice.
- *Jump:* a leap into the air named by the take-off position and the number of revolutions.
- *Lift:* a pair movement in which the male partner raises his female partner above his head.
- *Neutral position:* a position where the shoulders are square to the hips.
- *Spin:* a rotation of the body around the vertical axis. Spins can be performed in a vertical or horizontal position.
- *Stroking:* forward or backward skating movement.

CATEGORIES IN COMPETITIVE FIGURE SKATING

Figure skating (and speed skating) is governed by the International Skating Union (ISU), which was founded in 1892. The first ISU-sanctioned figure skating event was held in 1898. In 1908, because events could be held indoors, figure skating was added to the Summer Olympic Games. It eventually was moved to the Winter Games in 1924.

There are four Olympic Figure Skating events: ladies singles, men's singles, pairs, and ice dancing. In addition to these Olympic events, the United States Figure Skating Association (USFSA) also recognizes precision (synchronized team) skating. Each category has its own unique requirements and elements.

Singles: Men's and Women's

Singles skating consists of a short program and a free skate. The short program is comprised of eight prescribed elements including jumps, spins, and combinations. In the free skate program, the skater performs an original arrangement of elements and techniques to music.

Pair Skating

The pair skating event also consists of a short program and free skating. In addition to the standard elements seen in singles skating, pair skating involves overhead lifts and throws. The pair skating performance requires that the skaters also demonstrate strength, grace, and harmony.

Ice Dancing

Ice dancing is similar to ballroom dancing and consists of three sections: compulsory, original, and free dance. In the compulsory dance the couples perform two predetermined dances; original dance must follow selected rhythms, although the couple may choose their own music and steps. In the free dance, the pair is free to expresses their own interpretation of their selected music. The moves are limited to footwork, small lifts, and short spins.

Precision Skating

Precision (synchronized) team skating involves approximately 20 skaters who occupy the ice at the same time. The team performs intricate choreography involving footwork, speed, and close complex connecting moves. There are no jumps or spins, however; owing to the number of simultaneous participants, the risk of collision with a teammate is the highest of the four forms of skating.

DEMOGRAPHICS AND EPIDEMIOLOGY

Figure skaters often start at young ages and soon begin practicing long hours. Many skaters go on to compete at high levels before the age of 14. The sports medicine physician therefore must be familiar with the medical, growth, nutrition, and behavioral concerns in children and adolescents.

Although little injury data exists, in a study of elite Danish figure skaters, Kjar and Larsson (1992) reported an injury rate of 1.4 injuries per 1000 hours of competitive skating. Like many sports, the rate and severity of injury rise with higher levels of competition. Despite this, the overall incidence of injury in skating is lower than many other sports including gymnastics and dance.

Long practice hours predispose skaters to overuse injuries. The lower extremities are most commonly involved and the boot is responsible for a significant percentage of these injuries (Block, 1999; Smith, 2000). The remaining injuries are traumatic and occur from falls or collisions with other skaters or the boards that surround the ice surface. Collision between skaters is becoming more common with the increasing popularity of precision skating. Also, because precision skaters frequently hold onto each other, injuries to the upper extremities occur more frequently than in the other skating disciplines.

Environmental Concerns

The skater faces several potential environmental hazards in the ice rink. Many rinks have inadequate heating and ventilation systems subjecting the skater to cold conditions and poor air quality. Carbon monoxide (CO), nitrogen dioxide (NO_2), and other potentially toxic gases are produced by the internal combustion engine of ice resurfacing equipment (e.g., Zamboni). The use of an electric resurfacing machine can solve this problem; however, many facilities cannot afford this more expensive equipment.

Physicians covering events in ice arenas should become familiar with the symptoms of CO and NO_2 sickness. Symptoms of CO poisoning may include headache, dizziness, weakness, tachypnea, nausea, vomiting, and loss of coordination. Symptoms of NO_2 exposure include cough, hemoptysis, chest pain, dyspnea, profuse sweating, dehydration, weakness, anxiety, and nausea. Recognition and prompt treatment is imperative.

MEDICAL CONDITIONS

Exercise-Induced Bronchospasm

Exercise-induced bronchospasm (EIB) is frequently encountered in athletes who participate in cold, dry climates and is present in about 10% of the population. EIB is a separate and distinct entity from asthma, although 90% of those with underlying asthma demonstrate an exercise-induced component. Individuals with environmental allergies are also at increased risk for the development of EIB.

Individuals with EIB experience airway hyperreactivity beginning 6–10 minutes after the onset of intense activity. Most commonly, the athlete presents with a history of cough, shortness of breath, wheeze, and/or chest tightness. The cardiopulmonary examination is often normal. Exercise challenge pulmonary function testing (PFT) may provoke symptoms. However, if performed in the office setting, the ambient temperature, humidity, and physical challenge may be insufficient to trigger the skater's symptoms.

Although many physicians feel it is appropriate to treat based on history, diagnosis and treatment is more precise when PFT is obtained prior to initiating treatment. Testing may identify an individual with underlying asthma who may derive greater benefit from long-term asthma treatment as opposed to pre-exercise EIB treatment. Other conditions such as cardiac disease, other lung disease, vocal cord dysfunction, and gastroesophageal reflux disease, to name a few, may mimic EIB. A baseline PFT should be performed followed by a postexercise (6- to 10-minute exercise challenge at 85% of maximal predicted heart rate) test. A 15% drop in forced expiratory volume in 1 second (FEV_1) is diagnostic. If your testing facility does not have the ability to perform an appropriate exercise challenge, a methacholine challenge test may be used instead.

Short-acting, inhaled beta-2 agonists (e.g., albuterol) used 15–30 minutes prior to exercise is the treatment of choice for EIB. Other medications such as long-acting beta-2 agonists (e.g., salmeterol), leukotriene inhibitors, and inhaled mast cell stabilizers (e.g., cromolyn sodium) are also effective. In patients with underlying asthma, inhaled corticosteroids should be considered a mainstay of long-term therapy. Newer agents like leukotriene inhibitors are proving to be very helpful in the treatment of asthma and their effectiveness in the treatment of EIB is showing promise.

Eating Disorders

The figure skating athlete is believed to be at increased risk for the development of eating disorders. Figure skating is judged on both athletic abilities and aesthetic qualities. This external validation together with heightened body awareness and pressures to be thin, increase the potential for eating disorders in figure skaters.

An estimated 0.5–3.7% of women in the general population suffer from anorexia (APA, 1994). *Anorexia nervosa* is characterized by a symptom complex including (1) refusal to maintain body weight at or above a minimally normal weight for age and height; (2) intense fear of gaining weight or becoming fat, even though the patient is underweight; (3) altered body image, and (4) amenorrhea in postmenarchal females (APA, 1994).

Bulimia nervosa is believed to have a lifetime incidence of 1.1–4.2% of all females (McCrea et al., 1998). The diagnostic criteria for bulimia nervosa include (1) recurrent episodes of binge eating characterized by eating a larger than "normal" amount of food in a discrete period of time and a sense of lack of control over eating during the episodes; (2) recurrent inappropriate compensatory behavior to prevent weight gain (e.g., self-induced vomiting, laxative use, etc.); (3) the above activities occur, on average, at least twice weekly for 3 months; (4) self-evaluation is unduly influenced by body shape and weight; and (5) the disturbance does not occur exclusively during episodes of anorexia nervosa (Collins et al., 1999).

Parents and coaches may unwittingly make remarks that foster the development of an eating disorder. A seemingly simple comment like "your skating dress is getting a little tight" in the intensely competitive young athlete may cause them to experience feelings of self-doubt and fear of losing acceptance in their sport because they perceive their weight is outside the acceptable range.

Once an eating disorder is recognized, the nutritional status and the overall health of the individual are paramount. Anorexia nervosa and bulimia nervosa are considered potentially life-threatening conditions and treatment needs to be initiated immediately. The mortality rate for anorexia is approximately 12 times higher than the annual death rate due to all causes among females ages 15–24 in the general population (Sullivan, 1995).

Treatment strategies for eating disorders in general include (1) restoring weight loss and elimination of disordered eating patterns; (2) treating psychological disturbances; and (3) achieving long-term remission and rehabilitation.

Menstrual Irregularities

Young female athletes commonly experience menstrual irregularities. Menstrual abnormalities may be seen as an isolated entity or may be associated with other conditions such as eating disorders and osteoporosis, which together are known as the *female athlete triad.* Both primary and secondary amenorrhea may be the result of many exhaustive hours of training. Because of the potential long-term problems associated with amenorrhea, a physician should evaluate athletes with menstrual irregularities.

Concussion

Concussion, or mild traumatic brain injury, may occur due to direct or indirect trauma. Direct head trauma in figure skating usually occurs when the head strikes the ice or the boards during a fall. Head injury can also occur indirectly as a result of a hard fall onto the buttocks that transmits the force of the fall along the spinal column to the head, causing concussion.

A general, although not universally, accepted definition of *concussion* is traumatic brain injury causing alteration in mental functioning with or without loss of consciousness. Accelerative and deccelerative forces create movement of the brain within the skull causing direct injury to the brain tissue, which subsequently affects neurochemical brain function.

Any mild traumatic brain injury should be evaluated fully before return to athletic participation is allowed. Evaluation of the conscious athlete includes a general neurologic evaluation and tests to determine level of mental functioning. This testing includes a combination of many of the following: general orientation questions (person, place, time), long-term and short-term memory evaluation, general knowledge questions, math story problems, item recall, and ability to recite the months of the year in reverse order. The presence of associated symptoms such as dizziness, nausea, and headache, and signs such as confusion, poor concentration, and agitation should also be documented.

Grading the severity of concussion is difficult in that there is no agreed upon system. Currently, it is recommended that clinical evaluation with serial follow-up and neuropsychological testing be used to assess injury severity and individually guide return to play decisions (Johnston, 2002). Recently, several neuropsychological testing models have been developed as a way to follow patients after concussion to help determine severity of injury and when it may be safe for an athlete to return to play (Collins et al., 1999; McCrea et al., 1998; Wentzell et al., 2001). There are several computer-based programs that can be used to test skaters annually to establish a baseline for post-concussion testing to help with the return to play recommendation. Currently, the return to sport decision is made more on physician experience and level of comfort than on scientific evidence.

MUSCULOSKELETAL INJURY

Spondylolysis and Spondylolisthesis

In adults, most back pain is due to either muscular strain or intervertebral disk pathology. Because of this, empiric treatment can often be safely initiated. If symptoms fail to improve, then further work-up is begun. Back pain in a child or adolescent, however, should prompt an early, aggressive work-up to identify the underlying cause prior to the initiation of significant therapeutic intervention. This more aggressive approach arises from the fact that back pain in young athletes is often caused by other potentially more serious conditions (Micheli and Wood, 1995).

Spondylolysis is the most common cause of low back pain in active adolescents who seek medical attention for their pain (Micheli and Wood, 1995). It is believed that repetitive hyperextension activity is the primary cause of this injury. The stress of landing jumps and the layback position (Fig 36-1) places the posterior elements of the young spinal column at risk for injury. Although spondylolysis is more likely to occur in men, spondylolisthesis (bilateral spondylolysis that results in anterior/posterior slippage of the adjacent vertebral segments) is more common in women. A family history of spondylolysis or the presence of spina bifida occulta are considered additional risk factors for the development of this condition.

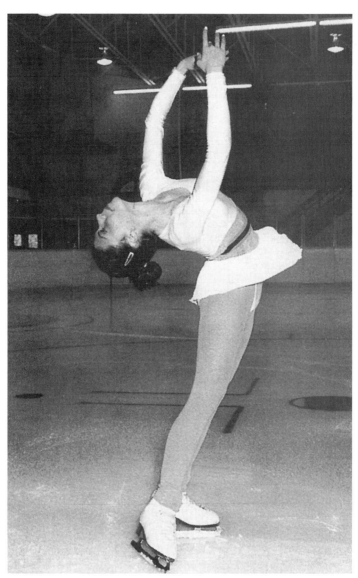

FIG 36-1 The layback position.

Athletes with spondylolysis usually present with unilateral low back pain. Less often, they may experience bilateral symptoms. In most cases, there is no radiation of the discomfort, no radicular symptoms, no bowel or bladder control issues, and no history of fevers, sweats, chills, or unexplained weight loss. There may be a history of trauma due to the athlete's physically active lifestyle, but often the onset is insidious. The pain is typically worsened by activity, especially activity that involves an upright position or hyperextension. The discomfort is often at least partially relieved by rest.

Physical examination often reveals tenderness in the paravertebral muscles. Lateral bending, rotation to the side of the injury, and hyperextension of the lower back, especially while the athlete is standing on one leg (Fig 36-2), all may increase the patient's pain. When the history and physical examination are consistent with spondylolysis, radiographs should be obtained. Many lesions can be identified on the AP and lateral projections alone; however, oblique views are classically obtained to look for radiolucent changes at the neck region of the Scotty dog (Fig 36-3). AP views are also helpful in determining the presence of spina bifida occulta and the lateral view is necessary for diagnosis spondylolisthesis. A radiolucent defect on standard radiograph examination does not determine whether the lesion is active (recent) or is inactive (old). To determine if the injury is active, a radionucleotide bone scan should be obtained (Fig 36-4). Computed tomography (CT) or magnetic resonance imaging (MRI) may provide additional information; however, they need not always be obtained. CT scanning is useful in determining the exact location and extent of the injury as well as pro-

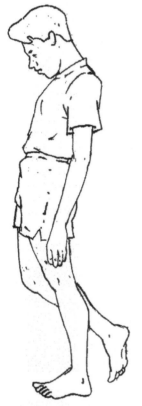

FIG 36-2 The "Stork" test.

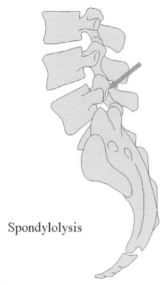

Spondylolysis

FIG 36-3   Pars interarticularis stress fracture.

viding some insight into healing, and MRI is useful in identifying any associated soft tissue involvement.

Active spondylolysis is managed conservatively. Initial treatment involves
rest, especially from lower back hyperextension. Ice and/or heat may provide
comfort and can be used alone or in a contrast pattern. Acetaminophen or nonsteroidal anti-inflammatory drugs (NSAIDs) can also alleviate the discomfort.
A rehabilitation program incorporating lower extremity flexibility together
with an abdominal strengthening and trunk stabilization should be initiated. If
these initial measures are unsuccessful, bracing, although now falling somewhat out of favor, may be needed (Moeller and Rifat, 2001). Bracing should
be used in conjunction with the rehabilitation regimen. Following successful
rehabilitation, activities should be introduced at a very low intensity with a

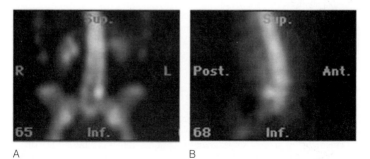

A   B

FIG 36-4   Abnormal bone scan L5 on left. **(A)** Coronal view. **(B)** Sagittal
view.

slow progression to full activity. Physicians who do not regularly treat spondylolysis should consider referring these patients to a sports medicine physician.

Spondylolisthesis presents with clinical symptoms similar to spondylolysis. The lateral radiograph is utilized to determine the degree of anterior/posterior displacement of the adjacent vertebral bodies. The progression of spondylolisthesis should be monitored closely during an adolescent's maximum linear growth stage owing to the increase risk of vertebral body displacement during this period. Many patients with a grade I (less than 25% displacement) injury are asymptomatic and can compete normally without symptoms or long-term problems. Larger degrees of displacement may require a thoracolumbar orthosis, and if the degree of displacement increases or neurologic compromise develops, surgical intervention may be necessary.

Fibular Stress Fractures

Stress fractures in the lower leg are common in many sports. In the lower leg, the tibia bears the majority of force in comparison to the fibula. For this reason, tibial stress fractures are very common in upright sports that involve running and jumping. The fibula is most often spared.

In figure skating, however, the fibula is often subjected to increased stress caused by the top of the skating boot. The compressive force of the boot at this location is believed to be significant. Additionally, figure skaters, unlike other jumping athletes, do not jump straight up and down. Take off and landing occur on either the inside or outside edges of the skate blade. Outside edge activities place increased stress on the peroneal musculature and fibula, which contributes to the risk of fibular stress fracture. Other potential risk factors for development of stress fractures in skaters include poor nutrition, abnormal mechanics, poor jumping/landing technique, improperly fitting boots, and menstrual irregularities.

Skaters with fibular stress fractures present with lateral lower leg pain that is worsened by activity and relieved by rest. There usually is no specific history of trauma. In more severe cases, routine daily activities may cause local discomfort and the patient may report soft tissue swelling. Palpation reveals fibular tenderness, which may mimic isolated peroneal muscle/tendon injury. Manual muscle strength testing may be painful, and may not be helpful in differentiating between a fibular stress fracture and soft tissue injuries. Use of a tuning fork to elicit tenderness with vibratory stimulus may be helpful as additional evidence.

Radiographs should always be obtained when fibular pain is present. Periosteal elevation and/or cortical thickening visible on radiographs indicate a stress fracture. Unfortunately, radiographs often do not reveal stress fractures. Therefore, if symptoms persist or the index of suspicion remains high, a bone scan should be obtained. A definitive diagnosis confirming the presence or absence of a stress fracture of the fibula is very important because the treatment for stress fracture is drastically different from the treatment of muscle strains and tendinopathies. If unrecognized, a fibular stress fracture may progress to a completed fracture. If this occurs, a prolonged period of immobilization is usually required.

Treatment of fibular stress fracture includes removing the athlete from activities that result in harmful stress to the injured bone. If the patient has pain with routine activity, non-weightbearing or partial weightbearing is indicated. To facilitate healing, however, crutches should be weaned as soon as pain permits because weightbearing stimulates bone metabolism. The boot should be examined for the presence of a pressure point that may cause undue stress to the fibula. If an excessive pressure point is found, the boot should be taken to the boot maker to stretch or pad the boot appropriately. During this rest period, the skater should be encouraged to remain as physically active as possible by engaging in activities that do not cause pain to the injured area. This continuing physical activity should be performed to prevent muscular and cardiovascular deconditioning. Activities may include bicycling, swimming, water running, and some resistance training. As symptoms improve, the athlete may begin a gradual progression to more vigorous physical activity. Activities should start at low intensity with slow progression back to full activity, leaving the most demanding weightbearing activities to the end.

Muscle Strains and Tendinopathy

Muscle strains and tendinitis are common overuse injuries among figure skaters. Although a great deal of the power for skating and jumping is generated from the hip, buttock, and thigh musculature, the foot and ankle muscles also play a large role in speed development and fine control of jumping and landing. Furthermore, the high repetitions and eccentric activity predispose to injury. The gastrocnemius, soleus, tibialis posterior, flexor hallucis, flexor digitorum, peroneal longus, and peroneal brevis muscles together with their associated tendons are all at increased risk.

Many muscle and tendon injuries can be treated aggressively with rehabilitation while the athlete continues to skate at a decreased level of intensity. A general program of muscle stretching and endurance training is initiated as soon as pain permits. Pain and swelling can be treated with a combination of compression, elevation, ice, and NSAID use. Activities should be performed below the soreness threshold (REST = *r*esume *e*xercise below the *s*oreness *t*hreshold). In more severe cases, electrical stimulation and ultrasound may be of benefit. In cases where the signs and symptoms of injury are severe and more refractive to these interventions, iontophoresis or phonophoresis may prove helpful.

Ankle Bursitis

Bursitis over the bony prominences of the ankle is an interesting entity described almost exclusively in figure skaters. Bursae do not typically develop over the bony prominences of the ankle; however, adventitial bursae may develop if the ankle is exposed to consistent stress and frictional forces. Long hours and tight boots lend to the formation of bursa over the malleoli and anterior aspect of the ankle. These bursae can grow large enough to cause improper fit of the skating boot, which worsens the friction and creates a vicious cycle. Many skaters with ankle bursitis see their physician complaining of swelling rather than pain.

The diagnosis of adventitial ankle bursitis is usually straightforward. There is no history of trauma to the affected area and no significant history of pain. The bursa is usually swollen, sometimes red, and fluctuant. Radiographs are of limited value in making an accurate diagnosis. If infection of the bursa is suspected based on clinical signs and symptoms (pain, fever, erythema, local warmth, adenopathy), a fluid analysis may be helpful.

Adventitial bursitis often does not respond well to simple, conservative treatment. Boot stretching and padding may be helpful, but may not entirely solve the problem. Aspiration of the bursal fluid may be both diagnostic and therapeutic. After the area is appropriately prepped, a large gauge needle is used to aspirate the thick, gelatinous fluid. Sometimes, the viscosity of the fluid may make it difficult or impossible to aspirate. If the fluid is clear and no clinical evidence of infection exists, a small amount of corticosteroid can be injected in an attempt to decrease inflammation within the bursa. A pressure wrap should be applied and the athlete should be advised to ice and take NSAIDs. If the fluid appears infected (cloudy), appropriate antibiotic therapy should be initiated. In refractory cases, surgical excision of the bursa may be required.

Apophyseal Avulsion Injuries of the Hips and Pelvis

Any acute injury to the hips or pelvis in the young skater should raise suspicion of apophyseal injury. In the skeletally immature the apophysis is often the weakest link in the musculoskeletal system. Specifically, the muscle tendon unit is often stronger that it's boney attachment. As a result, injuries that typically cause a muscle strain (pull) often cause avulsion injury or fracture in the skeletally immature (Table 36-1).

Skaters with an avulsion injury usually present complaining of acute onset of pain. Typically they report difficulty with movement of the affected muscle group. On examination pain with active range of motion and weakness with resisted movement are present. All skeletally immature individuals with a clinical suspicion of this injury should have x-rays performed.

Individuals with small, minimally displaced avulsion injuries should be treated with ice, analgesics, and sometimes given crutches if they have difficulty ambulating. The athlete should be removed from competition until they have regained normal range of motion and strength. Radiographic healing should also be present before full activity is resumed. Rarely, more significant (>2 cm displacement) avulsion injury occurs. Although controversial, some recommend surgical repair (Wooten et al., 1990).

Ischial Bursitis

Ischial bursitis is a painful condition that often occurs in the skating athlete as the result of repeated falls onto the ice surface. Symptoms include buttock pain and decreased range of motion at the hamstring on the affected side. On physical examination the individual is tender at the buttock over the ischial tuberosity. There is often also marked loss of hamstring flexibility on the affected side. Treatment usually consists of relative rest and protection of the affected area. Ice, anti-inflammatory medications, stretching, and sometimes physical therapy are helpful. If these measures do not seem to help, a local corticosteroid injection may be of benefit.

TABLE 36-1 Sites of Potential Avulsion Injuries at the Hips and Pelvis in the Skeletally Immature

Location of bony attachment	Muscle(s)
Anterior superior iliac spine	Sartorius
Anterior inferior iliac spine	Rectus femoris
Ischium	Hamstring
Lesser trochanter femur	Iliopsoas
Greater trochanter femur	Piriformis
Iliac crest	Abdominal oblique muscles

REFERENCES

American Psychiatric Association. *Diagnostic and statistical manual of mental disorders*, 4th ed. Washington, DC: American Psychiatric Association; 1994.

American Psychiatric Association Work Group on Eating Disorders. Practice guideline for the treatment of patients with eating disorders (revision). *Am J Psych.* 2000;157:1–39.

Bloch RM. Figure skating injuries. *Phys Med Rehabil Clin N Am.* 1999;10:177–188.

Collins MW, Grindel SH, Lovell MR, et al. Relationship between concussion and neuropsychological performance in college football players. *JAMA.* 1999;282:964–970.

Johnston KM (Chair). Summary and Agreement Statement of the 1st International Symposium on Concussion in Sport, Vienna 2001. *Clin J Sport Med.* 2002;12:6–11.

Kjar M, Larsson B. Physiological profile and incidence of injuries among elite figure skaters. *J Sports Sci.* 1992;10:29–36.

McCrea M, Kelly JP, Randolph C, et al. Standardized assessment of concussion (SAC): On-site mental status evaluation of the athlete. *J Head Trauma Rehabil.* 1998;13:27–35.

Micheli LJ, Wood R. Back pain in young athletes: Significant differences from adults in causes and patterns. *Arch Pediatr Adolesc Med.* 1995;149:15–18.

Moeller JL, Rifat SF. Spondylolysis in active adolescents. *Phys Sportsmed.* 2001;29:27–32.

Smith AD. The young skater. *Clin Sports Med.* 2000;19:741–755.

Sullivan PF. Mortality in anorexia nervosa. *Am J Psych.* 1995;152:1073–1074.

Wentzell T, Leclerc S, Johnston K. Sports medicine simplified? The challenge of combining ease of use with diagnostic capability in an on-field concussion assessment tool. *Med Sci Sports Exerc.* 2001;5(suppl 1):S198.

Wooton JR, Cross MJ, Holt KW. Avulsion of the ischial apophysis. The case for open reduction and internal fixation. *J Bone Joint Surg Br.* 1990;72:625–627.

37 | Dance Injuries

Jim Macintyre

Ballet is a demanding activity that requires a unique balance of athleticism and artistry. Ballet developed hundreds of years ago and the traditional positions and movements have changed very little over time. Dancers reaching the highest levels of performance must meet specific, rigorous demands for body type, strength, flexibility, balance, and mental concentration. Meeting these demands can place significant stress on the dancer, with attendant potential for injury.

Participation in ballet declines with age for a variety of reasons, but injury is frequently implicated. There are numerous epidemiologic studies of dance injuries, with injury incidence 40–80% depending on the level of participation and a lifetime incidence of up to 90% for all dancers (Liederbach, 2000). Many studies document injury patterns, with the lower leg, foot, and ankle making up roughly 35–50%, the knee 10–20% and hip about 10% of injuries (Liederbach, 2000). Injuries generally are classified into two types: acute traumatic injuries and overuse injuries.

ACUTE TRAUMATIC INJURIES

Acute injuries result form single episodes of overstress or trauma, and account for 40–50% of injuries; and male dancers tend to have more traumatic injuries than female dancers. Several factors predispose the dancer to acute traumatic injuries. High-level ballet involves a number of difficult maneuvers involving jumps, landings, twists, and lifts with partners. These movements are performed in positions determined by tradition rather than biomechanical efficiency and failure to perform these movements correctly can lead to acute injuries.

Following an acute injury, conservative treatment begins with the usual RICE (*r*est, *i*ce, *c*ompression, and *e*levation) therapy to treat the immediate symptoms of injury. Knee or ankle braces are useful for returning dancers to activity, and can be worn at all times by the lower-level dancers, but not in performances by professional dancers. Crutches may be needed for the first few days if the dancer is unable to ambulate normally. Strengthening of the supporting musculature is initiated, progressing to eccentric retraining to allow the affected limb to handle deceleration loads. Training of core stability and centering is essential. Balance and proprioception activities are emphasized and retrained. The dancer should begin activities at the barre, initially in flat foot with progression to demi-pointe, and full pointe as symptoms and strength improve. In some instances, depending on the injury site, the injured leg can be worked at the hip and/or knee while standing on the uninjured limb. At other times, when the injury does not permit working the injured leg, if the patient can stand on the injured leg at the barre they can work the contralateral uninjured limb. Once the dancer can perform at the barre, they can be slowly reintroduced to center floor with progressive turns, jumps, and pliés.

Ankle Sprains

Many traumatic injuries result form the loss of balance during landing from a jump. Dancers frequently perform complex spins in the air and must decelerate and stop rotation suddenly on landing. Complicated maneuvers such as the entrechats six, which requires the dancer to jump into the air and rapidly alternates the feet from front to back six times before landing on the floor, must be performed perfectly to avoid injury. If the dancer is fatigued and does not obtain adequate height of the jump or speed of the foot movements, there is significant risk for injury on landing. Additionally, fatigue or ongoing weakness of the peroneal musculature may prevent adequate stabilization of the ankle. Inversion ankle sprains are most common when a dancer loses balance while landing from a jump with the ankle in plantar flexion. The exact ligament injured depends on the position of the ankle at the time of landing. The anterior talofibular ligament (ATF) is the most commonly injured. In full pointe, the ankle is relatively stable because the posterior lip of the tibia rests and locks on the calcaneus and the subtalar joint is locked with the heel and forefoot in varus. The dancer is more likely to suffer a midfoot than an ankle sprain in this position. With slight dorsiflexion this complex releases, leaving the ankle vulnerable to inversion injury. As the ankle progressively inverts, further pressure is placed on other ankle ligaments. The talus is wider anteriorly and narrower posteriorly. This makes the ankle most vulnerable to inversion in plantarflexion due to the inherent instability of the narrow portion of talus within the ankle mortise, and the vertical alignment of the ATF. In this position the ankle derives minimal support from the calcaneofibular and distal tibiofibular ligaments.

Pain and swelling are the usual presenting complaints. The absolute inability to bear weight is suggestive of a fracture. Tenderness over the individual ligaments is indicative of injury to that ligament. Bony tenderness may be present even in the absence of fracture, but should alert the examiner to rule out fracture. Ankle instability can be demonstrated by laxity on the anterior drawer test, or by medial or lateral tilting of the talus within the mortise. Although these tests are useful in the chronic case, they add little to the acute management of the injury and are significantly painful to the injured dancer.

The Ottawa Ankle Rules (Pigman et al., 1994; Stiehll et al., 1993) and subsequent modifications (Leddy et al., 1998) recommend ankle radiographs if the patient is unable to walk for three steps (limping is okay) after the injury and in the emergency department, *or* there is tenderness over the midportion or crest of the medial or lateral malleolus from the tip to 6 cm proximally. Foot radiographs are needed if the patient is unable to walk for three steps (limping is okay) after the injury and in the emergency department *or* there is tenderness over the navicular or the base of the fifth metatarsal. Young dancers with open physes may require radiographs more frequently. Radiographic findings include fractures, widening of the ankle mortise, and avulsion fragments from the malleoli. Special attention should be paid to rule out easily overlooked fractures, including the medial or lateral domes of the talus, the lateral process of the talus, the os trigonum, the anterior process of the calcaneus, and the proximal fifth metatarsal. In adolescents, soft tissue swelling overlying the physis is suggestive of an epiphyseal fracture.

There are a number of other injuries that can mimic or accompany an ankle sprain. Ankle sprains failing to resolve should be investigated to rule out other causes of persistent disability. Occult fractures of tarsal bones can be easily missed on initial or even subsequent radiographs. If a patient has significant swelling and remains unable to bear weight after an injury despite apparently negative radiographs and symptomatic treatment for 4–5 days, a CT scan of the ankle and midfoot is indicated.

Inversion injury can cause tearing of the syndesmosis, diastasis of the distal tibiofibular joint, and a fracture of the proximal fibula, known as a *Maisonneuve fracture.* Examination reveals significant tenderness and swelling over the proximal fibula, as well as a positive squeeze test, which should be done in all ankle injuries to avoid missing this significant injury. Standard ankle radiographs may show widening of the mortise, but will not reveal the fracture. If clinically indicated, long leg radiographs should be performed.

Osteochondral injuries to the talar domes occur with inversion injuries. They are usually located on the posterior aspect of the medial talar dome or the anterior aspect of the lateral talar dome. They can result in persistent deep ankle pain, ankle effusions, and catching or a loose body sensation within the ankle. Some osteochondral injuries are evident on plain radiographs, but may require CT or MRI for diagnosis and staging. Talar dome injuries with an intact chondral cap usually heal with cast immobilization; higher grade injuries with partial or complete separation of the chondral surface generally need surgery.

Peroneal tendon disorders can cause persistent lateral pain, swelling, clicking, and a sense of something moving out of place. These injuries include longitudinal in-substance tears as well as anterior subluxation of the tendons. Resisted eversion with the examiner's fingers over the posterior aspect of the lateral malleolus can provoke and demonstrate tendon subluxation. MRI can demonstrate in-substance rupture or persistent tendinopathy. These injuries frequently require surgical repair.

Subluxation of the cuboid is common in dancers, and may occur in association with inversion ankle sprains or with repetitive plantar-dorsiflexion as a dancer goes up and down en pointe. The medial border of the cuboid generally subluxates in a plantar direction, resulting in dorsal displacement of the fourth metatarsal (MT) base, and plantar displacement of the fourth MT head. Cuboid dysfunction interferes with the function of the peroneus longus tendon pulley, and should always be a prime consideration in any dancer with peroneal tendonitis.

Cuboid subluxation presents with persistent lateral midfoot pain, often following a sprain that does not respond to the usual treatments. Dancers may be unable to bear weight or walk normally, and frequently have difficulty rolling through the foot onto pointe or with pushing off. Physical findings include significant tenderness over the cuboid bone, reduced mobility of the cuboid when compared to the opposite foot, reduced lateral midfoot mobility on passive pronation/supination, a step-off at the base of the fourth metatarsal, and a plantarflexed fourth MT head. Treatment is directed at mobilizing the rear and midfoot, including the subtalar and distal tibiofibular joints, adducting the forefoot, and then reducing the cuboid using a squeeze technique as described by Marshall and Hamilton (1992).

Early and aggressive treatment of ankle sprains is essential in dancers. Dancing on pointe requires maximal mobility of all joints of the lower leg, ankle, and foot, with restricted motion leading to difficulty with technique and further injury. Swelling contributes to loss of motion and must be minimized. Ice, massage, and compression taping with horseshoe pads are employed. The subtalar joint and the talocalcaneal ligament are frequently injured in inversion sprains. Subtalar sprains have been linked to chronic giving way and limitations of ankle motion (Tochigi et al., 1998), which can result in significant disability for dancers. Range of motion is therefore started early to maintain and restore mobility of both the ankle and subtalar joints. Dancers who have difficulty fully weightbearing should be placed on crutches for a few days along with aggressive treatment for swelling and motion to prevent stiffness and loss of function in the non-weightbearing foot. Strength training with specific emphasis on the everters should be performed both in the neutral position and with the foot in the plantarflexed pointe position. Flexibility of the gastrocnemius and soleus is critical. Retraining of balance and proprioception is very important. Functional mobility drills should be employed first at the barre, and subsequently on center floor before returning to full dance.

Midfoot Sprains

Dancers can suffer midfoot sprains and injuries to the Lisfranc joint, which may require prolonged recovery if the foot is to regain its normal stability and mobility. The second MT base articulates with the short intermediate cuneiform and is stabilized in a mortise formed by the longer medial and lateral cuneiform bones. This Lisfranc joint is essential to the stability of the midfoot, and the longitudinal and transverse MT arches. Severe Lisfranc injuries result in diastasis of the tarsometatarsal joint between the first and second MT bases. There may be associated avulsion fracture of the Lisfranc ligament between the lateral aspect of the medial cuneiform and the base of the second metatarsal. Less common midfoot sprains are injuries to the dorsal ligaments between the talus and navicular, or the calcaneus and cuboid.

Midfoot sprains usually result from a loss of balance while on pointe performing spins or upon landing from a jump, leading to a hyperplantarflexion injury, with or without rotation. Many dancers will be unable to roll through the foot onto demi- or full pointe, and some may be unable to bear weight. Physical findings include significant midfoot swelling, ecchymosis, tenderness to palpation over the injured structures, and pain on passive pronation and supination of the foot.

With significant midfoot sprains, radiographs should be performed in a standing, weightbearing position, including comparison views of the uninjured foot. Avulsion fragments from the talus, navicular, or cuboid may be visible. In Lisfranc, injuries anteroposterior (AP) and oblique radiographs demonstrate diastasis between the first and second metatarsal bases, and possibly an avulsion fracture of the Lisfranc ligament. Comparison weightbearing laterals will show collapse of the longitudinal arch and an abnormal relationship between the plantar aspects of the fifth metatarsal and the medial cuneiform. A side-to-side difference of greater than 4mm and/or a negative relationship whereby the base of the cuneiform is below that of the fifth metatarsal are indicative of more serious injuries often requiring surgery and associated with greater long-term disability (Faciszewski et al., 1990). CT scans may be useful in demonstrating instability and avulsion fractures not visible on plain films.

Delayed treatment frequently produces unsatisfactory results, so early recognition of the severity of these injuries is essential. Failure to diagnose and treat these injuries in a timely manner may threaten a dancer's career. Treatment depends on the severity of the injury, with non-weightbearing cast immobilization recommended for simple sprains with no radiographic instability and significant pain. They are allowed to resume weight bearing and activity as their symptoms improve. Some surgeons recommend open reduction and internal fixation (ORIF) if any diastasis is present, but more recent work has indicated that some degree of diastasis is acceptable so long as there is no collapse of the longitudinal arch on lateral weightbearing radiographs, although this study was in athletes and not specifically in dancers (Faciszewski et al., 1990). Dancers present a treatment dilemma due to the necessity of balancing adequate healing and midfoot stability with the maintenance and restoration of the mobility essential for dance.

Fractures of the Fifth Metatarsal

Dancers are susceptible to fractures at a number of sites within the fifth metatarsal, with treatment dependent on the location. When acute, all of these fractures present with tenderness, swelling, and ecchymoses over the base or shaft of the fifth metatarsal, and it is often difficult to differentiate them based on physical examination. Weight bearing is usually possible, but painful. The exact diagnosis is based on careful examination of the radiographs to determine the anatomic site of the fracture, and the presence or absence of antecedent stress reaction.

Avulsion fracture is the most common proximal fifth metatarsal fracture, and commonly presents accompanying a lateral ankle sprain. Avulsion fractures have a fracture line through the tuberosity of the proximal metatarsal, most commonly perpendicular to its long axis. They are occasionally intra-articular and involve the most proximal 1 cm of the metatarsal. They are treated symptomatically, with a hard-soled shoe, walking cast immobilization, or rarely ORIF if the fracture involves greater than 30% of the articular surface and is significantly displaced. Activity is advanced depending on the level of symptoms. Avulsion fractures have an excellent prognosis and usually recover well enough to return to dance within a moderate period of time.

Jones fractures are acute fractures at the metaphyseal–diaphyseal junction without extension to the medial side of the metatarsal at the fourth and fifth metatarsal articulation. The mechanism of injury is adduction of the fifth metatarsal, often while the foot is plantarflexed. Although acute, nondisplaced Jones fractures can be non-weightbearing and casted for 6–8 weeks, the high-performance dancer may elect to proceed with early operative management to avoid the negative effects of prolonged immobilization. Acute displaced Jones fractures should undergo early ORIF.

Diaphyseal stress fractures are often confused with the acute Jones fractures. They occur as result of repetitive adduction forces, which occur in cutting or pivoting. Patients often present with an acute event that was preceded by a prodrome of chronic pain to the lateral side of the foot. Radiographic features resemble acute fractures, but have associated signs of antecedent bone stress including periosteal reaction, cortical thickening, widening of the fracture line, and intramedullary sclerosis. The diaphyseal–metaphyseal junction is a vascular watershed zone; therefore, both acute and stress fractures in this area are prone to delayed or nonunion. Accordingly, diaphyseal stress fractures should be treated with bone graft and/or intramedullary screw fixation.

The *Dancer's fracture* is an oblique or spiral fracture of the mid- to distal portion of the fifth metatarsal that occurs when the dancer twists and inverts the foot while en demi-pointe. Although it was once thought that

ORIF was necessary, a large series has shown that conservative/symptomatic therapy is almost universally successful in treating this fracture (O'Malley et al., 1996).

Other Acute Foot and Ankle Injuries

Acute fractures and other bony impaction injuries can occur if the foot or ankle is forced beyond its maximum range of motion. Hyperplantarflexion can result in fracture of the os trigonum. This results in significant swelling and tenderness in the retrocalcaneal region and pain on forced passive plantarflexion. Additionally, soft tissue impingement can occur and may involve the flexor hallucis longus (FHL) tendon and its sheath.

Similarly, acute impingement injuries of the talar neck or the anterior ankle capsule can occur during an overaggressive grand plié with forced dorsiflexion. Hyperdorsiflexion in a landing or an eccentric load during push-off can result in an Achilles tendon rupture.

Acute Knee Injuries

Patellar Dislocation

The knee is vulnerable to acute injuries with spinning and twisting movements. If the dancer pushes off for a jump, torque is generated in the take-off leg as the body is rotated and the knee comes into full extension. When landing on an externally rotated foot, overrotation can lead to internal rotation of the femur on the tibia, as the body continues to rotate. Both of these mechanisms can result in patellar subluxation/dislocation. If the rotation to the knee is severe, or combined with valgus, this can progress to further injury including tears of the anterior cruciate ligament (ACL) and menisci. The clinician must be alert to this possibility, and not miss these more severe injuries once the patellar injury has been discovered. Contributing factors include fatigue and weakness of the hip abductors, which allows the knee to collapse further into valgus, overloading the support structures. Increased recurvatum of the knee reduces the stability of the patella within the sulcus and predisposes to dislocation. Tightness of the lateral retinaculum and iliotibial (IT) band will increase the lateralizing forces and tendency to dislocation. Core stability to control trunk movement and rotation is an essential factor in preventing traumatic injuries to the knee.

Diagnosis is based on a history of the mechanism of injury combined with the dancer's report that the patella moved or dislocated. Immediate hemarthrosis is common, although some dancers with marked ligamentous laxity do not experience much swelling. Examination reveals tenderness of the medial patellofemoral ligament, adductor tubercle, and medial patellar facet. In more severe cases, there can be tenderness of the lateral femoral condyle associated with osteochondral injuries. The uninjured contralateral knee should be examined to determine patellar glides and tilting, and the tubercle-sulcus angle, which will be helpful in planning any operative intervention. Imaging should include standard AP and lateral radiographs as well as a Merchant view of both knees to look for osteochondral fractures and to assess the anatomy of the sulcus, the degree of patellar tilting, and determine whether the patella is centralized symmetrically within the sulcus.

Indications for early operative treatment are significant osteochondral injury, loose bodies, and failure of the patella to centralize symmetrically in the sulcus. Conservative treatment includes the usual RICE therapy to treat the immediate symptoms of injury. Patellar stabilization braces with lateral buttress can be useful. These can be worn at all times by the lower level dancer, but cannot be worn in performances by the professional dancer. Strengthening of the quadriceps and hip abductors is initiated including a graduated program of eccentric quadriceps retraining. Training of core stability and centering is essential.

Acute Knee Ligament Injuries

Tears of the ACL are relatively uncommon in dance due to its very controlled choreography. The most frequent mechanism is hyperextension upon landing from a jump. ACL injury is often associated with a pop or snap and a sense that the knee has moved out of place. Early (within 6–12 hours) hemarthrosis is common. The dancer often has a sense of knee instability afterward. Examination findings include increased AP translation and a positive Lachman test. Pivot shift may be present. The ACL is an intra-articular ligament and does not heal, making surgical reconstruction mandatory for high-level dancers. Surgical decision-making in ACL tears is beyond the scope of this chapter, but should be made in consultation with an experienced surgeon.

Medial collateral ligament (MCL) injuries occur with a valgus force, but are relatively uncommon in dance. Examination reveals local swelling and tenderness over the course of the MCL, as well pain and instability with valgus stress testing. The MCL is extra-articular and heals with appropriate conservative therapy and bracing.

Meniscal Injuries

The menisci are vulnerable during the performance of a grand plié, especially if any twisting or loss of balance and position occurs. They can be injured with ballistic squatting such as in Russian dancing. Dancers with inadequate turnout can leave their menisci vulnerable to injury through the practice of screwing the knee by forcing turnout from the floor up and not the hips down. This occurs when the dancer flexes their knees and then takes advantage of the slight rotatory laxity of the knee to excessively externally rotate the lower leg to achieve greater turnout. As the dancer fully re-extends the knee on a fixed foot, the menisci are compressed and vulnerable to injury.

Acute Hip, Thigh, and Spine Injuries

The hip and thigh are susceptible to a number of acute injuries. Sudden hip flexion/extension movements can lead to muscular strains of the hamstrings, adductors, or hip flexors (quadriceps and iliopsoas). These are more frequent in the fatigued or deconditioned dancer with poor core stability. Treatment is the usual RICE for control of initial symptoms, followed by strengthening and restoration of flexibility. Acute hip strains will frequently be accompanied by sacroiliac joint dysfunction (SIJD), and correction of the functional asymmetry will help in pain relief.

Skeletally immature dancers are vulnerable to apophyseal avulsion, and these may be present in some female dancers in their late teens because of delayed menarche. These avulsions can occur at the ischial tuberosity (hamstrings), lesser trochanter (iliopsoas), anterior superior (sartorius), and inferior (rectus femoris) iliac spines, the iliac crest (quadratus lumborum and obliques), and the pubic ramus (adductors). The injury can be confirmed by radiographs, which show widening or displacement of the apophysis. Treatment is symptomatic and may require crutches in the early stages. Progressive functional rehabilitation is essential prior to return to dance.

Intra-articular injuries are uncommon, but can have significant morbidity for the dancer. Awkward, high-impact landing can produce shearing stress on the articular cartilage leading to chondral flap tears, osteochondral injuries, and labral tears. Dancers often have shallower hips with acetabular dysplasia. They are at greater risk of labral tears even without trauma. Intra-articular hip pathology is characterized by sudden, sharp anterior hip pain with a sense of catching or a loose body within the joint. Hip range of motion may be restricted, with the log-rolling test very sensitive for intra-articular pathology. Diagnosis depends on a high index of suspicion, and can be confirmed with MRI arthrogram. It is important to have an experienced radiologist interpret the arthrogram, as the findings may be subtle. Treatment is surgical removal or debridement of the offending structure. This can frequently be done through the arthroscope, which is best performed by surgeons with considerable experience with the procedure.

Dancers are vulnerable to a number of other pelvic and spinal injuries. Musculoligamentous sprains and strains are common, as are SIJD. These are often due to sudden ballistic hyperflexion, hyperextension, or twisting movements, or poor lifting technique during partnering. Acute intervertebral disk injury including annular tears and frank herniations are less common, but can occur and are often related to lifting technique. Acute mechanical thoracic spine and rib dysfunctions can occur with twisting and lifting. Cervical spine dysfunctions can occur due to the practice of spotting. To lessen dizziness during repeated spins, a dancer focuses their gaze on a distant spotlight and maintains their neck position and gaze stationary while the body is spinning. The dancer then quickly spins their neck to catch up with and then pass their body and refocus on the same spot. These rapid rotations can cause neck injuries.

Upper extremity injuries are relatively uncommon, but can occur, usually with partnering. Overhead lifting can result in rotator cuff tears. Loss of control during spins leading to abduction and external rotation of the shoulder can result in subluxation/dislocation. Poor lifting or dropping of the partner can lead to shoulder fractures, separations, and dislocations.

OVERUSE INJURIES

Overuse injuries account for 50–60% of all dance injuries, depending on the study methods and population. In contrast to traumatic injuries, overuse injuries result from repetitive microtrauma to bony, ligamentous, or musculotendinous structures. They generally arise from the inability of the body to absorb the forces generated by the repeated cyclical loading of the musculoskeletal structures during the performance of dance. Although it might seem that these injuries occur randomly, it is possible to identify numerous factors involved in their causation. Factors extrinsic to the athlete include the biomechanical demands of dance, and the dancer's training methods, training shoes, and training surfaces. There are several intrinsic factors related to the dancers themselves. These include primary intrinsic factors such as overall fitness, strength and flexibility, biomechanics and alignment, and individual variations in bony and ligamentous structures. Secondary or acquired intrinsic factors also play a significant role, including previous injuries that have been incompletely rehabilitated and lead to imbalances, functional asymmetries, and gait abnormalities.

Extrinsic Factors

One of the most frequent causes of overuse injuries is inappropriate training methods, usually in the form of excessive volume and intensity of training. Dancers generally take several classes per day, in addition to their rehearsal schedules, teaching, and performing. Some dancers also cross-train with running or aerobics after their dance work in an attempt to control their weight. Professional dancers feel an intense pressure to perform to maintain their jobs, and often attempt to dance through pain. This can result in delayed diagnosis and more severe injuries at the time of presentation. Financial pressures may also keep dancers from seeking medical care, as many aspiring dancers or performers with lower level companies have no health insurance coverage. Novice dancers are particularly vulnerable to acute overuse injuries when they rapidly increase their volume and intensity of training when they attend intensive summer dance training camps.

The characteristics of the dance floor are important in dance injuries. Most professional companies have specially designed and suspended floors that allow for good shock absorption with jumping and landing. Injuries can occur when dancers are on location and train on excessively hard surfaces, or in young dancers performing in small studios with poorly constructed floors.

Dance shoes can be the source of injuries. Unlike running shoes, which provide both shock absorption and support, ballet toe shoes are primarily designed to adequately support the foot on the pointe position, with little of either feature. Improperly fitted toe shoes can cause corns and calluses, as well as blistering. The ribbons used to tightly fasten the shoes can cut into the skin and have also been implicated in the development of Achilles tendonitis (Hamilton, 1996).

Intrinsic Factors

Intrinsic factors play a critical role in the etiology of overuse ballet injuries. The primary factors are those related to the individual dancer's physical characteristics. Secondary or acquired intrinsic factors are those that result from postural and movement dysfunctions arising from previous, incompletely rehabilitated injuries.

Primary Intrinsic Factors

Inadequate Strength and Flexibility. Muscles are the shock absorbers for joints. They are required to absorb the forces involved with the repeated impacts and movements associated with dance. Dancers have been found to have only 77% of weight-predicted norms for leg strength, which may predispose to injury (Reid, 1988). If there is inadequate strength or endurance of the muscular structures, fatigue results and overload can occur to the muscles, ligaments, tendons, or bones. Inadequate flexibility can cause relative tissue tightness, leading to the improper mechanics or imbalances of the forces acting on the joints. Imbalances in muscle strength between antagonist groups may lead to a tendency to acute muscle tears and injuries.

Dancers with excessive joint laxity may be predisposed to injury unless muscular support and balance are optimized.

Hormonal and Nutritional Status. Ballet demands a very specific body type to progress to its highest levels, yet many individuals who are not ideally suited still attempt to meet these rigid esthetic standards. Thinness is considered essential in high-echelon dance and inadequate and inappropriate nutrition is common. Dancers are at significant risk for the development of the female athlete triad of disordered eating, amenorrhea, and osteoporosis. Lower circulating estrogen levels can lead to an increased risk of stress fractures. There is significant concern that dancers with delayed menarche, prolonged oligo/amenorrhea, and poor nutrition with inadequate calcium intake have higher rates of osteoporosis in their later years. Nutritional deficiencies can lead to loss of muscle mass and early muscle fatigue, predisposing to overuse injuries. Benson et al. (1989) demonstrated a significant relationship between dance injuries and both body mass index and menstrual function.

Biomechanics and Alignment. It has long been thought that intrinsic factors are important in the genesis of overuse injuries in running. Many people have studied injured runners and made pronouncements as to why these injuries have occurred, including theories that biomechanical factors, such as excess pronation and abnormalities of lower leg and knee alignment lead to injury. Unfortunately, most of these conclusions were obtained by examining injured runners only without a cohort of uninjured runners. Well-controlled studies have been unable to confirm that these factors are important in running injuries (Reid, 1993; Wen et al., 1997).

In contrast to runners, however, biomechanics and alignment probably do play a significant role in dance injuries. The nature of the discipline demands that the feet must be placed in precise positions for the performance of specific closed-chain movements. There is nothing inherently dangerous about these movements if the body is allowed to perform them within its normal range of motion, and with less stringent foot positioning. Injuries occur when individuals who are not naturally gifted with the necessary alignment and turnout cheat to achieve these positions, placing increased stress on other structures, and leading to injury.

A prime requirement of ballet is adequate turnout, with all positioning and maneuvers performed with the hips and lower legs externally rotated. This evolved because of the presumed esthetic appeal of the turned-out position. Total turnout is the sum of femoral neck ante or retroversion, femoral torsion, knee alignment and flexibility, and tibial torsion. Dancers generally have total range of hip motion similar to that found in the general population; however, it is orientated with a predominance of external rotation. Hip rotation appears to be determined by an early age, although small improvements may be made with early training. Many of the overuse injuries in dance occur because dancers attempt to force their bodies to assume positions that they are anatomically incapable of achieving.

In addition to turnout, ballet requires other movements that load the joints in extremes of range of motion including full pointe (maximum plantarflexion of the forefoot, midfoot, and ankle joints), grande plie (flat foot with maximum dorsiflexion of the ankle and full knee flexion), and arabesques and attitudes (hyperextension of the hip so that the thigh is parallel to the floor while balancing on the contralateral leg).

Dancers with less than optimal external rotation may try to achieve turnout from the floor up rather than from the hips down. This attempt to force external rotation leads to excess pronation of the feet, external tibial torsion, valgus knee stress, increased Q angle, lateral patellar tracking, hip flexion, and increased lumbar lordosis, all of which can predispose to overuse injuries. When turnout is forced from the floor upward, the resulting excess pronation can lead to difficulty in re-supinating the foot to go up on pointe. This can lead to overstress and injury to the FHL and tibialis posterior tendons. It can also lead to sesamoiditis when coupled with an exaggerated turned-out gait, due to rolling medially off the first metatarsophalangeal joint. Pronation can also lead to torsional stress and whipping of the Achilles as the dancer goes up on pointe, contributing to tendonosis. When the dancer is not dancing, gait normalization is an important adjunct to local treatments to reduce the stress on the foot and ankle. This is especially important in young dancers who want to demonstrate to the world that they are dancers, and walk around with a turned-out gait.

Ballet dancers require a significantly greater range of ankle and foot motions than is found in the general population in order to perform both pointe and grande plié. Ideally, in full pointe, the axis of the foot is parallel to that of the tibia. It is theorized that inadequate range of motion leads to the axis of the foot falling anterior to that of the tibia, increasing the load on the tendons posterior to the ankle (Achilles, FHL, and tibialis posterior) predisposing to injury (Solomon et al., 1993). The pointe axis should be checked in every injured dancer, and limitation of movement is frequently found on the injured side. Restoration of joint movement is an essential part of rehabilitation and side-to-side symmetry of the pointe axis should be restored.

Repeated hyperplantarflexion from pointe work can lead to chronic impingement of the os trigonum. Posterior impingement may also be worsened following ankle sprains where lax lateral ligaments permit the tibia to slide forward (anterior) on the fixed talus during relevé. Similarly, chronic and repeated hyperdorsiflexion during grande plie can lead to anterior impingement of the tibia on the talus. This too, can be worse following third-degree ankle sprain (Hamilton et al., 1996).

Forcing turnout can also lead to external tibial torsion and increased valgus displacement of the knee during closed-chain flexion. Further aggravation of patellar tracking can result from poor hip abductor strength and core stability, which can increase closed-chain valgus displacement of the knee. These factors result in an increased Q angle and lateral displacement forces on the patella, predisposing to patellofemoral pain and patellar tendonosis. Valgus stress can also lead to tensioning and overuse injuries to the medial ligaments and the pes anserinus tendons. Dancers turning out from the floor upward are also vulnerable to attritional meniscal injuries through repeated screwing the knee, as described.

Artificially increased turnout can also be achieved through anterior tilting of the pelvis and hip flexion, which allows for greater external rotation. This in turn results in increased lumbar lordosis and loading of the posterior spinal elements, predisposing the dancer to mechanical back pain, facet dysfunction, and spondylolysis. Limited hip extension similarly increases lumbar extension, especially during performance of arabesque and attitudes. Overhead lifting of partners can also result in significant stress on the posterior elements if the dancer uses poor lifting technique or lacks upper body strength.

Secondary/Acquired Intrinsic Factors. Acquired factors for overuse injuries are the result of mechanical movement dysfunctions, usually resulting from incomplete rehabilitation of previous injuries. Ballet demands the performance of complex movements in a precise and controlled fashion. These movements require the action of muscular forces on a series of rigid limb segments joined by mobile linkages, commonly referred to as the *kinetic chain*. The pointe position requires stability of the foot, ankle, and lower leg, yet wide mobility of the joints and segments in the proximal portion of the kinetic chain. Optimum performance requires that all segments of the kinetic chain be appropriately positioned to support the body's weight and allow for movement. Anything that interferes with normal joint mobility or stability necessitates compensatory postural and movement changes, which can lead to increased stresses on other sites in the kinetic chain. If the capacity of the chain to compensate is exceeded, tissue breakdown and injury occur. This failure may be at the site of the abnormal mobility; however, the overt injury can also occur at a site distant to the dysfunction. One could simplistically compare this to *culprit* and *victim* in the injury (Kibler et al., 1992). The presenting injury may merely be the victim that has suffered an injury as a result of an inability to compensate for a dysfunction at a distant site in the chain (the culprit). When a dancer presents with an injury, it is easy to assume that the injury has occurred in isolation; however, it is quite likely that the injury may be secondary to an underlying dysfunction.

Dysfunctions are characterized by abnormal joint positioning and/or joint mobility (either hypo or hyper). In dancers, the most common joint mobility dysfunctions are those involving the subtalar and sacroiliac (SI) joints. Strength is important in maintaining proper joint position and function. Poor core stability and hip abductor weakness may lead to increased load on distal structures and resultant injury. Fatigue from poor conditioning can lead to improper support and injury.

Kinetic chain dysfunction has been implicated in overuse dance injuries. (Macintyre, 1994; Weisler et al., 1996). In a retrospective study, Macintyre (1994) found that 11 of 16 (69%) injured dancers had kinetic chain dysfunctions including 9 of 12 with overuse injuries and 2 of 4 with acute injuries. Evaluation of a similar group of uninjured dancers revealed that only 44% of 108 uninjured dancers had dysfunctions (Macintyre, unpublished data). Of the 9 dancers with overuse injuries to the lower leg and foot, 8 had abnormal functional foot movements and 7 of these 8 reported a history of previous injury to the same region. Weisler. et al (1996) found a significant correlation between previous injury and a new injury in a prospective study, and that dancers with previous injuries had significantly less ankle and foot mobility than uninjured dancers.

It would appear that previous ankle sprains are significantly related to new overuse injuries. Ankle sprains have been shown to lead to a persistent reduction of subtalar and ankle motion (Denegar et al., 2002; Tochigi et al., 1998). Because the subtalar joint acts as a rotational transducer between the ankle and the lower leg and knee, persistent abnormal pronation or supination can result in increased compensatory stresses on the muscle tendon units attempting to stabilize the foot and ankle, leading to injury. Restriction of normal ankle and subtalar motion has been associated with navicular stress fractures (Torg et al., 1982). A prospective study of army recruits found that previous injury, specifically sprained ankles, was a significant risk factor for new injuries (Jones et al., 1993). Impaired balance and proprioception can follow ankle sprains, and have been shown to persist for several weeks despite active rehabilitation (Leanderson et al., 1996). Failure to restore neuromuscular coordination may contribute to repeated injuries.

Physicians and therapists have frequently focused exclusively on the injury site when dealing with overuse injuries, ignoring the fact that an injury may be a manifestation of a local or distant dysfunction in the kinetic chain. Thus, the entire kinetic chain must be screened to rule out any primary or underlying injury. This is especially important in individuals who have had recurrent injuries to the same site or limb, as there may be an underlying dysfunction that places increased stress on elements of that limb resulting in serial episodes of tissue breakdown and injury.

The role of SI joint dysfunction in back pain and other injuries is controversial and not completely understood, but is gaining acceptance. Due to the extreme positioning in dance, abnormal SI positioning and stability can lead to significant problems. SIJD can lead to compensatory changes, which may lead to secondary dysfunctions and injury. Similarly, problems at other sites can lead to gait changes and SIJD. In the absence of a clear-cut precipitating injury, the exact causation of the dysfunction can resemble the classic chicken and egg paradox, so that it is frequently difficult to determine which condition started the path toward injury. Only the identification and treatment of all dysfunctional sites will allow the dancer an injury-free return to activity.

The assessment of functional foot movements is an essential part of the examination of any dancer. Passive range of motion performed in a supine position is not as informative as having the patient demonstrate functional movements in which restrictions are more apparent to both the dancer and the examiner. Cardinal movements of plantarflexion, dorsiflexion, pronation, and supination are examined from both the front and rear. The dancer stands facing the examiner with their feet 6 to 8 inches apart in sixth (parallel) position. The dancer is then instructed to do a plié. Any asymmetry of the degree of pronation should be noted. The midpoint of the patella should be lined up over the second toe, and note should be made if one patella tracks more medially or demonstrates more valgus than the other during the plié. It is particularly important to ask the dancer to let their feet and knees move where they want to, rather than where they have been trained to move them while performing a plié. This maneuver is then repeated in first position to assess closed-chain mechanics in a turned out position. Careful attention to detect cheating and the resultant abnormal mechanics is important. It is essential to encourage dancers who are cheating at turnout to reduce their turnout to the degree where they can safely do a plié while maintaining proper mechanics.

Next, the dancer is asked to go up on relevé to assess the degree and symmetry of plantarflexion. The calcaneus normally swings into a slight degree of inversion during this maneuver, and any asymmetry of movement during this maneuver may indicate an underlying dysfunction.

To assess functional pronation and supination, the dancer is asked to rotate the trunk and hips to look first over one shoulder and then over the other, while maintaining their knees straight and their feet in sixth position. This causes one foot to supinate and the other to pronate. Careful comparison should be made of the symmetry and range of motion. Restricted or exaggerated motion, especially in the presence of asymmetry, can indicate a kinetic chain dysfunction. It is often useful to ask the dancer which direction the feet move more easily, and it is not uncommon that the dancer identifies an inability to move in the direction of the clinically apparent restriction.

The dancer is then asked to lie supine on the examination table with their hips and knees flexed to 90°. The foot and ankle are then maximally plantarflexed into the pointe position and side-to-side comparison of the pointe axis is undertaken. Asymmetric restriction of the pointe axis is followed by tests of joint movements in the lower leg to determine the site of dysfunction.

If abnormalities of functional movement are detected, then tests of individual joint play and glide are performed on the entire kinetic chain from the proximal tibiofibular joint distally to the forefoot to reveal the exact site of the dysfunction. The most common site of restricted motion is the subtalar joint, although the midfoot is also commonly affected in dancers. Treatment of the dancer should therefore be directed at both the symptomatic site and the restoration of normal foot mobility. Detailed description of the testing and mobilization of the individual joints is beyond the scope of this chapter, but can be found in a comprehensive text by Walsh and Nolan (1999).

Stress Fractures

Stress fractures represent the endpoint of a continuum of bony stress reactions to repetitive loading. When a mechanical load is applied to a bone, remodeling accelerates to maintain skeletal integrity. Early in this process, osteoblastic activity to lay down new bone generally lags behind osteoclastic resorption, resulting in a net loss of bone and the development of microfractures. In most instances, the bone is able to adapt to the new level of stress; however, when loading is increased too rapidly, the imbalance can be of sufficient magnitude to lead to a clinically significant weakening of the bone.

Etiology

The etiology of stress fractures is multifactorial. The primary factors are similar to those of all overuse injuries as described. Women seem to have a greater predisposition to stress fractures than men. Numerous reasons have been postulated, including differences in bone mass, lower muscle to body mass ratio, lower levels of musculoskeletal strength and cardiovascular fitness, and hormonal and endocrine factors. Although none of these theories has been properly validated in a prospective study, there is consensus that there is a significant relationship between stress fractures, reproductive hormone levels, and bone mass.

There is significant concern that women suffering from the female athlete triad are at a greater risk for stress fractures during their athletic career, and that they will have significant risk for premature osteoporotic fractures later in life. A combination of intense training and amenorrhea has been shown to significantly increase the risk of stress fractures (Kadel et al., 1992).

Presentation and Clinical Findings

Stress fractures usually present with pain, initially following dance activity, and with worsening, the pain may progress to be present during and after dance, and finally being present with the activities of daily living. Night pain is a common feature that should alert the clinician to the possibility of a stress fracture. The pain is frequently poorly localized, and may be easy to dismiss due to the lack of physical findings. A high index of suspicion is needed in order not to miss these fractures. It is especially important to diagnose a bony injury in the early phases to minimize recovery time and prevent progression to an acute fracture.

Radiographic findings are frequently negative in the early symptomatic stages of stress fractures. A negative x-ray does not rule out a stress fracture. Technetium radionuclide bone scans are quite sensitive for stress fractures, and can be positive as few as 3 days after the onset of the injury. MRI is very sensitive and may aid in differentiating soft tissue from bony injuries. In symptomatic individuals, activity should be curtailed until a bone scan or MRI has been performed to confirm or rule out fracture. Bone scans are very sensitive to abnormalities, but lack specificity, and must frequently be followed up by a CT scan. Many clinicians now use MRI as a first step, because it reveals soft tissue pathology in addition to bony problems, and the cost of an MRI is less than the combined cost of a bone scan and CT scan.

In dancers, stress fractures can occur in the lumbar spine and in virtually any bone of the lower extremity. The most common site is the metatarsals due to the significant loading during pointe work and jumping. Stress fractures of the shaft and neck of the femur, the proximal or anterior cortex of the tibia, the base of the second and fifth metatarsals, and the tarsal navicular are considered to be at high risk for complications if they are not diagnosed and treated with appropriate rest and rehabilitation.

It is important that the dancer understand the significance of their injury and its potential complications, in order to have compliance with treatment; dancers who participate with sufficient intensity to suffer a stress fracture are often reluctant to stop their activity. Stress fractures are treated with modified rest. Ambulation is permitted for the activities of daily living, but all other weightbearing activities and skeletal loading is ceased until symptoms have abated. Alternate forms of nonimpact activity are substituted. Cycling, swimming, and pool training are recommended. The dancer can participate in barre work, so long as this can be accomplished without pain at the affected site. During the period of relative rest, underlying factors are corrected and strength training is undertaken. Once the dancer has been pain free in normal daily activities for 14 days, they are allowed to gradually reintroduce weightbearing activities, so long as they can do so on a pain-free basis. Principals of safe return to activity were discussed previously.

Foot

One of the most common stress fractures in dancers is at the base of the second metatarsal due to the loading of the foot in the pointe position (Harrington et al., 1993). This can be difficult to differentiate from synovitis of the Lisfranc joint. Both have activity-related pain and local tenderness. Early imaging is necessary to diagnose the bony injury, because healing time is prolonged once the injury has progressed to a complete fracture.

Tarsal navicular stress fractures are relatively uncommon, but should always be considered in dancers with unexplained midfoot pain. They present with poorly localized dorsomedial foot pain, which may radiate along the medial longitudinal arch, first or second ray, or the dorsum of the midfoot. The hallmark physical finding is tenderness to palpation over the dorsum of the navicular. A CT scan or MRI is necessary for diagnosis, with treatment depending on the presence of a cortical defect. Navicular stress fractures with a cortical defect rarely heal with activity restriction only, and require 6 to 8 weeks in a non-weightbearing cast (Khan et al., 1992). Surgical treatment with screw fixation, bone grafting, or both are considered for initial treatment of complete or displaced fractures and as secondary treatment for failed nonsurgical treatment.

Leg

Tibial stress injury presents as a continuum ranging from diffuse tibial periostitis (medial tibial stress syndrome [MTSS]) to focal tibial fractures associated with a radiolucent defects on plain radiographs. MTSS presents with generalized anteromedial tibial pain. If impact activity is continued progressive injury may result in a focal stress fracture of the posterior medial tibial border, most commonly at the junction of the proximal two-thirds and the distal one third of the tibia. Fractures in this region are on the compression side of the tibia, and usually behave in a relatively benign manner without frequent or significant complications. They contrast with focal stress fractures of the anterior cortex of the midshaft of the tibia, or proximal shaft fractures that occur on the tension side of the bone. These tension side fractures have a high rate of delayed union and nonunion, can progress to complete displaced fractures, and must be treated with caution.

Activity-related anterior tibial pain is the usual presentation. The pain may initially be diffuse, but localizes with continued activity. Physical examination reveals focal areas of tenderness over the anterior tibia, associated with local thickening and periosteal reaction. Hop test is positive. Lower leg musculature is often weak. Radiographs reveal diffuse cortical thickening and periosteal elevation. Single or multiple transverse radiolucent lines extend about half way through the anterior cortex. In late cases, CT scanning may reveal sclerosis of the fracture edges suggestive of nonunion.

Patients with activity-related anterior tibial pain must reduce the level of impact activity until they are asymptomatic. Once a dancer has developed a radiolucent line on x-ray, it is essential that they discontinue loading activity to prevent the fracture from progressing to completion. Various conservative treatments have been proposed, including electromagnetic bone growth stimulators. Surgery is often necessary, and may consist of curetting or drilling out the fracture and area of fibrous nonunion followed by bone grafting or intramedullary rodding. ORIF is required for displaced fractures.

Hip

Femoral stress fractures are relatively uncommon, and can occur in the shaft or less commonly the neck of the femur. Femoral neck fractures are further subdivided to the superior or tension side, and the inferior or compression side. Femoral stress fractures, especially those on the tension side, can go on to completion, with devastating consequences including displacement and avascular necrosis of the femoral head. Unfortunately, some femoral stress fractures present acutely with displacement because the dancer or physician have ignored the warning signs of persistent and increasing pain.

Femoral stress fractures may produce dull aching in the anterior or lateral hip with pain radiating down the leg. There is usually no point tenderness, due to the overlying musculature, although this can occasionally be found in shaft fractures in thin women. Gentle hopping on the affected leg reproduces the hip pain, although this must be performed with caution in individuals who are acutely symptomatic. Femoral neck fractures can occasionally present with decreased hip flexion and internal rotation.

Early stress fractures have normal radiographs and positive bone scans. MRI is very sensitive and can demonstrate early stress fractures and differentiate other causes of pain.

The management of femoral stress fractures is controversial. Treatment options have included complete bed rest, crutches and non-weightbearing, or modified rest with avoidance of offending activities. Bone scan–positive, x-ray–negative fractures can be treated with activity modification to eliminate impact activity, but allow pain-free activities of daily living. X-ray–positive compression or tension side fractures can be treated similarly, but may require crutches until they are symptom free in daily activity. Tension side fractures should probably be treated more conservatively, although some studies have shown no displacement of either type with this treatment (Fullerton and Snowdy, 1988) It is essential that the dancer understand the significance and potential complications of their injury and adhere to the activity restriction. Surgical fixation of femoral neck stress fractures has been used in cases of both displaced and nondisplaced fractures. Clearly, diagnosis of femoral stress fractures is essential before the fracture completes or displaces. Physicians must maintain a high index of suspicion for stress fracture in any dancer with deep, activity-related hip, groin, or thigh pain.

Tendon Injuries

Tendinopathies are common in dancers and present difficult therapeutic dilemmas. Repetitive loading with inadequate recovery can cause breakdown of the affected tendon leading to pain and disability. Although commonly referred to clinically as *tendonitis*, there is little histologic evidence of inflammation in the affected tendons and they should more properly be called *tendinopathies* or *tendinoses*. Additionally, the tendon sheath can also become inflamed or thickened, leading to peritendonitis or tenosynovitis, which is a true inflammatory condition.

Treatment of tendinosis is difficult. Tendons have very poor blood supply thus the time course of healing can be prolonged, leading to frustration on the part of the dancer and the clinician. Early intervention may allow an earlier return to unrestricted activity. Because there is little evidence of inflammation, nonsteroidal anti-inflammatory drugs (NSAIDs) are of limited utility. They are helpful to control the symptoms of pain, but do not treat the underlying pathology. Corticosteroid injections have limited utility, except in cases of tenosynovitis. Eccentric tendon retraining has proven effective in a number of tendinopathies. Newer modalities, such as extracorporeal shock wave therapy (ESWT), have been widely used in Europe for over 10 years and have documented efficacy.

Flexor Hallucis Longus Tendon Dysfunction

Dysfunction of the FHL can result in pain at several sites in the foot and ankle. The tendon descends in the deep posterior compartment of the lower leg, passes through a tunnel between the medial and lateral tubercles of the posterior aspect of the talus adjacent to the os trigonum, and then through the tarsal tunnel, exiting under the flexor retinaculum. It then proceeds along the medial midfoot, passing under the tendons of the flexor digitorum at the master knot of Henry, at the level of the base of the first metatarsal. It can become entrapped at several sites, resulting in stenosing tenosynovitis, and can also develop partial longitudinal tears.

Dancers with FHL dysfunction experience pain with jumping and dancing en pointe, and may have triggering and occasionally crepitus. In neutral position, passive dorsiflexion of the hallux may be restricted, especially in dancers with triggering, and this can be relieved by plantarflexion of the ankle. There is reproduction of the dancer's pain with resisted FHL function. MRI can demonstrate tendon degeneration and fluid in the paratenon surrounding the tendon. Treatment is initially conservative, emphasizing restoration of normal foot and subtalar mobility. Dancers should be cautioned against forcing turnout, as this places the tendon under increased tension. If conservative measures fail, surgical exploration and release usually provides good relief (Kolettis et al., 1996; Sammarco and Cooper, 1998).

Achilles Tendonosis

Achilles tendonosis is a common problem in dancers, especially participants in classic ballet. Overuse is a contributory factor, with significant demands placed on the tendon while dancing en pointe. There is a watershed area of relative avascularity in the distal tendon 2–6 cm proximal to its insertion. This area is often subjected to torsional stress and whipping in athletes who pronate excessively. This local stress can theoretically be increased in dancers with loss of normal joint mobility who are unable to fully re-supinate the foot when going onto full or demi-pointe and in dancers who attempt to force turnout from the floor upward. Additionally, tight toe ribbons from the pointe shoes may compress the tendon sheath and lead to a local paratenonitis.

Achilles tendonitis presents with local pain, swelling, and occasionally crepitus in the acute phase. At this stage it is most likely to respond to symptomatic treatments such as rest, NSAIDs, heel lifts, and local physical therapy. Unfortunately, most dancers do not present in the acute phase and try to dance through the pain. Chronic cases are characterized by tendon degeneration and occasionally palpable nodules within the tendon. All cases require stretching of the gastroc–soleus complex, and restoration of normal mobility of the foot and ankle with emphasis on the subtalar joint, until the pointe axis shows side-to-side symmetry. Eccentric strengthening is generally effective (Alfredson et al., 1998); however, ESWT or rarely surgical debridement are sometimes needed.

Patellar Tendinosis

Patellar tendinosis can be a frustrating condition. It shares similar histologic, ultrasound, and MRI findings with the other chronic tendinoses. It leads to sharp, central, infrapatellar pain particularly provoked with landing from jumps. Dancers are predisposed to patellar tendinosis if they cheat on turnout, which leads to valgus positioning of the knee causing increased torsional wringing and stress loading of the tendon. Treatment is similar to other tendinoses—relative rest, restoration of joint mobility above and below the knee, eccentric retraining, ESWT, and rarely surgical debridement and stripping.

Rectus Femoris Tendinosis

The rectus femoris is a two-joint muscle, crossing both the hip and the knee. It can become irritated when it is used inappropriately as the primary hip flexor in place of the iliopsoas, which has a much better mechanical advantage. It presents with anterior hip pain on forward elevation of the leg, especially with the knee extended. Treatment is relative rest, strengthening, and correction of technique faults.

Foot Disorders

Sesamoid Disorders

Sesamoid injuries can result in prolonged disability in dancers. The sesamoids are situated in the tendons of the flexor hallucis brevis (FHB) and articulate with facets of the plantar surface of the first metatarsal just proximal to the MTP joint. They bear weight during gait, and increase the mechanical advantage of the FHB, and are thus subject to considerable force in dance, especially with rolling through the foot onto demi- or full pointe. The sesamoids are also subject to increased loading in dancers who walk day to day with significant out-toeing of gait, so that the line of force progression exits the foot medially under the first MTP rather than more laterally between the first and second toes. Bipartite or multipartite sesamoids are not infrequent. The sesamoids are susceptible to a number of disorders, including inflammation, contusion, acute or stress fracture, osteonecrosis, and osteoarthritis.

Dancers present with pain in the vicinity of the plantar surface of the first MTP joint. This must be differentiated from capsulitis, which results in more generalized pain around the circumference of the MTP. There is tenderness over the sesamoid, with the medial (tibial) more commonly involved than the lateral. Pain is provoked by resisted MTP flexion, and passive dorsiflexion may be painful and/or restricted. Functional foot movements may show loss of supination, with the more pronated foot position causing increased loading of the sesamoid. It is important to examine the dancer during normal walking gait to determine the presence of abnormal medial toe-off over the first MTP. Hip capsular tightness or SIJD might lead to unilateral out-toeing with increased loading. The dancer should also be observed performing plies and going en demi-pointe in first and second position. Dancers who force turnout from the floor upward often roll forward, increasing sesamoid loading.

Treatment of sesamoid disorders is usually symptomatic, and may require prolonged time away from dance. While symptomatic, work on demi-pointe should be restricted. Gait and dance modifications are important, especially avoidance of excessive or forced turnout. Hip and SI dysfunctions should be corrected, and ankle, subtalar, and midfoot mobility must be restored. C-shaped pads may be used to assist local offloading, and NSAIDs, local physical therapy, and occasionally corticosteroid injections to the sesamoid-MT joint are used. Cases that are refractory to conservative care may require sesamoidectomy as a last resort.

Plantar Fasciitis

Plantar fasciitis is a common overuse syndrome in dancers. The plantar fascia originates on the plantar aspect of the calcaneus, runs anteriorly along the arch, and inserts on the base of the proximal phalanges. It assists the foot in converting from the pronated, shock-absorbing position, to the supinated position, which provides a rigid lever for the push-off and going up on relevé.

The dancer complains of pain at the plantar aspect of the medial heel, worse with activity, especially going up on demi-pointe, and often particularly noticeable with the first few steps in the morning. Examination shows maximum tenderness at the origin of the plantar fascia from the medial calcaneal tuberosity. Examination should include an assessment of the pointe axis and the mobility of the ankle, subtalar, and midfoot joints, with comparison to the uninjured side.

The treatment of plantar fasciitis begins with the PRICE principles, along with heel cups to improve intrinsic heel pad cushioning, simple arch supports, and supportive shoes. Dancers, however, cannot perform in orthotics, so low-dye taping is sometimes employed. Mobility must be restored to the ankle, subtalar, and midfoot joints, and this alone may provide significant relief for many patients. Eccentric strengthening of the gastrocsoleus is useful. Dorsiflexion night splints sometimes help. In refractory cases, corticosteroid injections have been used, but controlled trials have produced temporary relief only. Well-controlled studies have shown that ESWT is effective in about 80% of chronic cases (Rompe et al., 2002). Surgical release is a last resort if all other measures have failed. Nerve entrapments, rheumatic disorders, and gout may predispose to or mimic the symptoms of plantar fasciitis, and should be ruled out prior to any surgical intervention.

Posterior Impingement Syndrome

Impingement of bony and soft tissue structures between the posterior lip of the tibia and the calcaneus can occur while the dancer is on full pointe (Kadel et al., 2000). This can produce swelling and inflammation of the joint capsule and soft tissues, and occasionally the FHL tendon and sheath. Chronic stress or single acute episodes of hyperplantarflexion can cause bone bruising to the posterior tibia, os trigonum of the talus, and the calcaneus, occasionally leading to fragmentation of the os trigonum.

The dancer presents with posterior ankle pain, swelling, and loss of motion and the ability to fully pointe. Examination reveals local tenderness and fullness in the retrocalcaneal region, and pain on passively hyperplantarflexing the foot. If the FHL is involved there may be pain with flexing and extending the great toe with the foot in dorsiflexion. Radiographs may show an os trigonum and bony fragmentation. MRI shows bony edema, soft tissue swelling, tenosynovitis, and occasionally cyst formation. Treatments include the usual conservative measures, and if these fail, fluoroscopically or ultrasound-guided aspiration of any cysts and corticosteroid injection. Surgical debridement is needed for recalcitrant cases.

Knee Disorders

Patellofemoral Pain Syndrome

Patellofemoral pain (PFP) represents a spectrum of disorders of the patellofemoral joint, resulting in activity-related anterior knee pain. There are numerous reported causes for patellofemoral pain, including bony problems such as dysplastic femoral condyles, and abnormalities of patellar size, shape, and height. It is felt that the underlying cause is poor patellar tracking with lateral tracking of the patella, leading to abnormal distribution of the patellofemoral joint reactive forces. Soft tissue factors include generalized ligamentous laxity with poor patellar tracking, reduced patellar mobility with tethering of the lateral facet leading to lateral patellar compression syndrome, tightness of the hamstrings leading to increased patellofemoral joint reactive forces, and deficiency of the vastus medialis, leading to lateralization of the tracking. Poor core stability and gluteus medius weakness leads to increased valgus displacement of the knee with closed-chain flexion, and lateral patellar overload. Cheating on turnout from the floor up leads to increased patellofemoral forces. Restrictions of hip, SI joint, or foot mobility frequently lead to patellar tracking abnormalities, reinforcing the notion that it is important to examine the entire kinetic chain in patients with overuse injuries.

The dancer complains of activity-related anterior knee pain, usually worsened by pliés and relieved with rest. With continued dance, the pain may become constant and plague the dancer even during activities of daily living. Reports of significant swelling are rare, and the dancer may occasionally complain of buckling, but not true instability.

On examination, patellar tracking should be checked by having the dancer plié in both first and sixth position. The center of the patella should track over the second metatarsal. Unilateral abnormal tracking should alert the examiner to the possibility of a kinetic chain dysfunction, with abnormal mobility of the foot, hip, or SI joint on the affected side. Local examination generally demonstrates tenderness over the medial or lateral patellar facets. Patellar mobility and tilting may be abnormal. The patellofemoral compression test, in which the patella is compressed into the sulcus while the quadriceps are actively contracted, should be avoided because it leads to pain in a high proportion of normal individuals, and can cause significant pain in susceptible patients.

Radiographs may show variations of patellofemoral anatomy such as lateral tracking and tilting of the patella, patellar subluxation, and a shallow femoral sulcus. In adolescents, it is always important to carefully examine the radiographs for evidence of osteochondritis dissecans, which can present in a similar fashion.

In general, treatment for patellofemoral pain follows the same principles outlined previously for all overuse injuries. Extrinsic factors, such as improper technique and cheating on turnout, should be addressed and corrected. Intrinsic factors such as muscle imbalances, inflexibility, and strength deficiencies should all be identified and remedied. Kinetic chain dysfunctions resulting in abnormal and asymmetric patellar tracking should be identified and treated. Restricted subtalar or talocrural joint motion should be restored. Tight hip capsules should be stretched and released. SI joint alignment and mobility should be normalized.

Stretching is used to improve the flexibility of the quadriceps and hamstrings. It is also important to stretch the IT band, which send insertions to the lateral retinaculum and may contribute to lateral tracking of the patella. The Achilles and heel cords should be stretched, as tightness decreases ankle dorsiflexion, resulting in increased pronation and patellofemoral joint reactive forces.

Strengthening is generally done using a graduated program of eccentric quadriceps strengthening drills in the form of a mini-squat. The dancer stands with the feet approximately 8 inches apart in parallel position and slowly does a squat. This initially is done to a very minimal flexion angle with the knee. As the patient's tolerance to the activity progresses, they can gradually deepen the angle of the squat as well as increase the velocity. Two cautions must be exercised. First, it should be stressed to the patient that the mid-point of the patella should be centered over the second toe throughout the entire squat. Tightening the buttocks may assist in maintaining patellar alignment. Second, the squats should be done with minimal or no pain. If the exercises cause significant pain, then they should reduce the speed in the angle of the drop. In addition to eccentric mini-squats, the dancer should focus on the hip abductors and gluteus medius that are essential to maintaining stability and proper patellar tracking during one-legged balancing activities.

Patellar stabilizing sleeves work well in cases where the individual has a hypermobile patella, especially if they have had problems with subluxations and/or dislocations. Higher level dancers are unable to wear these during performances, although they may utilize McConnell taping. Taping and bracing are not treatments in and of themselves; they are adjuncts to allow the patient pain-free mobility to improve the level of symptomatology while the rest of the treatment is undertaken.

Hip Injuries

When a dancer presents with hip pain it is essential to rule out serious injuries such as stress fractures. Other common complaints include the snapping hip. There are generally two forms, lateral and anterior, which must be differentiated through a detailed history.

The *lateral snapping hip* results from the tensor fascia lata and the proximal portion of the IT band snapping over the greater trochanter as the hip is extended. Just like its distal counterpart, IT band friction syndrome, the lateral snapping hip is a strength and stability problem more than an IT band tightness problem. Contributing factors include poor core stability, hip abductor weakness, and SI joint dysfunction. With repeated friction, the underlying trochanteric bursa may become inflamed and painful. The dancer often states that their hip is dislocating, because of the significant clunk heard as the band passes over the trochanter. Examination reveals tenderness over the greater trochanter, increased with Ober's maneuver, weakness of the hip abductors, and evidence of SI joint dysfunction. Treatment involves NSAIDs and ice for symptomatic relief then a rehabilitation program emphasizing hip strength and core stability, and correction of underlying SIJD.

The anterior snapping hip is caused by the iliopsoas tendon snapping over the femoral head as the flexed, abducted, and externally rotated hip is returned to a neutral position. Extension causes further snapping as the tendon moves from the lateral to the medial side of the femoral head. Underlying factors include poor technique including excess lumbar lordosis, iliopsoas tightness, and SIJD. The Thomas test reveals tightness of the iliopsoas; diagnosis is then confirmed with the patient remaining in the same position and the examiner reproducing the pain and snapping as the hip is internally rotated, adducted, and extended. Treatment is directed at symptom relief, correcting the underlying technique faults, core stability, and iliopsoas stretching and strengthening. Fluoroscopically guided injection of the iliopectineal bursa can be attempted in refractory cases. Surgical release is rarely indicated.

Low Back Pain

Low back pain is a very common phenomenon in dancers, affecting virtually all dancers at some stage in their career (Seitsalo et al., 1997). Management can be frustrating and depends on an accurate diagnoses and then treatment specific to that diagnosis. Fortunately, almost all back pain is self-limiting, and even in the absence of an accurate diagnosis, excellent treatment results are frequently obtained with conservative management.

The cause of low back is multifactorial. The pain can arise from any of the structures in the back, including the muscles, ligaments, facet joints, intervertebral disk, or SI joints. Chronic overuse syndromes can occur with the back. These are predisposed by poor posture, including increased lumbar lordosis, tightness of the hamstrings and iliopsoas, and poor strength of the abdominal and paraspinal musculature. Most back pain in dancers results from poor technique, including improper lifting and partnering. Increased lumbar lordosis from cheating at turnout, tight hip capsules, and SIJD can lead to increased load on the posterior elements. Two of the most common causes of low back pain in dancers are spondylolysis and pelvic instability SIJD.

Spondylolysis

Spondylolysis is a stress fracture of the pars interarticularis, and is thought to arise from repetitive extension and flexion of the spine. Both the pathology and the clinical presentation of spondylolysis are variable. A study of Finnish dancers revealed a 32% incidence of radiographic evidence of spondylolysis, which compares to a 6% incidence in the general population (Seitsalo et al., 1997). The specific pathology is on a continuum and may range from an asymptomatic fibrous defect discovered on an x-ray to a stress fracture with disabling pain. It is thus important to correlate the clinical findings with any imaging studies.

Spondylolysis usually presents with activity-related low back pain, usually exacerbated by extension or twisting, which load the posterior elements of the spine. It is often unilateral and relieved by rest, although night pain may occur in acute cases. Affected dancers usually demonstrate poor technique as well as defective posture with lumbar hyperlordosis, poor abdominal tone, tight hip flexors and hip capsule, and weak hamstrings. Unilateral extension frequently reproduces the back pain.

Radiographs frequently show the characteristic Scotty dog lesion on the oblique view, but their clinical significance must be interpreted with caution due to the high prevalence of asymptomatic lesions. The technetium radionuclide bone scan is the diagnostic test of choice, and improved diagnostic accuracy can be gained through the use of single photon emission computed tomography, which can accurately localize the lesion to the pars. MRI can be utilized, with best results from fat-saturated T2 sagittal images with thin cuts through the area of the pars. A positive x-ray with a negative bone scan or MRI should prompt the clinician to search for another cause of the patient's back pain, including SIJD, which is common in dancers. Some dancers undergo anterior slippage of a vertebrae on the one below through a spondylolytic defect, which is termed *spondylolisthesis.*

The treatment of spondylolysis is controversial, and depends on the stage of the pathology. Early stress fractures with positive bone scans and negative radiographs have the best chance of healing. Well-established fractures with sclerotic margins have little healing potential. There is general agreement that the offending activities in dance should be stopped. Some clinicians recommend cessation of all activities, but it seems more reasonable, and equally effective, to maintain motions that can be performed without pain. Long-term studies have shown that patients with spondylolysis and spondylolisthesis can perform at high levels of athletics without symptoms (Seitsalo et al., 1997). These findings suggest that activity modification and possibly soft bracing for symptomatic relief should be the treatment of choice. Early lesions with negative radiographs and positive bone scans should possibly be treated with more rigid activity restrictions.

Other rehabilitation should be undertaken while the dancer is in the restricted activity phase. Lumbar and core stabilization exercises have been shown to have beneficial results. The dancer should correct their technique, work at stretching the hip flexors and hamstrings, and correct lumbopelvic mechanics and hyperlordosis. Dancers are allowed a gradual return to activity when they are asymptomatic and have completed a posture and stabilization program. They should be allowed to gradually progress their activity so long as it can be accomplished without provoking an increase in pain.

Pelvic Instability and Sacroiliac Joint Dysfunction

SIJD is a common, frequently overlooked, and almost universally controversial condition. The pelvic ring is composed of the innominate bones, which meet at the symphysis anteriorly, and articulate with the sacrum posteriorly at the SI joints. Excessive mobility can lead to instability and lumbopelvic pain. The most common dysfunctions occur with rotational subluxation of the innominate and sacral torsions leading to an asymmetry in the pelvic ring structure. The intrinsic motions and positioning demands of dance frequently result in SIJD, in both symptomatic and asymptomatic dancers. Tightness of the hip capsule or hip flexors limits hip movement, thus transferring increased stress to the SI joints, leading to dysfunction. Acute trauma such as a fall onto the buttocks or an awkward landing producing an axial load onto one leg can provoke SIJD. Vigorous hip flexion or extension movements may also lead to SIJD.

The pain is often localized to the SI joint itself, but may be found in the buttocks, groin, pubic symphysis, lower abdomen, or lateral thigh. Occasionally there is pain referred to the posterior thigh and lower leg and foot. Pressure over the SI joint can also reproduce leg symptoms in some individuals. Movement is painful, with extension often more painful than flexion. Patients with SIJD often present with a secondary injury arising from gait alterations, but admit to underlying activity-related back pain. Patients may also complain that they feel as if they are out of alignment, and that their gait is abnormal, but many do not admit to this sensation unless specifically questioned. Dysfunction of the SI joint leads to compensatory changes at other sites in the axial skeleton, including sacral torsion, rotation of the lumbar vertebrae, and frequently secondary rotations of thoracic and even cervical vertebrae.

The most common finding on physical examination is that of tenderness over the SI joint. Examination is also directed at the identification of functional asymmetries of the levels of the anterior and posterior superior iliac spines in the frontal plane and tilting of the sacrum. Additional clues are asymmetrical leg lengths and change when the patient goes from a supine position to a long sitting position in which the patient sits upright on the examination table with the hips flexed to 90° and the knees extended. An asymmetric range of hip motion may be found, with one hip having predominant range of external rotation and the other predominant range of internal rotation. The dancer is often be aware that turnout is restricted on one side. SIJD is a diagnosis of exclusion, and neurologic examination including nerve tension signs must be normal.

It is important to stress to the dancer that there is no magic treatment for back pain and that the responsibility for treating their back pain lies with them. All treatments ultimately require the patient's active participation and cooperation, and the performance of regular program of maintenance exercises. The treatment of lumbosacral problems is directed toward relief of symptoms, followed by restoration of strength and flexibility, specifically to the hamstrings, quadriceps, hip flexors, and hip capsule. Specific treatment of SIJD and pelvic instability consists of correcting the underlying dynamics and positional defects of the pelvis. The scope of this chapter does not allow a full discussion of this, but good reference texts are available (Lee, 1989).

CONCLUSION

Acute traumatic injuries are common in ballet dancers and are similar to the acute injuries in other athletes. A careful history, thorough examination, and appropriate imaging should allow for the diagnosis of most problems. The clinician must have a high index of suspicion for occult bony injuries, especially if the patient fails to recover as expected. Aggressive treatment of the sprained ankle is essential to maintain foot and ankle mobility and prevent prolonged disability and subsequent overuse injuries.

Overuse injuries are common in dance, and frequently result from technique problems as the dancer tries to perform within the rigid positioning demands of dance. Kinetic chain dysfunctions are common in ballet dancers with overuse injuries. They may represent a secondary phenomenon that developed in response to the compensatory movement changes caused by the presenting injury. It is important to remember, however, that these dysfunctions may have been longstanding and a causative factor in the injury. Regardless of the time of onset of the dysfunction, residual kinetic chain dysfunction associated with incomplete rehabilitation of an injury may predispose the dancer to further injuries. Untreated dysfunctions at one site in the kinetic chain may predispose to compensatory dysfunction at other sites in the chain. Accordingly, when dealing with an injured dancer, it is essential to thoroughly examine the entire chain while performing functional ballet movements. Identification and treatment of the kinetic chain dysfunction is critical in the rehabilitation of the dancer.

Rehabilitation of the injured dancer depends on identifying and correcting the underlying causes of injury. Restoration of strength and endurance, with the emphasis on core stability, is essential. The clinician must correct specific kinetic chain dysfunctions and flexibility deficits. A knowledgeable and thorough team of physicians and therapists should be able to return most dancers to normal dance activity.

REFERENCES

Alfredson H, Pietila T, Jonnson P, Lorentzon R. Heavy-load eccentric calf muscle training for the treatment of chronic Achilles tendinosis. *Am J Sports Med.* 1998;26:360–366.

Benson JE, Geiger CJ, Eiserman PA, Wardlaw GM. Relationship between nutrient intake, body mass index, menstrual function and ballet injury. *J Am Dietetic Assoc.* 1989;89;58–63.

Bolin DJ. Evaluation and management of stress fractures in dancers. *J Dance Med Sci.* 2001;537–542.

Conti SF, Wong YS. Foot and ankle injuries in the dancer. *J Dance Med Sci.* 2001;543–550.

Denegar CR, Hertel J, Fonseca J. The effect of lateral ankle sprain on dorsiflexion range of motion, Posterior talar glide, and joint laxity. *J Orthop Sports Phys Ther.* 2002;32:166–173.

Faciszewski T, Burks RT, Manaster BJ. Subtle injuries of the Lisfranc joint. *J Bone Joint Surg* 1990;72;1519–1522.

Fullerton LR, Snowdy HA. Femoral neck stress fractures. *Am J Sports Med.* 1988;16:365–377.

Hamilton WG. Ballet. In: Reider, ed. *Sports Medicine—The School Age Athlete.* Philadelphia: Saunders; 1996.

Hamilton WG, Geppert MJ, Thompson FM. Pain in the posterior aspect of the ankle in dancers. Differential diagnosis and operative treatment. *J Bone Joint Surg.* 1996;78:1491–1500.

Harrington T, Crichton KJ, Anderson IF. Overuse ballet injury to the base of the second metatarsal—A diagnostic problem. *Am J Sports Med.* 1993;21:591–598.

Jones BH, Cowan DN, Tomlinson JP, Robinson JR, Polly DW, Frykman PN. Epidemiology of injuries associated with physical training among young men in the Army. *Med Sci Sports Exerc.* 1993;25:197–203.

Kadel NJ, Teitz CC, Kronmal RA. Stress fractures in ballet dancers. *Am J Sports Med.* 1992;20:445–449.

Kadel NJ, Micheli LJ, Solomon R, et al. Os trigonum impingement syndrome in dancers. *J Dance Med Sci.* 2000;4:99–102.

Khan KM, Fuller PJ, Brukner PD, Kearney C, Burry HC. Outcome of conservative and surgical management of navicular stress fracture in athletes. Eighty-six cases proven with computerized tomography. *Am J Sports Med.* 1992;20:657–666.

Kibler WB, Chandler TJ, Stracener ES. Musculoskeletal adaptations and injuries due to overtraining. In: Holloszy JO, ed. *Exercise and sports science reviews,* vol. 20. Baltimore: Williams & Wilkins; 1992.

Kolettis GJ, Micheli LJ, Klein JD. Release of the flexor hallucis longus tendon in ballet dancers. *J Bone Joint Surg Am.* 1996;78:1386–1390.

Leanderson J, Eriksson E, Nillson C, Wyckman A. Proprioception in classical ballet dancers: A prospective study of the influence of an ankle sprain on proprioception in the ankle joint. *Am J Sports Med.* 1996;24:370–374.

Leddy JJ, Smolinski RJ, Lawrence J, Snyder JL, Priore RL. Prospective evaluation of the Ottawa Ankle Rules in a university sports medicine center—With a modification to increase specificity for identifying malleolar fractures. *Am J Sports Med.* 1998;26:158–165.

Lee D. *The pelvic girdle: An approach to the examination and treatment of the lumbo-pelvic-hip region.* New York: Churchill Livingstone; 1989.

Liederbach M. General considerations for guiding dance injury rehabilitation. *J Dance Med and Sci.* 2000;4:54–65.

Macintyre J. Kinetic chain dysfunction in ballet injuries. *Med Prob Perf Art.* 1994;99;39–42.

Marshall P, Hamilton W. Cuboid subluxation in ballet dancers. *Am J Sports Med.* 1992;20:169–175.

O'Malley MJ, Hamilton WG, Munyak J. Fractures of the distal shaft of the fifth metatarsal—"Dancer's fracture." *Am J Sports Med.* 1996;24:240–243.

Pigman EC, Klug RK, Sanford S, Jolly BT. Evaluation of the Ottawa clinical decision rules for the use of radiography in acute ankle and midfoot injuries in the emergency department: An independent site assessment. *Ann Emerg Med.* 1994;24:41–45.

Reid DC. Prevention of hip and knee injuries in ballet dancers. *Sports Med.* 1988;6;295–307.

Reid DC. The myth, mystic, and frustration of anterior knee pain. *Clin J Sport Med.* 1993;3:139–143.

Rompe JD, Schoellner C, Nafe B. Evaluation of low-energy extracorporeal shock-wave therapy application for treatment of chronic plantar fasciitis. *J Bone Joint Surg Am.* 2002:84A:335–341.

Sammarco GJ, Cooper PS. Flexor hallucis longus tendon injury in dancers and nondancers. *Foot Ankle Int.* 1998:19:356–362.

Seitsalo S, Antila H, et al. Spondylolysis in ballet dancers. *J Dance Med Sci.* 1997;1:51–54.

Solomon R, Micheli LJ, Ireland ML. Physiologic assessment to determine readiness for pointe work in ballet students. *Impulse.* 1993;1:21–38.

Stiehll IG, Greenberg GH, et al. Decision rules for the use of radiography in acute ankle injuries. *JAMA.* 1993:269;1127–1132.

Stone D. Hip problems in dancers. *J Dance Med Sci.* 2001;5:7–10.

Teitz CC. Hip and knee injuries in dancers. *J Dance Med Sci.* 2000;4:23–29.

Tochigi Y, Toshinaga K, Wada Y, Moriya H. Acute inversion injury of the ankle: Magnetic resonance imaging and clinical outcomes. *Foot Ankle Int.* 1998;19:730–734.

Torg JS, Pavlov H, Cooley LH, et al. Stress fractures of the tarsal navicular: A retrospective review of twenty-one cases. *J Bone Joint Surg Am.* 1982;64A:700–712.

Walsh MC, Nolan M. *Clinical assessment and treatment techniques for the lower extremity.* Vancouver: Kilkee Publishing; 1999.

Weisler ER, Hunter DM, Martin DF, Curl WW, Hoen H. Ankle flexibility and injury patterns in dancers. *Am J Sports Med.* 1996;24:754–757.

Wen DY, Puffer JC, Schmalzried TP. Lower extremity alignment and risk of overuse injuries in runners. *Med Sci Sport Exerc.* 1997;29:1291–1298.

38 | Gymnastic Injuries and Prevention

Mark Bouchard

QUICK LOOK

- Both acute and chronic injury patterns occur.
- Men tend to develop more upper extremity injuries (rotator cuff) and women more lower extremity injuries (ankle).
- Distal radial physeal injuries and spondylolysis of the lumbar spine are also common injuries.
- Treatment of the female athletic triad requires a team approach, which includes coaches, parents, nutritionists, and physicians.
- Prevention should include adequate strength and flexibility along with adequate rehabilitation of past injuries.

Gymnastics has grown dramatically in popularity and in the number of participants over the past several years. Competition has pushed the sport to progressively more difficult maneuvers, increasing the acute injuries in number and severity. Longer training hours have also led to an increase in overuse injuries. Although experts have noted increases in the injury rate of gymnasts who train more than 15 hours per week, highly motivated gymnasts train from 4–5 hours per day, 5–6 days per week to develop the skills required at higher levels of competition.

MEN'S GYMNASTICS

Although the floor exercise and vaulting events in men's gymnastics are essentially the same as in women's, the men's sport differs significantly because it includes rings, parallel bars, high bar, and pommel horse. The six events in men's gymnastics contrast to the four in women's gymnastics. It follows that there are differences in injury patterns, with more lower extremity injuries in women and more upper extremity injuries in men. Wrist problems occur with the pommel horse, rings, and high bar. Elbow problems occur with triceps, especially with the parallel bars and high bar. Misses from releases on the high bar can lead to significant injury. The same forces exist in men's and women's vaulting and floor exercise, with similar injury risks. All of the flying events share a risk of head and neck injuries if falls occur and also share a risk of knee and ankle injury with unsuccessful dismounts.

Pommel Horse

The pommel horse event consists of continuous motion of trunk and legs while maintaining support on hands and arms. It requires good balance and upper body strength. This event has the lowest risk of injury of all the men's apparatus. Overuse of the wrists is the primary risk; traumatic injury to the wrists occurs occasionally. Bruising of lower extremities from contact with the pommels is also common.

Rings

This event combines swing and strength elements, with strength becoming increasingly prominent. The shoulders sustain a great deal of stress with this event. Gymnasts are required to have enough strength to lift and hold their body weight through various positions while maintaining the flexibility to perform *inlocates* and *dislocates* for the swing elements. Shoulder tendinitis and back problems are common in both elite and lower level athletes. There is also some risk of injury to the lower extremities from dismounts on this apparatus which is 255 cm above the top of the mats.

High Bar

This apparatus consists of a single metal bar placed 255 cm from the top of the mat. Elements consist of continuous motion around the bar with various directions of swing. It also incorporates release elements that require the gymnast to release the bar and recatch after performing a somersault, twist, or both. These are the elements that make high bar the riskiest of all events. The most traumatic and serious injuries are related to the height of the bar and the rotation or twisting on contact with the ground if the bar is not recaught. Risk of injuries to the lower extremities is associated with dismounts from this height. It is also common for skin to be torn from the hands. These rips, however, are considered of minor importance to the gymnasts.

Parallel Bars

The parallel bars are two fiberglass rails located parallel to the ground at a height of 175 cm from the top of the mat. This event consists of swing, balance, and strength elements. The greatest risk of injury seems to be contact with the bar. Bruising is common around the upper arm from landing somersaulting elements in an underarm position. Injuries are uncommon, but they can occur to the lower extremities from incorrect landing or dismounts.

Floor

This exercise is 50–70 seconds long, performed on a 12 × 12 m carpeted wooden floor with either springs or, more commonly, foam cubes underneath. This event combines tumbling with at least one balance and strength element. Tumbling sequences should consist of both forward and backward tumbling. Overuse and traumatic injuries to the lower extremities are common in this event owing to landing forces and improper form on landings.

Vault

The sheer velocity in this event makes injuries common, especially for the lower level athletes who do not have the experience to control falls. Lower extremities are once again the most affected because of the speed and height. The horse is set at 135 cm from the floor but most vaults are performed 2–4 feet above the horse.

WOMEN'S GYMNASTICS

Female gymnastics involves activities of high velocity, impact, and torsion. Scoring is based on a system of 10 and involves the following:

1. Expression
2. Extension

3. Difficulty
4. Dance
5. Deductions

Four basic activities constitute women's gymnastics: floor exercise, uneven parallel bars, vault, and balance beam.

Balance Beam

The balance beam routines, performed on a 4-inch wide, 4-foot high apparatus, require intense precision and balance. There is a time limit for each routine of 1 minute 30 seconds. Skills performed on the beam are similar to floor exercise. The difference is in the exact placement of the foot on the beam. The skills are also performed at a lower speed than the floor exercise. This event has the highest frequency of injuries, most of which are from falls or dismounts. These injuries are less severe, for the most part, because of the lower velocity at which they occur.

Floor Exercise

Floor exercise combines tumbling skills with dance skills. Each routine has a time limit of 1 minute 50 seconds. The routines are done to music and need to have varying tempos within. The gymnast must have three passes: one mount, one dismount, and one middle pass. In addition to these passes, the athlete must use different speeds, heights, directions, and difficulties of skills. This event has the highest rate of injuries. Most injuries in this event are due to miscalculations of landings, and the lower extremities are most affected. McNitt-Gray (1993) did a study on peak vertical reaction forces. A vertical jump landing exerts two to four times the body weight. Double backs (two backward somersaults in the air) exert a force up to 18 times the gymnast's body weight.

Uneven Parallel Bars

This event requires a continuous fluid motion from one bar to the other while the gymnast executes various twists, releases, and hip rotations. It requires extreme upper torso strength, more so than any other event, but the momentum within the routine usually masks this. Injuries occur from falls or faulty dismounts. Other factors that the gymnast has to overcome are rips of the protective callus on the palms, and bruises of the pelvis and thighs from contact with the bars. Injuries due to apparatus failure are also seen in this event.

Vault

Vaulting is a high-velocity event. There is great potential for injury, because it combines the speed of the vault with increasingly more difficult dismounts. This event is less demanding on the gymnast in terms of duration, fewer moves, and so on. The injuries, however, tend to be more serious because of the speeds and vault height involved. The lower extremity is the most affected because of the landings and the speed at which the gymnast hits the springboard. The spotter is available, as in any event, but in vaulting they typically are not in a good position to help should anything go wrong.

EPIDEMIOLOGY

According to Chambers (1979), the rate of gymnastic injuries ranks behind football and is similar to basketball. Soccer, baseball, and swimming typically have much lower injury rates. Gymnastic injury rates also vary with the nature of the competition. Injury rates increase as a gymnast goes from club to high school, to collegiate, and on to elite competition. Many high schools and colleges have dropped gymnastics because of the high injury rates. Private clubs now are receiving more emphasis. There are approximately 30,500 high school participants each year, but only 2200 collegiate participants, the majority being female (70%).

A 10-year study of elite gymnasts in Australia showed injury rates of 1.1 injuries/gymnast/year for male versus a rate of 0.6 for female gymnasts. Male gymnasts were more likely to suffer from upper extremity injuries (especially rotator cuff lesions) and females were more likely to sustain lower extremity injuries (ankle sprains most common). There were no catastrophic injuries reported and rarely did an injury require more than 2 months away from training (Dixon and Fricker, 1993).

PATHOPHYSIOLOGY

Studies of injuries per participant-hour typically show high rates compared to other sports. Equipment failure, such as forgetting to tighten the beam, vault, or bar hinges, leads to injury. Mat thickness is also a problem. It is thin during competition for easier landing techniques, but this leads to higher impact on the lower extremities. It is thick during practice for softer landings, but the foot may become caught during twisting skills with resultant injury.

One must not evade the nutritional and psychological issues related to gymnastics. Striving for thinness may lead to nutritional deficiencies, decreased metabolic rate, and disordered eating. Low iron stores, electrolyte disturbances, and in extreme cases, multi-organ pathology may occur from anorexia and bulimia. There is a need to make gymnasts, coaches, and parents aware of unhealthy methods of weight loss and their prevention. Striving for the perfect 10 may be difficult psychologically.

Gymnastics shares several common injuries with other sports. These include ankle sprains, knee injuries, strains, overuse injuries, and fractures. However, there are injuries more unique to gymnastics, and we will examine this group. This uniqueness stems from two factors:

1. Gymnasts, primarily female, start training at a very early age, usually 5 or 6 years.
2. Greater stresses are placed on the upper extremities and lumbar spine than in other sports, and both upper and lower extremities are weight-bearing.

These factors lead to abnormal stresses on an immature, growing skeleton. Gymnastics involves activities of high velocity, high impact, and high torsion (Fig. 38-1). Combine these factors with the immature growing skeleton and you have a high risk for chronic as well as acute injuries. Female gymnasts begin training at age 5 or 6 and train up to 5–6 hours daily, 5 days per week, reaching peak performance at age 15 or 16. This amount of training places unusual stresses on the growth plates of the wrist and on the pars interarticularis of the lumbar spine. Eating disorders, amenorrhea, and sub-

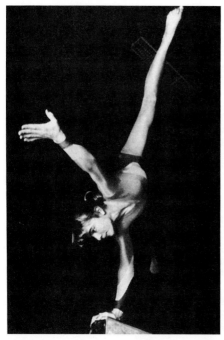

FIG 38-1   The *Rankin* puts considerable load on the entire upper extremity. (*Courtesy of Janine Rankin, Canadian National Gymnast.*)

sequent osteoporosis may aggravate this and affect health in later life. The emphasis on smallness in gymnastics tends to promote this triad. There is evidence to show that such a training schedule may affect skeletal growth. Intensive gymnastics—over 18 hours per week—beginning before and continuing throughout puberty has been shown to reduce adult height.

Stresses to an immature skeleton may lead to several orthopedic problems. Repeated hyperextension of the lumbar spine in floor exercise and on the dismount lead to stress on the pars interarticularis of L5–S1. Stress fractures can occur in this area, either unilateral or bilateral. Repeated stress on the distal radial epiphysis leads to changes in the growth of the distal radius with retardation and positive ulnar variance. This is related to the pronation and extreme dorsiflexion of the wrist, common to gymnastic activities and has several different but related entities. *Positive ulnar variance* is a disorder of the wrist in which the radial growth has been affected, leading to shortening of the radius. This makes the ulna either equal to or longer than the radius. This contrasts with the normal situation in which the radius is longer at the wrist than is the ulna.

Compression forces to the wrist that occur in vaulting, beam, and floor exercise can also lead to damage to the distal radial physis (growth plate). There is disagreement as to whether or not distraction forces lead to stress injury, and although this may occur, the injuries due to distraction seem to be less common and less serious than compression injuries.

GYMNASTIC INJURIES

Wrist Injuries

We first consider the progression of overuse or stress injuries of the wrist. With increased training of growing gymnasts, increased stresses have occurred in the wrist. Symptoms of wrist pain occur in specific areas of the wrist according to weightbearing and torsional activities such as pronation and ulnar deviation. With torsional stresses, symptoms of ulnar impaction syndrome predominate on the dorsal ulnar side of the wrist. Repetitive loading of the distal radius, which occurs with vaulting and floor exercise, can lead to a stress injury of the distal radial physis (Fig. 38-2). Subsequent growth of the distal radius may be affected, as mentioned, leading to a series of wrist problems.

Evaluation

When a young gymnast presents at the office with wrist symptoms, a careful history and physical examination are essential. Age of onset of training, present age, duration and intensity of training, type of training, recent changes in training schedule, site and duration of symptoms, as well as when symptoms occur, are all important in determining the diagnosis and treatment. Careful examination of the injured extremity is necessary. Palpation

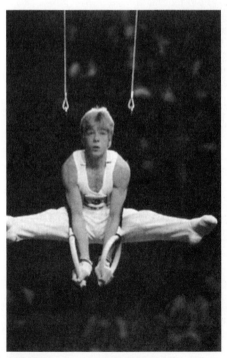

FIG 38-2 Repetitive stress injuries of the wrist. Repetitive loading of the distal radius may alter subsequent growth or damage the triangular fibrocartilage.

of the distal radial physis, radial-ulnar joint, distal ulna, and collateral ligaments should be done carefully to localize the area of maximal tenderness.

With a stress injury of the physis, there is usually limitation of dorsiflexion, mild swelling, and tenderness of the physis to palpation. X-rays may or may not be helpful in the diagnosis because the injury may be to soft tissue only. The main reason for x-ray is to rule out changes in the distal radial physis. These changes include irregular widening of the distal radial physis. This may be difficult to assess in a gymnast because the changes may be bilateral, and there is therefore no normal wrist with which to compare. However, widening should be readily appreciated if present and is evidence of a longstanding stress injury. If signs and symptoms of a stress injury of the epiphysis are present but x-rays are normal, the injury is of shorter duration and the prognosis is generally better.

Management

Treatment consists of relative rest with restriction of vaulting and floor exercise until the patient is pain free and nontender to palpation. This may take as long as 3 months with more severe injuries.

Confounding Conditions

In many cases of stress injury to the physis, distal radial growth is impaired, resulting in a positive ulnar variance. This may lead to other wrist problems if the athlete continues in gymnastics.

Positive ulnar variance and a subsequent malalignment of the distal radiocarpal joint may lead to an overload of the triangular fibrocartilage complex (TFCC). The TFCC fills the space between the distal ulna and carpus. Chronic overload leads to degeneration and tearing of this complex. Diagnosis is made by a history of ulnar-sided wrist pain, with tenderness and clicking with motion over the TFCC. Weak grip strength is often present and should be measured. Wrist MRI can confirm diagnosis. Initial treatment consists of rest, nonsteroidal anti-inflammatory drugs (NSAIDs), forearm strengthening, and splinting to eliminate maximal dorsiflexion on return to sport. Surgical intervention may be necessary if conservative management fails. A surgeon experienced in wrist arthroscopy can confirm the diagnosis and treat the injury arthroscopically, considerably shortening rehabilitation and time from sport.

Dorsal wrist ganglia are more common in gymnasts than in other athletes. Diagnosis is made by palpation of a tender mass of the dorsal wrist. Aspiration and steroid injection may give temporary relief, but ultimately surgical excision is necessary to remove the ganglion.

Elbow Injuries

Triceps Tendonitis

Evaluation. A rather unique injury to gymnasts is triceps tendonitis. It is characterized by elbow pain localized to the olecranon tip. Tenderness is present over the distal triceps insertion, and is an injury analogous to jumper's knee.

Management. Treatment consists of relative rest, a triceps flexibility and strengthening program, and oral anti-inflammatories as needed for pain relief. Steroid injections should be avoided.

Elbow Dislocation

Another frequent gymnastics injury is elbow dislocation. This is common because of the use of the upper extremities in many of the gymnastic maneuvers, and in a fall or miss, the elbow is at risk.

Management. Treatment consists of careful neurovascular examination, immediate reduction, postreduction x-ray examination to rule out associated fractures, vigilant checking for instability of the joint, a complete neurovascular examination following reduction, and early mobilization. Splinting is usually necessary for 7–10 days, but then gentle range of motion should be started. Once full painless range of motion with good strength has been achieved, then a return to gymnastics may be allowed. This may take 6–12 weeks.

If a suspected fracture is present, then comparison films with the opposite elbow may be helpful. Anatomic reduction is necessary to ensure the peak performance of gymnasts. This generally requires an open reduction with internal fixation, followed by early mobilization and rehabilitation. In the growing child an MRI may be indicated to identify a medial epicondylar fracture that is mainly cartilaginous.

Lumbar Spine

Lumbar spine problems are common in gymnasts, figure skaters, and ballerinas because of the hyperextension activities common to these sports (Fig. 38-3). It is most common, however, in gymnastics, especially in floor exercise, balance beam, and vaulting with associated hyperextension during dismount. This dismount loads the posterior elements of the spine, especially the pars interarticularis of L5–S1.

Spondylolysis is considered to be a stress fracture of the pars interarticularis. This condition is due to the repetitive microtrauma seen in gymnastics.

Evaluation

The young gymnast who presents with low back pain will usually have a normal range of motion with no pain on straight leg raising to 90°. Neu-

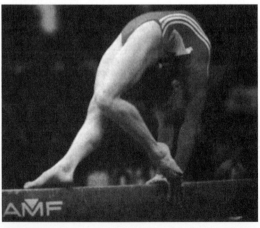

FIG 38-3 Hyperextension injuries. Repetitive hyperextension injuries of the lumbar spine may cause a stress fracture of the pars or *spondylosis*.

rologic examination is normal. There may be lower lumbar tenderness, but the most reliable test is the one-legged lay back or stork test. This test is done with the athlete standing on one leg, opposite knee flexed. While supported, the patient is then asked to do a lay back, or hyperextend the lumbar spine. If this movement reproduces low back pain, it is considered positive. If positive, or if low back pain has been present for longer than 3 weeks, then x-rays, including AP and lateral views of the lumbar spine are indicated.

If plain films are normal, then a single photon emission computerized tomography (SPECT) bone scan is indicated. A SPECT bone scan is effective in diagnosing a stress fracture of the pars. If spondylolysis is present, a limited CT scan at the level of the SPECT abnormality with thin slices is used to stage (early, progressive, terminal) the pars lesion. Staging has been shown to help predict prognosis for healing, which will affect the treatment plan (Standaert, 2002).

Management

Treatment consists of hamstring flexibility exercises and lumbar bracing. Bracing is done with a molded polypropylene brace with 0° lordosis. Initial rest is necessary until the athlete is asymptomatic in the brace. Gradual return to practice and competition is then allowed, avoiding any back hyperextension activities initially.

It may take 6–9 months for complete healing to occur. Terminal defects seen on CT scan have very little chance of healing. For early and some progressive lesions, a follow-up limited CT scan is helpful in showing healing of the pars defect. If a grade 1 spondylolisthesis is present, treatment is the same. However, some athletes do not become asymptomatic despite a prolonged, conservative course of therapy and lumbar fusion may be necessary. Standaert (2002) has written an excellent review on imaging and treatment of low back injuries in gymnastics.

Confounding Conditions

Recent studies have shown a high incidence of degenerative disk disease in young male and female gymnasts. In the event that sciatic symptoms are present or studies for pars interarticularis defects are negative, MRI imaging may be necessary to evaluate for disk degeneration or herniation.

Prevention of lumbar injuries is important in gymnasts, and there seems to be a direct correlation between the number of training hours per week and lumbar problems. Those athletes training more than 15 hours per week are at risk for developing spine problems. At times of rapid growth, attention must also be paid to hamstring tightness and tight lumbodorsal fascia.

It should be noted that, in female gymnasts, a 1991 study showed MRI abnormalities of the lumbar spine in the following categories: pre-elite (9%), elite (43%), and Olympic (63%) (Goldstein, 1991). The most common change was that of disk degeneration owing to the continued stresses on the lumbar spine; hence, more common in the more advanced gymnast.

Lower Extremity Injuries

Medial Tibial Stress Syndrome

Evaluation. Medial tibial stress syndrome (MTSS) or periostitis is a common problem in gymnastics, and deserves careful differentiation. The classic syndrome is caused by inflammation of the origin of the posterior tibial muscle on the medial edge of the tibia, and is referred to as a *posterior tibial periostitis*. This condition can be confused with a stress fracture of the tibia or with an anterior compartment syndrome. A careful history and physical examination should give the examiner clues as to the correct diagnosis.

MTSS is characterized by medial tibial aching pain that gets progressively worse as the season progresses. There is significant tenderness over the medial tibia at the origin of the posterior tibialis. X-rays are negative and a bone scan may show some uptake along the medial tibia, but this is markedly different from a stress fracture.

Management. Treatment consists of ice, relative rest, and elastic band strengthening of the posterior tibialis, and if possible, orthotics for the pronated foot. Vaulting shoes with orthotics may be used to continue training.

Confounding Conditions. Two conditions point to a diagnosis of intermittent *anterior compartment syndrome*: (1) A history of increasing pain with swelling of the anterior compartment, and (2) tenderness with relative tightness of the anterior compartment after activity. Definitive diagnosis can be made by measuring pre- and postexercise compartment pressures. An increase in pressure greater than 25–30 mm Hg or a resting pressure greater than 10–15 mm Hg is suggestive of anterior compartment syndrome. If conservative measures such as ice, rest, and flexibility are not helpful, then a compartment fasciotomy may be necessary for continued competition.

A *tibial stress fracture* gradually worsens with time. Pain is progressive, constant, and may make walking difficult. Tenderness is often thumb width and present over the front of the tibia at the junction of the middle and distal third of the tibia. X-rays are often negative, but a bone scan localizes and defines the stress fracture. Absolute rest of the extremity is necessary to heal the fracture, and the athlete should not be allowed back to impact loading practice until the bone is symptom free and the tibia is nontender. A lower leg length clam shell splint may allow earlier return to activity. Strength and flexibility should be continued during the rehabilitation phase. Healing of the stress fracture can be confirmed with MR or CT imaging.

Ankle and Foot Injuries

Anterior Impingement Syndrome and Turf Toe

If a gymnast underrotates during backward tumbling, springboard vaulting, or dismounts, the landing may occur with the ankle hyperdorsiflexed or with the great toe hyperdorsiflexed. This can lead to an anterior impingement syndrome of the ankle or to a turf toe.

The *anterior impingement syndrome of the ankle* is due to chronic irritation of the anterior capsule and other soft tissues. Rest, ice, and oral anti-inflammatories are helpful. *Turf toe* can be more difficult to treat and is often disabling. It is caused by a capsular strain, which may also involve the flexor tendon of the great toe. Rest, ice, taping, and oral anti-inflammatories are again helpful. Immobilization of the toe may be necessary until pain is relieved.

In the treatment of turf toe, consideration should be given to the use of a vaulting shoe in practice along with an orthotic. The orthotic can be designed to support the foot in a neutral position for gymnasts with a pronated foot and posterior tibial periostitis. A more rigid forefoot support can be designed for those with a first metatarsal phalangeal joint synovitis or sprain. The orthotic is worn during practice, but not during competition.

Ankle Sprains

As in many other sports, ankle sprains are the most common injury in gymnastics. Because success in this sport demands time and the need for near constant training, ankle sprains are often inadequately rehabilitated.

Athletes are too commonly seen at emergency rooms or emergent care facilities where proper evaluation of an ankle sprain is unavailable. In other instances, the coach or athlete may elect to treat a sprain without evaluation. Because the degree of injury to the lateral ligaments of the ankle varies, a sports medicine specialist should evaluate all ankle sprains. The evaluation and management of ankle sprains is discussed in Chapter 26. Proper treatment of an ankle sprain in a gymnast may be difficult. It should be discussed with the athlete, coach, and the parents, especially if the gymnast is a minor. With a grade 1 injury, rest, ice, compression, taping, and gradual return to use is appropriate. With a grade 2 injury, the same treatment applies with the addition of a double upright rigid splint such as an air cast. The cast should be worn 24 hours a day for 3 weeks. Activity can usually be resumed in 2–3 weeks.

With a grade 3 injury, a comparison of the opposite side is important to determine if this is a new injury or if a natural ligamentous laxity exists. If laxity is present bilaterally, then minimal treatment may be necessary. If it is unilateral, then the same treatment for a grade 2 injury is necessary. Protection such as taping, bracing, or a combination may be necessary over several months or permanently, if instability is present. As with all ankle sprains, rehabilitation to correct any proprioceptive and strength deficits should be performed in order to prevent recurrent injury.

Confounding Conditions. A rather common but somewhat unknown syndrome, *sinus tarsi syndrome* may develop after an ankle sprain. The gymnast complains of continued discomfort in the injured ankle. At times it is severe enough to interfere with training. The pain is aching in nature and aggravated by activity. Another typical complaint is ankle instability while walking on uneven surfaces. It generally gets worse with time in contrast to a sprain, which generally improves with time. On examination, the key finding is tenderness over the sinus tarsi of the foot. This discomfort is in the soft spot just anterior to the lateral malleolus and it does not usually respond to physical therapy or NSAIDs.

Sinus tarsi syndrome is usually diagnosed after 3 months or more of chronic pain. Treatment consists of a steroid injection deep into the sinus tarsi; resolution of symptoms immediately postinjection is diagnostic. The injection is done with a mixture of 2–3 cc of bipuvicaine and 1 cc of methylprednisolone (or equivalent) with a 25-gauge 1.5-inch needle. Occasionally, a repeat injection is required on follow-up examination in 1–2 weeks. The gymnast can sometimes return to practice within 1 week, but some experts prefer to rest or immobilize the foot in a boot walker after an injection, keeping the athlete out of impact loading practice for up to 3–4 weeks post injection.

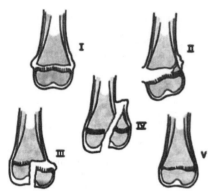

FIG 38-4 Epiphyseal fractures with growth plate damage: Salter-Harris classification. (*Reprinted with permission from Salter RB, Harris WR. Injuries involving the epiphyseal plate. J Bone Joint Surg. 1952;34:711.*)

Salter Fractures of the Ankle

Type I and Type II Fractures. These are low-risk fractures, which usually reduce readily and heal without incident. They can take full stress by 4–8 weeks, depending on the site and clinical and x-ray union.

Type III Fractures. These involve the epiphyseal plate and are serious (Fig. 38-4). Type III injuries damage the growing cells and can cause a growth arrest. They often lead to incongruity of the articular surface, and are usually treated with an open reduction and pin fixation.

Type IV Fracture. These are even more serious because they cross the epiphyseal plate and cause even greater damage to the growing cells. It is important to reduce these accurately, most frequently with open reduction.

Type V Fracture. These fractures are characterized as crushing of the epiphyseal plate, which may cause permanent damage, requiring late correction.

THE FEMALE ATHLETE TRIAD

The term *female athlete triad* was introduced at the American College of Sports Medicine Conference in Washington, DC, in 1992. The problem has been studied since the 1970s and involves excessive training regimes and low body mass. It is characterized by the triad of disordered eating, amenorrhea, and osteoporosis.

Eating Disorders

Eating disorders in gymnasts can take the form of 800-calorie diets, bingeing and purging by vomiting, overuse of laxatives and diuretics, and anorexia nervosa and bulimia nervosa. Diet pills, stimulants, and obsessive exercise also contribute to the problem.

Behavioral clues include intense fear of becoming fat, self-criticism, anxiety, hyperactivity, and inability to relax. Physical clues include variable athletic performance, fat and muscle loss, dry thin hair and dry skin, cold hands and feet, enlarged parotid glands, swelling of ankles, knuckle scars, and bloodshot eyes from repeated self-induced vomiting.

Amenorrhea

The average age of menarche in nonathletes is 12.8 years $\pm$ 1–2 years. The average age in athletes can be delayed 0–4 years for each year of premenstrual training. In athletic females, low body mass and overtraining are thought to be the main etiologies for amenorrhea.

Primary Amenorrhea

The diagnosis of primary amenorrhea at age 14 consists of absence of secondary sex characteristics absent and menses; at age 16, presence of secondary sex characteristics, no menses. Many female gymnasts have a prepubertal physique until ages 16, 17, or even 18 years.

Secondary Amenorrhea

Absence of menstrual periods for 3–6 consecutive months, in a woman who had previous established cycles is termed *secondary amenorrhea*.

Osteoporosis

Osteoporosis is a decrease in bone mass and strength, which can lead to bone pain and an increased risk of fractures. Women typically reach peak bone density at age 25–30 years and then it decreases gradually until menopause, after which the decrease is more rapid. This paradigm is altered when young female athletes have inadequate calcium intake and low levels of estrogen (amenorrhea).

Management

Management involves a team approach: athlete, parents, coach, psychologist, family doctor, and nutritionist. A complete metabolic workup is advised if decreased training and increased calories and weight do not solve the problem. For osteoporosis, the use of oral calcium supplements and the avoidance of nicotine, caffeine, alcohol, and steroids may help. After age 16, low-dose contraceptive pills also help to increase estrogen levels and hopefully bone density. Selective serotonin reuptake inhibitors are now used quite frequently to treat the obsessive-compulsive traits of this disease.

PREVENTION

Prevention of injury should be paramount in the minds of coaches, parents, and physicians. Although it may be impossible to prevent accidental injury, proper equipment, padding, and spotting during difficult techniques should minimize accidental injuries. Chronic or overuse injuries, on the other hand, may be lessened by the following:

- *Flexibility* of both upper and lower extremities and the lumbar spine is essential. Strength of the preceding has been shown to be important in prevention of overuse injuries.
- *Periodization* of training and modifying training schedules to accommodate symptoms of pain may be necessary.
- *Taping and splinting* of wrists and ankles may be helpful in alleviating and preventing injuries.

Gymnasts, in general, do most of their training while still growing. Because bone grows more rapidly than muscle and tendon, growth spurts may cause tightness in areas where a gymnast was previously flexible. Attention must be paid to gymnasts during this time of rapid growth to ensure that flexibility and strength are maintained. It may be necessary to spend more time on flexibility during a growth spurt.

Strength training is also an essential part of a gymnast's daily program. Therapy and exercises can be very helpful in strengthening both the upper and lower extremities. Strengthening of the peroneals on the lateral aspect of the ankle is helpful in preventing ankle sprains, especially if there is some instability present. Strengthening of the posterior tibial muscle on the medial side of the ankle is helpful in preventing shin splints. Strengthening of the extensors and flexors of the wrist is also important in the prevention of wrist injuries. This is also true for the scapular stabilizers and rotator cuff injuries. Strengthening the abdominals and the extensors of the spine is important in prevention of injuries to the lower back. Tightness of the lumbodorsal fascia has been associated with back pain and can be helped by stretching the fascia. Hamstring flexibility is essential in the prevention of back pain. Classic slow gradual stretching is preferred.

SUMMARY

Gymnasts, as a group, have astounding maturation, dedication, and confidence. They are capable of phenomenal zeal in their training. Because of their skeletal immaturity, their growing bones are subjected to stresses beyond normal tolerance. This stress can lead to irreversible complications. Thus, prevention of serious injuries is the key factor in dealing with gymnasts.

REFERENCES

Chambers R. Orthopedic injuries in athletes (ages 6–17). *Am J Sports Med.* 1979;7:195–197.

Dixon M, Fricker P. Injuries to elite gymnasts over 10 yr. *Med Sci Sports Exerc.* 1993;25:1322–1329.

Goldstein JD, Berger PE, Windler GE, Jackson DW. Spine injures in gymnasts and swimmers: An epidemiologic investigation. *Am J Sports Med.* 1991;19:563–468.

McNitt-Gray JL. Kinetics of the lower extremities during drop landings from three heights. *J Biomechanics.* 1993;26:1037–1040.

Nutzenberger F, Nutzenberger K. Men's gymnastics. Personal communication.

Standaert C. New strategies in the management of low back injuries in gymnasts. *Curr Sports Med Rep.* 2002;1:293–300.

United States Gymnastics Safety Association. *Certification course instructor's guide.* Reston, Va: United States Gymnastics Safety Association; 1997.

Weiker G, Ganim R. *Cleveland Clinic gymnastics injury survey, 1982.* Cleveland: Cleveland Clinic; 1982.

Wettstone G, ed. *Gymnastics safety manual,* 2nd ed. University Park: Pennsylvania State University Press; 1979.

Wettstone G. What is gymnastics safety? *Int Gymnast.* 1982;36.

39 | Track and Field Injuries

Robert Quinn and William Roberts

Track and field or *athletics* is immensely popular at all levels in Europe; however, elite-level interest in North America seems limited to the Olympic years and for the most part is of limited spectator interest. Track and field encompasses running, jumping, and throwing events. The pole vault is the most dangerous of the field events and may be the highest catastrophic risk activity within the mainstream of sports. Some events like the javelin and hammer throws have been dropped from high school competition due to risk to spectators. Participation in running, particularly distance running and road racing, remains strong with millions of North Americans taking to the roads on a daily basis, participating in fitness activities, road races, triathlons, and track events. The focus of this chapter is distance running-related injuries; however, we also address throwing, jumping, and sprinting issues. Injuries that arise suddenly, like acute muscle strains, joint sprains, and fractures, are far more common in sprinting and jumping. Conversely, the great majority of distance running injuries reflect overuse and repetitive injuries from high-volume, intense training.

Assessing problems associated with track and field begins with a detailed review of the onset (acute or insidious), mechanism, aggravating conditions, and alleviating factors. Specific attention should be paid to changes in training frequency, intensity, and duration; training surface; shoes; stretching; nutrition; cross-training; and weight training. Include a constitutional history looking for weight loss or gain, fevers, chills or night sweats, and in young women careful attention to history of eating, weight fluctuation, menses, and possible pregnancy.

Review the past history for prior sports-related injuries and indications of inflammatory or joint-related issues including inflammatory bowel disease, psoriasis, and family history of arthritis. Finally, a number of systemic complications can arise from sports training. In young or elite athletes the issue of performance-enhancing drugs should be addressed.

Shoes should always be examined for wear patterns and support. If at all possible the patient should be observed performing the activity as a part of the examination. If the symptoms are not present at the time of the examination, ask the patient to run from the office and return in an effort to reproduce the symptoms.

MECHANICS OF RUNNING

A brief overview of the biomechanics of running is necessary to understand common injuries. Bipedal ambulation can be analyzed by looking at either leg: the supporting leg on the ground is in *stance phase*; the other (moving) leg is in *swing* phase. During walking, 40% of the gait cycle is in swing, and 60% is in stance. In walking, there is a 20% overlap—double stance—when both feet are on the ground. Faster walking decreases double stance and increases swing time, but by definition there must always be a double stance period. Failure to do so results in *lifting*—a penalty in race walking.

Running is defined as ambulation without double stance, that is, both legs are in the air at the same time during part of the gait cycle. (*Jogging* often represents a running motion but insufficient swing time to eliminate the double stance phase.) Stance phase can be further broken down into stages, starting with heel strike.

Stance Phase

Heel strike is the initial contact of the foot with the ground. The extended leg (hip flexed, knee extended, ankle slightly dorsiflexed) prepares to take the weight of the body. Strike should occur on the outer aspect of the heel (this can be verified by checking sole wear), indicating the foot is slightly dorsiflexed and inverted (the subtalar joint is in slight supination).

Foot flat occurs after heel strike when the foot is plantarflexed by an eccentric contraction of the dorsiflexors (tibialis anterior, toe extensors). The entire foot comes into contact with the ground and the entire weight of the body is transmitted to the foot (while running, forces generated equal two to three times body weight). While plantarflexion is controlled by the eccentric contraction of the anterior compartment calf muscles, the subtalar joint rolls into pronation with increasing weight onto the longitudinal arch. Proximally, the tibia rotates internally with pronation, while the extended knee is controlled into a more flexed position by an eccentric contraction of the quadriceps. Runners often report maximum soreness with shin splints or quadriceps soreness after a long run at this stage. Similarly, iliotibial (IT) band pain may initially present with a sharp pain immediately after heel strike.

Midstance occurs at the point when the body weight is passing directly over the pronated midtarsal area, in front of the neutrally aligned ankle, just behind the slightly flexed knee. Suboptimal arch/pronation support results in excess weight along the medial aspect of the foot; inadequate heel cup/rear foot pronation support flattens the arch. This can be seen in the medial arch wear on the sole of the shoe, or a twisting of the shoe upper inward over the sole of the shoe.

Heel-off is the stage when the body has passed forward over the foot; weight is shifted forward to the metatarsal heads as the subtalar joint supinates, the ankle is slightly dorsiflexed (and about to powerfully plantarflex), the knee slightly flexed, and the hip extended. *Toe-off* initiates the swing phase as the foot plantarflexes and thrusts the body forward; the knee and hip are extended.

Once the foot leaves the ground, the leg is accelerated forward under the moving body by the iliopsoas to be extended in front of the body in preparation for the next heel strike. Injuries also occur in swing phase, particularly in sprinters. Toe-off is also crucial in jumpers, and is modified by the activity; long- and triple-jumpers exaggerate the motions of heel- and toe-off to extend the jump; high jumpers twist during a prolonged heel-off stage to capture centripetal force as part of their acceleration. The *airborne cycle* of the leg can be subdivided.

Swing Phase

In *acceleration* the toe leaves the ground, the hip flexes the leg forward and upward, the knee flexes, and the foot is behind the body. The powerful iliopsoas flexes the hip; initially the hamstrings help flex the knee, then contract eccentrically as the quadriceps begin to extend the knee. During *swing through* the hip flexes past neutral, clearing the flexed knee. At this point, the other foot is in midstance.

In *deceleration*, the knee extends and foot dorsiflexes in preparation for the heel strike. Hamstring injuries in sprinters often occur during acceleration or deceleration; the powerful hip concentric actions of the iliopsoas and quadriceps overcome the eccentric contraction of the hamstring, resulting in a pulled hamstring.

SYSTEMIC COMPLICATIONS OF DISTANCE TRAINING

In recent years increasing attention has been paid to the total body effect of distance running training. Most frequently, these only occur in elite level athletes running upwards of 100 km/week, with intensity in their training.

Anemia

Although anemia is fairly common in distance runners, exact incidence and etiology remain unclear. Suspicion should be aroused when performance begins to tail off, and specific questions such as the presence of hematuria after long runs should be raised. Some "tea-colored" urine after a long run is frequently related to muscle breakdown, and 14% of runners in the Comrades marathon in South Africa developed myoglobulinuria (Schiff et al., 1978). Although hematuria is usually not cause for concern, it should invariably clear within 72 hours; if not, a work-up is indicated.

Factors contributing to anemia can include microscopic or occult gastrointestinal (GI) loss; some have speculated this can be due to GI trauma on the long run or relative GI vascular insufficiency with shunting away from the splanchnic bed. Mechanical trauma has also been indicated. The use of nonsteroidal anti-inflammatory drug (NSAIDs) as a contributing factor should be considered.

Diet deficiencies are rare in those who eat a well-rounded, energy-sufficient diet that includes red meats. Vegetarian distance runners, particularly vegans, must be very conscious of their nutritional intake and are at risk for inadequate nutrient intake, especially iron. Relying on mean corpuscular volume (MCV) and hemoglobin indices can be misleading as these can change slowly. Any reasonable suspicion should trigger specific tests of serum ferritin, serum iron, and iron saturation studies.

Iron supplementation can be given orally dosed at 325 mg PO TID, ideally on an empty stomach. Oral iron is often poorly tolerated and can be taken with food. IM or IV iron can be given in those who do not tolerate PO or have malabsorption, but IM injection is painful. Hemoglobin should be rechecked in 3–4 weeks, with an appropriate response being a correction halfway to normal; full correction takes 2–3 months.

Folate and vitamin B_{12} deficiencies can occur and are associated with an increased MCV. Serum levels make the diagnosis. Folate can be replaced with 1 mg PO QD and vitamin B_{12} with 100 mg IM weekly for 4 weeks, but subsequent monthly injections will be needed if B_{12} malabsorption is the cause. In both cases reticulocytosis should occur within the week, and hemoglobin should normalize within 2 months.

Menstrual Dysfunction

Altered and absent periods occur frequently in female distance runners, and delayed onset of the menarche and secondary sexual characteristics is common in teenage female athletes engaged in intense training for distance running, ballet dancing, and gymnastics. All female athletes should be questioned regarding menstrual status, eating habits, body weight, recent changes in weight, and the use of prescription and over-the-counter medications. One should always be mindful of the *female athlete triad* of disordered eating, menstrual dysfunction, and osteoporosis. The identification of menstrual dysfunction should always trigger a review of thyroid, adrenal, and ovarian function. Pregnancy needs to be ruled out. Detailed physical examination including Tanner staging, pelvic examination, and signs of anorexia (lanugo hair, dry skin and nails, hypotension, lower extremity edema) or bulimia (parotid gland hypertrophy, dental caries, conjunctival petechia) should be performed. Relevant laboratory work includes complete blood count, electrolytes, BUN and creatinine, Ca^{++}, Mg^{++}, cholesterol, protein, albumin, follicle-stimulating hormone, luteinizing hormone, thyroid-stimulating hormone, serum prolactin, and pregnancy tests.

Although there is no uniform agreement, altered periods during intense training or competition for one or two cycles per year is acceptable, provided body weight and nutritional intake are adequate. Delayed menarche (age 16 years or 1 year beyond average of mother and sisters), amenorrhea (absence of 3–6 periods), any signs of anorexia or bulimia, or a history of stress fracture necessitate a thorough review including nutritional status, moderation/cessation of training, body weight goals, and nutritional counseling. Consultation with a psychologist with expertise in eating/body image should be sought early.

In the post-teen, athlete suppression of the menstrual cycle can happen with intense training and needs to be monitored; many athletes choose to use birth control pills to maintain control over their period, as a menstrual cycle concurrent with a significant athletic event can interfere with optimal athletic performance.

Osteopenia and Osteoporosis

Weightbearing exercise is paramount during the premenopausal years for optimal muscle bulk and bone density; women who have suppressed menses can have increased risk of osteoporosis, which can be seen in young, amenorrheic distance runners. Amenorrhea as defined above, recurrent stress fracture, stress fracture in an axial bone (stress fractures have been seen in the ribs of a female marathoner), or incidental radiologic findings of osteoporosis are definite indications for metabolic work-up, alteration of training, improved nutrition, and calcium supplementation.

PERFORMANCE-ENHANCING DRUGS

Although these have traditionally been limited to elite and international level athletes, their use continues to grow at national and collegiate levels in track and field.

Anabolic Steroids

There is evidence that the use of anabolic steroids continues to grow in high school—among both boys and girls. Most commonly, one sees the use of anabolic steroids in sprinters and jumpers to increase muscle mass, decrease recovery time, and enhance performance. These agents carry multiple complications to the user and should be discouraged; the question of whether to medically observe someone using substances illegally remains an ethical Catch 22. Signs of possible steroid abuse include facial swelling, acne, sudden increase in muscle mass, and irrational temper outbursts. Side effects are legion, including electrolyte imbalance, liver function test abnormalities, hirsutism, acne, mood disorders, cardiovascular problems including hypertension, altered lipid profile, decreased testicular size, and oligospermia.

Other performance-enhancing drugs are also routinely used, including human growth hormone (with the same desired effects as the anabolic steroids) and various amphetamine and amphetamine-related substances to increase performance. Nutritional supplements like creatinine are used to increase muscle mass and power.

Agents to Increase Red Cell Mass

The use of erythrocyte stimulating medications such as erythropoietin (EPO or Procrit) and darbypoietin has grown in the distance running, Nordic skiing, and cycling communities. Recombinant hormones can effectively increase red cell mass, thereby increasing oxygen delivery capacity to the tissues. This technology is as effective as *blood boosting* without the risks and difficulty of transfusion, but the potential complications include fatal polycythemia due to hyperviscosity and is now known to be the cause of death in several European international cyclists in the late 1980s and early 1990s. The deaths decreased after the athletes learned the upper limit of the "safe" range.

Autologous transfusion of red cells also increases oxygen-carrying capacity and significantly improves performance. Use was widespread several years ago; however, the perfection of erythropoietin use has made this practice obsolete. Anti-doping control testing technology has made the use of both techniques easier to detect.

Altitude training, altitude houses or chambers, and live high–train low techniques are designed to expose the athlete to lower oxygen concentration, naturally stimulating increased red cell production. All have been effective in performance enhancement.

Clenbuterol

Clenbuterol is a beta-2 agonist used as a bronchodilator. It is used in Europe and Asia, but not approved by the Food and Drug Administration in the United States. Six Olympians were disqualified in 1992 for its use, and Clenbuterol is banned by the International Olympic Committee (IOC) and National Collegiate Athletics Association (NCAA) (and in thoroughbred racing). Reputed benefits of Clenbuterol include anti-catabolic effects, which increase muscle mass and reduce fat.

Caffeine

Caffeine is widely used as a CNS stimulant in athletics and elsewhere; many athletes drink coffee before training, and caffeine tablets are widely available. Caffeine is rapidly absorbed and reaches peak activity within 1 hour, the half-life is 3.5 hours. Mechanism of action is by adenosine antagonism and potentiation of Ca^{++} release in muscle. This results in vasoconstriction, diuresis, CNS stimulation, gastric secretion, and increased lipolysis in adipocytes. Anecdotal evidence is highly suggestive, but published studies

TABLE 39-1 Caffeine Equivalency of Common Caffeine Preparations

Substance	Approximate urinary equivalency per dose (mg/mL)
Coffee	1.5–3.0
Tea	1.5–3.0
Cola	1.0–1.5
NoDoz	3.0–6.0
Anacin	2.0–3.0
Midol	2.0–3.0

are in conflict regarding its effectiveness in performance enhancement. Caffeine is banned by the IOC at levels above 12 mg/mL and by the NCAA above 15 mg/mL. The caffeine equivalency of common caffeine preparations is presented in Table 39-1.

GENERAL PRINCIPLES OF TREATING THE RUNNER

Specific treatment strategies for specific injuries will be addressed; however, certain overriding principles allows the sports medicine physician to establish and maintain a therapeutic relationship with the athlete. The desire to stay active or "not lose fitness" is often nonnegotiable. It is imperative that when activities are limited or curtailed, alternate activities be assigned; although this is particularly difficult for sprinters and jumpers, cross-training activities such as weightlifting, stationary cycling, or water running can be used to maintain muscle strength and fitness (without exacerbating the injury in question). For distance athletes, a number of options exist, including swimming, running in the water, stationary cycle, road cycling, and cross-country exercise machines.

Running in the pool is an extremely attractive alternate activity to distance running because the motions are sport specific; however, the athlete needs to be familiar with monitoring his or her heart rate because exercising at a subtraining rate threshold is a frequent mistake. A good rule of thumb is to estimate maximum heart rate (220 – age), and calculate target heart rates (65–85% maximum heart rate [MHR]) from there. It requires considerable mental effort to reach training rates running in the water. Perceived exertion levels also work well in the water for athletes attuned to their on-land training levels.

When analgesia and inflammation control are needed the use of oral anti-inflammatories is generally safe and effective in the short term; their side effects including gastric intolerance should be reviewed in detail. Simple guidelines include the prescription of inexpensive and readily available first-line agents: ibuprofen 600–800 mg TID or naproxen 375–500 mg BID. If one agent fails, a second agent from another family can be tried. Both efficacy and side effects can vary between agents. Gastric side effects can be reduced by administration with food. Oral sulcrafate 1 g BID or misoprostyl 200 mg BID are helpful in reducing side effects. Acetaminophen can also provide good analgesia for injured athletes.

Local steroid injection, usually with a long-acting local anesthetic agent, can be very useful. These injections are best used when an athlete can be away from training for at least 1 week because the connective tissue is temporarily weakened by the corticosteroid. A steroid injection alone without identification and correction of aggravating factors, modification of training and footwear, and incorporation of appropriate stretching and strengthening is inappropriate.

GENERAL CARE PROTOCOL

The classic paradigm of PRICE (protection, rest, ice, compression, elevation) should be applied to acutely traumatized areas.

Phase 1: Identification of the Problem(s)

Treatment of any injury begins with accurate diagnosis. This includes the appropriate laboratory work and x-rays, identification of contributing factors (physical and mental), and analysis of training and racing schedules. Diagnostic and therapeutic interventions, including injections, should be undertaken. During this time treatment is symptomatic, avoiding all aggravating activities.

Phase 2: Pain and Inflammation Control

This is usually the period of maximum rest, icing, physical therapy intervention, and assisted exercises. During this phase, correction of training errors and biomechanical problems with new shoes or orthotics should be completed. Cross-training should be established, with heart-rate training goals established.

Phase 3: Resumption of Modified Training

This period consists of return to modified activities as tolerated within the limits of tissue strength; that is, up to minor discomfort but *not* reproducing symptoms. The goal of this phase is to increase strength and endurance, test new training techniques and equipment, and set boundaries on training. Self-exercise and strengthening, self-icing, and careful monitoring of a gradually escalating training program.

Phase 4: Return to Sport

This phase consists of reintegration into full activities, monitoring for signs of overtraining or recurrence. Training modifications, stretching, warm-up, and strengthening must be maintained. Most athletes wish to truncate these stages as much as possible; however, phases 2 and 3 can frequently be done concurrently, provided alternate exercises and activities are prescribed. The transition to stage 4 should not be rushed, because many injuries that become chronic have simply not been allowed to heal. Repetition of the same errors—too much road running, too intense, inappropriate footwear—guarantees another trip to the clinic.

SPECIFIC INJURIES

Low Back and Buttock Pain

Back pain and sciatica are fairly common complaints in both distance and sprint runners. A careful history is needed to determine if the pain originates in the lumbar spine or elsewhere, if the pain radiates, and if the pain radiates below the knee. The latter, in combination with tingling, numbness, or perceived weakness, strongly suggests a radicular component.

The majority of back pain, however, occurs in the lumbosacral area and is related to mechanical factors; addressing this issue hinges on careful history and physical as outlined in Chapter 16. The pelvis should be assessed for abnormal rotation by inspecting for level iliac crests, anterior superior iliac spine (ASIS), and posterior superior iliac spine (PSIS). Lumbar spine, hip, knee, and ankle range of motion and kinetic chain motion should be assessed. Gaenslen's sign for assessment of the sacroiliac joints and Schoeber's test should be performed.

Most low back pain in runners is related to poor body mechanics and muscle tone. Instruction in proper body mechanics and posture, appropriate warm-up, and a specific core trunk and abdomen strengthening exercise program often addresses most back pain. In athletes with hyperlordotic spines, developing abdominal and core strength is key to preventing low back pain.

Although more common in gymnasts and football linemen, spondylolysis with or without spondylolisthesis may represent a stress fracture and cause of back pain, particularly in the throwing and jumping events. Classically, these injuries worsen with activity and are alleviated somewhat with rest; the physical examination may be completely benign or show tight hamstrings; on occasions this injury can lead to nerve root irritation.

Diagnosis hinges on lumbar spine films with lateral looking for the classic Scotty dog collar. Nuclear bone scan imaging can determine if the bone lesion is hot and active, or old. Treatment, unfortunately, means avoiding traumatic activities for a period of several months. In hot lesions, a rigid thoracolumbar corset may help to provide support.

Back pain that seems atypical or does not respond to treatment should always prompt a search for other etiologies, as unfortunately athletes are not exempt from other back conditions including Scheuermann's disease, Reiter's syndrome, and ankylosing spondylitis.

Sacroileitis (SI) represents a diagnostic challenge: The history is difficult to tease apart from other types of mechanical back pain. When suspected, sacroiliac views should be checked, as well as an erythrocyte sedimentation rate, rheumatoid factor, antinuclear antibodies, and possibly HLA-B27. Rheumatologic consultation is needed when an inflammatory etiology is suspected. For SI joint pain, NSAIDs, joint mobilization, a trial of a stabilizing belt, and occassionally intra-articular injections under fluoroscopy, are useful.

Sciatica

Athletes frequently present with symptoms of back or buttock pain with radiation down the leg. Clinical testing for disk disease, as well as palpation in the sciatic notch and tests stressing the piriformis muscle help to differentiate the cause of the radicular pain. Radicular signs can arise from irritation at the nerve root (often due to degenerative changes or disk protrusion) or compression along the course of the sciatic nerve, frequently owing to a tight piriformis muscle. It is always a challenge to separate piriformis muscle strain syndrome from hamstring origin inflammation.

Piriformis Syndrome

Buttock pain associated with sciatic symptoms suggests the diagnosis of piriformis syndrome. Usually the pain starts as a dull ache late in the run; with ongoing training the pain comes sooner in the run, becomes sharper, and is associated with a radiating pain or burning down the leg. Pain may be reproduced by prolonged sitting.

The piriformis muscle originates on the ventral side of the sacrum, exits via the sciatic foramen deep to the iliopsoas muscle, and tracks deep to the gluteus medius to insert on the superior aspect of the greater trochanter. The muscle serves as an accessory hip abductor and external rotator. In Grant's (1972) series of dissections, the tibial and peroneal divisions passed immediately below the piriformis in 87% of dissections; in 12% the peroneal division passed through the piriformis; and in 0.5% the peroneal division passed above the piriformis.

Palpation in the sciatic notch should reproduce pain, and may cause symptoms down the leg. With the patient lying on the unaffected side, hip flexed to 90°, adducted to allow the knee to rest on the bed, the gluteus muscles must be relaxed. A line drawn from the cephalad edge of the greater sciatic notch (just distal to the PSIS) to the greater trochanter roughly parallels the piriformis, and can be palpated at the one-third and two-third distance for tenderness. Piriformis tenderness can be confirmed by bimanual examination, with the muscle being palpated from within the pelvic floor rectally or vaginally. Provocative measures include resisted hip abduction/external rotation from the above position. Two simple stretches reproduce the pain of piriformis syndrome. The first is done sitting with the ankle of the affected side placed on the opposite knee. The ipsilateral knee is pressed down toward the floor and with back straight and chin tucked in, the athlete flexes forward at the waist putting a tight stretch on the piriformis and associated muscles. The second provocative stretch is started in the supine position by pulling knee of the affected leg toward the opposite shoulder and then with the knee flexed 70–100° pulling the lower leg cephalad. The provocative stretches also cure the problem. In addition to the usual physical examination, one needs to measure leg lengths.

Treatment is stepwise. Running should be avoided until symptoms are under control. Stationary cycling often reproduces symptoms by direct mechanical compression; therefore, water exercise during phase 1 is best. Saddle height and alignment should be checked carefully if the athlete is a cyclist. Correcting pelvic rotation and if true leg length discrepancy is found, correcting about half of the leg length difference initially is a good rule of thumb. Return to running must be on *level* surfaces.

Topical ice is helpful acutely, as are NSAIDs. A physical therapy program of prolonged stretching, friction massage, and steroid phoresis may be helpful. If these measures fail, direct injection with 1% lidocaine (without epinephrine) and a long-acting steroid can be attempted, but is a difficult and painful injection. Positioned as above, the tender area is palpated. The internal finger localizes the most tender area, and a spinal needle is introduced using the tender area as a target. The needle must be introduced deeply, depending on the amount of soft tissue. Care must be taken not to produce any neurologic symptoms. Surgical release has been described for refractory cases (Barton, 1993).

Chronic Hamstring Tendinitis

A difficult differential diagnosis is that of sciatica, piriformis syndrome, hamstring injury, and chronic hamstring origin tendinitis, often associated with an ischial bursitis (weavers bottom). The latter is common but often goes unrecognized. Symptoms are insidious in onset but become better defined: a dull pain in the low buttock/proximal hamstring, that worsens with prolonged activity. Pain may radiate to the knee, not lower. Pain may start to occur with prolonged sitting.

Physical examination reveals tight hamstrings, often reproducing pain. Discrete tenderness can be elicited at the proximal hamstring, often with a palpable band of tight muscle. A bursal inflammation is occasionally felt at the ischial tuberosity. Treatment is rest; cycling with progressive raising of the seat to further extend the hip or water running; stretching of the hamstring, then strengthening; and local deep heat with ultrasound, and deep friction massage (crucifixions per Noakes [1991]). Extracorporeal shock wave therapy may be effective in refractory cases.

Pelvic Pain

Pelvic pain is a frequent problem in distance runners and sprinters and can arise from a variety of sources including the sacroiliac joints, the symphysis pubis, and the origins of the large thigh muscles. Atypical pelvic pain from visceral pathology can occur. When assessing pelvic pain, particular attention should be paid to the presence of fevers and chills and changes in bowel and bladder habits, and the possibility of pregnancy or ectopic pregnancy must be addressed. Causes of refractory pelvic pain in athletes have included subacute appendicitis, fibroids, and even ectopic pregnancy.

Osteitis Pubis

Irritation and inflammation of the symphysis pubis is common in distance runners. Symptoms include pelvic pain and pain at the base of the penis, or the urethra in females; pain can be reproduced with resisted leg adduction and forceful abdominal muscles contractures or endurance activities.

Diagnosis is based on history, physical findings, and investigations. X-rays of the pelvis often show sclerosis and widening at the symphysis pubis, and bone scan may be hot to the area. Treatment includes avoidance of stressful activities, including weightbearing and running; mobilization of the symphysis pubis and SI joints, gradual strengthening of the adductor musculature; and anti-inflammatories. Refractory cases can be injected under fluoroscopy.

Thigh Pain

Quadriceps Rupture

The quadriceps muscle is subject to rupture, particularly with traumatic jumping or landing events. The history is usually straightforward, and often one finds a palpable knot of muscle (most commonly the rectus femoris). Immediate surgical repair is indicated in athletes, however, people can function at a reasonably high level with a chronic rupture, although this can lead to early fatigability and often muscle pain.

Muscle Soreness

Quadriceps soreness is common after extreme effort, such as a marathon and can be the rate-limiting step in return to fitness. It is felt to arise from damage related to repeated eccentric contractions and damage is to the area near the Z-band of the sarcomere. Cell damage and muscle fiber necrosis may persist for weeks. Activity should be curtailed during the recovery period. Appropriate activities during the reduced training period include slow jogging (avoiding hills), stationary bike at low resistance, intermediate speed, and swimming.

Knee Injuries

Approximately one third to one half of all running injuries occur around the knee. The most common is patellofemoral syndrome.

Patellofemoral Syndrome

Patellofemoral syndrome pain is felt to arise from poor dynamics between the patella and the femur and is discussed in Chapter 20. A variety of terms have been used including *chondromalacia patella;* however, pathologic terms should be avoided when the diagnosis remains a syndrome.

The typical presentation in distance runners is that of a dull aching knee pain; often worse with initiation of the activity, then frequently a period of letting up once the person is sufficiently warmed up, but the pain almost invariably recurs if the activity is maintained. Downhill running is particularly stressful and increases the pain during and after activity. Pain also occurs at rest when the knees are in a flexed position. The *aisle sign* is typical: the athlete prefers to sit with the knees extended and frequently opts for the aisle seat on planes and in movie theaters. Chronic problems can lead to degenerative changes in the patellofemoral joint.

Physical examination includes standing posture assessment for inward looking, high- or low-riding patellae; genu recurvatum; examination of the feet looking for pronation; and inspection of quadriceps muscle bulk, particularly vastus medialis. A small knee effusion is common, particularly after activity. The athlete should be observed doing a squat watching for pain and patellar tracking. Pain can be reproduced by pressing the patella into the femoral groove or by palpating under the edges of the patella. The *apprehension sign*, assessed by compression of the patella into the femoral groove with concurrent contraction of the quadriceps, causes a sharp pain in affected runners, but is associated with many false positives and should not be used. Commonly, the pain is due to poor tracking of the patella, with the patella tracking laterally in the groove and producing pain. Often distance runners fail to fully extend the leg during swing phase such that the final muscle contractors for knee extension is underutilized, resulting in deficiency of vastus medialis (VMO) and asymmetrical tracking. The VMO tends to be less developed than other components of the quadriceps; further, the patella is pulled laterally by the vastus lateralis, lateral retinaculum, and the IT tract. McConnell has described measuring distance from the condyles to the mid-patella (should be centered); tilt can be assessed by palpating the relative borders of the patella.

Imaging is often not needed, but skyline views can be helpful. X-rays are indicated when treatment fails and symptoms persist past 4–8 weeks. Standard knee films rule out other causes of knee pain; patella alta or baja can be best seen on lateral view, and axial views with the knee flexed 20–45° allow visualization of the patellofemoral joint.

Treatment and rehabilitation start with rest, ice, and core and pelvis stabilization exercises. Cross-training activities include swimming, water jogging, and cross-country skiing (or a ski machine). Stationary cycling can be done, with care to raise the seat to an appropriate height and with avoidance of pain. Exercise focused specifically on building the vastus medialis and gluteal muscles using closed-chain techniques with partial squats and low rise step-overs are indicated. High repetition, relatively low weight exercises requiring concentric and eccentric quadriceps and hamstring activity are needed, for example, leg presses (controlled rate; flex and extend, avoid flexion past 90°), drop squats, and lunges. Self-mobilization of the patella can be quickly taught by a physiotherapist and done several times daily.

McConnell taping techniques can help with tracking and hasten return to running. A nonirritating tape is applied to the patella and taped medially, the tape can be moved proximally or distally on the patella based on the riding angle. A strong tape is then applied to hold the patella medially. Some trial and error is needed to find the best taping alignment. A well-fitted patella stabilization orthosis can also hasten return. A Protonics device can help stabilize the pelvis and improve muscle imbalances that prolong the syndrome. Surgical options are a last resort for refractory cases and do not have good long-term outcomes.

Bursitis

Many bursae exist around the knee and can become inflamed due to overuse or poor mechanics related to muscle tightness. These are clinical/bedside diagnoses and imaging studies are rarely needed.

Pes anserinus bursa fills the potential space between the medial hamstrings and their insertion on the medial tibial plateau. History is that of a vague pain becoming sharper with continued activity, usually well localized to the area distal to the medial joint line. Pain can be reproduced by palpation distal to the medial joint line, by following the line of the hamstring tendons to the medial tibial flare. There is often swelling and localized tenderness. Treatment includes local ice, NSAIDs, and aggressive hamstring stretching. Ultrasound and steroid phoresis can be helpful. A local injection of lidocaine and steroid can provide immediate relief, and allow the athlete to train through the rehabilitation stage.

Prepatellar and deep infrapatellar bursae lie in front of and posterior to the patellae. Both can present with similar symptoms to patellofemoral syndrome, but usually there is no pain at rest. Prepatellar bursitis can usually be well localized by patient and examiner by a swelling directly in front of the patella; infrapatellar bursitis presents with more distal pain and fewer findings. For both, treatment is local ice, NSAIDs, and hamstring stretching. The prepatellar bursae can be easily aspirated and injected if needed. Refractory infrapatellar bursitis may require injection, which needs to be done behind the patellar tendon.

Jumper's Knee (Patellar Tendinitis)

Pain of jumper's knee occurs at the proximal patellar tendon just below the inferior pole of the patella. Common in jumpers and sprinters, it also occurs in distance runners. Often the athlete comes in having made the diagnosis; the challenge is to identify and correct training errors. Excessive bounding, bounding onto a hard surface, and inappropriate footwear are common triggers. Mechanical knee problems, poor patellar tracking, weak ankle dorsiflexors, and tight hamstrings also predispose the athlete to this injury.

Physical examination reveals tenderness at the inferior patella pole in the midline of the tendon. Assessment of quadriceps and hamstring tightness, strength, and range of motion, along with dorsiflexion at the ankle, help to determine the rehabilitation plan. X-rays may show degenerative changes at the inferior patella pole, and MRI may show a degenerative change of tendonosis in the midtendon.

Treatment includes ice acutely, NSAIDs, and avoidance of bounding/jumping. Ultrasound with steroid phoresis may be helpful. Hamstring, quadriceps, Achilles tendon stretching, and flexibility exercises combined with eccentric strengthening of the quads and ankle dorsiflexors (the major braking muscles of heel strike) often cure the problem. Extracorporeal shock wave therapy has been effective in recalcitrant cases.

Iliotibial Band Syndrome

The IT tract runs from the pelvic brim to the proximal lateral tibia at Gerdy's tubercle extending anteriorly to the patella and is in the tendinous continuation of the gluteus maximus and tensor fascia lata. Lateral knee pain in distance runners often suggests IT band syndrome, with the pain occurring in the last few degrees of extension as the IT band rides over the lateral femoral condyle and the proximal fibular complex. Pain occurs initially as a poorly localized ache, and with continued running it becomes sharper and more localized to the lateral aspect of the knee. With increasing severity, the pain may radiate proximally to the tensor fascia causing diagnostic difficulty. Pain is almost always limited to running, with little pain between episodes. Diagnosis is generally based on the history; physical examination of the knee is often unremarkable. However, tenderness sometimes occurs over the lateral femoral condyle. Pain can be sometimes be reproduced by pressure over the area while the patient fully extends the knee and a palpable click over the condyle may be felt. Ober's test for IT tightness is usually positive, reflecting the tight tissues that induce the problem. The test involves laying the patient on the unaffected side with both limbs flexed at hip and knee in a sitting position. The involved side leg is cradled with the examiner's arm with the knee flexed and the hip is extended, abducted, and allowed to drop to the table in adduction. Failure of the hip to adduct past horizontal is a positive test for IT tightness. Imaging studies offer little to confirm the diagnosis.

Treatment starts with the usual: rest, ice, and aggressive IT band and hamstring stretching. Check the running log to see that the downward crown of the road is not always on that side. Remove pronation control from the shoes to allow the lateral compartment to unload and loosen with extra pronation until the area is healed. Localized ultrasound with phonophoresis can hasten recovery. Unfortunately, any running must be avoided. Cross-training activities to maintain fitness should focus on swimming and stationary bike, with care being taken to have the seat a little lower than normal to avoid the last 15° of knee extension. Localized corticosteroid injection may provide relief and allow the athlete near peak to continue; however, athletes earlier in their training should take the time off, cross train, and aggressively stretch the area because these injuries can be problematic. Rarely, surgical release is indicated for refractory cases.

Plica Syndrome

The plica is an embryologic remnant appearing as a fold of synovium that may impinge on the joint space as a fold near the underside of the quadriceps tendon, or along the free edge of medial patellofemoral joint. The diagnosis is suggested by episodic pain/snapping/instability felt at the anterior edge of the knee. If conservative treatment with ice, stretching, steroid injection, and physical therapy fails, consider arthroscopy for definitive diagnosis and treatment.

Posterior Knee Pain

Runners often present with pain poorly localized to the posterior structures and popliteal fossae, occurring initially after the run and later in the course of the pain during the run. History should focus on mechanism of injury and aggravating factors recalling that both the hamstring (hip and knee) and plantarflexor (knee and ankle) groups span two joints. Pain may be caused by muscle tightness/strain in one of the groups, a posterior strained joint capsule, or Bakers cyst. A cyst can usually be easily visualized and is usually associated with a meniscus tear. In addition to the usual knee examination, the athlete must be viewed from behind standing, rising on toes, and squatting, and the posterior structures should be palpated to localize the pain. Knee extension with flexed hip and dorsiflexed ankle helps to determine muscle group tightness.

Strain of the popliteus and plantaris muscles are difficult to differentiate. Treatment is nonspecific with ice and ultrasound to the area, concerted stretching of the gastrocnemius/hamstrings, and modified training. Sprinting, downhill running, and forceful knee extension are to be avoided.

Shin Pain

Shin pain is common in all track and field athletes; the differential diagnosis necessitates a thoughtful work-up to differentiate tibial stress syndrome from stress fracture, chronic exertional compartment syndrome, and vascular entrapments. The key determinants of severity of injury are persistence of pain beyond running and imaging patterns on bone scan and MRI (not always needed).

Tibial Stress Syndrome (Shin Pain)

Beginning runners and established runners increasing mileage or intensity are at risk to develop *tibial stress syndrome*. A dull aching anterior shin pain occurring after running and then at ever-shortening intervals into runs suggests the diagnosis, which if untreated, may lead to a stress fracture. The exact etiology of tibial stress syndrome is unclear, but is felt to stem from inappropriate loading on the dorsiflexors of the foot (maximally eccentrically strained during the heel strike), inappropriate loading on other calf muscles related to controlling excessive foot pronation, and resultant strain at the origin on the bone. The bone site can arise posteriorly or medially on the tibia, or the lateral aspect of the fibula. Bone scans in asymptomatic, high-mileage runners can show increased remodeling in these areas.

Diagnosis is based on the history and physical examination. Unlike stress fractures, there is a wide area of bony tenderness, but no rest pain. Pain may be reproduced by resisting dorsiflexion of the foot. Bone scanning is more sensitive than plain x-ray, although frank stress fractures show upon plain films. In tibial stress syndrome, the bone scan or MRI shows diffuse periosteal changes along the tibia, but not the focal changes seen in a stress fracture. Treatment of tibial stress syndrome hinges on identification and correction of aggravating factors:

- Reduce training volume and intensity, especially downhill running, sprints, and overstriding.
- Use appropriate footwear with good heel cushioning and pronation control to minimize eccentric forces on the posterior tibialis.
- Athletes with chronic/recurrent stress syndrome should be assessed for orthotics to correct foot strike abnormalities like overpronation.
- Assess the training surface and contour for biomechanical stresses.

All athletes with tibial stress syndrome should have calf, anterior compartment, and lateral compartment stretching reviewed. Ice rubs to the affected areas 3–4 times daily can give good pain relief. Shin pain occurring early in a training program or after resumption of intense intervals often require only supportive shoes, reduced training intensity, and time.

Stress Fracture

A dull ache, initially similar to tibial stress syndrome but occurring with any activity and localizing to a small area, suggests stress fracture. Differentiation from other aches is difficult, and a frequent delay to diagnosis although athletes often suspect but fear the diagnosis. In runners, stress fractures occur most commonly in the lower leg (approximately 50% in the tibia and 15% in the fibula), followed by the tarsal and metatarsal bones (25%), and occasionally in the femur, femoral neck, and pubic arch.

Diagnosis is based largely on history. There is no history of trauma. The runner initially reports a localized ache only after exertion, but later with any weightbearing. The history should focus on recent training changes with particular attention to shoes, type of interval, running surface, mileage, intensity, and long runs. The final precipitating event can often be identified by the runner.

Physical examination demonstrates point tenderness and sometimes warmth and erythema over the area. Tenderness with vibration suggests the diagnosis. X-rays are usually normal for 2–6 weeks. A fine periostitis may be seen. Nuclear bone scanning is most helpful in confirming the diagnosis. The scan is hot in all three phases; tibial stress syndrome (periostitis) is hot only in the delayed phase. MRI with fat suppression technique is sensitive and useful for documenting healed stress fractures in critical areas of the femoral neck and pelvis. Treatment is frustrating for the athlete and requires removing the offending stresses until the fracture is healed. Rest, alternate activities, increased calcium intake, adequate nutrition, and estrogen for females are the common interventions. Electromagnetic bone stimulators may be of benefit in speeding the healing of stress fractures. The most common treatment failure is premature return to the offending activity, and recurrences are common if the training errors are not corrected.

Phase 1 focuses on establishing the diagnosis, identifying training errors to be avoided in the future, and correcting biomechanical deficiencies. Relative rest for the fracture site including crutch walking if pain is present with walking, ice packing, analgesics for pain (it may be prudent to avoid NSAIDs early in the fracture), and stretching of the muscles about the affected area. Conditioning is limited to pain-free activities like swimming, deep water running, and biking. Initially most runners with leg and foot stress fractures cannot even tolerate stationary cycling.

Phase 2 starts with slow-paced every other day running for 10–20 minutes on a soft surface after the resolution of bony point tenderness and ends when the athlete can progress to near-normal distances at a slow pace without pain. Progressive stretching and strengthening (concentric and eccentric) should be pain free. Alternate activities can be increased as tolerated.

Phase 3 starts when alternate day training on soft surfaces is tolerated by increasing running time, pace, and days per week. Intense interval training is the last activity to be reintroduced for runners and bounding the last for jumpers.

Compartment Syndrome

Chronic exertional compartment syndrome is probably underdiagnosed because the testing is painful and not done routinely until treatments for other conditions have failed. An inability of the fascia to accommodate the expanding (working) muscle results in abnormally increased intracompartmental pressure that retards arterial and venous circulation, leading to muscle ischemia, and inhibits neurotransmission. The pain may be due to the pressure phenomena along with the accumulation of the metabolic products of muscle activity. This usually occurs in the lower leg anterior, lateral, deep posterior, or superficial posterior compartments.

History is somewhat similar to claudication pain, but with more cramping, neuropathy, and myopathy. The pain is always related to exertion reaching a peak at a fairly reproducible point in a run and usually subsides 10–20 minutes after stopping the run. The athlete may report muscle cramping or spasms, an unusual firmness to the muscle, foot numbness related to compromise of the nerve coursing through the affected compartment, or foot drop. Physical examination is often normal when the athlete is asymptomatic; following exertion, the affected area may be firm and tender and the neuropathies are evident. In late phases, the changes may become evident at rest or with minimal exertion.

Intracompartmental pressure monitoring using either a solid state intracompartmental catheter or slit catheter remains the gold standard for diagnosis, but is not widely available. Often the diagnosis is made on clinical grounds and failure of conservative treatment (which will always fail). Treatment is surgical release fascia or severe restriction of activity to allow the muscle to fit the fascial compartment. There is probably some irreversible muscle change that occurs and surgical treatment is not universally effective, especially in the posterior compartments.

Ankle Pain

The majority of ankle pathology in track and field athletes is due to trauma; most frequently an inversion injury resulting in a first-, second-, or third-degree tear of the collateral ligaments. In severe cases accompanying injury to the peroneal nerve and/or avulsion fractures of the tibia occur. Treatment depends on the severity of the injury.

Achilles Tendinitis

This injury dates to the antiquities is relatively common in distance runners. Achilles tendinitis can occur anywhere from the insertion on the os calcis proximally to the muscle. The Achilles injury is common in runners for a number of reasons: the gastroc and soleus muscle complex is used each step both eccentrically at heel strike and concentrically at toe-off with forces well above body weight. An area of friction can arise at the heel collar leading to a pump bump, which can be confused with Achilles tendinitis. Women who wear heels during the day foreshorten the calf muscles and may be at increased risk for tendinitis. Clement et al. (1984) described a bowstring effect of the Achilles in runners who overpronate with the tendon being further stretched about the os, increasing the risk for tendinitis.

The symptoms are usually self-evident to the athlete and early injury is manifest with pain/tightness in the heel cord first thing in the morning. Early tendon symptoms can be treated with NSAIDs, icing for 20 minutes every 3–4 hours, lower leg stretching, decreasing intense training and hill running, supportive shoes, and a soft heel insert of 5–10 mm.

With pain that occurs during running, physical therapy for more aggressive stretching, friction massage, ultrasound, and night splints can be added. All intense training is held, and running should be stopped before discomfort occurs. At the end of each workout, the athlete should pinch the heel cord to assess for decreasing pain, which reassures, or increasing pain, which necessitates further reduction in training.

Once pain interferes with running or changes the gait, all running must stop and cross-training activity should begin. Even swimming can irritate the ankle with forceful kicking (plantarflexion). In addition to calf stretching, eccentric and concentric strengthening are needed. A simple at-home remedy has the athlete stand on the edge of a step with weight on the balls of the feet utilizing slow toe rises and with return to *below* neutral for strengthening through the full range of motion. When this is well tolerated for several sets of 15, three times daily, the same exercise can be done on one leg or with slowly increasing weight on the leg press.

Achilles tendon rupture also occurs and may be the end result of untreated tendinitis/tendonosis. The treatment, immobilization in a plantarflexed position versus operative repair, depends on the activity level, expected outcome, and time frame of the individual athlete. Most competitive athletes opt for surgical repair. Complete rupture can be determined by the immediate onset of pain and swelling, palpable deficit in the heel cord, impaired gait, and failure to move the foot with passive squeezing of the calf. Orthopedic consultation is needed for surgical repairs.

Tenosynovitis

Although the Achilles tendon is the most common injury, similar injuries can occur acutely or insidiously at other sites around the foot and ankle. Frequent sites are at the extensor retinaculum across the dorsal aspect of the ankle, laterally where the peroneal tendons track beneath the lateral malleolus, and medially in the posterior tibialis tendon. More proximal tendons at the origin and insertions of the hamstrings, the hip flexor origins, and the calf muscle origins are also frequently involved.

The history is usually straightforward with dull pain proceeding to sharp pain with activity that is often well localized. If addressed early, local icing, aggressive stretching, and biomechanical correction can prevent time away from training. Gait dynamics and shoe wear should also be checked. If ignored, chronic changes can be very difficult to reverse.

Foot Injuries

Foot injuries are extremely common in all track and field athletes.

Plantar Fasciitis

Plantar fasciitis typically presents as a well-localized pain at the distal calcaneous where the plantar fascia originates that is worse on arising in the morning and diminishes through the day. The pain may get better or worse with activity. Although the history is usually quite diagnostic, physical examination can confirm it with direct local pressure over the plantar fascia origin. Pain is also reproduced with forceful dorsiflexion of the toes and foot. X-ray of the heel is not routinely needed.

Symptom improvement can usually be obtained by supporting the longitudinal arch with foot orthotics and support sandals (even at night when up to the bathroom), strengthening exercises of the foot including the towel roll, stretching the plantar fascia and calf muscles, and night splints. Appropriate longitudinal arch support and foot wear cushioning are key to successful management. More refractory cases can be injected locally with lidocaine and corticosteroids, and utilization of extracorporeal shock wave therapy. Surgical intervention is a last resort.

Black Toe

Hematoma beneath the great toe is almost always related to repetitive trauma. Either the shoes are too small or too loose in the toe box causing the toe to strike against the inside of the shoe or the shoe top to slap the nail. Prolonged downhill running also causes shoe-to-nail trauma in a poorly fit shoe. This seemingly trivial injury can be quite painful. In acute cases, the hematoma can be drained by piercing the nail with a sterilized hot lancet or paper clip, or by drilling through the nail with a needle. The hole allows evacuation of the hematoma and pain-free return to activity.

Pole Vault and Jumping Events

Jumps forcefully load the leg muscle groups and increase the incidence of acute sprains and strains. Acute strains of the hip flexors and the hamstring muscle-tendon-bone units are common and should be treated conservatively, with aggressive physical therapy and alternate activities. Pole vaulters propel themselves to fatal heights and rule changes at the college and high school levels have been implemented to increase the size of the landing zone and pad the pole box. Some leagues now require helmets, but the helmets are not standardized, nor do they protect the cervical spine. A lack of qualified coaches to improve technique and safety at the high school level may cause the demise of pole vaulting for this level of competition.

Weight Events

Participants in weight and throwing events have shoulder problems similar to all throwing athletes. Training programs and rehab programs must emphasize the core strength and mobility that is key to successful throwing mechanics. The participants at higher levels of competition may be at increased risk for anabolic steroid use.

SUMMARY

The medical care of track and field athletes is based on an understanding of the underlying mechanics of the sport. Although track and field is not a popular spectator sport in North America, the athletes are dedicated and need the same dedication from medical providers to keep them in action.

REFERENCES

Barton TM. Pyriformis syndrome: A rational approach to management. *Pain.* 1991;45:347–352.

Baxter DE, ed. *The foot and ankle in sport.* St. Louis: Mosby–Year Book; 1995;84.

Clement DB, Taunton JE, Smart GW. Achilles tendonitis and peritendinitis: Etiology and treatment. *Am J Sports Med.* 1984;12:179–184.

Cumming DC: Exercise and reproduction in women. *J Surg Obstet Gynecol.* 1991;9–17.

Fredericson M. Common injuries in runners: Diagnosis, rehabilitation and prevention. *Sport Med.* 1996;21:49–72.

Grant JCB. *Grant's Atlas of Anatomy.* Baltimore: Williams & Wilkins; 1972.

McBryde AM. The foot and ankle in sport. In: Baxter DE, ed. *Book of Sports Medicine.* St. Louis: Mosby–Year Book; 1995;81–93.

Noakes T. *Lore of running.* Champaign, Ill: Leisure Press; 1991.

O'Conner RG, RP Wilder. *Textbook of running medicine.* New York: McGraw-Hill; 2001.

Schiff HB, MacSearraigh ETM, Kallmeyer JC. Myoglobulinuria, rhabdomyolysis and marathon running. *Q J Med.* 1978;47:463–472.

40 | Swimming

Peter J. Fowler and Lorie Forwell

Swimming is enjoyed by an enormous number of participants. Although accurate figures are not available, estimates of up to 100 million participants (Americans) at both recreational and competitive levels have been quoted. The current popularity of programs for master swimmers and triathlons contributes to both the continued growth of the sport and to the increasing age range of competitors. Swimming has relatively few inherent risks of injury. However, the intensely repetitive nature of the sport, particularly at the elite level, can result in overuse problems in the shoulder primarily, but also in the elbow, knee, foot, and ankle, and back.

The fundamental components of an accurate diagnosis and successful management of these problems are a good history, systematic physical examination, knowledge of anatomy and biomechanics, understanding the sport, review of the training program, and education of the coach and athlete. The role of an informed coach in treatment, and more importantly prevention, cannot be overemphasized. Preventative measures are essential to a successful training program and should be incorporated from the outset.

In the majority of athletes with overuse injuries, conservative treatment that includes relative rest, technique modification, and physiotherapy intervention will be sufficient to restore function. Surgical intervention is a consideration when all nonoperative treatments have failed. This chapter reviews the causative factors in swimming injuries, physical examination, treatment options, and a comprehensive discussion of shoulder rehabilitation.

THE SHOULDER

Injury to the shoulder is the most common problem facing the competitive swimmer regardless of age. The term *swimmer's shoulder*, first used in 1974 by Hawkins and Kennedy (1974), describes symptomatology that frequently results from of a combination of anatomic and biomechanical factors rather than from a single causative agent. The contributing factors include overuse, anatomic features, shoulder joint laxity, fatigue, impingement, and stroke mechanics. Recent literature has identified an increase in the incidence of swimmer's shoulder from 3% in 1974 and 50% in 1981 to between 47 and 73% in 1986 (Kennedy et al., 1974; Lo et al., 1990; McMaster et al., 1993). Rigorous training programs for swimmers that compete on the national level that typically demand at least nine 4000- to 8000-m sessions per week may be a factor in this increased incidence.

Swimming Strokes

In three of the four competitive strokes, the front crawl (freestyle), butterfly, and backstroke, 75% of propulsion is provided by the arms. In the breaststroke, the arms and legs contribute equally. With respect to arm action, the biomechanics of all four strokes are deceptively similar. The phases common to each stroke are the reach, the catch, the pull, and the recovery. During the reach or entry, the arm reaches forward to enter the water. In the catch phase, which is alike for all competitive strokes, the swimmer begins to pull or scull the water. Here, the swimmer flexes the elbow to 100° and begins to extend, horizontally abduct, and slightly medially rotate the

637

shoulder. In the pull phase, which is the propulsion or power phase, the glenohumeral joint of the shoulder is in adduction and internal rotation, with the exception of in the breast-stroke. The arm is at maximum elevation at the start of the pull and in full extension at its completion. During the recovery phase, when the arm returns to start another pull, the glenohumeral joint is in abduction and external rotation. Again, excluding the breast-stroke, the recovery is performed out of the water.

Anatomic and Biomechanical Features

The shoulder joint is a highly mobile joint with little bony support. The stability necessary for the arm to function with power and precision through its range of motion is provided by the shoulder capsule, ligaments, rotator cuff muscles (supraspinatus, subscapularis infraspinatus, and teres minor), and larger muscles such as the pectoralis major and the serratus anterior.

Dynamic stability for containment of the humeral head in the glenoid fossa is provided by the rotator cuff muscles working in a force couple combination with the deltoid and the long head of the biceps. The supraspinatus helps resist upward displacement of the humeral head; the infraspinatus works in combination with the supraspinatus and subscapularis to depress the humeral head. The subscapularis also resists anterior or inferior displacement of the humeral head in the glenoid fossa. The subscapularis as well as serratus anterior are continuously active throughout the freestyle stroke. Their constant use combined with their essential function increases their susceptibility to fatigue (Pink et al., 1991). The long head of the biceps is active in forward flexion and as a humeral head stabilizer. This dual function should also be assessed in the shoulder biomechanics of swimming.

Factors in Tendinopathy

Overwork

As the most mobile and least stable joint, the shoulder is most vulnerable to injury in the overhead position. To keep up with the continuous, repeated demands of competitive swimming, the muscles of the rotator cuff may be required to work excessively to contain and stabilize the humeral head. Such a workload can lead to fatigue of the muscles and the onset of a chronic condition. Superior migration of the humeral head may occur, and with this, a subsequent increase in subacromial loading is seen that can trigger a tendinopathy. In addition to rotator cuff fatigue, scapular muscle fatigue can alter the mechanics of the entire shoulder complex. In swimmers with painful shoulders there is a decrease in muscle activity of both the serratus anterior and subscapularis (Scovazzo et al., 1991). This could be explained by fatigue. In the case of the serratus anterior, an increase in activity is seen in the rhomboid muscles in an attempt to control the scapula. Fatigue and lack of control of the periscapular muscles can alter the glenohumeral joint mechanics and may contribute to the onset of impingement tendinopathy. Infraspinatus activity also increases as subscapularis activity decreases. This is likely to externally rotate the humerus to avoid the excessive internally rotated position and impingement. With an unstable scapula, these muscles, which move the glenohumeral joint, will also be somewhat disadvantaged or inefficient.

Hypovascularity

Rathbun and Macnab (1979) demonstrated that the blood supply to the supraspinatus and the biceps tendons is affected by arm position. An area of avascularity occurs close to the musculotendinous junction during adduction and internal rotation. In this position at the end of the pull phase, the tendons are stretched tightly over the head of the humerus. This repeated avascularity, known as the "wringing out" mechanism, occurs in the area of the tendon most vulnerable to loading. Repeated interruption of the vascular supply may contribute to early degenerative changes and increase the potential for rotator cuff damage. Circulation to the area is restored during abduction.

Subacromial Loading

The supraspinatus and biceps tendons insert on or across the humerus directly below the coracoacromial arch, which is formed by the coracoid process, the rigid coracoacromial ligament, and the anterior acromion. The anatomic arrangement of these tendons makes them particularly susceptible to impingement. When the arm is in abduction, forward flexion, and internal rotation, a position assumed in the catch phase of all competitive strokes, the humeral head moves under the arch, where the tendons may be repeatedly impinged. If scapular mechanics have been altered, the tendons may be pinned against the arch, causing a mechanical irritation and inflammatory response that can further compromise the available space beneath the arch. Untreated, this may progress to involve the subacromial bursa and acromioclavicular ligament.

Three acromial shapes have been identified by Bigliani and colleagues (1986): type I, flat; type II, curved; and type III, hooked. A competitive swimmer with a hooked (type III) acromion or a master swimmer with degenerative spurring of the acromion may be predisposed to impingement due to the decreased dimensions of the coracoacromial arch. In these situations, a tendinopathy that is resistant to treatment may develop.

Stroke Mechanics

During the entry phase and the beginning of the pull phase, the shoulder is in forward flexion, abduction, and internal rotation. The head of the humerus is forced under the anterior acromion and the coracoacromial ligament and may impinge the supraspinatus and biceps tendons, particularly if fatigued.

Lateral impingement may be associated with the recovery phase of the freestyle and butterfly strokes. To return to the entry position, the arm must abduct. With associated horizontal abduction and internal rotation, the head of the humerus comes up against the lateral border of the acromion. This is particularly true when the shoulder leads the rest of the arm. When the head leads the arm through recovery, there is less potential for lateral impingement. As mentioned previously, during the end of the pull phase, the shoulder is in adduction and internal rotation, a position that leads to the wringing out mechanism.

An analysis of the arm position in the freestyle stroke of swimmers experiencing pain appears to correlate the occurrence of the pain with the biomechanical factors implicated in rotator cuff tendinopathy. Almost 50% of the swimmers experienced shoulder pain during entry or the first half of the pull phase, 14% felt pain during the second half of the pull phase, 23%

during the recovery, and 17.8% during the entire pull or recovery. Some swimmers in this last group experienced pain throughout the entire stroke (Webster-Bogaert, 1981).

There are subtle signs of injury that are evident in the stroke. Dropping the elbow in the recovery phase of the freestyle stroke may be a mechanism by which the swimmer is trying to limit the amount of humeral internal rotation, possibly to avoid pain. In order to drop the elbow the swimmer may pull the hand out early in the recovery phase. This may also be associated with excessive body roll. A wider hand entry may be used to decrease the need for scapular upward rotation or retraction if its control is challenging. An asymmetrical pull may be seen if the injured shoulder cannot generate the same amount of torque or force than the other. This may also alter the beat of the kick (Pink et al., 2000).

Increased Laxity

Increased laxity should not be overlooked as a contributing factor in the athlete with resistant tendinopathy. In the individual with loose or lax shoulders, the rotator cuff muscles are already working excessively hard just to contain the humeral head. The rigor of training makes additional demands on fatigued or fatiguing muscles. In 1982, Fowler and Webster-Bogaert (1991) investigated the association between rotator cuff tendinopathy and shoulder laxity. They assessed 188 competitive swimmers between the ages of 13 and 26 years for positive signs of tendinopathy and for posterior, inferior, and anterior instability or increased laxity. Fifty recreational athletes without shoulder pain were used as a control group. A formal history was taken of each subject, and any episodes of shoulder pain were recorded.

The apprehension test was used to assess anterior instability. Any sign of pain or anxiety was recorded as a positive response. Inferior instability was assessed using the sulcus sign. The load and shift test to evaluate posterior laxity was conducted with subjects both sitting and supine. Excursion of the humeral head relative to the posterior glenoid fossa was the index for posterior laxity. In many normal asymptomatic individuals, the proximal humerus can be translated posteriorly 50% of the glenoid width; therefore any movement greater than this was classified as excessive posterior laxity.

Fifty percent of the 188 swimmers had a history of shoulder pain. Some degree of posterior laxity was present in one or both shoulders in 55% of the swimmers and in 52% of the control group. This suggested that swimming does not predispose an athlete to increased laxity. Twenty-five percent of the swimmers had a history of tendinopathy and increased posterior laxity. The tendinopathy was consistently present in the lax shoulder, indicating that there is a relationship between shoulder pain and increased laxity.

Shoulder Strength Imbalance

Manual testing performed on these same swimmers demonstrated external rotator weakness in one or both shoulders of 40 subjects, with 33 having both weakness and a history of tendinopathy in the same shoulder. Based on these findings, a second study was conducted to measure rotation strength about the shoulder. One-hundred nineteen swimmers and 51 controls (participants in activities not requiring arm rotation strength primarily) were tested on the Cybex II dynamometer. Internal and external rotation strength was measured in three arm positions: neutral, 90° of abduction, and 90° of flexion. A significant difference was found in the rotation torque ratio between swimmers and controls in neutral and 90° of abduction that was attributed to the greater strength of the internal rotators. External rotation strength between the two groups was not significantly different.

In the pull or power phase of the swimming stroke, the glenohumeral joint is in adduction and internal rotation. Many swimmers selectively train their internal rotators to improve speed and endurance. This may explain the resulting imbalance between the internal and external rotators that may contribute to the onset of shoulder pain.

Clinical Evaluation

An accurate history to define the pain is essential. This should include onset, duration, location, activity causing the pain, and position of maximum pain. A review of the complete training program, including the dry-land and weight-training components, will provide important additional information. A systematic physical examination should include inspection, palpation, and assessment of range of motion, joint laxity, motor strength, and neurologic status. The history and physical examination are augmented by provocative and stability testing as well as appropriate imaging when indicated.

As a tendinopathy progresses, generalized pain about the shoulder is often present at night or at rest. The athlete avoids painful positions and those which aggravate the symptoms. To minimize pain during swimming, subtle changes in stroke mechanics may develop. Over time, a gradual loss of shoulder range of motion along with muscle weakness may occur. Wasting of the supraspinatus and infraspinatus muscles may become apparent. In the mature athlete, this may be an indication of gross degeneration of the rotator cuff tendon or of a partial tear. Such changes are seldom seen in age-group swimmers, and in fact are rare in athletes younger than 25 years.

Clinical classification of tendinopathy is based on Blazina's categories (1980) for jumper's knee that associate pain with level of activity. In grade I, there is pain after the activity; in grade II, there is pain during and after activity, but it is not disabling; in grade III, there is disabling pain during and after the activity; and in grade IV, there is pain with activities of daily living.

Physical Examination

Successful treatment of shoulder girdle dysfunction is based on a detailed and thorough assessment. Circumspect observation of the athlete prior to a hands-on assessment will reveal important information. The individual's posture or the resting position of soft tissue structures can affect patient function. The adaptation of muscle and soft tissue to these positions may cause resting and/or functional imbalances in flexibility or strength. In flexibility imbalances, one group of muscles is shortened and the antagonist(s) are lengthened. In strength imbalances, there is a weakness differential between muscle groups. For example, a muscle resting in its lengthened position will be most effective in that position and somewhat weaker in the shortened position. In this situation, because muscles require more energy to function in the lengthened position, they may be prone to fatigue and dysfunction (Astrand and Radahl, 1977). Similarly, a shortened muscle is weaker in its lengthened position and often will lack the ability to achieve its full length. These imbalances will become more obvious with time and stress. Although we will focus on muscle imbalance, it is important to keep in mind that for every muscle there is surrounding connective tissue that plays an important role.

Posture and Alignment

Although the alignment of the entire body should be assessed, the areas of primary importance for the function of the shoulder girdle are the cervical spine, the thoracic spine, the scapulae, and the humerus. Following a thorough history, a visual inspection of these areas and a quick screening test will indicate the degree of their involvement in the patient's problem (Table 40-1).

The Cervical Spine

In most cases, patients will attempt to correct their posture if they know that it is being assessed. Therefore, this is best done when the patient is unaware that his or her posture is the focus of the therapist's attention. It is important to keep in mind that the effect of small but habitual deviations such as head tilt or rotation on soft tissue, disks, and facet joints can become significant.

The cervical spine should be inspected from sagittal, anterior, and posterior views. Sagittally, the presence or absence of a lordosis as well as the location of the curve should be noted. A headforward position (when the ears are in a plane anterior to the shoulders) predisposes to a lengthening of the neck flexors coupled with a shortening of the neck extensors and the posterior cervical-scapular muscles (eg, levator scapulae and upper trapezius). In this case, since the levator scapula also elevates and downwardly rotates the scapula, the force may exceed that of its antagonists and influence

TABLE 40-1 Overview of Shoulder Rehabilitation

• Assess posture (resting position) of soft tissue structures	
• Assess involvement of supporting structures	
• Quality of movement	
Cervical and thoracic spine	Correct alignment
	Instruction
	Stretching, strengthening
	Functional exercises
	Assess joint function
	Quality of movement
	Mobilization
Scapula	Periscapular muscle retraining
	Assess static, dynamic, functional status
	Biofeedback
	Control of strength and power
	Training modification
	Involve coach
Glenohumeral joint	Joint function assessment
	Muscle balance
	Specific strength training
	Speed
	Type of contraction
	Open versus closed chain
	Joint/muscle position
	Control of movement
	Proprioception

scapular function. The result may be a weakness and lengthening of the lower trapezius, which depresses and upwardly rotates the scapula. This in turn will exaggerate the imbalance of that force couple.

Anteroposterior (AP) observation may reveal a rotated or side-flexed cervical spine that will result in shortening of the corresponding muscles and lengthening of their antagonists. Unilaterally, the levator scapulae can rotate the cervical spine, and imbalances similar to those cited earlier may be due to an entirely different cause. The assessment of cause and effect is essential. Muscle contour and bulk are assessed anteriorly and posteriorly. Asymmetries can be indicative of problems with the function of the surrounding soft tissue. Comparing paravertebral and periscapular muscle bulk with suprascapular muscle bulk will provide important information. A slight person should be proportionately slight; a muscled person should be proportionately muscled. Asymmetries in this situation may indicate a recruitment preference caused by strength training routines or neurologic deficits.

A cervical spine scan should include quick tests of range of motion, strength, dermatomes, and myotomes, as well as a history of complaints. Any abnormal findings should be followed by further investigation. For instance, if range of motion is limited or excessive, an in-depth assessment of the mobility of the intervertebral joints should be undertaken. Any limitation or pain with mobilization of these joints will affect the function of the cervical spine and those muscles attached to it.

The Thoracic Spine

The thoracic spine should be observed for normal alignment. Lordosis, kyphosis, scoliosis, and rotation can be noted with sagittal and AP observations. As in the cervical spine, any deviation from optimal function of the thoracic spine will affect the surrounding soft tissue. Rhomboids, for example, can be inhibited with pain or dysfunction of the midthoracic spine. As rhomboids downwardly rotate and adduct the scapula, the patient may present with an abducted and/or upwardly rotated scapula. This in turn will shorten the serratus anterior, pulling the scapula further into the abducted, upwardly rotated position. The thoracic spine is often ignored when treating the shoulder girdle. However, its function and integrity are important to much of the soft tissue that stabilizes the scapula. Again, a scan similar to that of the cervical spine should be undertaken and followed up as indicated.

The Scapula

The scapula is the base of support for the upper extremity as the pelvis is for the lower extremity; therefore its position and stability have a great influence on upper extremity biomechanics. The common scapular movements are elevation, depression, abduction, adduction, upward rotation, and downward rotation. The resting positions of the scapula can be altered in severe cases. However, dysfunction in milder cases is more easily noticed with movement. Scapular position will dictate the position of the glenoid fossa and the ability of the periscapular muscles to control its movement.

The position of the glenoid fossa is a critical element to the reloading of the scapulohumeral muscles. If the glenoid fossa is tipped such that it is facing more inferiorly, the humerus will sit in a relatively abducted position, thereby functionally shortening supraspinatus and other abductors. Associated lengthening of the teres major and other adductors and rotation of the humerus may then occur. The stronger, shorter muscle will be preferentially recruited, predisposing the humerus to return to its resting position. When movement does occur, the facility of recruitment will favor the shortened muscles and place them at risk for fatigue and overuse.

Similarly, if the scapula rests in a upwardly rotated position, causing the glenoid to face superiorly, the glenohumeral joint will sit in a relatively adducted position. This in turn will shorten the adductors and lengthen the abductors. The muscle contraction occurring when the swimmer abducts the shoulder will be initiated from a lengthened position. The muscle then goes through a greater range of motion, which increases the eccentric contraction required for the return movement. This creates more work for the muscle, resulting in fatigue and overuse.

It is important to keep in mind that rarely does a joint as mobile as the glenohumeral joint selectively shorten one set of muscles without the added element of rotation. This should be assessed. For example, in many swimmers, in addition to shortened adductors, there is often a shortening of the internal rotators. This imbalance of flexibility and frequently strength between the internal and external rotators of the shoulder has been documented (Fowler et al., 1991). Once established, such a muscle imbalance can progress due to abnormal stresses on the muscles stabilizing the scapula. This creates a vicious cycle. Patients with an elevated or depressed scapula present a challenge that can to a great extent become an anatomy review for the physician and therapist. If the upper trapezius is tight, the clinician is likely to note an elevated or upwardly rotated scapula or a scapula that elevates and/or upwardly rotates with the initiation of humeral movement. The affect of this on the lower trapezius is one of lengthening and weakening, which again compounds the problem. With this force couple acting on the scapula, its control and stability are compromised. Since the scapula is the insertion for many muscles controlling the glenohumeral joint, these cease to have a stable base, resulting in less-than-optimal function. The added stress placed on the muscles as they attempt to compensate, especially during sporting activities, can be the source of pathology.

The Glenohumeral Joint

Tenderness elicited by palpation of the supraspinatus tendon medial to its insertion of the greater tuberosity suggests a tendinopathy. If the long head of the biceps is involved, there will be tenderness over the bicipital groove. Those with supraspinatus involvement often demonstrate the classic *painful arc syndrome,* which causes pain with active abduction between 60 and 100°. Symptoms of a biceps tendinopathy can be reproduced by resisting forward flexion of the straight arm while the forearm is supinated. Biceps tendinopathy can be associated with refractory rotator cuff tendinopathy.

Placing the shoulder in the impingement-aggravated position often will reproduce clinical pain. In the test described by Neer, the examiner resists forward flexion of the raised straight arm while the forearm is supinated. This drives the head of the humerus against the anteroinferior border of the acromion. In a second test, the examiner internally rotates the arm, which is forward flexed to 90°.

It is important to determine if muscle weakness, particularly in the external rotators, is present. With the patient's arm in external rotation and adduction and the elbow flexed to 90°, the examiner applies an internal force, which the patient is instructed to resist. Gross weakness will be conspicuous. Pain may accompany this test.

Increased laxity or frank instability may contribute to the progression of tendinopathy or may be the absolute cause of pain. The relocation test assessing anterior instability has two components. First, the arm is stressed in external rotation and abduction, and the patient is observed for a reaction to pain. Then the examiner, by applying posteriorly directed pressure on the proximal humerus, either relocates or supports the humeral head, allowing increased external rotation with less pain. The patient with anterior glenohumeral instability will experience apprehension and/or pain when the humeral head is slightly subluxated during external rotation and abduction. When it is reduced or supported, the pain and/or apprehension is lessened.

Anterior and posterior glenohumeral translation is assessed with the patient in both the supine and upright positions. In order to assess the amount of translation, the humeral head must be reduced at the start of the test. In the technique for carrying out the test with the patient sitting, the examiner stabilizes the shoulder girdle with one hand, and grasping the humeral head between the thumb and forefinger, applies anterior and posterior stress, noting the amount of translation. When the test is performed with the patient supine, the arm is positioned in 90° of abduction, and anterior and posterior translation is assessed. With respect to posterior translation, movement of the humeral head to 50% of the glenoid width is considered to be within normal limits. Although movement greater than 50% is not necessarily abnormal, this would increase the workload of the rotator cuff and influence shoulder mechanics. If the shoulder is unstable, applying an axial load may reproduce the symptoms experienced during swimming. This would be pain caused by instability itself. Inferior instability is indicated by the presence of a sulcus between the acromion and the head of the humerus with inferior traction.

Treatment

Treatment is directed at reducing pain and correcting biomechanics. This should incorporate relative rest, which means rest from aggravating factors rather than complete rest. The cornerstone of treatment is to retrain soft tissue and muscle to resume normal function. Patient education, which requires a great deal of time on the part of the clinician, is the key. In addition, communication with the athlete and the coach will assist in working out a program to minimize the detraining effect of reduced training. If the patient does not understand the importance of correct biomechanics and resting positions, treatment will be only temporarily effective. Much of what the patient is required to do will be in the form of exercise and functional retraining. The function of the spine and scapula is just as critical in activities of daily living as during sport. In most cases, in any given day individuals spend 1–3 hours at sport but 12 hours or more "at life." This does not take into account positions assumed during sleep! Patient education is the most important aspect of treatment.

Cervical and Thoracic Spine

The first step is to correct the alignment and posture of the cervical and thoracic spine. The use of a mirror and mimicking by the therapist is very effective. In most situations, instruction and demonstration will be sufficient. However in some cases muscles are already too tight and/or weak to sustain normal posture. Here appropriate stretching and strengthening are required before the patient can find or maintain correct posture successfully. Frequency is more important than intensity when performing functional exercises. For example, five times per hour throughout the course of the day is more advantageous than exercising for a 45-minute period. The patient should develop a constant awareness of body position, and to this end, work and daily activities must be taken into account when prescribing a rehabilitation program. As is the case in any learned motor skill, repetition is the key to neuromuscular retraining.

If this approach is unsuccessful, a more thorough evaluation of the spine may be indicated. An assessment of joint mechanics may demonstrate a need for mobilization of a specific segment. Sometimes a patient presents with all the classic signs of an overuse problem of the shoulder, and the underlying culprit is dysfunction of the cervical or thoracic spine.

Scapula

Scapular function and control directly influences the function of the glenohumeral joint. Retraining the periscapular muscles can be particularly challenging. A muscle such as the lower trapezius, which the patient can neither see nor relate to a specific activity, can be retrained using biofeedback. Visual or auditory feedback is provided by means of electrodes when the correct contraction is performed (Fig. 40-1). Patients can then repeat the correct contraction until they are able to recruit the muscle with ease. Initial progression will include exercises to incorporate simple arm movements, such as forward flexion, while receiving feedback. Then more complex or sport-specific movements can be added. Rehabilitation is completed when exercises for strength, speed, and power can be performed with scapular stability. This final step will ensure that the patient does not return with the same problem in the near future. Mirrors and videotaping can also be effective teaching tools. Retraining takes time, and more importantly, repetition. It is essential that the patient understand the process in order to achieve long-term success. In the case of excessively weak scapular stabilizers, taping the

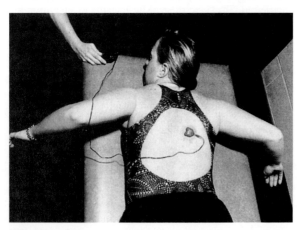

FIG 40-1   Biofeedback allows the retraining of a specific muscle with visual or auditory input by means of electrodes when the correct contraction is performed.

scapula to facilitate the muscles may help to limit pain in the overhead and impingement positions (Host, 1995). As the muscles are specifically retrained for the activity, strength, and endurance, the swimmer can gradually be weaned from the tape. This is particularly useful to keep an athlete training during rehabilitation.

Pathology or habitual improper posture may be due to or encouraged by technique that is less than optimal. Coaches and/or parents should be encouraged to observe the patient's swimming stroke for compensation or inefficiencies. Viewing a videotape together with the physiotherapist, coach/parent, and athlete often can shed much light on the problem. This may mean a total revision of the training program to realize long-term gains.

Glenohumeral Joint

As in patellofemoral joint, the glenohumeral joint is largely controlled by soft tissue. Therefore most pathology is found in these structures, and they should be the focus of treatment. Optimal soft tissue function is paramount if injury during sports is to be prevented.

Grade I Tendinopathy

A grade I tendinopathy responds well to conservative management. Swimmers are instructed to increase the time spent in both prepractice stretching and in-the-pool warm-up. Stretching to increase blood flow, restore range of motion, and decrease the potential for impingement should involve all components of the shoulder, including the anterior structures. In-the-pool warm-up with pain-free strokes should be prolonged and slow paced. Additional warm-ups should be continued after kicking sets. A swimming warm-down is recommended after the training session. Icing the shoulder with ice cups or bags for a maximum of 15 minutes after practice often will reduce pain.

Strengthening the external rotators is important to improve control of the glenohumeral joint, which in turn maximizes muscle efficiency and improves performance. The external rotators are initially worked in adduction and then in varying degrees of abduction. External rotation strength should be progressed to more functional positions, speeds, intensities, and repetitions. If one stroke causes symptoms, it should be discontinued until symptoms subside. Then gradually, when functional strength improves and faulty mechanics have been corrected, the stroke can be re-introduced. Physiotherapy assessment at this early stage may prevent the inevitable progression of pathology. If the faulty mechanics are not rectified, pain will likely return in time. Often treatment will be an independent exercise program for the re-education of correct mechanics.

Grade II Tendinopathy

In addition to the preceding measures, a grade II tendinopathy requires relative rest, physiotherapy, and medication. Relative rest is not abstinence from sport. The athlete is encouraged to use strokes that do not cause pain and to emphasize leg work. Kick-boards place the shoulder in a pain-provoking position and should not be used. For aerobic training, running (on dry land or in water) and cycling can augment the limited swimming workouts. Anti-inflammatory medication often will provide symptomatic relief.

At this stage, physiotherapy is indicated. Proper functioning of this joint depends on optimal soft tissue function. Treatment is based on the therapist's evaluation. All the basic assessments of range of motion, strength, sensation, stability, joint mobility, and neural tension, as well as additional appropriate special tests, must be considered. This will include the cervical and thoracic spines, scapula, and glenohumeral joint mechanics. Any specific findings should be addressed with the specific treatment techniques. For example, if capsular restriction is evident when assessing glenohumeral joint mobility, it should be treated with mobilization techniques in order for functional activities and muscular exercises to be successful.

Observation is once again an effective assessment tool. Note the resting position of the humerus: abduction, adduction, internal rotation, external rotation, and the position of the head of the humerus in the glenoid. One role of the subscapularis is to stabilize the head of the humerus anteriorly. An anterior position in the glenoid may indicate some subscapularis dysfunction.

At this point, the glenohumeral joint can be addressed in more detail. Full range of motion at the expense of other structures is unacceptable and should be guarded against. When assessing the movement of the glenohumeral joint, it is important to note the presence and degree of any associated movements. For example, normal abduction requires some external rotation of the humerus to allow the head of the humerus to pass under the acromion. Limited or excessive rotation will necessitate some compensation. Once again, the quality of the movement must be considered.

Accessory movements (ie, those that cannot be performed voluntarily by a given muscle but must occur for normal joint function) also can be compromised with dysfunction. An example is the inferior glide of the head of the humerus on the glenoid during flexion or abduction of the glenohumeral joint. If this inferior glide does not occur, the subacromial space will be smaller due to the position of the head of the humerus and potentially exacerbate impingement problems.

Muscle Balance

As mentioned earlier, muscle imbalance can be in the form of flexibility or strength. A tight or shortened muscle can greatly influence the integrity of the joint, capsule, and connective tissue as well as its own function and that of its antagonists. Also, in a tight muscle there is a shortened distance between its origin and insertion. The joint will accommodate by rotating the humerus, thereby shortening the functional distance for a given muscle. Eventually, one rotator will be shortened and its antagonist lengthened, thus compounding the problem. The two-joint muscles, such as the biceps, are common culprits. If shortened, the biceps can choose one of many functions (or a combination of all) to alter the position of the scapula, humerus, and forearm. For instance, the biceps is a powerful supinator, elbow flexor, and glenohumeral joint flexor. If tight, especially during forearm pronation, the elbow and perhaps the shoulder will experience less resistance in a slightly flexed position. This in turn may elevate the scapula, affecting the function of all scapulohumeral muscles.

With most activities, the prime movers of a given joint can be isolated to allow the task to be performed. However, with every movement an equal and opposite force is required to stabilize the base structure and facilitate optimal movement. In many instances, especially in sport, the movers develop to a greater extent than the stabilizers, creating an imbalance. Swimmers tend to develop the internal rotators of the glenohumeral joint. When this occurs without adequate strengthening of the scapular stabilizers, the internal rotators (many of which have a scapular origin) will pull the scapula into an abducted position. This will disadvantage the scapular adductors that stabilize, and a vicious cycle will be established. Many swimmers augment their training with weights. If poorly designed, these programs can add to the problem and inhibit rather than enhance performance. Programs should be designed with the length and strength balance of the movers and stabilizers in mind.

Strength Testing

Strength testing as part of a complete assessment should address quality and specificity in addition to force. Testing a particular muscle isometrically in neutral may demonstrate normal strength but will not identify deficits through range or at higher speeds. A circumspect history will give the clinician insight as to where attention should be focused. The patient may complain of pain only when force is required in a given position (eg, in overhead or abduction/external rotation). Eccentric and high-speed testing may be necessary to reveal any biomechanical compromise. Any compromise in scapular action or in the thoracic or cervical spine function during testing should be noted. In addition, strength is very specific, and its many aspects need to be considered. These include speed, type of contraction (eccentric versus concentric), type of biomechanical chain (open versus closed), and position of the joint/muscle. For example, a swimmer who rehabilitates the shoulder musculature up to 90° of abduction, at speeds less than 300° per second, and always open-chain concentrically will not have prepared the muscles with adequate specificity to return to the sport. Such a swimmer requires strength and control overhead, at speeds in excess of 1000° per second, both eccentrically and concentrically. This specificity must be addressed for the movers and stabilizers to be adequately trained to prevent recurrence. Many of these exercises can be incorporated into a home program or training regime using free weights and/or tubing. Pain during strengthening should be avoided at all costs, since the result will be a reflex inhibition of the muscle instead of activation.

Proprioception

Control of movement is also an essential part of rehabilitation. In a joint with the mobility of the glenohumeral joint, control of the joint movers and stabilizers is accomplished through range by proprioception of the shoulder girdle. Kinesthesia or proprioception of the glenohumeral joint is difficult to assess objectively. However, providing the patient with controlled tasks may identify specific difficulties. Ease of performance, comparison with the other side, and reproduction of joint position (eyes closed) can be assessed subjectively. These exercises can be progressed to more challenging positions, such as overhead or abduction with external rotation. In patients with recurrent glenohumoral joint dislocation or instability, it has been shown that once visual feedback has been removed, patients perform control tasks much differently from those with a normal capsular structure (Forwell, 1994). This compensation comes at a cost. As with the lower extremity, it is important to perturb the stability to demand a controlled reaction of the musculature. This can be done using physiotherapy balls, a Body Blade, tubing, water exercises, balance boards, and Profitters. Once the concept is defined and understood, the exercises are limited only by the imagination of the therapist. Again, proprioceptive exercises should be progressed through gradations of difficulty of speed, position, and type of contraction required. They also should be progressed to include a functional component that is individualized according to each patient's needs. In swimmers, ball exercises done overhead against a wall are appropriate (Figs. 40-2 and 40-3). They can be progressed to use tubing through a simulated swimming stroke and weights to isolate different specific muscles.

Hydrotherapy

Water as a medium for exercise and retraining is valuable and underutilized. Buoyancy allows the therapist to devise a variety of exercises and activities

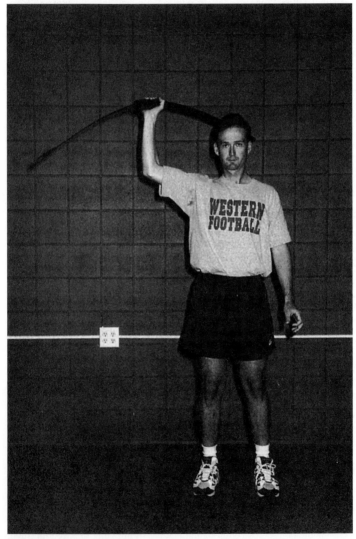

FIG 40-2   Functional proprioceptive training with a Bodyblade.

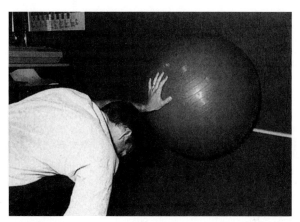

FIG 40-3 A proprioceptive ball exercise in a functional position for swimmers.

to enhance range of motion, strength, and proprioception. In water, resistance is not isolated to one plane, and no muscle can act independently without sufficient trunk stability. The neuromuscular reeducation that occurs when these exercises are performed correctly can effectively accelerate the rehabilitation process. These exercises can be progressed using paddles, water wings, air mattresses, or pool noodles (Fig. 40-4). Unfortunately, the availability of this medium in the clinic setting can be limited. However, with adequate instruction and demonstration on land, compliant patients can benefit from unsupervised pool activities outside the clinic.

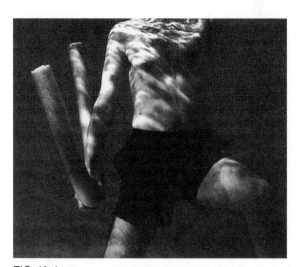

FIG 40-4 The use of hydrotherapy to train for strength and control of the glenohumeral joint (abduction/adduction) with a pool noodle providing resistance.

Additional Areas of Consideration

Other important areas are pain, modalities, and neural tension. The topic of pain alone can overtake any discussion of rehabilitation. Pain not only will inhibit activity, but also will influence the quality of the movement at any time. Appropriate treatment of pain should be included with the primary purpose of allowing the patient to perform a given task. Normalizing the biomechanics of the glenohumeral and scapulothoracic joints will assist in pain relief. If this indeed eliminates the cause of the problem, local management of pain should be much more successful. However, the vicious cycle of dysfunction-pain-dysfunction needs to be broken before rehabilitation can be successful.

A number of modalities are available for use by therapists. Ultasound, laser, electric current, heat, and cold are important and effective adjuncts. These applications should be thoughtfully applied to enhance the effect of retraining.

Neural tension and connective tissue are other important areas believed to have far-reaching effects on both metabolic and musculoskeletal problems. However, our understanding of these is limited, and while many physiotherapists and massage therapists have treated these areas successfully, more knowledge is needed about their role. It is an ongoing challenge to develop a more complete understanding so that treatment can be more effective. No single structure acts in isolation, and therefore assessment and treatment of interactive as well as individual function will meet with greater long-term success.

Follow-up is also a concern. It has been shown that swimmers with shoulder injuries have still not returned to full peak power output 8 weeks after their return to training (Swaine, 1997). In this case it might be suggested that those swimmers could be at risk of recurrence during this time frame. Closer observation of stroke mechanics and ongoing clinical follow-up should be considered.

A steroid injection into the subacromial space should be considered only if there is no response to treatment and if impingement-aggravated tests still elicit pain. The swimmer's load should be decreased after injection, and return to previous levels should take place over a 4- to 6-week period. Steroid injections should not be used routinely.

Grade III Tendinopathy

If tendinopathy progresses to grade III or beyond and becomes refractory despite conservative measures, the swimmer may have to choose between a change of sport and surgical intervention. Most young athletes select the former, a wise decision in most instances. However, if a career at the national or international level is possible, the athlete can be faced with a difficult dilemma. With guidance from both coach and physician, the swimmer can carefully examine the implications of each alternative.

Surgical options may include resection of the diseased segment of tendon along with the involved adjacent subacromial tissue and/or decompression of the same area. Before surgery is planned, the swimmer must understand that the postoperative period demands a commitment to a rehabilitation program and that the success of any procedure is contingent on compliance with this program. Typically, a postoperative regimen is a progressive exercise program geared to restoring range of motion and balanced muscle strength.

In the early stages when shoulder movement may be restricted, more attention may be paid to the cardiovascular fitness of the swimmer. Using primarily lower extremity workouts like bike, stairmaster, and running in water, there need not be a loss of conditioning despite the lay-off. Return to the pool should begin with slow swimming over limited distances, which advances to interval training and guided stroke modification. In addition, there should be an overlapping period between formal rehabilitation and return to the sport.

This functional rehabilitation stage should include exercises that work the muscles of the shoulder girdle in the position and manner in which they are needed for the performance of the swimming stroke. Overhead exercises with the ball, tubing, pulleys, and wobble boards will incorporate trunk control and specifically retrain the neuromuscular system to accept additional training. Attention to the number of repetitions and sets can mimic the need for anaerobic and aerobic work. These needs will depend on the events in which the athlete competes.

Grade IV Tendinopathy

A grade IV tendinopathy is seen most often in the mature athlete and may indicate a torn rotator cuff. Imaging techniques such as arthrography, ultrasonography, and magnetic resonance imaging (MRI) will help confirm the clinical diagnosis. Lesions such as partial-thickness tears and a thickened subacromial bursa can be identified by arthroscopy of the shoulder joint and subacromial space. In the younger swimmer, anterior and posterior superior quadrant labral tears can cause pain, although this is not a common occurrence. These may be treated successfully with arthroscopic excision. Bursectomy alone followed by appropriate rehabilitation can provide relief in the younger swimmer, but a more radical decompression, which includes resection of the anteroinferior acromion and a portion of the coracoacromial ligament, is generally recommended. Return to preinjury level of participation is unlikely, a fact that should be understood before plans are made for surgery. Postoperatively, range of motion is often low, and muscle strength, endurance, and power, particularly in the abductors and external rotators, deteriorate. Physiotherapy, as described previously, that rehabilitates all the muscle groups and biomechanics of the shoulder girdle plays a significant role in the postoperative period.

Prevention

Overuse syndromes of the shoulder in the swimmer are much easier to prevent than to treat. Four components are fundamental to a preventive program: balanced muscle strengthening, flexibility, technique modification, and avoidance of overwork. Again, the importance of an informed coach cannot be overstated. Ongoing stroke analysis, advice concerning stroke errors, careful planning of practice/training sessions, and regular monitoring of performance to prevent rotator cuff fatigue are among the responsibilities of the coaching staff.

Training

Overwork is a primary cause of tendinopathy and is often the result of increased intensity of training sets. Increases in workload should take place gradually. Rigorous training sets before the athlete is ready, or "extra hard" practices at the beginning of a training regimen can trigger the onset of shoulder pain. The use of paddles and special devices to enhance the upper extremity component of the stroke can also contribute to overwork. Workouts should be designed so that the difficult portion is completed early in the practice when the swimmer is rested. These should be organized so that there is relative rest for structures at risk. For example, after the difficult work has been completed, the practice can continue with stroke drills, with alternating stroke and leg work or with emphasis on start and turn techniques. With proper instruction, the swimmer will learn to guard against fatigue. Rest days also can be planned to follow a practice with an increase in intensity.

Strengthening

As mentioned previously, in competitive swimming, both pool and dry-land training focuses on strengthening the internal rotators, extensors, and adductors important to propulsion. Little emphasis is placed on strengthening the antagonists that play a significant role in containment of the shoulder. The imbalance in strength that may result can contribute to tendinopathy. Therefore awareness and early correction of any imbalance are important in prevention. External rotators are strengthened by performing both concentric and eccentric exercises to improve power and control of the primary mover/antagonist muscle action. The training program should not neglect the scapular and triceps muscles. When doing weight training, subacromial loading positions should be avoided. Paddles can produce increased leverage, which may overload the rotator cuff muscles and should be used with caution.

Flexibility

Regardless of sex or the stroke most frequently used, those swimmers with restricted flexibility were more likely to develop a tendinopathy than those who maintained and improved their flexibility with a stretching program (Griep, 1986). Stretching should be included in the daily warm-up routine. When teaching and demonstrating stretching techniques, it is important to emphasize that overstretching of the soft tissue can be harmful, especially for patients with instability. For this reason, pairs stretching is not recommended, particularly for younger swimmers who may not appreciate the risks of overstretching. Individual stretching is appropriate for this group.

However, if chosen, the stretching techniques employed by pairs can be either passive or proprioceptive neuromuscular facilitation. In the first, the partner very slowly and gently stretches the swimmer to the pain-free limit and then holds this position. In the second, the swimmer stretches to the pain-free limit. This position is maintained by the partner while the swimmer contracts against the resistance provided. These are repeated a variable number of times.

Technique Modification

Poor technique can slow a swimmer down and cause injury. Ongoing stroke analysis and recognition of breakdown in stroke mechanics will help the swimmer adjust technique and limit excessive subacromial loading. It is particularly important to analyze stroke mechanics during fatigue. In freestyle or backstroke, lateral shoulder impingement can be a result of insufficient body roll. A high elbow position during the recovery phase of freestyle must be achieved by body roll. Attempting to force the elbow into a higher position with muscle activity rather than sufficient body roll can induce subacromial impingement.

Overreach with excessive internal rotation during the catch phase of all swimming strokes may result in undue subacromial loading and extra work by the cuff muscles to contain the humeral head. In addition, excessive internal rotation may intensify the wringing out phenomenon. Changes to body roll, the amount of reach, and shoulder rotation will reduce the frequency and length of time that the shoulder is in the precarious position.

Although evidence of the effect of breathing patterns on the incidence of tendinopathy is contradictory, breathing to alternate sides does prevent constant leaning on one shoulder. It is a learned skill and should be taught in the early stages of training.

Shoulder Instability

Anterior Instability: Prevention and Treatment

Anterior instability is not often the cause of pain in competitive swimmers but is usually secondary to a traumatic incident in another sport. Primary conservative treatment of anterior instability includes controlling the head of the humerus in the glenoid and balanced strengthening exercises. The subscapularis controls the head of the humerus anteriorly on the glenoid. A thorough assessment of its function in a variety of positions and conditions should be done early. This training should be the basis for progression of any exercise regime. Once return to the pool is indicated, stroke analysis and correction is essential. If symptoms do not subside, examination under anesthesia and/or arthroscopy will confirm intra-articular lesions such as a Bankart or Hill-Sachs lesion. An anterior stabilizing procedure can provide relief, and the athlete can return to preinjury levels of performance if motion and strength are regained.

Multidirectional Instability: Prevention and Treatment

Swimmers with frank posterior instability may have pain from dislocating their shoulders during the swimming stroke cycle. The at-risk position of forward flexion and internal rotation is a component of all strokes. Pain in swimmers with congenital or acquired multidirectional instability must be differentiated from that experienced by those suffering from tendinopathy who have concomitant increased laxity.

Persistence with a nonoperative program is recommended in swimmers who have experienced instability over a long period. Again, controlling the head of the humerus in the glenoid is important. The patient should be taught how to recruit both subscapularis and supraspinatus in neutral and instructed to practice this to fatigue. In some patients, this could involve as few as three repetitions. Teaching this new recruitment pattern is easiest with the patient supine and the scapula stabilized. Progression to sitting must start with the coordination of both the scapular and glenohumeral stabilizers. Recruitment of one without the other will be ineffective. The use of biofeedback is helpful to allow the patient to monitor more than one muscle group at a time. These exercises requiring control should then become more and more challenging and sport specific with respect to strength, endurance, speed, and position. In most cases, stroke modification, correction of biomechanics and strength deficits, as well as adjusting training programs to minimize the magnitude and incidence of abnormal motion can be successful.

Surgical intervention such as an inferior capsular shift, "a reefing procedure" to the posterior cuff and capsule, or a glenoid osteotomy should be considered only when all nonoperative treatments have been exhausted. These procedures are intended to provide symptomatic relief for daily activities, perhaps for recreational swimming and other sports, and occasionally for highly competitive swimming.

THE ELBOW

The arm pull in the butterfly stroke and breaststroke and less frequently in the freestyle is the main cause of stress syndromes about the elbow. Most competitive swimmers use a form of "elbow up" pull in which the elbow is bent and held higher than the hand throughout the first part of the pull. This position permits maximal backward thrust of the hand by allowing the swimmer to push the water back at the most efficient angle. The elbow then bends to about $100°$ as the arm is pulled under the body. The upper arm is rotated medially, and the forearm is pronated. The high-elbow position is likened to reaching over a barrel. Dropping the elbow is a common fault in the swimmer's stroke pattern. This results in a less efficient angle to push the water backward, requiring more force in the common extensor muscles.

Lateral epicondylitis, frequently referred to as tennis elbow (described in detail by Nirschl) can ensue (Nelson et al., 1991). There is inflammation of the extensor carpi radialis brevis and extensor communis aponeurosis at the lateral epicondyle of the humerus. The prime etiologic factor in swimming appears to be overwhelming moments of force combined with repetition. This results in a combination of extrinsic overload in conjunction with excessive muscle contraction.

Treatment

The treatment of this condition includes relief of acute and chronic inflammation; increase in forearm extensor power, flexibility, and endurance; a decrease in the moments of force placed against the elbow by altering stroke; and rarely surgery. Relief of acute inflammation is aided by the application of ice and the judicious use of anti-inflammatory medication and physiotherapy modalities such as ultrasound. Extracorporeal shock wave therapy is approved for lateral epicondylitis and provides pain relief in 80% of patients after three treatments. Stroke alteration is essential in most cases for long-term management.

The physiotherapy approach is similar to that for the shoulder, which includes a thorough assessment of the biomechanics of the upper quadrant and muscle imbalances, as well as range of motion, strength, and stability. Joint function of the radio-ulnar, radio-humeral, and ulnar-humeral joints is also assessed, corrected if necessary, and then controlled. Two-joint muscles, the biceps and triceps which cross the shoulder and elbow joints, should be considered when assessing the elbow. If the resting position of the shoulder predisposes the biceps to shorten, the elbow is free to rest or function in a biceps-lengthened position at the elbow (pronation). As both these muscles take their origin on the scapula, its position and stability is important. As for the shoulder rehabilitation previously mentioned, stabilizing the scapula and maintaining stability throughout elbow retraining is essential. Once pain and inflammation have been treated, progressive strength, endurance, and power training to the elbow must include specifically designed exercises with special attention paid to the extensor carpi radialis. These exercises should address concentric, eccentric, and low and high speed as well as positional and functional specificity. Sometimes the elbow may develop an overuse syndrome because of a particular weakness more proximal. Therefore the elbow will attempt to compensate and thereby become fatigued and overused.

In resistant cases, there is a place for steroid injections. These should be used with caution and infrequently. Kennedy and Willis (1976) have verified evidence of collagen disorganization and weakening for up to 6 weeks associated with steroid injections.

In refractory cases, surgical excision of the degenerative lesion most frequently found in the extensor carpi radialis brevis is carried out. Surgery is followed by slow, methodical return to the swimming training program.

THE KNEE

Medial knee pain is not infrequent in breast-stroke swimmers and is related to the whip kick. Although this is the superior kick in terms of speed and propulsion, it subjects the knee to abnormal motion. Faulty technique can cause problems; however, because of the nature of the kick, the intensity, and the number of repetitions performed, even proper execution does not preclude knee injury. Medial synovial plica syndrome, medial collateral ligament stress syndrome, and patellofemoral syndrome are the common diagnoses attributed to the high valgus and outward rotational stresses necessary to achieve the maximum propulsive effect of the whip kick.

In medial synovial plica syndrome, pain is secondary to the inflammation caused by the friction produced as the plica snaps across the medial femoral condyle during repeated knee flexion and extension. The diagnosis is made by eliciting local tenderness and palpating the thickened synovium as it crosses the medial femoral condyle.

During the whip kick there is increased tension in the medial collateral ligament (MCL) as the knee moves from flexion to extension. This is further increased with a valgus stress and dramatically increased when external rotation forces are applied to the knee. Medial collateral stress syndrome is suggested by point tenderness along the course of the ligament. Often this is located at the origin of the MCL at the adductor tubercle of the femur, but just as frequently it occurs where the superficial fibers cross the upper tibial margin. The pain often can be reproduced by applying a valgus external rotation force to the knee flexed to 20–30°.

The clinical findings of patellofemoral syndrome do not differ in the swimmer and may include abnormal alignment of the lower extremity as well as hypermobility or frank instability of the patellofemoral joint. This may be associated with patella alta. There will be tenderness when the patellar facets or femoral condyles are palpated. Symptoms may be reproduced by the patellofemoral compression test or by laterally deviating the patella. In our experience, the more serious patellofemoral problems occur in age-group swimmers. This may be due to improper execution of the whip kick. However, an inherently unstable patellofemoral joint, because of the forces generated by the whip kick, often will preclude the achievement of elite levels in the breast-stroke.

In the age-group swimmer, other knee pathologies not related to swimming must be ruled out. Chronic ligamentous instability, a torn medial meniscus (uncommon in the stable knee in this age group), and osteochondritis dissecans are among the possibilities. Osteochondritis dissecans should be sought radiographically, particularly if there is any chronicity to the complaints. It is important to keep in mind that a multifactorial etiology may be present in many knee problems.

Treatment

Identifying the cause is critical to successful long-term treatment. Improper technique should be recognized by the coach and corrected. In many cases this will eliminate the knee pain. However, anatomic problems such as significant patellofemoral or ligamentous instability may be incompatible with the repetitive stress inherent in the whip kick, and a prolonged treatment program in these athletes may be doomed to failure. Physiotherapy assessment of the functional mechanics of the lower quadrant may be necessary. The muscle imbalances around the pelvis, hip, and knee can greatly influence the recruitment pattern of the muscles around the knee. Assessing gait and dry-land function can demonstrate what muscles are short and weak such that the kinetic chain of the lower extremity is altered. The correction of these faulty movement patterns and the subsequent functional training should ensue. In the short-term, taping the patellofemoral joint can be helpful in order to continue training. The tape will assist the muscles in control of the patella. When those muscles are specifically trained for speed, activity, strength, and endurance, taping can be gradually discontinued. Communication among the coach, swimmer, physician and physiotherapist is important to avoid frustration and disappointment and to provide realistic direction. Therapeutic measures depend on the diagnosis and include anti-inflammatory medication and ultrasound to control acute symptoms.

FOOT AND ANKLE

Foot and ankle pain can be a problem in swimmers regardless of the stroke performed. Tendinitis of the extensor tendons of the ankle and foot where they are firmly bound over the ankle dorsum by the extensor retinaculum is the most common cause. In both the flutter and dolphin kicks, the ankle and foot are brought into extreme plantar flexion and then back to neutral. There is little room for inflammation under the tight retinaculum. The diagnosis is obvious in most cases. Crepitation may be palpable and audible as the foot is brought from plantar flexion into dorsiflexion.

Treatment

Local therapeutic modalities such as ultrasound and ice as well as anti-inflammatory medications and wrapping of the foot and ankle are often of benefit. Preventive stretching prior to practices is important. Less vigorous kicking or no kicking will allow swimming to continue. Resumption of normal kicking is achieved gradually. If persistent, physiotherapy intervention may be necessary to assess the biomechanics of the foot and lower extremity. Locally, plantar-flexors and toe flexors may be tight and the antagonists relatively weak. This will affect the way the foot contacts the floor in gait and may aggravate the problem. Specific exercise to correct this imbalance and subsequent retraining is indicated. In more severe cases, a pedorthist should assess for orthotics. As with the knee, the function of the foot and ankle during the nonswimming hours of the day may predispose the use-pattern of the muscles of the foot and ankle in the water.

THE BACK

Diagnosis and Treatment

During the breast-stroke, many swimmers pull with an early elbow flexion and increased arm abduction. This prolongs the elbow-up position and propels the upper torso above the water. This aggravates the already lordotic attitude of the lower back. This stress can cause a variety of lower back problems, including stress fractures of the pars interarticularis or even frank spondylolisthesis. More often, accentuation of a mildly symptomatic spondylolisthesis or a mechanical low back pain from posterior facet irritation occurs and limits the competitive breaststroker's training. Such back complaints also may occur in butterfly stroke swimmers. Here, inefficient and incorrect mechanics are often the cause.

An accurate and precise diagnosis is important. In most cases the primary complaint is pain with some radiation into the buttocks. Hamstring tightness may occur with a diagnosis of spondylolisthesis. Positive findings that are frequently identified include palpation of a step deformity at the spine of L5 and the sacrum, and an abnormal gait with a backward-tilting pelvis. The diagnosis is confirmed radiographically. If x-rays are normal, a bone scan will help in the diagnosis of a pars stress fracture. A recent stress fracture must be treated with a prolonged period of rest.

Spondylolisthesis is treated symptomatically according to the severity of the complaints. Rest from training may be indicated. In severe cases this may last for 3–6 months and may include a lumbar brace or corset. Following any rest, slow return with a carefully planned program is prescribed. Hamstring stretching and abdominal strengthening are of particular importance in the ongoing treatment and for prevention. The function of the spine is somewhat more complex than that of the peripheral joints. A physiotherapy assessment of the dysfunction should include an in-depth assessment of joint mechanics. The position and function of the pelvis, hip, and lower extremity will complete the story of the kinetic chain. In the water this chain is open. When standing on land, the kinetic chain is closed. The differing mechanics that ensue have to be well understood for full rehabilitation. Lumbar extension (passive or active) should be avoided. Joint mobilization is often not indicated as the joint has more movement than desired. Control of L5-S1 is the priority. Once symptoms are relieved and abdominal and erector strengthening has begun, positional and functional strength is important. This should include the position of the pelvis and hip as well as the lumbar spine. At no time should symptoms recur with exercise. Once training has mimicked the pool work-out, water work-outs can begin. Similar exercises should be included in dry-land and off-season training.

Mechanical low back pain often will respond to a similar program. More resistant cases may require prolonged treatment that can incorporate modalities such as transcutaneous electrical nerve stimulation or repeated mobilizations to the affected area. Occasionally, a steroid injection to the inflamed facet is necessary.

When returning to the pool, it is important to asssess stroke mechanics and monitor the intensity and duration of practices. Also of concern is the use of special devices for isolating a leg or arm workout. Many such devices that limit the lower extremity work will require the upper body to come out of the water further (Nyska et al., 2000). This in turn will stress the lower lumbar area into extension and thereby potentially cause a recurrence. This should also be considered when looking at causative factors, especially in younger swimmers.

The term *adolescent swimmer's* back was coined by Wilson and Linseth. Three adolescent patients with backache aggravated by swimming the butterfly stroke were diagnosed with Scheuermann kyphosis. The authors were not certain whether the forceful contraction of the chest and abdominal musculature during the power phase of the butterfly stroke caused the vertebral abnormalities or merely was an aggravating factor. Two of the three swimmers experienced dramatic relief once they had stopped performing the butterfly stroke, which suggests that these patients should confine their swimming to the backstroke and freestyle. Strengthening of the antagonist musculature is also helpful.

SUMMARY

Prevention, diagnosis, and treatment of injuries depend on an understanding of the basics of swimming strokes and practice techniques as well as interaction and communication among professionals charged with the care and training of swimmers. With respect to physiotherapy, biomechanics and control of motion are two areas of growth with the potential to enhance and accelerate rehabilitation programs. As few injuries are traumatic in nature, retraining is a common solution.

REFERENCES

Astrand P, Radahl K. Neuromuscular function. In: *Textbook of Work Physiology: Physiological Bases of Exercise*, 2d ed. New York: McGraw-Hill; 1977;55–128.

Blazina ME. Jumper's knee. *Orthop Clin North Am*. 1980;4:65.

Bigliani NU, Morrison DS, April EW. The morphology of the acromion and its relationship to rotator cuff tears. *Orthop Trans*. 1986;10:216.

Forwell LA. Proprioceptive deficits associated with recurrent shoulder dislocation. Thesis, University of Western Ontario, Department of Physical Therapy, 1994.

Fowler PJ, Webster-Bogaert MS. Swimming. In: Reider B, ed. *Sports Medicine: The School-Age Athlete*. Philadelphia: Saunders; 1991;429–446.

Griep JF. Swimmers shoulder: The influence of flexibility and weight training. *Orthop Trans*. 1986;10:216.

Host HH. Scapular taping in the treatment of anterior shoulder impingement. *Phys Ther*. 1995;75:803–812.

Kennedy JC, Hawkins RJ. Swimmer's shoulder. *Phys Sports Med*. 1974;2:35.

Kennedy JC, Willis RB. The effects of local steroid injections on tendons: A biomechanical and microscopic correlative study. *Am J Sports Med*. 1974;4:11.

Lo YPC, Hsu YCS, Chan KM. Epidemiology of shoulder impingement in upper arm sports events. *Br J Sports Med*. 1990;24:173–177.

McMaster WC, Troup J. A survey of interfering shoulder pain in United States competitive swimmers. *Am J Sports Med*. 1993;21:67.

Nelson M, Leather GP, Nirschl RP, et al. Evaluation of the painful shoulder: A prospective comparison of magnetic resonance imaging, computerized tomographic arthrography, ultrasonography, and operative findings. *J Bone Joint Surg*. 1991;73:707–716.

Nyska M, Constantini N, Calé-Benzoor M, Back Z, Kahn G, Mann G. Spondylolysis as a cause of low back pain in swimmers. *Int J Sports Med*. 2000;21:375–379.

Pink M, Perry J, Browne A, et al. The normal shoulder during freestyle swimming: An electromyographic and cinematographic analysis of twelve muscles. *Am J Sports Med.* 1991;19:569–576.

Pink MM, Tibone JE. The painful shoulder in the swimming athlete. *Orthop Clin North Am.* 2000;31:247–261.

Rathbun JB, Macnab I. The microvascular pattern of the rotator cuff. *J Bone Joint Surg.* 1979;54A:540–553.

Scovazzo ML, Browne A, Pink M, et al. The painful shoulder during freestyle swimming: An electromyographic and cinematographic analysis of twelve muscles. *Am J Sports Med.* 1991;19:577–582.

Swaine IL. Time course of changes in bilateral arm power of swimmers during recovery form injury using a swim bench. *Br J Sports Med.* 1997;31:213–216.

Webster-Bogaert SM. Swimmer's shoulder. University of Waterloo, Waterloo, Ontario, Canada, 1981.

41 | Cycling

Jonathan T. Finnoff

QUICK LOOK

- A majority of injuries are due to overuse.
- Severe injuries are usually traumatic.
- Most fatal injuries are a result of head trauma.

Factors that contribute to overuse injuries include:

- Poor bicycle fit
- Bad bicycling technique such as pushing a gear that is too hard
- Inadequate training program

Treatment of overuse injuries:

- Modification of bicycle fit
- Reduce the size of gear used, and increase the pedaling speed (cadence)
- Review the bicyclist's training program

Prevention of traumatic injuries:

- Ride with appropriate protective equipment, particularly a helmet
- Ride at a reduced speed over unfamiliar terrain and in adverse conditions
- Pre-ride race courses
- Learn to fall in a tuck-and-roll fashion
- Use a light and reflective gear when riding at night
- Do not ride while intoxicated

Treatment of "road rash":

- Cleanse the area with an antiseptic solution and topical local anesthetic to reduce pain
- Remove gravel and dirt using a sponge or brush
- Dress with antibiotic ointment, nonadherent dressing, and gauze wrap or netting
- After healing, be sure to use sunscreen over the affected area

Prevention of environmental injuries:

- Drink adequate fluid to replace sweat losses
- Fill one water bottle with water and the other with a sports drink
- Wear sunscreen with an SPF of at least 15
- Wear lightweight clothing with breathable fabric in hot weather
- Wear several layers in cold weather with a base layer that wicks moisture away from the skin and a water-repellent and windproof outer layer
- Extra covering for the feet is required if the temperature is below 40°F

INTRODUCTION

Bicycling is a common form of aerobic exercise for both competitive and recreational athletes. For some people, bicycles are used as a primary form of transportation. Estimates suggest that there are more than 45 million bicyclists in the United States, and that 45% of the population bicycles at least occasionally (National Safety Council, 1999). As the popularity of bicycling increases, so too does the incidence of injury. Injuries may be related to poor

663

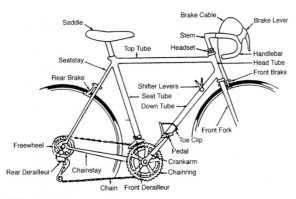

FIG 41-1 The bicycle.

bicycle fit, overuse, direct trauma from collisions or falls, faulty equipment, or environmental factors. There are also injuries specific to the type of bicycling, such as mountain biking or road biking. This chapter will provide the sports medicine clinician with an overview of the physiologic, biomechanical, and medical aspects of bicycling.

THE BICYCLE

The bicycle is composed of a frame with various components including handlebars, brakes, wheels, pedals, gears, and a saddle (Fig. 41-1). There are some differences in the equipment on a mountain bicycle and a road bicycle. Mountain bicycles often have front and/or rear shock absorbers to reduce the impact of uneven terrain on the rider. The frame of a mountain bicycle tends to be smaller so the bicyclist has more clearance between the pelvis and the top tube. Mountain bicycles have three front chain rings, whereas most road bicycles only have two. This allows for a wider range of gears for the mountain bicyclist. The handlebars of a mountain bicycle are straight across, thus maintaining the biker in a more upright position. Road bicycles have curved handlebars, known as the "drops," that lower the position of road bicycle handlebars. These handlebars allow the road bicyclist to choose between sitting upright or leaning forward in a more aerodynamic position.

PHYSIOLOGY AND BIOMECHANICS OF BICYCLING

While subsets of bicyclists, such as track cyclists, predominantly rely on anaerobic metabolism and fast-twitch muscle fibers, most bicyclists are far more dependent on aerobic metabolism and slow twitch muscle fibers. Research has demonstrated a higher proportion of type I (slow twitch) muscle fibers in professional bicyclists than in sedentary controls (Ryschon, 1994). Bicyclists also have a much lower average body fat percentage than the general population. Elite road cyclists have between 6 and 9% body fat for males, and 12 to 15% body fat for females (Burke, 1980).

Competitive bicyclists have high maximum oxygen uptakes (VO_{2max}), which reflects the aerobic nature of this sport. A study of national team road and mountain bike racers in the United States by Wilber and colleagues

(1997) revealed the VO_{2max} of female cyclists to be between 57.9 and 63.8 mL O_2/kg/min, while male cyclists were between 70 and 70.3 mL O_2/kg/min.

Although VO_{2max} is important, the lactate threshold appears to have a stronger correlation with performance. The lactate threshold is defined as the percentage of VO_{2max} at which point there is an exponential increase in the concentration of blood lactate beyond baseline values. If two cyclists compete, and cyclist 1 has a lower VO_{2max} than cyclist 2, but a higher lactate threshold, cyclist 1 will outperform cyclist 2. Other strong predictors of cycling performance include the volume of training and years of competitive experience (Sanner et al, 2000).

Pedaling technique is another important determinant of bicycling performance. There are two phases of the pedal cycle. The phase from the top of a pedal stroke (called 0° by convention) to the bottom of the pedal stroke (called 180° by convention) is the power phase of the pedal cycle (Sanner et al, 2000). From the bottom (180°) to the top (360°) is called the recovery phase (Sanner et al, 2000).

Pedals have been designed to improve pedaling efficiency and increase force production. The initial design, which used toe clips, held the foot onto the pedal using an external strap system. This was followed by the development of a cleat on the bottom of the cycling shoe that could attach directly to the pedal and release when the cyclist twisted their foot to the side. This system was called the clipless pedal. Most competitive cyclists now use clipless pedals. Toe clips and clipless pedals allow the cyclist to pull up on the pedal during the recovery phase of the pedal cycle. However, the majority of power produced during pedaling is still attributable to the power phase (Coyle, 1995).

The total sagittal plane joint movement during one full pedal cycle is approximately 45° at the hip, 75° at the knee, and 20° at the ankle (Gregor, 2000). The knee is affected more than the hip or ankle by changes in seat height. Knee joint excursion is 20° more than the ankle or hip when the seat is relatively low, and 50° more than the ankle or hip when the seat is relatively high. The knee flexes more when the seat is low than when the seat is high. About 6 cm of frontal plane movement occurs at the knee during a pedal cycle. During the power phase of the pedal cycle, the knee moves medially due to femoral adduction, the tibia internally rotates, and the foot pronates. Raising the seat exaggerates these motions, while lowering the seat reduces them (Gregor, 2000).

Transverse and frontal plane movements in the lower extremity contribute to the development of knee pain in cyclists (Gregor, 2000). Cyclists with knee pain have a larger degree of frontal and transverse plane motion than cyclists without knee pain (Gregor, 2000). There have been many anecdotal reports of reduced knee pain with the use of clipless pedals that allow unrestricted transverse plane motion of the foot during the pedal cycle. Video feedback, pedal adjustments, and orthotics have all resulted in reduced frontal plane movement and knee pain among elite cyclists (Gregor, 2000).

Coordinated contraction of trunk and extremity muscles is required for an efficient pedal cycle. The paraspinal and abdominal muscles stabilize the trunk and pelvis, allowing the extremities to generate power (Sanner et al, 2000). During the pedal cycle, the quadriceps and gluteal muscles are active in the first two thirds of the power phase, while the hamstrings are active during the last three- quarters of the power phase (Sanner et al, 2000). During the power phase, the hamstrings and gluteal muscles act as hip extensors, and the quadriceps as knee extensors (Sanner et al, 2000). This indicates that active hip extension occurs throughout the entire power phase, while active knee extension only occurs for the first two- thirds of the power phase.

The importance of the hip extensor muscles during the power phase of the pedal cycle was demonstrated in a study by Coyle and associates (1995). The power generated per pedal stroke was evaluated in a group of elite cyclists with identical lean body weight and VO_{2max}. One group of cyclists was able to produce 11.2% higher power per pedal stroke than the other cyclists. The increased power resulted from an increase in hip extensor muscle activity during the power phase of the pedal cycle. The additional recruitment of hip extensors during the power phase of the pedal stroke increased the total cross sectional area of muscle active during the pedal stroke. Spreading the force production over a larger muscle mass reduced the metabolic demands on individual muscles and led to an increase in the lactate threshold. Therefore, increased hip extensor muscle recruitment may significantly improve cycling performance through increased power production and an increase in the lactate threshold. Consciously thinking about using the hip extensor muscles while pedaling or creating a biomechanical advantage for the hip extensor muscles during the pedal cycle by moving the seat further backward or lengthening the handlebar stem are two ways to increase hip extensor muscle recruitment.

The quadriceps muscles are also active during the transition from the late recovery phase into the power phase, thereby propelling the pedal over the top of the pedal stroke (Sanner et al, 2000). The hamstring muscles are active during the transition from the power phase into the early recovery phase thus helping to propel the pedal through the bottom of the pedal stroke (Sanner et al, 2000). The hamstring muscles also provide an upward force on the pedal during the early recovery phase.

The soleus and gastrocnemius muscles are both active during the middle half of the power phase (Sanner et al, 2000). The gastrocnemius muscle continues its activity through the remainder of the power phase into the recovery phase (Sanner et al, 2000). During the power phase, the gastrocnemius and soleus muscles provide downward force on the pedal and resist ankle dorsiflexion. This improves the power transfer from the lower extremities into the pedals. The gastrocnemius contraction during the early recovery phase causes plantar flexion of the foot and improves the ability of the hamstring to flex the knee and pull up on the pedal.

The number of pedal revolutions per minute is called the cadence. For competitive cyclists, the optimal cadence for racing appears to be between 80 and 110 rpm and during leisure riding between 60 and 90 rpm (Ryschon, 1994).

Factors that contribute to the resistance of forward propulsion during cycling include rolling resistance, air resistance, and gravity. Rolling resistance contributes less than 10% to the overall resistance of cycling and is minimized through use of narrow tires with high air pressure (Ryschon, 1994). Gravitational resistance is most important during uphill cycling and places the larger cyclist at a disadvantage during hill climbs (Ryschon, 1994). Since small cyclists are unable to generate as much power per unit of transported mass as larger cyclists, bicycle weight is very important for lighter bicyclists (Ryschon, 1994). Air resistance accounts for nearly 90% of the resistance to cycling while on a flat surface, therefore aerodynamics is very important in cycling. While small cyclists have an advantage on hills, large cyclists have an advantage on the flats due to the larger power generation per unit of frontal area (Ryschon, 1994). Thus large cyclists are not as affected by air resistance as small cyclists.

EPIDEMIOLOGY OF BICYCLING INJURIES

There are approximately 900 deaths, 580,000 emergency room visits, 23,000 hospital admissions, and 1.2 million visits to physician offices per year in the United States attributable to bicycle accidents (Thompson et al, 2001). Bicycle injuries result in an estimated health care cost of more than $8 billion per year (Thompson et al, 2001). Bicycle accidents are the second most frequent cause of serious recreational injuries (Thompson et al, 2001).

It has been proposed that a majority of bicycling injuries are due to overuse, training errors, or poor bicycle fit (Mellion, 1991). However, most epidemiologic studies of bicycling injuries have been performed in emergency rooms or by medical personnel at bicycle races or tours, so these studies have a significant bias toward traumatic injuries. The following epidemiologic review reflects this bias. Prospective studies of bicycling injuries, both traumatic and atraumatic, are needed.

For road bicyclists, the most common traumatically injured areas are the extremities followed by the head, face, abdomen/thorax, and neck (Mellion, 1991). A majority of the injuries are abrasions, contusions, and lacerations (Mellion, 1991). Injuries to the head most commonly occur from collisions between cyclists and automobiles (Mellion, 1991). Over 60% of bicycling deaths and most cases of long-term disability are due to head injuries. Children and adolescents sustain head injuries more frequently than other populations (Eilert-Petersson et al, 1997). Facial trauma includes injuries to the eyes from airborne objects, contusions, abrasions, and fractures (Mellion, 1991). Blunt trauma is the predominant cause of abdominal and thoracic trauma in road bicyclists (Mellion, 1991).

One study performed by Dannenberg and associates (1996) did provide some information on the incidence of traumatic and atraumatic injuries in bicyclists participating in a tour across Maryland. Injury data were collected at the first-aid stations, and via a pre- and post-ride survey. There were 1638 participants; two-thirds were male, and the age range was from 7–79 years old. Helmets were required for participants. There were 85 traumatic injuries, 76 atraumatic injuries, and 37 medical problems. The types of traumatic injuries were not described. The atraumatic injuries included knee pain, numbness in the hand or wrist, and blisters. Other medical problems included insect bites or stings, heat-related illness, and dehydration.

Mountain biking is becoming increasingly popular in the United States, and mountain bike sales account for 62% of the bicycle market (Pfeiffer et al, 1995). During competition, the incidence of injury per race for cross-country racers is 0.40–0.49% and for downhill racers it is 0.51% (Kronisch et al, 1996a; Kronisch et al,1996b). Women tend to sustain injuries more frequently than men (Kronisch et al, 1996a; Kronisch et al, 2002). Injuries sustained by falling over the handlebars result in more severe injuries than when the cyclist falls off the side (Kronisch et al, 1996a; Kronisch et al, 1996b). Mountain bicyclists tend to wear helmets more frequently than road cyclists, and appear to incur fewer head and facial injuries (Chow et al, 1993; Rivara et al, 1997). Over a 1-year period, 51% of mountain bicyclists report sustaining an injury (Chow et al, 1993). While most injuries occur off road (87.6%), those sustained on road are more severe (Chow et al, 1993). Most injuries sustained by mountain bicyclists are relatively minor such as abrasions, lacerations, and contusions, but up to 26% of injuries reportedly require medical evaluation (Kronisch et al, 1996b; Chow et al, 1993).

Injuries sustained during motocross (BMX) bicycle racing were reported at the 1989 European Championship (Brogger-Jensen et al, 1990). While only 6.3% of participants sustained an injury, 52.5% of those injured required medical evaluation, and 3.3% were admitted to the hospital for further care. A majority of the injuries were reported as minor (72.1%), with the most commonly sustained injuries being abrasions followed by contusions. Approximately 7% of the injured riders sustained fractures. Interestingly, women sustained twice as many injuries as men, reflecting the findings of mountain bike racing research.

A significant number of injuries to the abdomen have been caused by mountain bike and BMX bicycle handlebar ends. The injuries sustained by this mechanism have included ruptures or contusions to the spleen and/or liver (Erez et al, 2001; Clarnette et al, 1997; Nehoda et al, 1998; Richmond, 1994), injuries to major arteries (Sarfati et al, 2002; Roth et al, 1999), bowel perforations or eviscerations (Clarnette et al, 1997; Lovell et al, 1992), pancreatic injuries (Clarnette et al, 1997; Lovell et al, 1992; Koestner et al, 1999), renal contusions (Clarnette et al, 1997), iliac wing fractures (Krishnan et al, 2002), and abdominal wall disruption resulting in a "handlebar hernia" (Kubota et al, 1999). Bicyclists who sustain an abdominal injury by this mechanism need to have a thorough evaluation to rule out significant internal injury.

There are many risk factors for bicycling accidents. Accidents occur most frequently to male cyclists between 9 and 14 years old (Thompson et al, 2001). Bicycle accidents are more common in the summer during the afternoon and early evening in urban areas (Thompson et al, 2000; Eilert-Petersson et al, 1997). Cyclists are more likely to be involved in an accident if they don't wear a helmet, ride in an unsafe environment, or are intoxicated (Thompson et al, 2001). Other risk factors include an unstable family environment and preexisting psychiatric condition (Thompson et al, 2001). Mechanical failure, excess speed, bicyclist or motorist errors, and environmental hazards also appear to contribute to bicycle accidents (Thompson et al, 2001; Eilert-Petersson et al, 1997). Risk factors for bicycle accidents in mountain biking include excessive speed, unfamiliar terrain, inattentiveness, riding in a competition, and riding beyond one's ability (Pfeiffer et al, 1995; Kronisch et al, 1996b).

Two special populations deserve mention. The first are children riding in bicycle-mounted seats and bicycle-towed trailers. Two studies have addressed injuries to this pediatric population. Tanz and colleagues (1991) found that 55% of those injured in bicycle-mounted child seats were male, with a peak incidence at 2 years old. Most injuries were due to falls. All serious injuries were associated with trauma to the head or face, while mild injuries occurred to the extremities. Powell and Tanz (2000) reported 6 injuries associated with bicycle trailers. Two of the injuries were due to collisions with motor vehicles, three were caused by falls, and one involved the spokes of the trailer wheel. Five of the injuries were to the head or face, and all six children sustained contusions or abrasions.

The second special population is those aged 65 or older. Many of the elderly use bicycling as a form of low-impact aerobic exercise, and bicycling is also frequently used as a form of transportation by this population (Ekman et al, 2001). The risk of death due to a bicycle accident is 3.7 times greater in the elderly than in children 14 years old or younger. While the number of injuries sustained in the pediatric population may actually be decreasing, the incidence of injuries in the elderly appears to be increasing significantly (Ekman et al, 2001). With a trend toward increasing longevity and a growing population of people over 65 years of age, bicycle-related injuries in the elderly may become a significant public health concern in the near future.

PROPER BICYCLE FIT

Proper bicycle fit is an integral part of bicycling. Not only does a properly fit bicycle improve the comfort and enjoyment of bicycling, it is also important in preventing and treating injuries. In fact, it has been suggested that improper bicycle fit is the leading cause of overuse problems in bicyclists (Mellion, 1991). For avid bicyclists, the best bicycle fit is achieved through a measurement system known as the Fitkit, which is available at top bicycle shops. The following are general guidelines for proper bicycle fit that can be used in the clinical setting.

In order to determine the correct frame size, the bicyclist should straddle the frame with both feet flat on the floor, and determine the clearance between the crotch and the top tube. For road bicycles, the appropriate frame will have 1 to 2 inches of clearance between the crotch and the top tube, while mountain bikes should have a clearance of 3 to 6 inches.

There are several ways to determine saddle height. A simple method is to place the bicycle on a wind trainer. The bicyclist mounts the bicycle, sits on the seat, and places the heels of the feet on top of the pedals. The bicyclist then rotates the pedals backward. The proper saddle height is indicated by the bicyclist's knees becoming fully straight at the bottom of the pedal stroke without the hips rocking from side to side on the seat. At this height, when the bicyclist places the ball of their foot over the pedal, the knee will be in slight flexion at the bottom of the pedal stroke.

Another method of determining saddle height is by ensuring 20–25° of knee flexion when the pedal is at the bottom of the stroke. The angle is measured using a line from the greater trochanter to the lateral femoral condyle, and a line from the lateral femoral condyle to the lateral malleolus.

The choice of saddle is important since many disorders may be caused by inappropriate saddles. Recently, saddles with a groove down the center have been introduced, thus alleviating pressure on the perineum. This helps to prevent pudendal neuropathy, male impotence, vulvar trauma, and traumatic urethritis. If a cyclist uses the bicycle infrequently, it is important that the saddle have adequate cushioning such as gel inserts under the ischial tuberosities. Competitive cyclists frequently choose a saddle based on its weight, but improvements in design and materials allow the racer to purchase a lightweight seat without sacrificing comfort.

The correct fore and aft position of the saddle can be determined by placing the pedals in the 3 and 9 o'clock position with the bicyclist seated comfortably on the saddle. The appropriate fore and aft seat position is found when a plumb line placed on the tibial tubercle of the forward leg drops down through the middle of the ball of the foot and shaft of the pedal. Some bicycle racers prefer to have the seat set back approximately 1 cm from this distance. This allows better traction for the rear wheel during climbing (mountain bikers), improves gluteal muscle recruitment, and permits the cyclist to use larger gears while remaining in the saddle.

The saddle tilt should be parallel to the ground. This can easily be determined using a level. A downward tilt may help relieve pressure on the perineal area, while an upward tilt may lead to urologic and neuropathic problems, as well as perineal skin lesions. One study has suggested that having a 10° anterior depression of the seat may change the lumbar spine orientation, resulting in a decreased incidence of lumbar pain (Salai et al, 1999). This may be tried in patients with low back pain.

The handlebar reach is defined as the distance from the saddle to the handlebars. The appropriate handlebar reach can be found by placing the bicycle on a wind trainer, and having the cyclist sit comfortably on the saddle. The pedals should be at the 3 and 9 o'clock positions, while the hands are placed on the lower part of the handlebars (drops). In this position, the knee on the side of the 3 o'clock pedal position should be within 1 inch of the elbow on the same side. Competitive bicyclists may choose to have a longer handlebar reach, resulting in a more aerodynamic position, while recreational bicyclists often prefer to have a shorter handlebar reach to maintain a more upright position.

The handlebar height should be level with or 1 to 2 inches below the height of the saddle. Novice bicyclists may prefer to have a higher handlebar height in order to maintain a more upright position, while competitive bicyclists often choose to have a handlebar height below the level of the saddle.

The handlebar should be the width of the bicyclist's shoulders measured from acromion to acromion. Mountain bikers frequently mount bar ends on their handlebars. Bar ends are handgrips that extend anterior to the distal ends of the handlebars. These allow the bicyclist to change positions, improve aerodynamics, and alter the biomechanical stress placed on the upper and lower body. Room to place bar ends on the handlebar should be considered when determining the appropriate handlebar width for mountain bikers.

The standard crankarm length is 175 mm. This is appropriate for bicyclists between 5 feet 5 inches and 6 feet tall. Shorter and taller bicyclists should talk to their bicycle dealer about changing to a shorter or longer crankarm, respectively. A longer crank arm provides more leverage and allows bicyclists to push larger gears at a lower cadence and is often used for hill climbing. If the crankarm length is changed on the bicycle, remember to adjust the saddle height.

The proper shoe-pedal interface involves placing the ball of the foot directly over the pedal axle. It is important to adjust the cleats so that the foot is in a neutral position relative to internal and external rotation, in order to prevent knee pain. Many newer pedal systems have built in "float," which allows 15–30° of resistance-free internal and external rotation of the foot in a transverse plane. This permits the bicyclist's foot to find the most biomechanically appropriate position during the pedal cycle, and has been demonstrated to reduce forces across the knee (Gregor, 2000). This may translate into a reduced incidence of overuse knee injuries in bicyclists.

OVERUSE INJURIES

Overuse injuries are a common malady of bicyclists (Mellion, 1991). The most frequent cause of overuse injuries is poor bicycle fit, but other factors include improper training and poor bicycling technique (Mellion, 1991).

When evaluating the bicyclist with an overuse injury, it is important to determine the underlying cause so the appropriate treatment can be instituted. Have the bicyclist bring their bicycle, and set it up on a trainer in the clinic to review the bicycle fit. Discuss their training program and/or review their training log. Finally, ensure that they are using an appropriate gear ratio to maintain an appropriate pedal cadence while riding.

The initial treatment for most overuse injuries includes relative rest, appropriate physical modalities, and anti-inflammatory medications. Relative rest is a very important concept in sports medicine. When treating a bicyclist for an overuse injury, it is important to either find a level of bicycling that the athlete can perform pain-free during the rehabilitation process, or another activity that will maintain their aerobic fitness until they can return to bicycling. Commonly used physical modalities for overuse injuries include ice, heat, electrical stimulation, iontophoresis, ultrasound, and phonophoresis.

The following is a review of the common overuse injuries in bicycling by anatomic region. The discussion of treatments in this section will emphasize appropriate changes in bicycle fit and technique and correction of kinetic chain strength and flexibility deficits.

Foot and Ankle

Overuse injuries to the foot and ankle may include metatarsalgia, compressive neuropathies, plantar fasciitis, or Achilles tendinitis. Metatarsalgia is typically due to mechanical factors such as excessive pedal pressure and an inappropriate shoe-pedal interface. Treatments include adjustment of the shoe-pedal interface, use of a lower gear with a higher cadence, and placement of a metatarsal pad or cushioned orthotic in the cycling shoe (Mellion, 1991).

Compressive neuropathies result in foot paresthesias, often described as "burning feet." Risk factors include excessive pedal pressure, inadequate shoe cushioning, improper shoe size, or toe clip straps that are too tight. Management of compressive neuropathies in the foot begins with attention to footwear. Ensure that the shoe is not too tight. A cushioned orthotic may be placed in the shoe to reduce pressure on the sole of the foot. A metatarsal pad can be added to the shoe if the athlete has a fallen transverse arch. Strength and endurance exercises of the foot intrinsic and ankle support muscles may reduce abnormal foot and ankle biomechanics. Cyclists should adjust their pedaling technique to use a lower gear and higher cadence. If toe clips are being employed, either reducing the tightness of the toe strap or changing to a clipless pedal system may be suggested (Mellion, 1991).

Plantar fasciitis in cyclists may be caused by excessive foot pronation, tight Achilles tendons, weak foot and ankle musculature, or a seat that is too low. Treatments include correction of strength and flexibility deficits. The athlete should be instructed on proper stretching exercises for the Achilles tendons. Strength and endurance exercises for the hip external rotator and abductor muscles may reduce femoral adduction and internal rotation, thereby reducing tibial internal rotation and ankle/foot pronation. Strength and endurance exercises for the foot intrinsic and ankle support muscles should also be employed. Other treatments include using a lower gear with a higher cadence, raising the seat height, and placing a custom orthotic in the cycling shoe. Occasionally a corticosteroid injection is required.

The most common tendinitis in the ankle region of bicyclists is Achilles tendinitis (Cohen, 1993). Achilles tendinitis may be due to training errors, using an excessively large gear, or riding with the seat too low, causing excessive ankle dorsiflexion (Mellion, 1991; Cohen, 1993). Initial treatment includes stretching the gastrocnemius and soleus muscles. Strengthening of the foot intrinsic muscles can begin immediately, while strengthening of the ankle support muscles should begin as the pain resolves. Eccentric strengthening of the calf musculature is an important component of the rehabilitation treatment. Raising the seat and using a lower gear with a higher cadence will both reduce stress on the Achilles tendon. Sport-specific training is the final phase of treatment.

Knee

There are a variety of bicycle-related overuse injuries about the knee. The most common cause of knee pain is patellofemoral joint arthralgia, or "bikers knee" (Sanner et al, 2000; Mellion, 1991; Conti-Wyneken, 1999). Other causes of knee pain may include meniscus injuries, iliotibial band friction syndrome, patellar tendinitis, quadriceps tendinitis, or pes anserine bursitis (Sanner et al, 2000; Mellion, 1991; Conti-Wyneken, 1999). Patellofemoral joint arthralgia in bicyclists has been attributed to excessive retropatellar compressive forces; malalignment at the hip, knee, or ankle; inflexible quadriceps and hamstring muscles; an inflexible iliotibial band; hypoplasia of the vastus medialis obliquus muscle; improper bicycle fit; and poor riding technique (Sanner et al, 2000; Mellion, 1991; Conti-Wyneken, 1999). Adjustments that can be made to the bicycle fit that reduce patellar compressive forces include raising the seat height and/or moving it posteriorly to decrease knee flexion during the pedal cycle. A higher cadence and lower gear should be used while riding. As Dr. Cohen suggests, "if the knees hurt, gear down" (1993). Flexibility and strength deficits in the hip, thigh, lower leg, and foot should be corrected. Strengthening exercises of the quadriceps muscles should emphasize the vastus medialis obliquus head. If the bicyclist has excessive pronation, an orthotic shoe insert may be helpful. Appropriate cleat adjustment on the cycling shoe may reduce patellar malalignment. Occasionally patellar bracing is employed. If the above treatments fail, then surgical consultation may be warranted.

Meniscus injuries may be caused by the twisting motion of the knee during the late power phase of the pedal cycle (Sanner et al, 2000). The bicyclist may complain of joint line pain, mechanical symptoms of locking and clicking, and effusion. While tradition suggests that meniscal injuries require surgical treatment, many peripheral tears are amenable to non-operative treatment. During the relative rest phase of treatment, isometric strengthening exercises for the lower extremity musculature and pain-free range-of-motion exercises can be used. As symptoms resolve, the athlete can begin isotonic followed by sport-specific exercises. When the bicyclist returns to bicycling, the bicycle seat may be lowered to reduce the amount of twisting that occurs at the knee during the late power phase of the pedal cycle. If mechanical symptoms and/or pain persist despite an appropriate non-operative treatment program, surgical consultation may be appropriate.

Iliotibial band friction syndrome is due to excessive rubbing of the distal iliotibial band across the lateral femoral condyle during repetitive knee flexion and extension. Biomechanical and bicycle fit factors that may contribute to this pathology include a tight gluteus maximus muscle, an inflexible iliotibial band, excessive femoral adduction or tibial internal rotation, excessive pronation, and a seat that is too high (Sanner et al, 2000). Treatments include lowering the seat height and possibly moving the seat forward, raising the handlebars, stretching the iliotibial band and gluteus maximus muscle, and using orthotic inserts in the cycling shoes if the cyclist pronates (Sanner et al, 2000). Occasionally, a local injection with steroid medication is necessary.

The pes anserine bursa lies over the anteromedial aspect of the proximal tibia, and reduces friction between the tibia and the distal tendons of the sartorius, gracilis, and semitendinosus muscles. Inflexibility of these muscles or external tibial torsion can cause pes anserine bursitis. Appropriate treatment entails lowering the seat; stretching the sartorius, gracilis, and semitendinosus muscles; strengthening the gluteus maximus, hip external rotator, ankle support, and foot intrinsic muscles; and occasionally a steroid injection.

Patellar and quadriceps tendinitis can also cause anterior knee pain in bicyclists. Treatments include raising the seat and/or moving it backward, stretching the quadriceps muscles, and possibly using a patellar tendon strap or neoprene knee sleeve. Strengthening of the quadriceps muscle should emphasize eccentric exercises. Corticosteroid injections should be avoided due to the risk of tendon rupture.

Hip

The most common overuse injuries in the hip region include greater trochanteric bursitis, iliopsoas tendinitis, and proximal hamstring tendinitis (Mellion, 1991). Greater trochanteric bursitis can be caused by the same factors as iliotibial band friction syndrome. The incidence of greater trochanteric bursitis is higher in female cyclists than male cyclists due to their gynecoid pelvis (Sanner et al, 2000). Treatments for greater trochanteric bursitis are similar to those for iliotibial band friction syndrome. A steroid injection into the greater trochanteric bursa may be helpful.

Iliopsoas tendinitis manifests as pain in the anterior hip and is often seen in bicyclists whose seats are too high (Mellion, 1991). Repetitive rubbing of a tight iliopsoas muscle across the pubic bone may result in a psoas or iliopectineal bursitis. Treatments include stretching the iliopsoas muscle and lowering the seat height.

Many bicyclists develop muscle imbalances with excessively strong quadriceps muscles and relatively weak hamstring muscles (Cohen, 1993). The biomechanics section of this chapter discusses the importance of the hamstring muscles during the pedal cycle. In fact, the hamstring muscles are active during a larger part of the pedal cycle than any other muscle (Sanner et al, 2000). Despite this information, the hamstrings are often neglected in training programs. Overload of the hamstring musculotendinous unit may manifest as pain in the posterior proximal thigh while bicycling. Predisposing factors include weak and inflexible hamstring muscles, training errors, a seat that is too high or too far back, or handlebars that are too low. Treatments include stretching the hamstring muscles, lowering the seat and/or moving it forward, and raising the handlebar height. As the pain resolves, the hamstring muscles should be strengthened using both knee flexion and hip extension exercises. The knee should be kept straight during hip extension exercises to optimize the hamstring muscle's length–tension curve for this movement.

A rare but significant cause of buttock and hamstring pain is related to endofibrotic disease of the femoral or external iliac arteries (Bradshaw, 2000). Cycling causes repetitive hip flexion that can lead to intimal damage and eventual endofibrotic changes in the femoral or external iliac arteries. Symptoms include a feeling of deadness or numbness in the buttock or calf during exercise. The symptoms are relieved by a reduction in the intensity of exercise. Examination may reveal a bruit of the femoral artery with the hip in a flexed position. Pre- and post-exercise ankle-brachial indexes may reveal abnormalities, while the definitive diagnosis is made with angiography. Treatments include activity modification, angioplastic balloon catheter dilation and stenting, bypass surgery, or endarterectomy.

Pelvis

Several different injuries are related to saddle pressure on the buttock and perineum, including ischial tuberosity tenderness and bursitis, buttock and perineal chafing (saddle sores), folliculitis and furuncles, yeast and fungal infections, subcutaneous perineal nodules, pudendal neuropathy (Alcock's syndrome), male impotence, traumatic urethritis, and vulvar trauma (Mellion, 1991; Cohen, 1993).

The early season ischial tuberosity tenderness experienced by most bicyclists is usually self-limited (Mellion, 1991). In some, continued pressure and chafing may progress to skin breakdown commonly referred to as "saddle sores," or subcutaneous perineal nodules. Appropriate seat height, angle, and fore–aft position should be reviewed. The bicycle seat should be approximately 1–2 inches wider than the distance between the ischial tuberosities. If the bicyclist is experiencing significant pressure-related symptoms, then a seat with a gel cushion should be considered. Ensure that the bicyclist is riding with padded bicycling shorts. Using a cream over the perineum reduces friction between the skin and bicycling shorts. This type of cream can be found at bicycle shops. The bicyclist should use a clean pair of bicycling shorts with each ride. This prevents the build up of sweat, dirt, and oils in the clothing that reduces breathability of the bicycle shorts. Sitz baths are also used as an adjunct to treatment. Duoderm can be placed over the area of skin breakdown to provide protection and an appropriate environment for wound healing. The area should be cleansed and the dressing changed daily. Occasionally surgical removal of painful subcutaneous perineal nodules is required.

The cause and treatment of perineal folliculitis and furuncles are similar to those of skin chafing and ulceration. Sitz baths appear to be helpful. Occasionally incision, drainage, and antibiotic medications are required (Mellion, 1991).

If fungal or yeast infections develop, antimicrobial therapy should be instituted. Review proper hygienic practices including showering daily, towel drying the perineum after showering, and wearing clean bicycle shorts on each ride (Cohen, 1993).

Pudendal neuropathy occurs due to compression of the pudendal nerve between the bicycle seat and the pubic symphysis in the area of the Alcock canal (Oberpenning et al, 1994). Symptoms include numbness or paresthesias in the penis or scrotum, or male impotence (Mellion, 1991). Up to 22%

of male long-distance bicyclists report numbness and paresthesias in the genital region, while 13% report impotence (Andersen, 1997). If male impotence occurs, then discontinuation of bicycling until the symptoms resolve is appropriate (Mellion, 1991). Treatment should also begin with a review of appropriate saddle position. Ensure that the seat is level. An upward seat tilt increases perineal pressure. Specially designed bicycle seats with a central groove reduce perineal pressure and symptoms of perineal neuropathy (Keytel et al, 2002). Padded bicycle shorts and bicycle seats with a gel insert also reduce perineal pressure.

Neck and Back

The incidence of neck and back pain in bicycling has been reported to be anywhere from 10–95% (Mellion, 1994). Neck and back pain in bicycling may be related to myofascial pain, repetitive microtrauma to the ligaments, local muscular ischemia, or disc pathology. The positioning of the bicyclist on the bicycle is very important in the etiology and treatment of neck and back pain. The following is a discussion of current causation theories and treatments of bicycle-related neck and back pain.

The lower back provides stability for the lower extremities during the pedal cycle. Having a strong and stable lower back improves the transmission of force from the lower extremities into the pedals. The ideal bicycle fit places the pelvis in a neutral position relative to the lumbar spine and the ischial tuberosities comfortably on the seat. During the pedal cycle, the pelvis and lower back should remain relatively motionless without rocking from side to side, or fore and aft.

A common cause of lower back pain in the bicyclist is poor bicycle fit. If the length of the top tube and stem is too great, then the bicyclist will be flexed too far forward (Mellion, 1991; Mellion, 1994). This places stress on the lumbar paraspinal muscles and the posterior elements of the lumbar vertebrae. If the distance of the top tube and stem is too short, the bicyclist will be sitting too upright, causing increased pressure on the intervertebral discs (Mellion, 1991; Mellion, 1994). Vibration transmitted from the road or trail to the bicyclist can add to the mechanical stress in the low back region.

Seat angle also plays a role in lumbar pain. A study by Salai and associates (1999) revealed that a level seat tends to place the pelvic/lumbar spine angle in hyperextension. By tipping the seat slightly downward, causing an anterior inclination, the pelvic/lumbar spine angle was placed in a more neutral position. The authors tested the clinical applicability of their finding by having a group of bicyclists with lower back pain tip their seats forward slightly. Greater than 70% of the bicyclists reported a reduction in the lower back pain.

Other factors that may contribute to lower back pain in bicyclists include muscular imbalance, muscle weakness, local muscular ischemia, leg length discrepancy, and stress on the lumbar intervertebral discs. Tight iliopsoas, quadriceps, and latissimus dorsi muscles tend to pull the pelvis forward, while tight hamstring muscles pull the pelvis posteriorly (Mellion, 1994). The abdominal muscles are significant pelvic stabilizers and weakness in this area can result in abnormal pelvic movement and positioning during bicycling (Mellion, 1994). All of the muscles providing pelvic stability must perform sustained isometric contractions, which may cause painful local muscular ischemia (Mellion, 1994). Leg length discrepancy can cause the pelvis to rock back and forth over the seat and may increase lower back stress (Mellion, 1994). The lumbar disc is an avascular structure that is dependent on movement to pump nutrients into the disc, and waste products out of the disc. A prolonged static posture could theoretically reduce this process and cause discogenic pain.

The treatment of lower back pain begins with a review of bicycle fit and evaluation of biomechanical contributors. Flexibility imbalances should be corrected. A conditioning program addressing the strength and endurance of the trunk and pelvic stabilizing muscles should be initiated. Any problems with bicycle fit should be corrected. A trial of tipping the front of the seat down may be appropriate. If a leg length discrepancy is identified, a spacer should be placed between the cleat and the shoe on the side of the shorter leg to correct the discrepancy. The bicyclist should be encouraged to change positions frequently while bicycling in order to maintain adequate disc nutrition and reduce the stress on the lower back region.

Neck pain in bicyclists is typically due to myofascial-type pain. Myofascial pain is characterized by tight muscular bands with exquisitely tender points called trigger points (Mellion, 1991). Myofascial pain is commonly found in the cervical and shoulder girdle muscles of bicyclists, and appears to be more common on the left than the right side (Mellion, 1991). This is probably related to riding on the right side of the road and looking more frequently over the left shoulder than the right (Mellion, 1991). While bicycling, the head tends to sit anterior to the thorax. Therefore the cervical and shoulder girdle musculature must constantly contract to prevent the head from falling forward. This results in postural fatigue and contributes to the development of myofascial pain. Errors in bicycle fit that may exacerbate this condition include a long top tube and stem, using the drop handlebars too frequently, and handlebars that are too low.

Morris Mellion has proposed an additional mechanism of cervical pain in bicyclists (Mellion, 1994). The transfer of force from the road or trail surface through the bicycle to the cyclist results in a repetitive vibrational stress to the cervical tissues. Dr. Mellion feels that this may result in a "multiple micro-whiplash" type of injury to the cervical spine causing musculotendinous strain, and contributing to the development of myofascial pain.

Treatment for this condition includes evaluation and correction of bicycle fit errors. These may include a smaller frame size, shorter stem, and/or raising the handlebar height. Using a larger diameter tire, padded handlebar tape or grips, and padded gloves can reduce the vibrational stress from the road or trail. Mountain bikes can reduce vibrational stress further with the use of front and/or rear shock systems. The bicyclist should initially reduce their riding frequency and duration to allow rest of the injured tissues. An exercise program that includes cervical and shoulder girdle strength, endurance, and flexibility exercises should be instituted. The bicyclist should be encouraged to change hand positions on the handlebars frequently, which will result in changes in neck position and reduce postural fatigue.

Upper Extremities

The main bicycle-related overuse injuries in the upper extremities are compression neuropathies. The median and ulnar nerves are both susceptible to injury in the bicyclist. Compression of the ulnar nerve occurs at or near Guyon's canal (Mellion, 1991). This canal is bordered by the pisiform bone

ulnarly, the hook of the hamate radially, the transverse carpal ligament posteriorly, and the pisohamate ligament anteriorly. Typically injuries to the ulnar nerve in Guyon's canal affect both the sensory and motor components of the nerve, but pure motor or sensory neuropathies can occur (Mellion, 1991). While compression is the usual etiology, traction can occur due to prolonged hyperextension of the wrist (Mellion, 1991).

Median neuropathy occurs less frequently than ulnar neuropathy in bicyclists because the carpal tunnel is less susceptible to direct compression injury (Conti-Wyneken, 1999). While prolonged hyperflexion or hyperextension of the wrist may contribute to median nerve injury in the carpal tunnel, other causes of carpal tunnel syndrome should be investigated due to the rarity of this condition in bicyclists.

Almost all compression neuropathies respond to a period of rest. Other treatments for compression neuropathies in the hand and wrist include raising the handlebars and reducing the seat-to-handlebar distance so that less pressure is applied on the hands while bicycling (Mellion, 1991). Padded gloves and handlebar tape or handgrips should be used (Mellion, 1991). The bicyclist should change hand positions on the handlebars frequently, and try to hold their wrists in a neutral position. If symptoms do not improve despite rest and appropriate modifications to bicycle position, technique, and equipment, then further work-up including electrodiagnostic studies and a search for other possible etiologies should be performed.

TRAUMATIC INJURIES

Traumatic and impact injuries range from minor abrasions to fractures and fatal head injuries. The high risk of injury among children emphasizes the need for improved safety measures.

Case-control studies indicate that helmets reduce the risk of head injury by 45–85%, of traumatic brain injury by 65–88%, of facial injury by 28–65%, and of loss of consciousness by 86% (Finnoff et al, 2001). The two accepted standards for bicycle helmets are the American National Standards Institute (ANSI) standard and that of the Snell Memorial Foundation, the latter being the stricter of the two. There is an ANSI or Snell sticker attached to the inside of helmets that meet these standards. A helmet without a sticker provides a false sense of security to the rider. In order for a helmet to be effective, it must be worn at all times for recreation, training, and competition, regardless of the distance to be traveled. It is estimated that 75% of cycling-related deaths are a result of head injury (Burke, 1988).

An approved helmet consists of:

1. A stiff, smooth outer shell that distributes the force of the blow and protects against penetration from sharp objects.
2. A foam liner made from expanded polystyrene that absorbs shock. It should be at least ½ inch thick.
3. A strong retention system should be in place that holds the helmet securely and comfortably against the head. Only about one-half of the forehead should be visible.

Once there has been an impact to the helmet, with or without any visible damage to the inner or outer shell, it is recommended that the helmet be replaced with a new one, as the integrity of the helmet may have been compromised.

A concussion is defined as "a trauma-induced alteration in mental status that may or may not involve loss of consciousness" (Quality Standards Subcommittee, 1997). While many authors suggest that grading concussion severity and determining return to sports activity should be based on a comparison between baseline and postconcussion neuropsychological and balancing testing, these tools are not readily available to most clinicians (Wojtys et al, 1999). The most commonly used clinical scale for determining concussion severity was developed by the American Academy of Neurology (Quality Standards Subcommittee, 1997). A grade 1 concussion was defined as a transient bout of confusion, no loss of consciousness, and resolution of symptoms within 15 minutes. A grade 2 concussion involved a period of transient confusion lasting greater than 15 minutes, and no loss of consciousness. A concussion was considered a grade 3 if any loss of consciousness occurred.

Treatment of concussion depends on severity (Quality Standards Subcommittee, 1997). Certainly any athlete who sustains a grade 3 concussion should be transported to the nearest emergency room for further evaluation. Athletes who sustain a grade 1 concussion can return to competition the same day, while those who sustain a grade 2 concussion should be withheld from sports participation for 7 days after their symptoms resolve. Any athlete who sustains a concussion and continues to have postconcussive type symptoms for more than 7 days should have further diagnostic work-up including imaging studies.

Traumatic injuries to the extremities include contusions, sprains, and fractures. These injuries tend to occur on the left side of the body (Bohlmann, 1981). This may reflect the fact that most cyclists find right-hand turns easier than left-hand ones, and tend to slow or hesitate when making fast left turns. With the derailleur and drive train or working parts of the bike on the right, cyclists prefer to fall to their left to protect these components. In competitive cycling, track races are run counterclockwise, whereas road races are run in both directions.

The most common fractures sustained in cycling are those involving the upper extremities. Clavicular fractures usually occur from a fall on the point of the shoulder or on the outstretched arm. Most fractures occur in the middle third of the clavicle. The diagnosis is usually obvious with a visible deformity, pain, crepitus, or fracture motion. Radiographs confirm the diagnosis. Clavicular fractures are described by the location of the fracture (middle, distal, or proximal third), amount of angulation, and displacement.

Treatment for the nondisplaced or minimally displaced fracture consists of symptomatic treatment with a sling or a figure-of-8 bandage for 6–8 weeks (until the fracture is healed), analgesics as needed, and early rehabilitation with gentle range-of-motion exercises of the shoulder to maintain mobility. The athlete should not ride or train for at least 1 week postinjury. Once the pain has subsided, he or she may train on a wind trainer or stationary bicycle while continuing to wear the figure-of-8 bandage until the fracture has healed. Follow-up radiographs should be taken at 6 weeks postinjury to confirm fraction union. Bicycling on the road or trail should not resume until the fracture is healed. If there is significant displacement or severe skin tenting over the fracture, then open reduction and internal fixation is recommended. In order to help prevent clavicular fractures, the cyclist should learn to fall with the arms held near the body, and to "tuck and roll." Beginners can practice this on soft grass.

Acromioclavicular (AC) joint sprains, also known as shoulder separations, usually result from a direct blow to the point of the shoulder when falling from the bike. Occasionally this injury can occur from a fall onto an outstretched arm, transmitting the forces up to the AC joint. The cyclist presents with pain, tenderness, swelling, and possibly deformity at the injury site.

There are three grades of AC joint sprains according to the extent of ligament injury. Clinical examination and radiographs are required for accurate diagnosis. Comparison views with the uninjured AC joint can be helpful. A stress view of the AC joint may assist in grading the injury. Radiographs also rule out fractures in the region of the AC joint.

A grade 1 sprain is a mild sprain of the acromioclavicular (AC) and coracoclavicular (CC) ligaments with no separation of the joint. There is tenderness and swelling over the AC joint with minimal decrease in shoulder movement. The AC joint is stable.

Treatment of grade 1 sprains is conservative with ice, analgesics, and antiinflammatory medications, a sling for support, and local physical modalities. Gentle range-of-motion and strengthening exercises can begin as the pain resolves. Road riding can resume as tolerated, preferably on smooth level terrain initially. The cyclist can return to racing when the AC joint is nontender and shoulder range of motion is full, usually 2–3 weeks postinjury. As a safety precaution when returning to cycling, the athlete may tape a 1-inch-thick rubber doughnut pad over the AC joint for protection.

A grade 2 sprain involves a complete tear of the AC ligament, with little or no injury to the CC ligaments. There is considerable tenderness and swelling over the AC joint and mild tenderness over the CC ligaments. Shoulder range of motion is significantly limited secondary to pain. Further injury may easily convert a grade 2 sprain to a grade 3 sprain.

Treatment involves early sling immobilization for comfort. The athlete should take the sling off several times a day and perform elbow and gentle passive shoulder range-of-motion exercises. As the pain resolves, the sling can be discontinued and more aggressive range-of-motion and strengthening exercises can be initiated. Riding a stationary bicycle or wind trainer can begin when the athlete can tolerate this activity. Bicycling on the road or trail is not recommended until the athlete has full pain-free shoulder range of motion, which usually takes 3–4 weeks.

A grade 3 sprain involves a complete tear of the AC and CC ligaments, and may be associated with injuries to the trapezius or deltoid muscles. There is marked swelling, tenderness, and obvious deformity of the AC joint.

Typically, treatment is conservative with the same progression as described for a grade 2 sprain. Return to outdoor riding may take as long as 10–12 weeks. The operative approach has been advocated by some for manual workers and elite athletes. However, recent research does not support the routine use of surgery for the treatment of grade 3 AC sprains (Schlegel et al, 2001). Referral to an orthopedic specialist may be warranted to assist in the management of this injury. Possible complications from this injury include degenerative changes of the acromion with osteophyte formation, soft tissue calcification, and osteolysis of the distal clavicle.

Traumatic wrist injuries generally occur from a fall on an outstretched hand. Fractures of the carpal bones should be ruled out when evaluating acute wrist injuries in bicyclists. Tenderness to palpation over the scaphoid in the anatomic snuffbox is highly suggestive of a fractured scaphoid. Radiographs of the wrist should include scaphoid views. Often the initial radiographs are negative despite clinical findings suggesting a fracture.

If a scaphoid fracture is suspected despite a negative radiograph, treatment should begin with immobilization using a plaster or fiberglass thumb spica cast with the wrist in slight radial deviation and dorsiflexion. Repeat radiographs should be performed in 2 weeks. If the radiographs remain negative despite a high clinical suspicion of a scaphoid fracture, a bone scan may be used to confirm the diagnosis. Usually the fracture heals within 8–12 weeks, but can occasionally take up to 20 weeks. Complications such as nonunion, delayed union, and avascular necrosis have been reported with scaphoid fractures. All displaced fractures of the carpals should be referred to an orthopedic surgeon for treatment.

Acute wrist ligament sprains are initially treated with rest, appropriate splinting, compression, ice, and elevation. As the pain resolves, gentle range-of-motion and isometric exercises may be added. Progression to more aggressive range-of-motion and strengthening exercises can be made as healing occurs.

Bicycle spoke injuries occur when a body part is trapped between the frame and the spokes of a bicycle (Helzer-Julin, 1994). This can result in laceration, crushing, and shearing injuries. Sometimes the true severity of the injury is not apparent for several days, so these injuries should be closely monitored. The bicycle should be equipped with a spoke guard if there is a child carrier attached to the bicycle. "Doubling," or giving another person a ride on a bicycle, should be prohibited.

Injuries to the abdomen can occur from bicycle accidents. These injuries can be quite severe, and insidious development of symptoms may delay appropriate diagnosis and treatment. A review of the literature regarding abdominal injuries from bicycle accidents was presented in the etiology section of this chapter. Health care providers involved in the initial evaluation of bicyclists who have sustained an abdominal injury should maintain a high index of suspicion regarding internal injuries and early diagnostic studies should be performed when indicated.

"Road rash," the term used for abrasions sustained while cycling, is the most common skin-related traumatic cycling injury. The severity of the wound is graded as follows:

1. First degree: involves just the epidermis
2. Second degree: extends through the epidermis and partially through the dermis
3. Third degree: extends through the epidermis and dermis to the subcutaneous tissue and/or muscle

It is imperative that the wound be thoroughly cleansed and embedded dirt particles removed soon after the injury has occurred to prevent infection and tattooing. Sterile water and antibacterial solutions or water-diluted hydrogen peroxide can be used. If these are not available, then use tap water and soap. If the cleansing is done within the first few minutes after the injury there is often decreased pain, possibly owing to numbness in the area from the trauma. As time from the injury elapses, there is increased pain and local edema. Topical or local injectable analgesics such as xylocaine can be used to reduce the pain during proper cleaning of the wound. A prepackaged surgical sponge/brush can be used to assist in wound cleansing.

After the wound is cleaned, a topical antibiotic ointment and a nonadherent dressing are applied and held in place with a gauze wrap or tubular netting. This dressing is changed 1–2 times a day until the abrasion has healed. An alternative dressing involves placing a hydroactive dressing such DuoDerm over the area and changing it every 2–3 days until the wound has healed. A tetanus shot should be given if the bicyclist is not up to date on their immunizations. Complete healing takes place in 10–12 days. To prevent further scarring and blistering, sunscreen should be applied over the healed area.

Abrasions are usually associated with contusions so the area should be treated with ice. Monitor for signs of compartment syndrome or myositis ossificans traumatica if a significant contusion occurs. Wearing a thin layer of clothing underneath the usual cycling attire can reduce the risk of road rash because the two layers of fabric slide over each other.

ENVIRONMENTAL INJURIES

Environmental injuries from sun, heat, or cold exposure can occur in bicyclists (Helzer-Julin, 1994). Solar injury includes sunburn and skin damage. Heat injuries include heat syncope, heat cramps, heat exhaustion, and heat stroke. Cold-related injuries include hypothermia and superficial or deep frostbite. A comprehensive discussion of environmental injuries is presented in Chapter 28.

Prevention strategies are effective for environmental injuries. Clothing should be appropriate for the weather. In the summer heat, clothing should be a lightweight synthetic fabric such as Lycra, which allows dissipation of heat. In cold weather, bicyclists should wear several layers of loose clothing starting with a base layer that maintains its insulation properties while wet with sweat. An example would be polypropylene. The outer layer should be water-repellent and windproof. It is also important to provide extra covering for the feet in temperatures at or below 40°F (Helzer-Julin, 1994).

Bicyclists riding in the sun should use sunscreen with a skin protection factor (SPF) rating of at least 15 (Helzer-Julin, 1994). Acclimatization to hot or cold weather can help reduce the incidence of environmental injury. It is extremely important to ensure adequate fluid and electrolyte intake during bicycling, particularly in hot weather. The bicyclist should drink adequate fluid to replace sweat losses with water or sports drinks. A half-hour ride with pre- and post-ride nude weights will provide an estimate of fluid losses based on the change in weight. Doubling the weight loss in one-half hour will give the fluid required to give adequate replacement during a bike ride.

It is also important to be aware of the relationship between certain medications and environmental injury. Medications with anticholinergic or antihistamine properties inhibit sweating. Beta-blockers reduce cardiac output. Diuretics may predispose to dehydration and electrolyte disturbances. Amphetamines mask symptoms of fatigue and predispose to heart failure and hyperthermia. Ephedrine and ephedra increase heart rate and interfere with heat homeostasis, increasing the risk of heat stroke during activity.

PREVENTION

Many principles of prevention have already been discussed in this chapter. It is important to ensure that the bicycle fits the bicyclist properly to reduce overuse injuries. The bicyclist should be educated to change positions frequently while riding, and to use an appropriate cadence. The bicycle should be tuned up regularly to prevent equipment malfunction or failure.

To prevent traumatic injuries, steps should be taken to reduce the chance of falling. First, ride under control. Bicyclists should ride slower over unfamiliar terrain to improve the chances of successful evasive maneuvering if an unexpected obstacle should appear. Constantly paying attention while riding helps prevent injuries since even familiar terrain can change from one day to the next, particularly in mountain biking. Competitive bicyclists should try to ride the course prior to the race day so the terrain is familiar. Consider practicing a tuck-and-roll fall on a grassy surface to help prevent traumatic upper extremity injuries. Never ride while intoxicated.

Appropriate clothing and protective equipment is essential. All bicyclists should wear a helmet that is approved by ANSI or the Snell Memorial Foundation every time they ride their bicycle. Clothing appropriate for the weather is important. Wearing a thin base layer of clothing underneath the jersey reduces the incidence and severity of road rash on the trunk after a fall. Padded bike shorts and gloves reduce compression-type injuries to these areas. Applying cream to the perineum can reduce injuries to the perineum caused by friction. Clean clothing should be worn on each ride. For mountain bicyclists who enjoy riding fast downhill, they should wear clothing that covers the entire arms and legs, and possibly additional padding over bony prominences such as the elbows and knees. A light and reflective gear should be used while riding in reduced light conditions and at night.

Eyewear should be worn to protect the bicyclist's eyes from mud, dirt, dust, rocks, wind, and rain. It is important to choose eyewear that is constructed from unbreakable material such as polycarbonate. Most eyewear also provides some protection from ultraviolet radiation.

Appropriate conditioning not only prevents injuries, but also increases the enjoyment of bicycling. Training can be thought of as a yearly cycle composed of three periods: preseason, in-season, and postseason. A brief discussion of each follows.

During the preseason, the bicyclist should maintain general conditioning through dynamic trunk stabilization exercises, proprioceptive exercise, circuit training, weight training, and aerobic exercise (Burke, 2000). In addition to the legs, bicycling (particularly mountain biking) is very demanding on the bicyclist's upper body and trunk, and these areas should not be neglected during this phase of conditioning. Resistance training should be performed 2 to 4 times per week, while aerobic conditioning should be performed 3–6 times per week. In the preseason, the emphasis of aerobic conditioning should be on long, slow distance activities that improve the body's oxidative capacity (Burke, 2000). If bicycling is used during this period, the cadence should be maintained between 90 and 110 rpm with a low pedaling resistance (Burke, 2000).

During the in-season phase of conditioning, the focus switches from general strengthening and long, slow aerobic workouts, to interval and race-pace (tempo) training designed to improve the body's lactic acid tolerance, and sprint training to improve the body's use of the ATP-phosphocreatine system (Burke, 2000). A maintenance program of general strength and trunk stabilization training may be performed two times per week during this phase. A sample program during the in-season phase would include:

1. Monday: easy 2- to 3-hour ride
2. Tuesday: interval training

3. Wednesday: tempo training interspersed with sprints and trunk and strength training
4. Thursday: easy 1- to 2-hour ride
5. Friday: easy 1-hour ride
6. Saturday: Race or race simulation
7. Sunday: Race or race simulation, trunk and strength training

The postseason is often called the period of "active rest." This time period should not be dedicated to deconditioning, but instead the postseason should involve activities other than biking that are enjoyable but maintain a moderate to high level of aerobic conditioning (Burke, 2000). During the postseason, it is important to recover emotionally and physically from the in-season phase while maintaining fitness for the upcoming season.

CONCLUSION

In summary, cycling injuries can result from overuse or trauma. Injury prevention strategies include proper bicycle fit, correct cycling technique, appropriate protective equipment and clothing, a good training regimen, and practicing a tuck-and-roll type fall. Despite these strategies, both traumatic and atraumatic injuries will still occur. Thus it is important for health care providers who work with bicyclists to be prepared to assess and manage these injuries.

BIBLIOGRAPHY

Andersen K, Bovim G. Impotence and nerve entrapment in long distance amateur cyclists. *Acta Neurol Scand.* 1997;95:233–240.

Bohlmann J. Injuries in competitive cycling. *Phys Sports Med.* 1981;9:117–124.

Brogger-Jensen T, Hvass I, Bugge S. Injuries at the BMX Cycling European Championship, 1989. *Br J Sports Med.* 1990;24:269–270.

Bradshaw C. Exercise-related lower leg pain: Vascular. *Med Sci Sports Exerc.* 2000;32:S34–S36.

Burke E. Physiology of cycling. In: Garrett W, Kirkendall DT, ed. *Exercise and Sports Science.* Philadelphia: Lippincott Williams & Wilkins; 2000:759–770.

Burke E. Safety standards for bicycle helmets. *Phys Sports Med.* 1988;16:148–153.

Burke E. The physiological characteristics of competitive cyclists. *Physician Sportsmed.* 1980;8:78–84.

Chow T, Bracker MD, Patrick K. Acute injuries from mountain biking. *West J Med.* 1993;159:145–148.

Clarnette T, Beasley SW. Handlebar injuries in children: patterns and prevention. *Aust NZ J Surg.* 1997;67:338–339.

Cohen G. Cycling injuries. *Canadian Family Physician.* 1993;39:628–632.

Conti-Wyneken A. Bicycling injuries. *Phys Med Rehabil Clin North Am.* 1999;10:67–76.

Coyle E, Feltner ME, Kautz SA, et al. Physiological and biomechanical factors associated with elite endurance cycling performance. *Med Sci Sports Exerc.* 1991;23:93–107.

Coyle E. Integration of the physiological factors determining endurance performance ability. *Exerc Sports Sci Rev.* 1995;23:25–63.

Dannenberg A, Needle S, Mullady D, et al. Predictors of injury among 1638 riders in a recreational long-distance bicycle tour: Cycle across Maryland. *Am J Sports Med.* 1996;24:747–753.

Eilert-Petersson E, Schelp L. An epidemiological study of bicycle related injuries. *Accid Anal Prev.* 1997;29:363–372.

Ekman R, Welander G, Svanstrom L, et al. Bicycle-related injuries among the elderly—A new epidemic? *Public Health.* 2001;115:38–43.

Erez I, Ludwig L, Gutermacher M, et al. Abdominal injuries caused by bicycle handlebars. *Eur J Surg*. 2001;167:331–333.

Finnoff J, Laskowski ER, Altman KL, et al. Barriers to bicycle helmet use. *Pediatrics*. 2001;108:1–7.

Gregor R. Biomechanics of Cycling. In: Garrett W, Kirkendall DT, eds. *Exercise and Sport Science*. Philadelphia: Lippincott Williams & Wilkins; 2000;515–537.

Helzer-Julin M. Sun, heat, and cold injuries in cyclists. *Clin Sports Med*. 1994;13:219–234.

Keytel L, Noakes TD. Effects of a novel bicycle saddle on symptoms and comfort in cyclists. *S Afr Med J*. 2002;92:295–298.

Koestner A, Hoak S. A 6 year old with a pancreatic injury from bicycle handlebars. *J Emerg Nurs*. 1999;25:84–87.

Krishnan S, Rathjen KE. Open iliac wing fracture caused by penetrating injury from a bicycle handlebar. *J Orthop Trauma*. 2002;16:277–279.

Kronisch R, Chow TK, Simon LM, et al. Acute injuries in off-road bicycle racing. *Am J Sports Med*. 1996b;24:88–93.

Kronisch R, Pfeiffer RP, Chow TK. Acute injuries in cross-country and downhill off-road bicycle racing. *Med Sci Sports Exerc*. 1996a;28:1351–1355.

Kronisch R, Pfeiffer RP, Chow TK, et al. Gender differences in acute mountain bike racing injuries. *Clin J Sport Med*. 2002;12:158–164.

Kubota A, Shono J, Yonekura T, et al. Handlebar hernia: Case report and review of pediatric cases. *Pediatr Surg Int*. 1999;15:411–412.

Lofthouse G. Traumatic injuries to the extremities and thorax. *Clin Sports Med*. 1994;13:113–135.

Lovell M, Brett M, Enion DS. Mountain bike injury to the abdomen, transection of the pancreas and small bowel evisceration. *Injury*. 1992;23:499–500.

Mellion M. Common cycling injuries: Management and prevention. *Sports Med*. 1991;11:52–70.

Mellion M. Neck and back pain in bicycling. *Clin Sports Med*. 1994;13:137–164.

National Safety Council. *Injury facts*. Itasca, Illinois: National Safety Council; 1999;101, 118.

Nehoda H, Hochleitner BW. Subcapsular liver haematomas caused by bar ends in mountain bike crashes. *Lancet*. 1998;351:342.

Oberpenning F, Roth S, Leusmann DB, et al. Alcock syndrome: Temporary penile insensitivity due to compression of the pudendal nerve within the Alcock canal. *J Urol*. 1994;151:423–425.

Pfeiffer R, Kronisch RL. Off-road cycling injuries. *Sports Med*. 1995;19:311–325.

Powell E, Tanz RR. Tykes and bikes: Injuries associated with bicycle-towed child trailers and bicycle mounted child seats. *Arch Pediatr Adolesc Med*. 2000;154:351–353.

Quality Standards Subcommittee. Practice parameter: The management of concussion in sports (summary statement). *Neurology*. 1997;48:581–585.

Richmond D. Handlebar problems in bicycling. *Clin Sports Med*. 1994;13:165–173.

Rivara F, Thompson DC, Thompson RS, et al. Injuries involving off-road cycling. *J Fam Pract*. 1997;44:481–485.

Roth J, Boyd CR. Recreational bicycling and injury to the external iliac artery. *Am Surg*. 1999;65:460–463.

Ryschon T. Physiologic aspects of bicycling. *Clin Sports Med*. 1994;13:15–38.

Salai M, Brosh T, Blankstein A, et al. Effect of changing the saddle angle on the incidence of low back pain in recreational bicyclists. *Br J Sports Med*. 1999;33:398–400.

Sanner W, O'Halloran WD. The biomechanics, etiology, and treatment of cycling injuries. *J Am Podiatr Med Assoc*. 2000;90:354–376.

Sarfati M, Galt SW, Treiman GW, et al. Common femoral artery injury secondary to bicycle handlebar trauma. *J Vasc Surg*. 2002;35:589–591.

Schlegel T, Burks RT, Marcus RL, et al. A prospective evaluation of untreated acute grade III acromioclavicular separations. *Am J Sports Med*. 2001;29:699–703.

Segers M, Wink D, Clevers GJ. Bicycle spoke injuries: A prospective study. *Injury.* 1997;28:267–269.

Tanz R, Christoffel KK. Tykes on bikes: Injuries associated with bicycle mounted child seats. *Pediatr Emerg Care.* 1991;7:297–301.

Thompson M, Rivara F. Bicycle-related injuries. *Am Fam Physician.* 2001;63:2007–2014, 2017–2018.

Wilber R, Zawadzki KM, Kearney JT, et al. Physiologic profiles of elite off-road and road cyclists. *Med Sci Sports Exerc.* 1997;29:1090–1094.

Wojtys E, Hovda D, Landry G, et al. Concussion in sports. *Am J Sports Med.* 1999;27:676–687.

42 | Racquet Sports: Tennis, Squash, Badminton, and Racquetball

Marc R. Safran

Tennis is by far the most popular of all of the racquet sports, especially in the United States. Over 20 million people participate in tennis in the United States at least once a year, with more than 5 million playing tennis at least twice a month. Tennis is an individual, non-contact sport played on a court 78 feet long with a net 3 feet in height dividing the court into two equal parts. The court is 27 feet wide for singles, with one player on each side of the net. Doubles is played with 2 players on each side of the net with the court 36 feet wide.

The racquets measure 27–29 inches long, though the maximum length allowed is up to 32 inches. There is no weight restriction on the rackets, though current technology has resulted in rackets weighing $7\frac{1}{2}$–13 ounces. Racquets which were once made of wood are now made of fiberglass, graphite, and titanium. Strings are made from resilient gut or nylon. The tennis ball is hollow, composed of inflated rubber and covered with fabric. The ball measures $2\frac{1}{2}$–$2\frac{5}{8}$ inches in diameter and weighs 2–$2\frac{1}{16}$ ounces. The ball may travel at a velocity of up to 140 mph with adult players on the serve and 85 mph on the return. The court surfaces may be hard court, clay (and har-tru), grass, or carpet. Tennis is usually played outdoors, though it may be played indoors, usually on carpet.

The International Badminton Federation estimates that 1 billion people play badminton worldwide. Badminton is a very popular sport, especially in China, Indonesia, and Malaysia. It is estimated that almost 10 million people in the United States played badminton at least once in 1998, though this number includes social backyard games. It is estimated that nearly 1 million people play badminton more than twice a month.

Badminton is an individual, noncontact sport played on a court 20 feet wide and 44 feet long with the court evenly divided in two lengthwise by a net 5 feet high at the center. Opponents are on opposite sides of the net. This sport is usually played indoors on a wood floor. The shuttlecock is made of 16 feathers with a fixed base. The shuttlecock is almost cone shaped, $2\frac{1}{2}$–$2\frac{3}{4}$ inches long with a diameter of $2\frac{1}{4}$–$2\frac{5}{8}$ inches at one end and 1–$1\frac{1}{8}$ of an inch around at the other; it weighs between 4.7 and 5.5 grams. The racquets are much lighter than those used in tennis (3–3.7 ounces). The rackets are $26\frac{3}{4}$ inches long. The head length cannot exceed $11\frac{3}{8}$ inches. The shuttlecock may travel up to 200 mph in world-class adult play.

It is estimated that 18 million people play squash worldwide, and in the United States 500,000 play at least once a year, and less than 150,000 play regularly. Squash is a sport played in an indoor enclosed court. The North American type court is more narrow than the international sized court and measures $16\frac{1}{2}$ feet by 32 feet, and is enclosed by a ceiling that is used in play. In the American game, a 15-point score wins, whereas in the English rules the server must score 9 points to win. The first player to win three games wins the match. The American ball is more solid and bouncy, and the English ball makes a "squash" sound when it hits. The player has more time to retrieve the ball in the English game. Racquets measure 27 inches in length and weigh 7½–9 ounces. The strung racquet head measures 7½ × 8½ inches, though racquets with larger heads are now available. The ball velocity has been measured at over 110 mph after direct contact. The players are in close proximity in singles and especially in doubles.

Racquetball was invented in 1949 by an individual who sought a fast-paced game that was easy to learn on a handball court. Racquetball has grown to approximately 7 million players a year in the United States, and 8 million worldwide. More than 1.5 million of the participants play at least twice a month.

The racquetball court is enclosed with a ceiling that is used in play. The court is 40 feet in length and 20 feet in width. The height of the front wall is 20 feet, while the back wall is equal to or greater than 12 feet. The racquet cannot exceed 22 inches in length. The ball is soft, weighs 1.4 ounces, and has a diameter of 2¼ inches. The ball travels consistently at 127 mph during highly competitive play after a direct hit. The players are in close proximity, both in singles and doubles.

Squash, racquetball, and badminton are faster games than tennis and more taxing on the joints. Sudden deaths, although rare, occur in squash and racquetball owing to the intensity of the cardiovascular workout.

Tennis is a very versatile game that allows people of all ages and physical statures to play satisfactorily against their peers. Players of different ability can rally well, although minor skill differences can result in large score differences in a game. Conditioning is vital for singles play, whereas doubles is more forgiving. To play well in singles, one usually needs additional cardiovascular training (ie, interval running), whereas a doubles player does not need that additional work. It can usually give senior players a satisfactory workout over the course of 1 hour.

This chapter reviews injuries in each of these racquet sports; however, the focus will be on tennis injuries and associated factors.

TENNIS INJURIES

Most injuries in tennis are classified as overuse injuries. Some series report injury rates as high as 74% in men and 60% in women in world-class players. The most common injuries are to the back, shoulder, and elbow in that order. Muscle cramps and strains of the ankle extensors (rupture of the medial head of the gastrocnemius [tennis leg] and Achilles tendon ruptures) frequently occur. Ankle sprains are the most common acute injury and occur most often on hard courts.

Upper Extremity Injuries

Shoulder

The shoulder girdle is especially prone to injury because it has to maximally accelerate and decelerate the arm while maintaining precise control over the racquet at ball strike. A tennis player performs repetitive motions that generate high-magnitude forces about the shoulder during the various tennis strokes. Due to the repetitious nature of these forces, it may be difficult to maintain the balance between motion and stability in the shoulder. The serve, high forehand and backhand volley strokes, and overhead smash also place large stresses on the shoulder and rotator cuff.

The shoulder is the most frequently affected part of the upper extremity, with rotator cuff inflammation being one of the most common injuries in tennis players of all levels. Rotator cuff inflammation usually occurs as a result of chronic repetitive swinging of the racquet, including overhead serving. Pain from rotator cuff inflammation is associated with shoulder abduction such as with serves, overhead smashes, high backhand volleys, and the follow through with the backhand stroke. As many as 50% of adult tennis players and 30% of junior players complain of shoulder pain at some time. It is usually the older players that may have rotator cuff impingement, rotator cuff tear, or shoulder degenerative arthritis of the glenohumeral and/or acromioclavicular (AC) joints. In contrast with the older player, the young player's rotator cuff symptoms are more often secondary to mild instability of the glenohumeral joint. Instability may result in labral degeneration or tears. Other shoulder injuries include humeral periostitis and bicipital tendinitis. To prevent and rehabilitate the tennis player's shoulder overuse syndromes, imbalances must be corrected. Specifically it is important to (1) improve glenohumeral internal rotation, (2) stretch the posterior capsule; and (3) strengthen the posterior rotator cuff and scapular stabilizing muscles.

Less common shoulder injuries have also been described in the young tennis player. Traction apophysitis of the shoulder is similar to Osgood-Schlatter's disease of the knee. It is an overuse injury caused by repetitive microtrauma at the insertion of the supraspinatus muscle into the greater tuberosity, or the subscapularis muscle into the lesser tuberosity of the humerus. Slipped capital humeral epiphysis occurs secondary to shear and distraction caused by rotational forces about the shoulder. Widening of the physis or slight slippage may be seen, but severe slippage is not usually present.

Tennis shoulder refers to a drooping, internally rotated shoulder caused by long-term overhead arm use contributing to generalized laxity of the shoulder capsule and musculature (Fig. 42-1). This is more common in professional players or those who have played for many years. Tennis shoulder may potentiate rotator cuff symptoms due to the protracted scapula not allowing the acromion to rotate sufficiently out of the way from the greater tuberosity. Drooping of the shoulder may also be associated with thoracic outlet syndrome.

Acute shoulder injuries are uncommon in tennis, though shoulder dislocations and AC joint separations may occur from collisions with the wall in squash and racquetball or as the result of a fall in any racquet sport.

Elbow

Lateral epicondylitis (tennis elbow), medial epicondylitis, and injury to the medial epicondylar apophyseal growth plate in skeletally immature players are common injuries about the elbow seen in tennis players. Up to 25% of elite junior tennis players complain of elbow pain. Due to the rapid, repetitive arm movements required in the other racquet sports, medial and lateral epicondylitis has been reported in badminton, squash and racquetball. On the lateral aspect of the elbow, epicondylitis involves the wrist extensors, and is thought to be the result of repetitive microtraumatic injury that results in microtears of the muscular origin. Focal degeneration and healing with vascular and fibroblastic proliferation suggests this is a degenerative process. Lateral epicondylitis occurs more frequently in recreational tennis players, particularly those with poor mechanics of the backhand. When the pain is

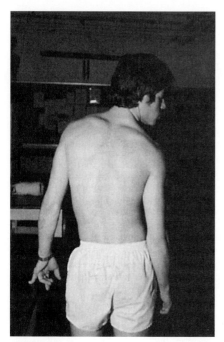

FIG 42-1 Tennis shoulder. Early one-sided training and excessive loading lead to tennis shoulder. The racquet arm has enlarged bones and muscles, and increased laxity of the joint capsule occurs. The shoulder is lowered and the arm is relatively lengthened. Also note an S-shaped scoliosis of the thoracic spine.

quite acute, physiotherapy is usually beneficial, including icing the painful area and stretching and strengthening of the wrist extensor muscles. Three steroid injections right into the periosteum over the lateral epicondyle and adjacent to the extensor tendon can be done. Additionally, counterforce bracing may be beneficial to reduce stress to the degenerative tendon while it is healing. Extracorporeal shock wave therapy can be effective for lateral epicondylitis.

Medially, the medial epicondylar growth plate, the flexor mass, or the medial collateral ligament may be involved. Medial epicondylitis occurs much less frequently than lateral epicondylitis, though it tends to occur in higher level tennis players. It has been noted that the incidence of tennis elbow in world-class athletes ranges from 35–45%. The incidence is much lower in elite junior athletes, supporting the opinion that tennis elbow is related to age. Again, stretching and strengthening of the wrist flexors and pronator are recommended, while bracing and steroid injections are also effective. Surgery is less effective in the medial aspect, whereas a lateral tennis elbow release is usually a satisfactory procedure in the 10% of cases that are resistant to conservative therapy.

In addition, small avulsion fractures may occur because of the anatomy of the adolescent elbow. Non-union of the medial or lateral epicondyle is rare. Ulnar collateral ligament injuries in the tennis player are uncommon.

Hand and Wrist

Hand and wrist complaints are common in tennis players, especially females, and can occur in either wrist. Tendinitis of the wrist may develop in elite players who put a lot of spin on their shots or in novices with mechanically improper technique. Wrist extensors are most frequently involved, but flexor tendons may be involved as well. DeQuervain's stenosing tenosynovitis is one of the most common tendon problems seen in the tennis player. This usually occurs due to shearing within the fibro-osseous sheath from repeated ulnar deviation. This can be treated by cortisone injection and physical therapy modalities, but often needs surgical release.

Insertional tendinitis of the extensor carpi radialis longus and brevis tendons commonly occurs in tennis players at the base of the second and third metacarpals and is usually associated with carpal bossing. Extensor carpi ulnaris tendinitis is primarily due to overuse or technical flaws, and often is associated with triangular fibrocartilage tears or ulno-carpal impingement. It is often seen in the non-dominant wrist of players with two-handed backhands, possibly due to the overuse during the backswing. Extensor digitorum communis tendinitis, particularly of the index and little fingers due to their oblique course across the wrist, is often seen in tennis players. Tendinitis of the extensor pollicis longus uncommonly occurs in tennis players as the tendon passes Lister's tubercle. Tendinitis at the insertion of the dorsal interossei into the proximal phalanges may occur in tennis players from repeated gripping. Occult dorsal ganglions may be the most common cause of radial wrist pain in the tennis player. Swelling associated with the different forms of tendinitis often improves with splinting, anti-inflammatory medications, and cortisone injection when necessary. Stretching and strengthening of the muscle-tendon units help prevent recurrence.

Recurrent dislocation of the extensor carpi ulnaris tendon is associated with hypersupination and ulnar deviation in tennis players, such as with a backspin slice or low forehand or slice, or topspin service motion.

The evaluation of the wrist also should include the possibility of a fracture of the hook of the hamate (from abutment with the bottom of the grip), injury to the triangular fibrocartilage complex (TFCC), ulno-carpal impingement, chondromalacia of the pisiform, ulnar nerve compression in Guyon's canal, ulnar artery thrombosis, median nerve entrapment in the carpal canal, and triquetro-lunate ligament injury; however, these are less common causes of wrist pain in tennis players. Wrist fractures and dislocations have been reported with all the racquet sports from falls, though collision with a wall may also be a mechanism of injury. It is important to order special x-ray views depending on the site of injury, including special hamate views if injury to this bone is suspected. TFCC injuries can be diagnosed by MRI or arthroscopically. These injuries are treated arthroscopically with debridement of the tear, though occasionally a repair may be performed. Debridement allows for return to tennis within 4–6 weeks. Chondromalacia of the pisiform may be treated with excision of the pisiform, and a fracture of the hook of the hamate may also be treated by removal of the fracture fragment. Carpal tunnel syndrome and ulnar nerve entrapment respond well to surgical decompression if conservative treatment including relative rest, anti-inflammatory medications, splinting, and therapy fail.

Digital nerve compression, particularly of the index finger, may occur at the radial digital nerve due to pressure between the metacarpal head and the racquet handle.

Forearm

Stress fractures of the ulna of the non-dominant forearm in adolescents, as well as distal radius and ulna fractures of the dominant wrist have been reported and should be kept in mind when evaluating the tennis player with forearm and wrist pain. These injuries to the non-dominant forearm occur in players who use a two-handed backhand.

Central Region Injuries (Back and Trunk)

Overuse injuries of the central region are common in the racquet sports athlete. It has been reported that 38% of professional male tennis players reported missing at least one tournament because of low back pain and up to 50% of elite junior tennis players noted a history of low back pain. There are several sources of low back pain in the tennis player. High demands placed on the lower back and trunk combined with low flexibility patterns result in frequent overuse-type injuries. The three areas most often involved are: (1) the posterior midline paraspinal musculature (used in the service motion, when charging the net or when dropping straight back for a volley); (2) the peripheral trunk musculature (ie, the quadratus lumborum or oblique muscles used during the service motion or in ground strokes); and (3) the rectus abdominis (tears in this muscle may be associated with hitting overhead strokes or serves). Other potential causes of low back pain include intervertebral disk degeneration and herniation, facet impingement, sacroiliac joint dysfunction, and spondylolysis due to the repetitive hyperextension and rotation of the spine.

Injuries to the abdominal muscles occur frequently during serves, particularly to the nondominant rectus abdominis muscle and obliques. Open stance forehand strokes are purported to be the cause of the increasing incidence of abdominal muscle injury as well. Strengthening of the abdominal muscles may help prevent pain and injury to the low back and abdomen.

Lower Extremity Injuries

Racquet sports place unique stress on the soft tissues of the lower leg. This is due to the amount of time players spend in the ready position (on the balls of their feet with their knees bent slightly), as well as the extreme ranges of motion that the ankle and foot must go through and the ballistic nature of these movements. In young tennis players, lower extremity overuse injuries are about twice as frequent as upper extremity or central region overuse injuries. This predominance has been identified in squash and badminton as well. Lower extremity injuries are common for two reasons. First, each of these sports involves repeated short bursts of activity with quick stop-start, and sharp lateral movements and accelerations that place high demands on the lower extremities. Second, athletes may be less flexible and weaker in specific anatomic areas, including the lower extremity, which may predispose them to overuse injuries.

Hip and Thigh

Leg muscle strains may be acute or chronic in nature. Acute injuries tend to occur later in the match, when the muscle is fatigued or when there has been inadequate warm-up and stretching. Chronic muscle strains usually occur secondary to inadequate rest or rehabilitation from an initial injury.

The most common areas for strains in the thigh are the adductor muscles (groin pulls) and the hamstrings. Adductor muscle strains usually result from sudden changes in direction, particularly when attempting to stop lateral movement by sliding or posting the lead foot. Slipping on clay courts, resulting in "the splits," may also strain the adductor muscles. Hamstring tears may occur at either end of the muscle and are usually associated with explosive acceleration, for example when sprinting or charging toward the net. Quadriceps strains, sometimes with full ruptures, occur in the older athlete, particularly when a player slides on clay courts with the knee flexed and then the player tries to extend the knee forcefully.

Knee

Nearly 20% of all injuries are knee injuries, with 70% of the injuries being traumatic and 30% due to overuse. Due to the sudden changes in direction, repetitive stop-start activity, and lunging and jumping involved in tennis, the patellofemoral joint is susceptible to overload and overuse injuries. This is commonly manifested as Osgood-Schlatter's syndrome (tibial tubercle apophysitis) in young racquet sports players, patellar (jumper's knee) and quadriceps tendinitis in adults, and patellofemoral syndrome or chondromalacia patellae.

Acute knee sprains and meniscal tears are less common in tennis and the other racquet sports, but can occur secondary to the twisting demands of the sport on the knee. Knee ligament and meniscal injuries are more common in squash, badminton, and racquetball than in tennis. This may be because of the frictional characteristics of the wood court in squash and racquetball as compared with the different surfaces in tennis. Medial collateral ligament injuries are the most common injuries, though ruptures of the anterior cruciate ligament have been reported. Patellofemoral pain is more common in tennis as compared with the other sports. Patellofemoral pain may be related to the sudden starts and stops of these sports as well as lunging and jumping. Patellar dislocations have also been documented in tennis, racquetball, and squash.

Less common causes of knee pain in tennis players include prepatellar bursitis, pes anserine tendinitis, semimembranosus tendinitis, and iliotibial band syndrome. Isolated popliteus musculotendinous injuries are uncommon in any sport including racquet sports. However, the mechanics of lunging with the trailing knee flexed and externally rotated puts the popliteus musculotendinous unit at risk for injury.

Leg

Muscle cramps of the calf are very common. Gastrocnemius muscle strains are common and occur during repeated, explosive accelerations of the leg, such as while sprinting or jumping. These strains and injuries to the Achilles tendon occur when a plantar flexed foot is suddenly forced into dorsiflexion while the knee is in full extension. This happens during the serve when the first step forward is made and during ground strokes as forward and lateral lunges are executed. "Tennis leg" is a strain or partial tear of the gastrocnemius at its medial origin. Tennis leg tends to occur in players 30–45 years of age. Less commonly, soleus injuries may occur with sliding on clay courts with extreme ankle dorsiflexion with concurrent knee flexion. Injuries of the gastroc-soleus are treated with limited weight bearing as necessary, ice, and stretching of the calf muscles to prevent shortening of the muscle due to scarring. Gradual strengthening precedes return to play, which may occur 4–6 weeks after injury. Wearing a ⅜-inch heel lift may be beneficial initially when practice and play are resumed.

Achilles tendinitis and Achilles tendon ruptures occur in tennis players, but not as frequently with racquetball and squash. A sudden increase in activity, including changing surfaces from hard court to clay, or the effect of long-term repetitive stress on the tendon may lead to the development of microtears or degeneration of the tendon. Achilles tendinitis can be chronically debilitating and is often associated with a recent change in the amount or intensity of play, especially on clay courts. Once again, most injuries are acute exacerbations of chronic injuries. Achilles tendon ruptures are common in older racquet sports participants, usually those over 40 years of age, due to the sudden bursts of speed that are necessary in each of the sports. Achilles tendon ruptures occur with an estimated incidence of 5.5%.

Medial periostitis is an overuse injury seen frequently in all the racquet sports, especially when participants play tennis on hard courts. Changes in training habits or an increase in play and running may also account for the high incidence of these injuries in tennis players. Stress fractures of the tibia and of the distal fibula also infrequently occur in tennis players.

Ankle

Ankle sprains are the most common macrotrauma injury in tennis as well as the other racquet sports. Each of these running-based sports demand frequent pivoting, stopping and starting movements, lunging, and jumping. As a result, high twisting forces about the ankle result. Most injuries occur during twisting while the ankle is in plantar flexion, resulting in lateral ankle sprains.

Foot

Foot injuries in tennis players may include stress fractures, plantar fasciitis, blisters, abrasions, heel bruises, calluses, corns, warts and "tennis toe." Stress fractures in racquet sport athletes occur most commonly at the base of the fifth metatarsal, the metatarsal diaphysis, the lateral process of the talus, and occasionally the navicular neck. Older racquet sports participants with poorly cushioned footwear and absent medial arch support may be prone to plantar fasciitis or rupture of the plantar fascia. Tennis players are particularly susceptible to this injury due to the great amount of time spent on the balls of their feet while making quick changes in direction. A heel bruise is an intracutaneous hemorrhage located at the plantar aspect of the heel and is more common in older players. The etiology of this injury is the increased impact seen during the landing phase of jumping or running activities. Hallux rigidus, degeneration of the first metatarsal phalangeal joint with dorsal exostosis, occurs frequently in tennis players due to the excessive dorsiflexion of the first toe during play. Players have pain during push-off.

Tennis toe is an injury to the great toe or second toe due to impaction of the toe onto the toe box of the shoe. The injury frequently occurs as the athlete makes a quick stop after charging towards the net. The impaction of the toe onto the anterior aspect of the shoe can lead to subungual hematomas, nail bed injuries or to jammed joints at the distal interphalangeal, proximal interphalangeal, or metatars ophalangeal joints. Shoes with a small, tight toe box may be associated with tennis toe. The court surface and shoe design determine traction and the impaction of the toes;

hard court and wood surfaces are associated with greater traction than grass or clay courts, and consequently toe impaction is more common with the former surfaces. Tennis toe is also associated with improperly sized shoes, loose fitting shoelaces, and long toenails or digits. Fortunately, tennis toe is infrequent in young racquet sports players. Calluses and corns develop due to increased pressure at the bony prominences of the foot. Soft corns develop between the toes as a result of toe condylar prominence and moisture of the feet. Fungal infections such as athlete's foot are common in tennis players due to the moisture that accumulates from prolonged play with rapid foot movement.

STROKE MECHANICS

Poor stroke technique may be the most important predisposing factor for upper extremity injury in the recreational player. This is not true in the elite or professional player. The following are important principles in understanding tennis biomechanics.

1. To be successful at tennis, a player must develop control, consistency, depth, and power. The successful player must not sacrifice control, consistency, or depth for increased power. This is a common error in all players. The professional game has certainly become a power game on both the men's and women's tour. Professional players spend as much time in the gym as they do on the court. Pros are bigger, stronger, and more powerful than ever. Advances in technology provide players with powerful racquets. The difference between pros and recreational players is that professional players can control the power, use appropriate mechanics, and do not produce as many abnormal forces for the body to absorb. Recreational players want to hit like their favorite pro, so they often purchase a much too powerful weapon for their ability, and then try to hit the ball as hard as they can, often with poor stroke mechanics.
2. The grip on the racquet is just as important. It becomes confusing, as there are three variations of tennis grip: the Western, Eastern, and Continental. In the past, most players used one grip (Continental) for all strokes. At present most tennis coaches teach different grip styles. The grip type depends on the player's ability, style of play, and shot selection.

   In patients complaining of any upper extremity injury, in particular wrist and elbow pain, the grip should be evaluated by their teaching professional. A common error seen in the amateur player is the attempt to place a lot of topspin on the ball in the forehand and to slice the backhand. These shots can produce tremendous forces on the elbow and wrist at the best of times, let alone when the grip mechanics are faulty.

   In those players wishing to continue to play or train while injured, recommend that they return to hitting the ball flat while recovering.
3. What happens to the ball when it leaves the racquet starts at the footground interaction. The forces begin at the ground, and move up to the lower limb, hips, trunk, upper limb, and finally the racquet. This is the kinetic chain principle. When you leave out any part of this system or the links occur in the wrong order, the athlete will place increased forces on the other links, and the result is injury.

   Biomechanically, a one-handed backhand requires more links working in sequence. The two-handed backhand requires fewer links as the trunk and upper extremities all move together as one segment. It is simple—

the fewer parts to worry about, the lower the percentage of error and abnormal force production.

In reality, the two-handed backhand is a forehand with the arm at the back of the racquet acting as the dominant force. The player must use body rotation to hit the ball, thereby reducing the chances of leading with the arms before the trunk. The essential body rotation also generates the much-wanted power of the stroke.

EQUIPMENT AND PLAYING SURFACE

Most of the advances in tennis technology, as well as in squash, have occurred in the racquet. Changes have been made in racquet size, composition, and playing characteristics. These changes have had a major impact on the nature of play at all levels.

Racquet

Metal (aluminum and steel) tennis racquet frames were introduced in the mid 1960s, ushering in an era that displaced the wood frame. Since the 1970s there has been an explosion of technological change in the composition of tennis racquets from metal to fiberglass, and then to graphite, boron, ceramic, magnesium, and Kevlar. The most recent entry is the titanium racquet, which is predominantly a graphite frame with small amounts of titanium at high stress points on the frame. Many modern racquets combine two or more materials. The goals for changing racquet composition include reducing the weight of the racquet while increasing its durability and strength, and to increase the power of the stroke as well as reduce injury. Theoretically, a racquet that dampens vibration and reduces shock impulse (force of contact at impact) to the athlete's arm may reduce injury. Dampening and force reduction is a function of the materials used in construction, and modifying the size of the head helps increase the sweet spot and reduce the effect of off-center hits. It has never been shown that injury rates or severity is reduced by racquets that dampen vibration or reduce the shock (impulse). However, metal racquets that do not dampen vibration well are an identified risk factor for developing lateral epicondylitis. The increased stiffness of racquets, including those with a heavy and wide-body design, reduces vibration, though the frequency of vibration to the forearm is increased and the increased impact shock transmission may be longer. Again, the effects of these elements on injury has not been scientifically proven.

The shape of the racquet has also undergone changes, including the head going from oval to a more square shape, head size from regular to mid to oversize heads, increasing the length of the racquet, changes in thickness of the frame resulting in a stiffer racquet, and tapering of the thickness along the frame affecting the flexibility and the vibration of the frame. These changes affect the stiffness of the racquet, which may reduce twisting with off-center hits and provide more power with each shot and reduce vibration; however, they may also promote shock transmission to the body and thus increase the susceptibility to injury, while flexible racquets tend to dampen the shock. Other changes include decreasing racquet weight and moving the center of the head and center of percussion toward the handle, increasing power. Unfortunately, there are currently no data that support or refute any effect of these changes on the risk of injury.

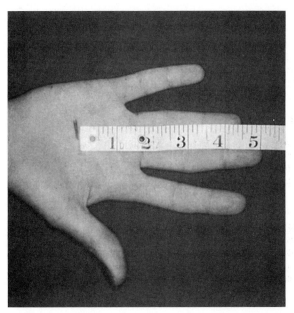

FIG 42-2   Racquet handle grip. Larger grips are more forgiving when elbow and wrist problems are present. A comfortable size can be selected by measuring the distance from the middle of the palm to the tip of the middle finger (shown here as 5 inches or 12.7 cm).

An important aspect of racquet selection involves the size of the grip. The recommended grip size should correspond to the distance between the tip of the ring finger and the proximal palmar crease with the ruler placed between the ring and long fingers (Fig. 42-2). Both grips that are too small and too large are related to the etiology of tennis elbow. Grips traditionally have been made of leather. Cushioned grips reduce impact shock and vibration transfer from ball impact and today have become more popular.

Although the effects of racquet changes on injury are not clear at this time, the author does recommend lighter, less flexible racquets for players rehabilitating from upper extremity injury.

Strings

Strings have undergone an evolution from steel strings to gut and nylon, and now the most popular string is synthetic gut. Steel strings were very durable, but the rapid destruction of tennis balls resulted in the decline of their use in competition and recreational tennis. Gut strings are more elastic and have a soft feel with decreased energy being transmitted to the forearm of the player. However, gut strings wear out rapidly and are costly. Nylon strings have intermediate elasticity, with some types of synthetic strings having properties very similar to gut strings, but they last longer. At higher string tensions, nylon strings lose their elasticity and have an effect of being more stiff longer. Multifilament synthetic strings are made up of many tiny filaments that have a softer feel and may result in reduced stiffness, reduced impact, and potentially less vibration transmission. Kevlar strings are relatively inelastic and are not as popular as the synthetic multifilament nylon strings. Titanium strings have been introduced to the market, although their purported benefit is unclear to the author. To the knowledge of the author, the effect of string types on injury patterns or incidence has not been studied.

String tension has been the subject of much research and debate. There is laboratory evidence that at lower string tensions (looser strings) the ball stays on the strings longer and comes off the strings at a higher velocity. It is thought that the force of impact of the ball is spread over a longer time. With looser strings, the strings will deform more and the ball will deform less. Thus less energy will be absorbed from the ball, which reduces the force exerted on the body and potentially reduces the risk of injury. However, the difference in terms of demands on the tennis player is negligible. Similarly, there has been no demonstrable evidence that string tension is a variable in cause or prevention of tennis-related injuries.

Dampers placed in the strings have no effect on elbow and forearm pain. While these string dampers quickly decreased the high-frequency string vibrations, the lower-frequency frame vibrations were not affected.

Shoes and Court Surface

Sports shoes have undergone as much a technological transformation as tennis racquets in the last 20 years. Tennis shoes are very important to the player due to the quick starting and stopping, cutting, pivoting, and jumping that are part of the game. Many of the innovations, such as sole cushioning systems (eg, air, special polymers), variable lacing patterns, deepened heel cups, reinforced toes, and additional supportive mechanisms, have no research data to prove the superiority of one type over another. However, tennis players may benefit from wearing shoes that are made specifically for tennis. The shoes should be properly fitted with the socks the player plans to use while playing. Often players use a thick pair of socks or two pairs of socks to afford padding and protect the underlying skin. The shoes should have a fairly wide heel and good heel counter for rear foot control, and a heel thickness of ⅝–1½". The traction surface of the heel should be shock absorbent and made of a non-slip material. The heel cup should fit snugly, which helps prevent the foot from slipping forward in the shoe. The shoe should have a medial arch support that is appropriate for the individual's arch. There needs to be good lateral support for the forefoot. The toe of the shoe must not create pressure and should conform to the general shape of the foot. The vamp (upper front) of the shoe must never constrict or cause pressure across the metatarsal area or instep. The rolled heel is an important innovation to absorb shock when the leg is stretched forward and the heel strikes the ground. The high heel counter is purported to reduce Achilles tendon rotation and thus injury.

Court surface, style of play, and foot structure should be considered when selecting a tennis shoe. A competitor who plays mostly from the baseline requires a shoe that has more sidewall support to stabilize the foot during the quick side-to-side movements. The baseline player also needs good support for forward and rear forces in addition to the extra sidewall support. The serve and volley player generates tremendous levels of forward forces in the forefoot or toe box area of the shoe. Without the appropriate shoe, these players are susceptible to developing tennis toe, subungual hematoma of the toe. Appropriate footwear for these players includes a large toe box to provide adequate room so the toe will not slam against the end of the shoe.

Custom orthotics are seldom necessary for the average player. Their shock absorption ability is not high, and flexible joints combined with muscle strength in the legs can better maintain foot control.

A natural rubber outer sole provides excellent traction on all court surfaces. Polyurethane soles do not provide as much traction as natural rubber, and are usually only recommended for high-traction court surfaces that provide exceptional footing, such as indoor carpet, where too much traction may result in injury. Lighter-weight shoes with less support are more applicable to clay or composite courts rather than hard courts.

Court surfaces have influences other than those regarding shoe wear and type. Different court surfaces can alter the demands placed on the tennis player. In general, clay courts and some synthetic courts slow the ball down and produce a higher bounce, allowing for longer points and longer matches. Because more strokes are hit in trying to impart more speed to a slower ball, there may be extra strain on the arm and back. The softer surfaces cushion the knees and legs, reducing knee pain, particularly for arthritic knees, and reduce the likelihood of shin splints and lower extremity stress fractures. However, since the softer surfaces result in longer matches, the extra running may put more demands on the legs, resulting in muscular fatigue, and there may be more muscle strains from sliding on the soft surfaces. Achilles tendinitis occurs more commonly when switching to clay courts after playing predominantly on hard courts. Most synthetic courts and hard courts speed the ball up and keep the bounce lower, creating shorter points. However, because of the speed of the ball, more impact forces may be placed on the racquet and arm. Similarly, the quick pace of the points on the harder surface may cause increased stress on the legs, such as shin splints and lower extremity stress fractures. This is particularly true when starting the hard-court season after playing on clay courts for a prolonged period of time. Grass courts place increased stress on the upper extremity due to the frequency of irregular bounces and an increased ball speed. The player must compensate for the fast-moving ball that may bounce awkwardly and change their stroke mechanics to hit the ball. During prolonged practices and match play, this difference in repetitive stress is evident.

Tennis Balls

Tennis balls have undergone less change than most of the other equipment. The tennis ball is hollow and pressurized, and is composed of inflated rubber covered with fabric. The ball measures $2\frac{1}{2}$–$2\frac{5}{8}$ inches in diameter and weighs 2–$2\frac{1}{16}$ ounces. Pressureless balls are preferred on clay courts and at high altitude, but they are very heavy and do not bounce well on hard courts at sea level. The tennis ball has had few recent changes, although there are some proposed changes. Softer balls with properties similar to those of current balls may reduce injury in a way similar to that of the softer strings, with the ball staying on the strings longer. Conversely, harder balls are being considered for play on clay courts. Harder balls increase the speed of play and the ball bounces higher on clay. Lastly, a larger tennis ball, approximately 7–8% larger than the standard ball, became legal on January 1, 2000, although it is not used in professional play. The goal of the larger ball is to slow the game on faster surfaces (hard court, grass), and potentially make tennis easier for recreational players by being easier to hit longer. The effect of these changes in the ball on injury is unclear at this time. Used or "dead" balls (balls that have lost some pressure) require more stroke energy to achieve a comparable amount of speed compared with new balls. Players have a tendency to stroke the ball harder and overhit their shots. This increases stress on the upper extremity and back and may result in an overuse injury.

It is most important to have your racquet restrung at the beginning of each season and again midway through your season by a certified racquet technician. The stringer can help you select the appropriate string type, tension, and racquet type for your game style.

SQUASH AND RACQUETBALL INJURIES

The demands of these two sports reveal many similarities to tennis. The major musculoskeletal demands in racquetball and squash in the upper extremity are to the shoulder, elbow, and wrist due to the repetitive fast swinging of the lighter racquets with more whipping or snapping motions to attain power for the swing. The squash and racquetball swings are swifter and more compact than the tennis swing. However, the lower extremities are most frequently injured, especially the knee and ankle, which are subjected to the greatest stresses due to the rapid starting, stopping, cutting, and pivoting on predominantly coated wood surfaces that provide excellent traction. Young players appear to sustain more fractures, while older players tend to sustain more cartilage and tendon injuries. More experienced players appear to sustain more serious injuries and more orthopedic injuries, while less experienced players sustain more numerous but less severe injuries, such as lacerations. Squash and racquetball participants are more likely to sustain acute injuries, as opposed to the predominance of overuse injuries seen with tennis and badminton.

Contusions and Abrasions

Due to the enclosed nature of the court and the close proximity of the players, there is a greater risk of acute contact injury as compared with tennis and badminton. Contusions, abrasions, and fractures can occur in racquetball and squash due to contact with the ball, the opponent, the opponent's or partner's racquet, the walls, and occasionally the player's own racquet. Contusions that occur to the trunk or extremities due to the impact by the ball sting and are painful, but usually are superficial. Local swelling is usually minimal. Early return to play is the rule.

Contusions that occur due to racquet impact may have damaging consequences involving deeper structures, and may actually tear muscle or cause fractures, especially around the face and head. Pain may be significant enough to stop play. Gradual return to normal use is usually advocated. This process may take 3–4 weeks and will result in excessive scar tissue if too much tension is placed on the repair site too early in recovery. Lacerations about the face, eyelid, and eye also occur due to contact with the racquet, either the opponent's or the player's own. Facial lacerations and eye wounds account for 36% of all squash injuries.

Eye

The most dangerous injury that occurs in all racquet sports is damage to the eye, from direct contact with the ball or the racquet. Eye injuries are more common with racquetball and squash as compared with tennis and bad-minton due to the confined nature of the court and because a net does not separate the players. Both the racquetball and squash ball function as mis-siles with high velocity and great kinetic energy. Both balls are capable of conforming tightly to the orbital cavity on direct impact, creating tremen-dous direct and concussive forces on the fragile eyeball and orbit. Eyeguards are mandatory in the United States and reduce the risk of eye injury in rac-quetball and squash. The mechanism of contact with the ball or opponent's racquet is usually the player looking back at the opponent or ball as the opponent hits the ball, though it may also occur from a bounce off the wall, such as when a ball is being played off the side or back walls. Another mechanism of eye injury occurs when a player rushes to the wall to chase a drop shot and immediately turns to run back. Experience does not reduce the risk of injury. Hyphemas, which result from direct contact between the racquet or ball and the eye, may be effectively treated in the acute stage, but may be associated with cataract, retinal detachment, or retinal hemor-rhages. Increased risk of future glaucoma may also occur with these injuries.

Regular glasses do not protect the eye in these sports, and may in fact increase injury to the eye either by shattering, or if they are shatter-proof, they may rotate out of the frame and lacerate the eye. The optimal eye guards are wrap-around polycarbonate lenses with eyeguard rims that are posterior to the orbital rim, are antifog coated, and have secure attachment to the back of the head. It is estimated that there is a 25% risk of eye injury in the life-time of a participant who regularly plays squash without eye protection.

Upper Extremity Injuries

Shoulder

Shoulder pain occurs less frequently in racquetball and squash players com-pared with tennis players. Though these sports do not require an overhead service motion, overhead shots, such as smashes or lobs, are needed in both sports. However, rotator cuff inflammation (impingement, tendinitis, or instability) occurs more commonly in racquetball due to lengthy ceiling ral-lies in this sport. The AC joint is susceptible to injury due to falling or impact with the wall, resulting in sprains and separations.

Elbow

Lateral epicondylitis is the most common upper extremity injury in rac-quetball and squash players. As with tennis, poor technique and a faulty grip may play a role in the development of this problem. Further, racquet tech-nology is changing in both of these sports and racquet type, size, and strings may also play a role in this malady, especially if a recent change was made prior to the onset of symptoms.

Medial elbow pain is very common in squash and racquetball due to the snapping mechanism of kill shots and to the lighter racquet. Contact with the wall may also cause extra valgus force. Injuries sustained include medial epicondylitis and ulnar collateral ligament injury with secondary findings of lateral and posterior elbow pain and ulnar nerve irritation.

Traumatic hemorrhagic olecranon bursitis may infrequently occur due to falling or diving for the ball. Repeated microtrauma may also result in non-hemorrhagic olecranon bursitis. Elbow sprains and fractures may also occur due to falling or contact with the wall.

Wrist

Racquetball and squash require a snapping motion of the wrist as part of the normal stroke. This puts stress on the tendons and ligaments of the wrist that may result in an overuse injury. The chronic overstretching or recent initiation of a new motion or technique will result in the wrist pain. This is often manifest as tendinitis about the wrist. The tendinitis is often in the wrist extensor tendons, either in the dorsal compartment or at the distal insertions. DeQuervain's tenosynovitis is also common among racquetball and squash players. Intersection syndrome, a peritendinous bursitis that occurs when the musculotendinous junction of the first extensor compartment overlaps, or intersects, with the second compartment is particularly common in squash players. Review of the player's stroke mechanics, particularly the backhand, may provide insight into the cause of this problem and help in the resolution of the symptoms. The stroke mechanics of these sports are also felt to be the etiology of anterior interosseous nerve syndrome of the forearm.

Ligamentous injuries and fractures are not as common as tendinitis and may occur as a result of a fall or being hit by a racquet. TFCC tears may result from a fall, though the stresses that occur during a squash swing have also been implicated in these injuries. Subluxation of the extensor carpi ulnaris tendons has been associated with both racquetball and squash.

Injuries including fracture of the hook of the hamate, ulnar artery compression and thrombosis, and chondromalacia of the pisiform-triquetral joint due to pressure from the butt of the racquet on the base of the hand may occur in these sports. Carpal tunnel syndrome has also been reported in racquetball players.

Back Injury

Overuse, over-reaching for the ball, hyperextension, and bending to hit the ball are motions that have been implicated in the high incidence of low back pain among squash players. These motions may produce flexion and rotation stresses to the spine, factors known to result in the commonly seen problem of intervertebral disc prolapse in squash players. These injuries often may be traumatic in origin and were identified in higher level players.

Lower Extremity Injuries

Hip

There is debate as to whether degenerative hip disease is increased in elite squash players by the third decade of life.

Knee

Knee injuries may occur in any racquet sport, but they are of particular concern in racquetball and squash, in which nearly every type of knee injury may occur.

Patellofemoral pain is the most frequently encountered condition in racquetball and squash players. This is usually insidious in onset due to the rapid starts and stops, cutting, pivoting, jumping, and lunging that define these sports. The frequent pivoting maneuvers in racquetball and squash, particularly on wood floors with excellent traction, predispose players to meniscal and ligamentous injuries. Older players are particularly susceptible to symptomatic meniscal tears due to propagation of degenerative tears. Ligamentous injuries are relatively uncommon in these sports; however, with increasing use of play on bare, unvarnished floors, the improved traction increases the risk of injury to knee ligaments, especially the anterior cruciate ligament.

Leg

The classic and most common injury in the leg is cramps of the calf musculature. The explosive bursts necessary in these sports, especially when ankle plantar flexion is combined with knee extension, places the gastrocsoleus group at risk. In players 30–45 years of age, this may result in a partial tear of the medial head of the gastrocnemius, or "tennis leg." Players usually feel a sudden onset of pain in the upper to middle third of the calf, and note it feels like they were shot or hit in the leg by the ball or a block of wood. Fortunately, these injuries are self-limited, and take about 6 weeks to heal. In older players over 40 years of age, Achilles tendon ruptures occur. This is a more severe injury. These patients note a snap and inability to push off on the affected foot. Return to play is delayed after this injury, regardless whether it is treated surgically or with a cast. Achilles tendinitis is an uncommon entity in racquetball and squash players. When Achilles tendinitis does occur, it is usually secondary to overuse or recent change in training or play habits.

Ankle

Ankle sprains are among the most common injuries in racquetball and squash due to the sudden changes in direction and jumping necessary for these sports. Chronic, recurrent ankle sprains usually occur secondary to incomplete rehabilitation. Ankle fractures have been reported.

Foot

Blisters, calluses, and tennis toe are common complaints of racquetball and squash players. Plantar fasciitis is the most commonly seen orthopedic condition of the foot in these athletes, and responds well to rest, stretching of the calves, and heel cups, and rarely necessitates injections or surgery. Less commonly, foot sprains occur due to the sudden changes in direction.

BADMINTON INJURIES

Most injuries in badminton are from overuse, though acute injuries, particularly to the lower extremity, are common. Overall, lower extremity injuries are the most common, followed by upper extremity injuries and then back injuries. Much of the power for play comes from the upper extremity— shoulder, elbow, and wrist,—placing greater strain on these structures, resulting in overuse injuries from repetition.

The badminton shuttlecock can travel over 200 mph, and as a result it may function like a missile, causing injury. In badminton, contusions, abrasions, and eye injuries have been reported from uncommon contact with the shuttlecock, the partner, or the partner's racquet. There have been reported cases of eye injury in badminton, though eye protection is not mandatory. It has been shown that the shuttlecock can produce an injury of severity equal to that of a squash ball, ranging from hyphema to retinal detachment. Due to the aerobic nature of badminton, with the sudden stops and starts and long play times, muscle cramps are common in male players.

Upper Extremity Injuries

Shoulder

Shoulder pain due to overuse occurs occasionally in the badminton player. Though this sport does not require an overhead service motion, overhead shots such as smashes or lobs are needed. As such, rotator cuff inflammation (impingement, tendinitis, or instability) does occur. Furthermore, it has been shown that the greatest force producing movement is internal and external rotation of the shoulder for the forehand and backhand. This biomechanical technique can result in stress fractures of the proximal humeral epiphysis in skeletally immature players.

Elbow

Lateral epicondylitis is a common overuse upper extremity injury in badminton.

Wrist

Badminton requires a snapping motion of the wrist as part of the normal stroke. This puts stress on the tendons and ligaments of the wrist that may result in an overuse injury. This is manifest as tendinitis about the wrist. Often this is in the wrist extensor tendons, either in the dorsal compartment or at the distal insertions as well as flexor tendon inflammation. DeQuervain's tenosynovitis also occurs in athletes in this sport.

Ligamentous injuries and fractures are not as common as tendinitis and may occur as a result of a fall or being hit by a racquet. Triangular fibrocartilage complex (TFCC) tears may result from a fall. Fracture of the hook of the hamate, chondromalacia of the pisiform-triquetral joint, and hypothenar hammer syndrome (occlusion of the distal ulnar artery at the level of the hamate bone) due to pressure of the butt of the racket on the base of the hand may occur.

Back Injury

Musculoskeletal back pain due to overuse, over-reaching and lunging for the shuttlecock, and hyperextension and bending to reach low have all been implicated in low back pain among badminton players.

Lower Extremity Injuries

Thigh and Groin

Quadriceps and groin strains are particularly common in badminton due to the leaping and lunging required in this quick sport.

Knee

Knee injuries may occur in any racquet sport, including badminton, due to the pivoting and jumping required. Patellofemoral pain is the most frequently encountered condition in persons playing badminton. This is usually insidious in onset and is due to the rapid starts and stops, cutting, pivoting, jumping, and lunging that predominate the sport. Knee ligament injuries do rarely occur due to the motions mentioned above. Uncommon acute knee injuries identified in badminton include patellar dislocation, patellar fracture, and meniscal tears.

Leg

Achilles tendon injuries in badminton may be due to a combination of factors. These factors include the special footwork required, which involves a fast forward movement and stopping with a forceful heel strike, eccentric work by the gastrocnemius alternating with concentric gastrocnemius work seen with backward or combined backward and sideways jumps, and backward running. These movements produce alternating, rapidly changing high tension in the Achilles tendon.

Achilles tendinitis is a particularly common entity in badminton players secondary to overuse or recent changes in training or play habits. As with racquetball and squash, the explosive bursts necessary for play places the gastrocnemius-soleus muscle group at risk, including partial tears of the medial head of the gastrocnemius, tennis leg, and Achilles tendon ruptures.

Ankle

Ankle sprains are among the most common injuries in badminton due to incorrect placement of the foot that occurs due to the sudden changes in direction and jumping that are necessary. Chronic, recurrent ankle sprains usually occur secondary to incomplete rehabilitation. Ankle fractures have rarely been reported to occur during play.

Foot

Blisters, calluses, and corns are common complaints of badminton participants, particularly due to the high-friction court surfaces and low shock absorption of the shoes. Plantar fasciitis is the most commonly seen orthopedic condition of the foot in badminton players.

PREVENTION OF INJURY

Flexibility is an important part of injury treatment and prevention. For stretching to be effective, it must be done on a regular basis. Always stretch when you are warmed up. It is important to stretch before and after activity. Stretching should not be painful. All stretches should be done in a slow, static manner, with no bouncing. Hold stretches for at least 30–60 seconds and repeat several times. For difficult problems, a therapist may have to assist you to improve your flexibility.

Weak or inflexible muscles of the arm are a major contributor to the problem of golfer's and tennis elbow. The exercises shown here will not only strengthen the damaged muscle tendon unit to prevent injury, but will also help improve your game.

Weak and inflexible muscles in the back of the shoulder may result in rotator cuff inflammation, pain, and limited function. Weak and inflexible abdominal and back muscles may predispose these muscles to being injured. Patellofemoral pain may be diminished or prevented by maintaining flexibility of the hamstrings and strength of the quadriceps muscles, particularly the vastus medialis obliquus. Achilles tendon and gastroc-soleus injuries may be prevented by stretching before play and maintaining good cardiovascular fitness to prevent fatigue.

HEAT ILLNESS

The racquet sports require sudden, sharp, side-to-side and front-to-back movement patterns and great endurance sometimes in a confined space, often in conditions of high temperature and humidity. Because of the highly aerobic nature, especially in indoor courts with poor ventilation, there is significant cardiovascular and thermal stress placed on the body. Heat-related illness, such as heat cramps, heat syncope, heat exhaustion, and heat-stroke may result.

Prevention of Heat Disorders

1. Identify susceptible individuals.
2. Gradually increase the practice time in the heat (conditioning). It takes several days to acclimatize to new hot, humid, environmental conditions.
3. Hydration is the most important preventive measure. Although an athlete can overhydrate, it is difficult to do so when sweating profusely, so ingesting cool fluids such as water, electrolyte drinks, and diluted fruit juice before, during, and after a practice or match to replace sweat losses is critical to performance and heat safety. In match situations, the athlete should drink approximately 1 cup of fluid at each changeover. If one waits until they are thirsty, it is too late. Avoid or limit caffeine and alcohol intake, as they act as diuretics. Athletes should monitor their body weight and urine (which should be light yellow like lemonade) when training and competing for several days or weeks in the heat. Dehydration most definitely leads to decreased physical performance.
4. Remember that cooling occurs by evaporation, so expose skin to air and avoid restrictive clothing, dark colors, nylon, spandex, and polyester blends.
5. Evaluate weather conditions in advance. The greater the humidity, the harder it is for the body to cool itself.
6. Towel off sweat. In match play, a player should towel off all exposed skin every changeover. The player must regularly change shirts and wear a hat. Fanning the athlete or using ice towels or packs on the neck, armpits, and abdomen will help cool the player unless the humidity is too high for effective evaporative heat loss.
7. The loss of emotional control in a match or during practice expends needed energy.
8. Educate athletes, coaches, and professionals. Certain issues are sensitive, and they should certainly be treated with respect and confidentiality.

Treatment of Muscle Cramps

Exercise-associated muscle cramps are one of the most devastating problems in racquet sports. This is due to a buildup of metabolites in the muscle associated with fatigue, salt loss, and dehydration. Poor conditioning also plays a major role in cramping. Emphasis must be on prevention through adequate hydration, salt replacement, nutrition, and conditioning.

If cramping occurs, the player should drink salted fluids, gently stretch the muscle, and apply ice to the muscle to help reduce the pain and spasm. Often gentle massage helps. The recreational player should stop playing until the cramp stops completely. The competitive player, particularly the elite player, may continue to play but must understand the following:

- Their performance will decrease as the cramping progresses.
- They risk injury to the cramping muscle or to another muscle or joint owing to the compensation (ie, the player will not want to explode with the legs in the service action and will therefore begin to serve more from the arm).
- Their performance will be reduced the next day.
- The more severe the dehydration and cramping, the greater the requirement for medical intervention such as intravenous treatment.
- The player must be educated as to why cramping occurs and make changes to his or her hydration and nutrition routine in order to prevent this most

disabling tennis injury. Conditioning also plays an important role in prevention. On the professional tennis tour, a trainer may assist a cramping player only once during a match.

REFERENCES

Berson BL, Rolnick AM, Ramos CG, Thornton J. An epidemiologic study of squash injuries. *Am J Sports Med*. 1981;9:103–106.

Chandler TJ, Kibler WB, Stracener EC, Zeigler AK, Pace B. Shoulder strength, power, and endurance in college tennis players. *Am J Sports Med*. 1992;20:455–458.

Easterbrook M, Cameron C. Injuries in racquet sports. In: Schneider RC, ed. *Sports Injuries*. Baltimore: Williams & Wilkins; 1985;553–571.

Hoy K, Lindblad BE, Terkelsen CJ, Helleland HE, Terkelsen CJ. Badminton injuries—A prospective epidemiological and socioeconomic study. *Br J Sports Med*. 1994;28:276–279.

Kibler WB. Concepts in exercise rehabilitation. In: Leadbetter W, Buckwalter JA, Gordon SL, eds. *Sports Induced Inflammation*. Park Ridge, IL: American Academy of Orthopedic Surgeons; 1990;759–769.

Kibler WB, Chandler TJ. Musculoskeletal adaptations in injuries associated with intense participation in youth sports. In: Cahill BR, Pearl AJ, eds. *Intensive Participation in Children's Sports*. Park Ridge, IL: American Academy of Orthopedic Surgeons; 1993;2–7.

Kroner K, Schmidt SA, Nielsen AB, et al. Badminton injuries. *Br J Sports Med*. 1990;24:169–172.

Lehman R. Racquet sports: Injury treatment and prevention. *Clin Sports Med*. 1988;7:211–457.

Levisohn SR, Simon HB. The knee and lower leg. In: Levisohn SR, Simon HB, eds. *Tennis Medic: Conditioning Sports Medicine and Treatment for Every Player*. St Louis: CV Mosby; 1984;150–155.

Livingston B, Chandler TJ, Kibler WB, Safran MR. Racquet sports. In: Ireland ML, Nattiv A, eds. *The Female Athlete*. Ho-Ho-Kus, NJ: Tage Publishing; 2002.

Nirschl RP. Sports and overuse injuries to the elbow. In: Morrey BF, ed. *The Elbow and Its Disorders,* 2d ed. Philadelphia: Saunders; 1993.

Rose CP, Morse JO. Racquetball injuries. *Phys Sports Med*. 1979;7:73–78.

Safran MR. Injuries sustained in tennis and other racquet sports. In: Fu FH, Stone DA, eds. *Sports Injuries. Mechanisms, Prevention and Treatment*. 2d ed. Baltimore: Lippincott, Williams & Wilkins; 2001;617–656.

Safran MR. Tennis injuries and strategies for prevention: Gender differences in the elite American junior tennis player. In: Crespo M, Pluim B, Reid M, eds. *Tennis Medicine for Tennis Coaches*. London: International Tennis Federation; 2001;44–46.

Soderstrom CA, Doxanas MT. Racquetball: A game with preventable injuries. *Am J Sports Med*. 1982;10:180.

43 | Golf

L. Tyler Wadsworth

QUICK LOOK

- The golf swing is an asymmetrical movement with different demands on the dominant and nondominant sides of the body.
- Most golf injuries are overuse injuries.
- Common injury sites for golfers include the lumbar spine and nondominant upper extremity.
- Definitive treatment may include relative rest, rehabilitation, and professional instruction in swing technique.
- Catastrophic golf injuries are usually related to lightning, carelessness in swinging the club, hitting toward other golfers, or driving a motorized cart.

INTRODUCTION

Golf is one of the fastest growing participation sports in the past decade and the number of American golfers has swelled to over 25 million participants. This growth phenomenon is mirrored by increasing references to golf in the sports medicine literature. Early references to golf in the medical literature primarily concerned case reports of interesting or unusual injuries. Over the past decade, studies demonstrating the health benefits of golf, epidemiology of injuries, and kinematic and electromyographic studies dissecting the golf swing have made their way into the sports medicine literature.

Golf appeals to participants on a number of levels. It can be played throughout the life span, and unlike many sports the skill and level of play of a golfer may increase through the fifth and even sixth decades of life. The game of golf provides a unique blend of physical and mental challenges. The wisdom and judgment of the experienced golfer can overcome the declining physical skills that accompany aging. In stroke play, the player competes with himself and with the course; in the rules of golf, playing companions are considered "fellow competitors" rather than opponents. Because of the United States Golf Association handicapping system, players of diverse skills can have a competitive contest. Golf provides an important social and physical outlet for seniors, and is an acceptable fitness activity for players who walk the course (Parkkari et al., 2000).

Clubs may be carried or pulled on a cart, a good option for golfers with back pain. Walking the course while carrying a bag requires the same caloric expenditure as walking 3.5–4.0 mph continuously (McArdle et al., 1991). Unfortunately, in the United States most golfers use motorized carts. The caloric expenditure for golf using a cart is less than that of walking 1–2 mph; it qualifies as a fitness activity only for the most sedentary individuals.

THE GOLF SWING

A variety of different swing techniques are used to advance the ball to the cup. The *full swing* refers to longer shots, in which the goal is to hit the ball to a target far down the fairway or to a putting green. Other techniques include putting, chipping, and pitching for shots of shorter distances. Most acute and overuse golf injuries occur as a result of the full swing, which is described below. In considering the mechanism of injury and treatment of golf injuries, it is useful to have a basic understanding of the golf swing.

709

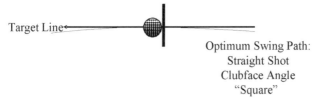

Optimum Swing Path:
Straight Shot
Clubface Angle
"Square"

FIG 43-1   Right-handed golfer. Creating backspin creates lift and increase distance.

Volumes have been written on countless theories, tips, and bits of advice regarding swing techniques. It is not unusual to leaf through a golf magazine and see swing tips proffered by various professionals that seem to be completely contradictory. For a more detailed description of the basics around which a good golf swing might be built, *Five Lessons: The Modern Fundamentals of Golf* by Ben Hogan (1957) and *Golf My Way* by Jack Nicklaus (1998) are recommended. These classic instructional books describe swing techniques and philosophies of two great champions who had very different swings. Although the golf swing varies considerably, even among professionals, the swing can be broken down into basic components common to all techniques: the pre-shot routine, setup or address, the backswing, the downswing, impact, and follow-through.

Similar to throwing and racket sports, golf is a very asymmetrical sport. Most sports involve facing the line of play, whereas in golf, one stands perpendicular to the line of play. There are differing demands on the right and left side of the golfer's body, regardless of dominance. Ultimately, golf is a sport of balance, and neither the right or left upper extremity should dominate. Many naturally left-hand dominant individuals choose to play golf right-handed. In fact, Phil Mickelson has been one of the PGA Tour's top money winners playing left-handed, despite being naturally right-handed. Sergio Garcia frequently plays nine holes left-handed during practice rounds in an effort to maintain balance of the trunk muscles. There are differences in firing patterns of the shoulder muscles from right to left (Pink et al., 1990). In discussing the biomechanics and physics of the golf swing, references to "dominant" versus "nondominant" refer to the side the golfer is playing from, right-handed versus left-handed, rather than right- versus left-brain dominance.

The golf swing begins with the large muscles of the legs, trunk, and shoulders, and allows the smaller muscles of the forearms to play a more passive role in gripping the club and allowing it to whip through the impact area. The clubhead follows a round, slightly elliptical path determined by such variables as the spine angle, the amount of hip and shoulder turn, and the hinging and unhinging of the wrists. Centrifugal force keeps the clubhead

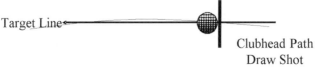

Clubhead Path
Draw Shot

FIG 43-2   Creating counterclockwise spin in a right-handed golfer produces draw. The ball flies lower and rolls farther.

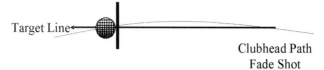

Clubhead Path
Fade Shot

FIG 43-3 Creating clockwise spin in a right-handed golfer produces fade. The ball flies higher and does not roll as far.

traveling in a single plane of movement, called the *swing plane*. The plane of the swing in relation to the target line is one of several factors that determine the flight of the ball. Ideally, the club approaches the ball slightly from the inside of a line drawn between the ball and its target (target line), with the clubface perpendicular (square) to the target line (Fig. 43-1). This produces a shot with backspin, which creates lift and increases distance.

Most shots also have an element of sidespin. The preferred swing path brings the club to the ball from slightly inside the target line, introducing backspin with slight sidespin (Fig. 43-2). For a right-handed golfer, this produces counterclockwise spin, causing the ball to curve slightly from right to left, termed a *draw*. Shots hit with this type of spin typically are the result of an efficient, well-timed release of the kinetic chain. The swing that produces this type of shot usually imparts slightly less backspin, so the ball flies on a somewhat lower trajectory and rolls significantly farther than a shot hit with clockwise, or *fade* spin. The swing path that leads to a fade, or slightly left-to-right ball flight for a right-handed golfer, causes the golf club to approach the ball from slightly outside the target line (Fig. 43-3). This typically causes the clubhead to take a steeper trajectory to the ball, imparting greater backspin. The resulting ball flies higher, with decreased roll. This trade-off can be useful in trying to hit shots to targets. Most low-handicap and professional golfers are comfortable hitting balls with draw spin and fade spin, and use these shots strategically around the golf course.

A swing path that is significantly off-plane increases sidespin, which will cause the ball to curve severely during its flight, much like a pitcher's curveball. The most common swing path fault for amateur golfers is the "out-to-in" swing path (Fig. 43-4). The resulting sidespin causes the ball to curve from left to right for the right-hander. The more off-line the swing, the greater the resulting sidespin and the farther the ball will curve off line. This type of swing path results from poor synchronization of the kinetic chain. Usually, the shoulders, arms, and/or hands begin to move ahead of the unwinding of the hips and trunk, causing the club to move away from the body and outside the target line. To make contact with the ball, the golfer must pull the club across the target line at impact, which imparts

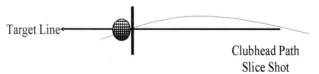

Clubhead Path
Slice Shot

FIG 43-4 Out-to-in swing path fault in a right-handed golfer causes the ball to curve in the air.

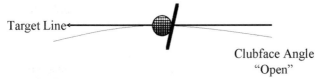

FIG 43-5 An *open club face* refers to the clubface pointing to the right of the target line for a right-handed golfer.

sidespin. Because the swing is poorly synchronized and inefficient, maximum clubhead speed is not achieved, and the ball flies a shorter distance. This effect is magnified by the loss in distance caused by sidespin. Aerodynamically, sidespin increases drag, which further hampers distance as compared to a shot hit with pure backspin. Golfers with this swing fault tend to swing harder to compensate, which tends to further disrupt the timing of the swing. Unfortunately, this frequently results in exaggeration of the original swing fault, and increased forces that can cause injury. These injuries can be acute, related to a single intemperate effort, but more frequently occur due to repetitive microtrauma, as the golfer hits scores or hundreds of balls on the driving range trying to find that elusive key to correct the swing path.

The *clubface angle* refers to the direction the face of the club is pointing relative to the target line at impact. An *open clubface* refers to the clubface pointing to the right of the target line for a right-handed golfer (Fig. 43-5). This will cause the same type of sidespin as the out-to-in swing path, resulting in a ball that curves from left to right. Several factors may contribute to this swing fault, most related to gripping the club. The position of the hands on the club at address is extremely important in determining whether the clubface is square at impact. Grip pressure, or how tightly the club is gripped, is another important factor. Gripping the club too tightly will prevent the club from swinging freely through the hitting area. A tight grip also leads to eccentric loading of the common extensor tendon of the dominant arm on follow-through, another prelude to overuse injury.

The swing plane, clubface angle, and clubhead speed at impact, and the location of impact of the ball on the clubface determine the flight of the struck ball. Errors in any of these factors can result in shots that are significantly off target. The clubhead travels approximately 27 feet during the golf swing, and errors of only a few millimeters or a few degrees can result in embarrassingly bad shots. Kinematic studies demonstrate the ability of professional golfers to repeat the swing in such a way that delivers the clubhead square to the target line, consistently striking the ball at or near the "sweet spot" of the clubface, where the ball will rebound at maximum velocity. One of the basic differences between amateur and professional golfers is the ability of professional golfers to generate increased clubhead speed. Newtonian physics dictate that, all things being equal (the club used, direction of club path, and impact at sweet spot with the clubface square), the faster the clubhead is traveling at impact, the faster the ball will rebound off the clubface and the longer the resulting shot. Inefficiencies common to the amateur golfer include swinging across the target line, failure to square the clubface at impact, and improper timing when "releasing" the club. Professional golf instruction can assist the golfer in improving the efficiency of the swing by identifying specific swing faults and giving the golfer specific drills and goals to work toward during practice sessions.

Pre-Shot Routine

The pre-shot routine refers to the preparations a golfer goes through before beginning the golf swing. This includes mental and physical preparation for striking the golf ball. Assessing how the ball lies on the fairway, in the rough, or in the sand, choosing a target, determining the type of shot to hit, selecting a club, aligning oneself, taking a practice swing, setting up over the ball, and perhaps a relaxation breath or mental recitation of a "swing thought" might all be part of the player's pre-shot routine. Consistency in the pre-shot routine is part of the foundation upon which a reliable, repeatable swing must be built.

Stance

The golf stance, also referred to as the *setup* or *address*, refers to the posture assumed by the golfer in preparation for hitting the ball. The proper setup should include several features, all related to balance. A good setup is similar to the "athletic ready position": feet approximately shoulder width apart, knees and hips slightly bent, torso upright and leaning slightly forward, good spinal posture, weight balanced on both feet, perhaps slightly toward the balls of the feet but certainly not the heels. The arms should hang free and relaxed at address. The hips and shoulders should be aligned along the target line (Fig. 43-6).

One of the most important components of the setup is the golf grip. The club should be gripped lightly. The end result of the golf swing is a chain of events that results in the club whipping through the hitting area at maximum velocity. This is a passive event, the end result of the unwinding kinetic chain, guided lightly by the hands and wrists, rather than an active

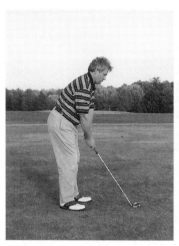
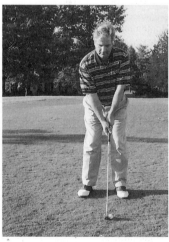

A   B

FIG 43-6   The hips and shoulders are aligned along the target line as seen from the front (A) and side (B).

swatting at the ball. A tight grip increases tension in the other muscle groups of the upper extremities. This restricts the club from swinging freely through the impact zone, reducing clubhead speed. Therefore, the grip pressure should remain light, just firm enough to prevent the club from flying out of the hands.

An additional consideration in the grip is the position of the hands on the club in relation to the clubface. A *neutral grip* involves no additional rotation clockwise or counterclockwise, resulting in the "V" between the thumb and index finger pointing roughly between the chin and dominant ear. Golfers who have difficulty squaring the clubface at impact are frequently advised to take a stronger grip. This does not refer to gripping the club more tightly, but to the rotational position of the hands on the club. A stronger grip involves rotating the hands slightly toward the dominant side (clockwise for a right-handed golfer). This preloads the hands and wrists and assists in the closing of the clubface through the impact zone.

Foot position plays a role in determining the shape of a golf swing. Again, balance and comfort are keys to consider. Generally, when using the driver, woods, and long irons, the stance should be slightly wider to promote a more stable base, and with shorter clubs, the feet should be slightly closer together. External rotation of the nondominant lower extremity will restrict the hip turn, but can allow a more full follow-through. Internal rotation of the nondominant lower extremity will allow a bigger hip turn and longer backswing, and might be advisable for individuals with chronic low back pain, as this will decrease the torque established by the differential between the hip and shoulder turn (see The X Factor on page 715).

Another consideration is the spine angle—the angle between the spine and the ground. The spine forms the axis around which the golf swing occurs. Good spinal posture should be maintained throughout the golf swing. Flexion should occur at the hips and knees rather than at the waist. Maintaining some lumbar lordosis is important in the prevention of lumbar disk injuries. The spine angle should be approximately 45° when viewed from behind, viewing down the target line. The spine angle is slightly less (more upright) for longer-shafted clubs such as the driver, and slightly more horizontal for shorter-shafted clubs such as the wedges. Because the club is gripped with the right hand lower on the grip than the left, the spine is tilted about 15° away from the target when viewed from across the ball. Therefore, the right shoulder is lower than the left shoulder on setup, but the shoulders remain perpendicular to the spine.

Backswing

During the backswing, the club is brought into a position from which the ball will be struck. This involves rotation or coiling of the upper body, loading the kinetic chain. The initial few feet of clubhead movement is termed the *take-away* (Fig. 43-7). EMG demonstrates increased firing patterns during take-away in the following muscles: bilateral lumbar paraspinals and supraspinatus; dominant infraspinatus and posterior deltoid; nondominant subscapularis, pectoralis major, anterior deltoid, latissimus dorsi, and abdominal oblique muscles. The club is brought back, away from the ball, starting along the target line, then rotating around the body as the shoulders and upper torso rotate (Fig. 43-8). The pelvis rotates, typically 30–45°, and the shoulders rotate

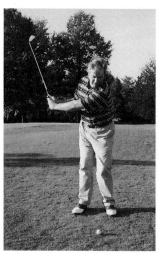 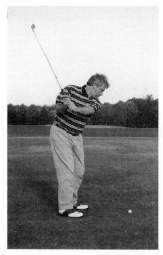

A   B

FIG 43-7 *Takeaway* is the initial movement of the clubhead as seen from the front (A) and side (B).

60–90° from the setup position. The weight should remain balanced, although as the club is taken back, the weight shifts toward the dominant side. Classic teaching encouraged golfers to keep the head from moving at all. However, current teaching fundamentals allow slight backward drift of the head as the club is taken back, to allow the spine to maintain good posture. During the backswing, the dominant shoulder is externally rotated in extension and slight abduction, and the dominant scapula is retracted. The nondominant shoulder is flexed, adducted, and internally rotated, bringing the biceps into contact with the chest wall. The nondominant scapula is protracted. This results in a coiling of the shoulders around the axis of the spine.

Cocking of the wrists during the backswing results in radial deviation of both wrists at the top of the backswing. The dominant wrist is extended. The nondominant wrist flexes slightly during the backswing. The golf swing is a two-lever system. The arms and shoulders turn around the axis of the spine, forming one lever, and the wrists hinge, forming the axis of the second lever. During the backswing, torque is generated as the shoulders rotate farther than the hips.

The "X Factor"

One of the findings in kinematic studies of the golf swing has been that professional golfers typically have a greater difference between the amount of hip turn and shoulder turn than amateurs do. This builds tension through the trunk, the uncoiling of which results in a powerful swing. The difference between hip and shoulder turn is called the *X factor*. Although a positive correlation between increased X factor and clubhead speed has been established, there is concern that increased trunk rotation causes torsional stress on the lumbar disks, which might predispose to disk injury. The classic golf

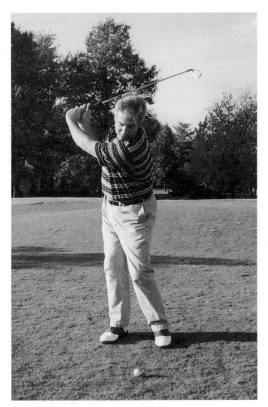

FIG 43-8 The club rotates around the body.

swing, on the other hand, allows more turning of the hips during the back-swing. This decreases the X factor and therefore is a safer technique for individuals with lower back problems. The drawback to this technique is primarily a loss of distance.

Downswing

The downswing in golf is analogous to the acceleration phase of throwing. The kinetic chain unwinds, beginning with rotation of the pelvis toward the target. The arms swing downward, on a path similar to the backswing, maintaining the cocking of the wrist until the last possible moment. The downswing represents the peak of activity for the latissimus dorsi and pectoralis major muscles. The dominant pectoralis major fires early in the downswing, joined by the nondominant pectoralis major closer to impact and through early follow-through (Pink et al., 1990). The external obliques and lumbar paraspinals fire bilaterally to assist in the unwinding of the trunk and shoulders (Hosea et al., 1996). Maximum clubhead speed results from the "release" of the club as the wrists unhinge while the arms and shoulders rotate through the hitting area. Premature unhinging of the wrists causes the clubhead to travel outside the target line and releases stored energy before

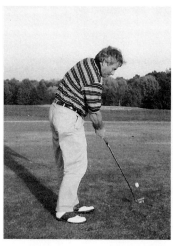
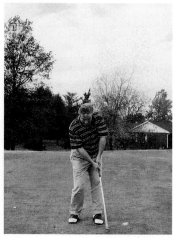

A   B

FIG 43-9 The position at impact as seen from the side (A) and front (B).

impact, typically resulting in a weak slice. Professional golfers consistently delay the release of the club until last possible moment, with the peak clubhead speed occurring through the impact zone.

Impact

The position at impact is similar to the position at address (Fig. 43-9). Subtle differences are worth noting. The lower body has rotated slightly toward the target, evidence that the lower body leads the swing. The hands remain slightly forward of the clubface at impact. The clubhead passing the hands before impact is a sign of a premature release of the wrists. In this situation, peak clubhead speed has occurred before impact. However, if the hands are too far ahead of the clubhead, peak acceleration of the clubhead has been delayed too long.

Follow-Through

The follow-through begins at impact and represents a gradual deceleration of the club. At the finish, the golfer should be balanced, most of the weight having shifted to the nondominant leg (Fig. 43-10). A smooth, full follow-through is necessary to ensure maximum clubhead speed through the impact zone. Many amateur golfers have a jerky, abbreviated follow-through. This results in increased stress on the musculoskeletal system as tense muscles are used to actively decelerate the club, rather than allowing a long, smooth, gradual deceleration of the club. Short follow-through is frequently a sign of deceleration through the impact zone. Follow-through is commonly inhibited by gripping the club too tightly. One favor the sports medicine physician can perform for the golfer with lateral elbow pain is to recommend a swing evaluation with a teaching professional, with specific attention to grip and follow-through.

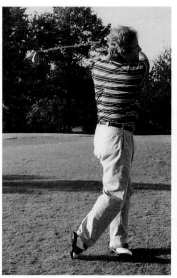 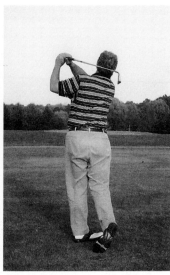

A B

FIG 43-10 The position at follow-through as seen from the side (A) and back (B).

EPIDEMIOLOGY

There are differences in injury rates and patterns between professional and amateur golfers. These differences appear to be related to differences in swing mechanics and time spent practicing and playing golf. Amateur golfers most frequently report injuries to the lower back (34.5%), elbow (33.1%), hand and wrist (20%), and shoulder (11.9%) (McCarroll et al., 1982; Batt, 1992). Professional golfers report a similar incidence of nondominant wrist (24%) and lower back (23.7%) injuries, with elbow injuries representing only 6.6% of injuries. Female professional golfers experience more injuries to the left wrist as compared to male professionals, whereas male professional golfers experience more injuries to the left shoulder than their female counterparts (McCarroll et al., 1982). Of elbow injuries, lateral epicondyle injuries were five times more common than medial epicondyle injuries in amateurs, but occur with similar frequency among professional golfers. Acute injuries to the eyes and head are the most common golf injuries reported among children and young people in the medical literature, and also occur in adults. A number of surveys have addressed factors contributing to golf injuries. Many of these implicate poor biomechanics and faulty swing techniques as contributing factors to golf injury. Overtraining, advanced age, and lack of physical conditioning have also been associated with golf injuries.

EQUIPMENT

Improvements in equipment technology have been ongoing throughout the history of golf. The latest technological advances in club design have focused on improving clubhead speed through use of lighter materials and improving the size of the sweet spot. Advances in ball design have focused on decreasing spin off the driver (sidespin results in hooks and slices), and improving aerodynamics. Shaft technologies have improved dramatically over the past 12–15 years. Graphite shafts are available over a range of flexes that can be tailored to a golfer's size and clubhead speed. Graphite shafts deliver less vibration to the hands and forearms at impact. An investment in new, custom-fitted clubs may improve performance and decrease risk of injury (Kohn, 1996).

INJURIES AND EVALUATION

Trauma

Acute traumatic injuries may occur as a result of being hit with the club or ball. Most catastrophic injuries are a result of being struck with the club, especially among children. Most pediatric golf-related head injuries occur in unsupervised children. In a prospective study in Scotland, half of the children presenting with head injury related to golf required surgery (McGuffie et al., 1998). Educating young golfers about golf etiquette and safety is an important strategy in preventing these injuries, most of which do not happen on the course.

Golf cart–related injuries are a cause of golf-related catastrophic injury and death, and are nearly always preventable. Golf cart injuries include including death, spinal cord injury, and various chronic disabilities of an extremity (Kelly, 1996). Driving on a sidehill, allowing arms and legs to leave the confines of the cart, driving the cart while intoxicated, and failure to secure the parking brake have all been implicated in cart-related injury and death.

Ocular Injuries

Injuries to the eye may occur as a result of being struck by the ball or club. In fact, there is a case report of a youngster who experienced a penetrating eye injury when his plastic tee flew into his eye during a swing (Mulvihill et al., 1997). Golf balls and clubheads are made of hard materials, easily penetrate the orbit, and travel at a high rate of speed, and so are capable of causing severe damage. Golf-related ocular injuries have been among the most serious eye injuries reported in published series of ocular injuries (Pollack et al., 1997). These injuries result in a high rate of enucleation. Definitive treatment requires ophthalmologic consultation. Prevention is key; as with head injuries, teaching young and beginning golfers to look before swinging and not to swing toward others is important.

Lightning

Death and injury from lightning strikes can be reduced but not entirely eliminated. There is always that first strike of lightning in a storm. However, many golfers seem to let a $60 greens fee interfere with good judgment. In some years, more golfers die from being struck by lightning than participants in any other sport, and most other years rank second only to people who fish, despite their much lower numbers. Rule 6-8 permits players to discontinue play if they believe there is a danger from lightning.

Golfers should know the proper precautions to take when lightning is potentially in the area. As a rule of thumb, the adage "if you can hear it, clear it" works well for lightning safety. Golfers should observe the 30:30 rule that requires seeking shelter if there is less than 30 seconds from a lightning flash to the thunder retort and staying in the shelter until 30 minutes after the last thunder clap is heard. Avoiding open areas, lone trees, power lines, bodies of water, golf carts, clubs, and umbrellas are important safety strategies (Cherington, 2001). Clubhouses, protected shelters, and closed vehicles are the best options. The National Fire Protection Association has published codes for construction of lightning protection systems for shelters. Courses vary in the protection afforded to players. Some are equipped with lightning detection systems and sirens to warn golfers of lightning; most do not. Familiarity with the protection at any course played during potentially inclement weather is a frequently neglected but important prevention strategy. Most courses that make the investment in lightning protection systems will have this information prominently displayed.

Heat and Solar Injury

Golfers who walk the course in hot weather are susceptible to heat injury. This is especially true of older individuals, who are more susceptible to heatstroke. Golf courses vary in providing opportunities for fluid replacement on the golf course. Educational strategies include encouraging golfers to increase fluid intake on hot, humid days and reviewing early signs and symptoms of dehydration. Likewise, repeated exposure to ultraviolet radiation increases the risk of sunburn and skin cancer. Protection of the skin with sunscreen is advisable to prevent sunburn, and may also protect against solar keratosis, although data regarding protection against skin cancer including melanoma are lacking.

Myocardial Infarction

Sudden cardiac death is the leading cause of mortality on the golf course. This is attributed to a number of factors, including the age of the golfing public and the remote location of players on the course, and sometimes the course itself. Stricken golfers may be more than a mile away from the clubhouse, so some form of communication is key. As in all cases of cardiac arrest outside the clinical setting, activating the emergency medical system and beginning cardiopulmonary resuscitation (CPR) are the initial steps. Ventricular fibrillation is the pathologic rhythm in 80–90% of cardiac arrests. Defibrillation is the definitive treatment for this condition. Survival diminishes by approximately 10% per minute of delay.

A charged cellular phone may be a lifesaver in this situation, although it is imperative to ensure that the phone has coverage over the entire course. Some courses have installed emergency phones on locations around the course. *Golf Digest* magazine, along with the American Heart Association, the National Safety Council and Medtronic Physio-Control, a manufacturer of automated external defibrillators (AEDs), established the Links for Life program in 1999. The goals of this program are to educate the golfing public about the risk of sudden death and to encourage golf courses to obtain AEDs and train personnel in CPR. Courses that have implemented this plan are also encouraged to provide radio or other communication ability with each of the groups on the course. Response times can be improved to 5 minutes or less with such a system. These programs have already been shown to reduce death from cardiac arrest on the golf course (Smith, 1999).

Prevention of cardiac death largely centers on lifestyle changes and appropriate screening. Often, a sports medicine physician provides entry to the medical system for golfers who would ignore their heart, but not their painful back or elbow. Remembering to consider the individual, not just the injury, is part of the practice of good medicine. It is wise to include screening for risk factors for coronary artery disease when obtaining the medical history.

Low Back Pain

Back pain is extremely common in America. Approximately 80% of Americans will experience back pain at some time, and golf is hardly protective against this phenomenon. Back injuries in the golfer include musculotendinous injuries (acute and chronic muscular strain and muscular spasm), acute disk injury, and exacerbation of the myriad causes of back pain unrelated to golf. Professional golfers typically have fluid, efficient, beautiful swings that are envied by most amateurs. These swings are reliable and repeatable under stressful conditions. They have been honed and maintained by countless hours on the driving range. This exacts a toll in the form of overuse injuries. In fact, golfers have the highest incidence of back injury of all professional athletes (Watkins, 2002). Unlike professional golfers, low back pain in the amateur is frequently associated with poor swing techniques. The "reverse C" finish is frequently seen in golfers with poor balance and golfers who have been instructed to keep their head still throughout the golf swing. A lurching, jerky swing is stressful to the back. Many golfers are otherwise sedentary, spending little time trying to improve strength, endurance, and flexibility. The rapid, sometimes violent swinging of a golf club represents an acute assault on the integrity of these weak, tight structures, frequently resulting in injury. This tendency is compounded by the average golfer's attempts to hit prodigious drives. Unfortunately, these attempts usually involve brute force rather than skill, and often cause injury.

Electromyographic studies have demonstrated that amateur golfers attain 90% of their peak muscle activity compared to 80% for professionals. During the downswing, peak trunk muscular forces occur, which correspond to peak spinal loading of the shear, lateral bending, and torsional forces generated by the golf swing. Additionally, amateur golfers have been shown to exhibit 80% greater torque and shear loads than professional golfers during the golf swing (Hosea et al., 1996). These findings are felt to be related to the muscular and biomechanical inefficiencies of the swings produced by amateur golfers relative to their professional counterparts. The combination of torsional, compressive, and lateral bending forces have been implicated in disk herniation (Adams et al., 1981). Repeated, near-maximal exertion coupled with the biomechanical forces involved in the golf swing stress the spine of the weekend golfer.

Fortunately, most of these injuries represent acute or chronic muscular strain and are self-limited. The golfer will typically recover from this condition within 2–4 weeks, as with most cases of back pain. Relative rest and supportive treatment with analgesics followed by a gradual return to activities is typically all that is required to manage these injuries. Pain lasting more than 2–4 weeks may be associated with a decrease in muscular strength and endurance. A visit or two with a physical therapist can help identify and address these imbalances when appropriate.

Chronic back pain in the golfer may have a muscular, discogenic, and/or spondylogenic component. A common diagnosis seen in spine care centers is myofascial pain syndrome, a condition that may coexist with other spine pathology. Painful localized trigger points are palpable, typically in the lumbar paraspinals, gluteals, and sometimes at the musculotendinous attachment (Travell et al., 1982). Fortunately, this condition responds well to the principles of sports medicine: working to regain range of motion, strength, endurance, and power, and implementing sport-specific drills as soon as practical. In chronic pain, changes occur at the spinal cord level that facilitate pain transmission. A number of medications can be useful in treatment of chronic pain, including low-dose tricyclics (nortriptyline, amitriptyline, desipramine, and doxepin), anticonvulsants (gabapentin, carbamazepine, and phenytoin), topical lidocaine patches, and opioid and related medications (Galer et al., 2000). Trigger point injection, manual therapy including myofascial release and other types of manipulation therapy, spray and stretch, acupuncture, and massage may all have a role in management of chronic back pain. Psychologists experienced in treating chronic pain might recommend biofeedback, relaxation therapy, self-hypnosis, cognitive-behavioral therapy, guided imagery, stress management, and other techniques to manage chronic pain. As a resumption of activities is a goal with all chronic pain patients, any measures that provide enough pain relief to allow the golfer to return to play should be considered.

A spectrum of disk injuries is observed in the golfer. The annulus fibrosus is a laminated ring of collagen surrounding the nucleus pulposus, a combination of water, protein, and glycosaminoglycans. Tears to the annulus fibrosus may occur with flexion and torsion (Haher et al., 1993). The annulus is well-innervated, and a tear of the annulus may cause central and referred low back pain. Acute disk herniation, on the other hand, occurs with the combination of annular tearing and protrusion of the nucleus pulposus. An age-related loss of hydration, accompanied by diminished viscoelastic properties, occurs throughout the lifespan. These changes may or may not cause pain, but likely increase the risk for disk injury by compromising the normal function of the annulus-nucleus complex (Oegema, 1993).

Disc herniation typically occurs in a posterolateral direction, threatening the contents of the spinal canal or neural foramen. If the herniation abuts the exiting nerve root, specific corresponding symptoms may occur along the affected dermatome. A thorough neurologic examination is paramount in the evaluation of individuals with low back and leg pain. Motor, sensory, and reflex abnormalities should be documented. In disk herniation with radiculopathy, the straight leg raising sign is usually positive. Pain is typically exacerbated by sitting and lumbar flexion. Initial management of discogenic pain, with or without radicular symptoms, is essentially the same for golfers as nongolfers. Up to 95% of patients with acute disk herniation can be treated successfully without surgery. As the annulus fibrosus is more likely to fail when axial loading is combined with rotation, a period of relative rest is useful after acute disk herniation. A period of 2–4 weeks of relative rest to allow healing of the annulus before returning to golf and vigorous physical activity is advisable. Resumption of activity is guided by symptoms. Walking is encouraged as soon as tolerated without worsening symptoms. In the presence of acute radiculopathy, oral corticosteroids may be useful. If radicular symptoms do not resolve within the first 1–2 weeks, further evaluation is warranted. Magnetic resonance imaging is a useful test to evaluate the intervertebral disks, although it must be remembered that a relatively high percentage of asymptomatic individuals have abnormal disk findings on MRI (Jensen et al., 1994). Symptoms caused by disk herniation documented by MRI and correlating with symptoms may respond to selective epidural steroid injection. Up to three of these injections may be necessary to treat radicular symptoms. Epidural steroid injection is generally not useful in treatment of central low back pain. Rehabilitation of disk injury may include passive therapies, such as manual or mechanical traction and extension-based exercises.

Facet arthropathy may occur as a result of trauma or degenerative change. Frequently, there is a progression from degenerative disc disease, with disc space narrowing causing increased facet loads and accelerating degenerative changes at the facet joints (Hosea et al., 1996). As the facets are typically loaded in extension, most individuals with facet pain experience increased pain with lumbar extension. A progression of degenerative changes in the joint may lead to spurring into the neural foramen, causing nerve root impingement. Treatment is similar to the above measures, as well as facet joint injection when necessary, which can serve diagnostic as well as therapeutic needs.

Surgery is reserved for individuals who do not respond to nonsurgical therapy and those with cauda equina syndrome (pain in the posterior thighs and legs, numbness of the buttocks, posterior legs, and soles of the feet, motor weakness of the legs and feet, and incontinence). The extent of surgical management is beyond the scope of this text, but may include lumbar microdiscectomy with or without laminectomy. Fusion surgery should be considered when a wide decompression is necessary for treatment of stenosis or when the posterior elements are disrupted, as lumbar instability can develop.

In addition to the usual musculoskeletal causes of back pain, non-orthopedic causes should be considered, including postherpetic neuralgia; pain referred from the kidneys, abdominal viscera, and prostate; aortic aneurysm; and lymphoma.

As symptoms improve, introducing abdominal and trunk strengthening are important in preventing recurrent injury. Trunk stabilization and muscular coordination is an important part of rehabilitation after spine injury. Motor control and coordination have become important components of trunk rehabilitation over the past decade. Exercises done on an exercise ball (Swiss ball) facilitate this. Exercises begin in a neutral, pain-free position. The specific injury, range of motion, strength, and endurance are all considerations in designing the specific rehabilitation program for the golfer with back pain. Rehabilitation coupled with lessons from a teaching professional allows most golfers with back pain to return and can actually improve performance. Frequently, a discussion of the specific injury with the teaching professional can be useful. For instance, golfers who are unable to tolerate rotation through the lumbar spine can learn to increase the hip turn to increase power. Professional instruction in swing mechanics can be useful to the amateur as well as the professional golfer who is recovering from low back pain (Grimshaw et al., 2000).

Suction devices are available that attach to the grip end of a putter to retrieve the ball from a cup. Teaching patients to bend at the knees rather than at the waist or hips to tee the ball can allow individuals with back pain to continue to enjoy playing.

Trunk

In addition to the abdominal wall muscles active in the golf swing, any of which may develop an acute or chronic strain, stress fracture of the ribs has been observed in golfers, and is felt to be related to weakness of the serratus anterior (Lord et al., 1996). These injuries typically occur on the nondominant side. Treatment includes relative rest and rehabilitation as for back injury.

Upper Extremity Injuries

Shoulder

Shoulder injuries in the golfer primarily occur in the nondominant shoulder. Determining the phase of the golf swing during which the patient experiences pain can be useful. At the top of the backswing, the nondominant shoulder is maximally horizontally adducted and internally rotated. This position may lead to symptoms from acromioclavicular (AC) joint arthrosis, impingement of the humerus on the anterior labrum, or tensile load on the posterior capsule or rhomboids of the nondominant shoulder. During the downswing, the nondominant rhomboids, pectoralis major, and latissimus dorsi fire maximally from a lengthened position, and acute or repetitive injuries may occur to these structures (Spinner et al., 1998). At follow-through, the nondominant shoulder is externally rotated and abducted, which may cause injury to the posterior labrum or impingement of the posterior cuff on the posterior labrum. Pain on follow-through and a positive relocation test would suggest injury to these structures (Jobe et al., 1996).

The rotator cuff fires at a low level during most of the golf swing, with a couple of exceptions. There is increased firing of the dominant supraspinatus and infraspinatus at take away. The supraspinatus of the nondominant shoulder shows increased activity as compared to the dominant shoulder throughout the golf swing, with the exception of take-away. Therefore impingement problems in the dominant shoulder are usually well tolerated by the golfer, whereas symptoms from the nondominant rotator cuff can limit participation. The nondominant subscapularis fires through all phases of the golf swing, assisting in take-away and firing to stabilize the humerus through downswing and follow-through (Jobe et al., 1986a). Most injuries to the rotator cuff respond to nonsurgical treatment, with rehabilitation emphasizing the rotator cuff, periscapular muscles, and kinetic chain. Diagnostic evaluation may include plain films to exclude degenerative changes, especially at the AC joint, and other causes of shoulder pain. MRI can be useful in determining impingement and rotator cuff tears, although one must be wary of false negatives and false positives. Judicious use of corticosteroid injection remains a widely used tool in treatment of rotator cuff injury. Surgical treatment is sometimes necessary in management of rotator cuff and labral injury, although return to golf is typically successful after this (Jobe et al., 1996).

Elbow

Although the term *golfers elbow* is frequently used to describe medial epicondylosis, injuries to the nondominant lateral humeral epicondyle are much more common in amateur golfers. A common fault of amateurs with this problem is to grip the club tightly. Grip tension significantly increases tensile load to the common flexor and extensor tendons, and is associated with medial and lateral epicondylosis. Golfers rarely admit to a tight grip. The intervention of a teaching professional is likely to benefit the golfer at least as much as the usual rehabilitation program described elsewhere in this book. Ideally, a rehabilitation program combined with golf instruction is utilized in helping the golfer recover from this injury. Because of the explosive tensile loading of the common extensor tendon during the golf swing, it may be advisable to avoid the golf swing to allow this injury to heal. This may be even more important after corticosteroid injection, if this becomes necessary for treatment of this condition.

Injuries to the medial epicondyle may occur in the dominant elbow as a result of contacting the ground before (or sometimes instead of) the ball, hitting off practice mats, or hitting off hard, packed earth, or overuse. Experienced golfers are more likely to sustain injuries to the medial epicondyle as a result of overuse.

Treatment of elbow injury in golfers includes all of the measures useful in nongolfers. Initial interventions include relative rest, use of a counterforce forearm band, nonsteroidals to treat symptoms, and physical therapy. Physical therapy may include physical modalities (iontophoresis, ultrasound, or phonophoresis), cross-friction massage, and stretching and strengthening exercises for the forearm muscles. Corticosteroid injection remains widely used and is frequently effective, despite a lack of evidence supporting its use (Boyer et al., 1999). Acupuncture has been shown useful in treatment of this condition (Fink et al., 2002). Extracorporeal shock wave therapy has recently been approved for use in the United States and has 80–95% effectiveness after 3–5 treatments. When the golfer is able to perform stretching and strengthening exercises without significant pain, a progression to the full swing can be introduced. Professional instruction can help prevent recurrence of this problem and sometimes hasten return to golf.

Wrist and Hand

DeQuervain's disease is seen in golfers in the nondominant wrist. Ulnar deviation of the left wrist occurs at impact, which may be an etiologic factor in the development of deQuervain's disease (Murray et al., 1996). This injury is seen in experienced golfers as a result of overuse. Additionally, golfers with an out-to-in swing path experience an acute ulnar deviation, which may also predispose to this condition. Treatment includes relative rest, which may include fabrication of a thumb spica splint. Injection of corticosteroid into the first dorsal compartment can also be useful in managing this condition. Symptoms persisting beyond 3 months might be amenable to surgical release of the first dorsal compartment, and referral to a hand surgeon should be considered. If the golfer typically hits a slice, professional instruction is advisable. Extensor carpi ulnaris, flexor carpi radialis, and flexor carpi ulnaris tendinitis occasionally occur in golfers as well, and usually respond to same strategies. Injuries to the forearm, wrist, and hand have been associated with a significantly greater arc of motion in the left wrist during the golf swing despite demonstrating decreased range of motion (Cahalan et al., 1991).

Acute and stress fractures of the hook of the hamate have been observed in golfers (Skolnick, 1998). This may occur acutely as a result of striking a solid object (hard packed earth or rock) or because of repeated microtrauma of the butt of the club against the nondominant hamate. Symptoms include pain in the ulnar side of the wrist, weakness of grip, painful grip, and ulnar nerve paresthesias (Bishop et al., 1988). Pain with direct palpation over the hook of the hamate should be further evaluated. Both acute and stress fractures can be difficult to diagnose on plain films, requiring special views. MRI, bone scan, and high-resolution CT can be useful in making this diagnosis. Treatment of acute injury includes immobilization in a short-arm cast for 6–8 weeks, followed by rehabilitation and a gradual return to activity. Unfortunately, a majority of these fractures present late with nonunion. These fractures respond successfully to surgical excision of the palmar fragment (Murray et al., 1996).

Lower Extremity Injuries

Hip

Trochanteric bursitis is not uncommon in golfers, usually involving the nondominant hip. Many individuals slide or shift the hips forward rather than rotating the hips during the golf swing. This creates an adduction moment at the nondominant hip, stretching tight tissues over the trochanteric bursa. Instruction and drills to teach the golfer to turn rather than shift the hips is key in treatment of this injury, along with measures useful in other individuals (NSAIDs, corticosteroid injection, cross-friction massage, strengthening of hip abductors, etc).

Osteoarthritis of the hip is a common condition among older golfers. Treatment includes the usual measures, and acetaminophen, NSAIDs, gentle range-of-motion exercises, and local muscular strengthening exercises can be useful. Most golfers are able to return to participation after total hip arthroplasty when this becomes necessary (Mallon et al., 1996).

Knee

Golf-related injuries of the knee may be acute or overuse in nature. These injuries may occur as a result of slipping on wet grass or other traumatic events. A survey of 35 golfers seen over a 2-year period showed similar numbers of injuries to right and left knees, while all the golfers in this study were right-handed (Guten, 1996). The most common location of injury was the medial meniscus, with osteoarthritis being the second most common diagnosis. Knee joint forces and moments generated during the golf swing are not large enough for golf to be considered an activity with a higher risk for traumatic knee injury (Gatt et al., 1998). Meniscal injury can respond to nonsurgical management, especially in golfers over 40 in whom degenerative tears of the meniscus are common. Osteoarthritis of the knee is a common condition in older golfers, and it responds to the same strategies used in nongolfers. Range-of-motion, flexibility, and strengthening exercises can increase tolerance for physical activities. Osteoarthritis and degenerative meniscal tears may respond to acetaminophen, nonsteroidals, glucosamine with or without chondroitin, acupuncture (Christensen et al., 1992), viscosupplementation, and corticosteroid injection. Symptomatic meniscal tears that do not respond to nonsurgical treatment can be treated arthroscopically, generally with good results. Osteoarthritis predominantly involving the medial or lateral compartment may respond to use of an unloader brace. Knee replacement surgery should be reserved for those with symptoms that do not respond to nonsurgical treatment. A return to golf can be anticipated after knee arthroplasty (Mallon et al., 1996).

MANAGEMENT

Professional instruction is useful in a number of skill sports, none more so than golf. The old adage "practice makes perfect" is the mantra of many amateur golfers on the driving range. A more accurate statement quoted by many golf professionals is "practice makes permanent." Unfortunately, a lot of golfers practice faulty techniques, ingraining poor swing mechanics while the overuse mounts. Among the best bits of advice sports medicine practitioners can impart to their golfing patients is to take a lesson, or ideally a series of lessons, with the goal of improving swing technique. Practicing an efficient golf swing will lead to a reliable, repeatable technique that is less likely to fall apart under the stress of competition and less likely to result in injury.

Principles of management of these injuries do not differ significantly for golfers than for athletes involved in other sports. Addressing kinetic chain issues remote from the injury site is important. Enlisting the assistance of a golf professional to help address swing mechanics benefits injured golfers greatly.

RETURN TO PLAY

Depending on the specific injury, the athlete may be able to putt and chip during the rehabilitation period. The putting and chipping motions involve a limited, pendulum-like motion of the shoulders and arms, requiring precision rather than force. These are extremely important parts of the game for shooting good scores, yet the majority of golfers neglect this part of practice. All golfers have heard the adage "practice the short game." Psychologically, it is useful to help any dedicated athlete find some component of the game to improve during recovery from injury, and golfers are no different. Many will be grateful for the opportunity to stay involved with the game, and they all know they play better if they practice their short game. Warm-up and stretching before practice sessions is a part of the overall treatment program. Golfers sometimes need to be reminded that resuming golf participation does not obviate the need for continued rehabilitation.

The address position for chips and putts is similar to the full swing with a bit more flexion in the hips. Because of flexion at the hips, the lumbar paraspinals are active and the disc pressure is increased, so individuals with low back injuries may not tolerate this. Putting and chipping for only a few minutes at first, or taking a 5-minute break between sets of putts and chips may allow the golfer to begin building endurance of these muscles. Golfers with upper or lower extremity injuries will usually tolerate these activities without difficulty.

A progressive return to the full swing is desirable for golf rehabilitation. In golf, *pitching* refers hitting a shot that flies farther than it rolls, but is less than a full swing. Pitching is part of the short game and is as important for scoring well as chipping and putting. While the chip is struck with a motion that is somewhat similar to putting, pitches are more similar to the full swing. In fact, working on pitching is a good way to develop a smooth, relaxed full swing.

As the golfer is allowed to resume the full swing, initial efforts should be made only with the wedges. These are the shortest clubs, require less force to swing, and do not carry the psychological impetus to hit a prodigious shot. Instruct the golfer to limit the initial session to pitches of no greater than 50% of their full wedge distance. For most golfers, this will be in the range of 40–60 yards. For some youths, women, and older golfers, 60 yards may represent a full swing with the wedge, so be sure to find out what the full wedge distance is for that individual, and begin with targets at half that distance. It is also important to limit the number of swings during the initial sessions to 10–20 of these shots. Initially, this can be combined with chipping and putting if the golfer desires more practice and tolerates this.

If the golfer tolerates the initial session, the next sessions should include shots of a longer distance. After stretching and warm-up, the golfer should begin with half-wedge distance for a few (5–10) shots. A progression to a few shots of greater distance, in the 75% range, is allowed next. If these are tolerated, the golfer should progress to a few full wedge shots. A gradual progression through the rest of the clubs is permitted after the golfer tolerates a few full shots with the wedge (Table 43-1). The golfer should avoid playing or practicing on consecutive days until he or she has worked up to the driver. As long as the golfer tolerates working through the sequence of clubs, increasing the workload each session is allowed. Depending on how often the golfer is able to practice, it will take 2–4 weeks to work through the progression.

If the golfer experiences recurrent symptoms after an increase, the workload should be reduced to the previous asymptomatic level after a few days of recovery as necessary. The workload should then be increased by approximately 10% per week until the golfer is able to hit the number of full shots on the range that one would expect to hit for 9 holes. A par shooter would be expected to take two putts per hole, or 36 putts per round of golf, leaving approximately 36 full shots to play 18 holes on a par 72 course. The average American golfer shoots in the low 90s on a par 72 course and roughly half of those shots would be full swings. When the golfer is able to hit 20–30 full shots with a selection of clubs, a nine-hole round is permitted. If recovering from a spine or lower extremity injury, use of a pull-cart may be advisable; occasionally a motorized cart is necessary. A return to walking the course should be encouraged as soon as practical.

Appropriate cross-training for the injured golfer should include walking whenever possible. A sports medicine physician who treats golfers without advising them to walk the course is missing a key opportunity for fitness counseling. Unless contraindicated, walking should be an integral part of the game. In the United Kingdom and Ireland, "buggies" are shunned by golfers, available only at the resort courses favored by Americans. Walking the golf

TABLE 43-1 Sample Rehabilitation Regimen for Golfers

Day	50% wedge	75% wedge	Full wedge	Short irons (PW, 8, 9)	Middle irons (7, 6, 5)	Long irons (4, 3, 2)	Woods (7, 5, 3)	Driver
1	10–20	0	0	0	0	0	0	0
2	5	5–10	5–10	0	0	0	0	0
3	5	5	5–10	5–10	0	0	0	0
4	5	5	5	5–10	5–10	0	0	0
5	5	5	5	5–10	5–10	0	0	0
6	5	5	5	5	5–10	5–10	0	0
7	5	5	5	5	5	5–10	5–10	0
8	5	5	5	5	5	5	5–10	5–10

course is an acceptable fitness activity, and has been shown to improve lipids and aerobic capacity (Parkkari et al., 2000).

SIDELINE TIPS

Probably the best advice for physicians on the golf course is to be a "safety monitor." The most serious injuries usually happen as a result of carelessness. Do not be shy about pointing out some of the data about cart and ocular injuries when it may be illustrative.

The cellular telephone is generally a bane on the golf course. Yet it may also be an important piece of safety equipment, especially for walkers who may be far from the clubhouse with no quick way back in an emergency. Silence the cell phone and keep it in the bag.

PREVENTION

Advice regarding prevention of golf injuries is largely based on recommendations from experienced physicians and researchers rather than hard scientific data. Proposed measures include proper swing mechanics, adherence to conditioning (strength and stretching) programs, adequate warm-up before both practice and play, adherence to safety rules and etiquette, seeking safety during storms, the use of proper equipment, sun protection, and the replenishment of food and drink (Sherman et al., 2000). For many recreational golfers coming off an injury, a few sessions with a golf pro for individualized instruction is well worth the time and effort to avoid future injury.

Flexibility

A number of body sites are amenable to flexibility training that can improve the biomechanics of the golf swing. Improvement in flexibility of the heel cords and hamstrings improves the stable base around which the golf swing occurs. Additionally, limitations of hamstring flexibility predispose to flexion occurring at the lumbar spine rather than at the hips during address. The combination of lumbar flexion and rotation predisposes to lumbar disk injury. Improving flexibility of the shoulders, with particular attention to the scapular protractors (serratus anterior, pectoralis minor) and retractors (rhomboids and middle trapezius) can enhance the shoulder turn and increase power and control. Flexible shoulders allow a more full backswing and follow-through no matter how little spinal rotation is permissible. Flexibility exercises for the muscles of the forearm can be useful in treatment and prevention of elbow injury.

Strengthening

Strength training is particularly useful for the trunk rotators (abdominal obliques, short spine rotators) and shoulder muscles. Swiss ball exercises have gained acceptance in golf performance programs around the country, and likely have a role in prevention as well as performance, although data are lacking. Shoulder strengthening exercises including the rotator cuff, pectoralis major, latissimus dorsi, and scapular stabilizers are recommended for prevention of shoulder injuries (Jobe et al., 1996). *30 Exercises for Better Golf* by Dr. Frank Jobe (1986b) is written for the layperson, and includes a combination of strengthening, flexibility, and sport-specific exercises for the golfer interested in prevention of injury or improving performance.

Warm-Up

Taking time to warm up can prevent acute injury. The merits of stretching have not been confirmed by research, but most sports physicians recommend stretching before golf. Stretching the shoulders and trunk takes only a few minutes, to be followed by some easy swings. Beginning with a few half-wedges, the golfer should gradually build up to a full swing with a wedge, then progress through the middle irons, woods, and/or driver. The first swing a golfer takes should not be a full swing with the driver.

Safety

Waiting for the playing area to clear, taking one last look around before taking a practice swing, and heading for appropriate shelter during thunderstorms are examples of golf injury prevention. Putting a charged cellular phone in the golf bag can be useful in an emergency if cellular service is available on the golf course.

SUMMARY

Golfers primarily experience overuse injuries. Acute injuries are also seen, usually a result of ambitious swings by deconditioned individuals. Catastrophic injuries are rare, and usually result from carelessness. Accurate diagnosis and a targeted rehabilitation program combined with professional instruction will allow most golfers to return to participation. Adjustments to the swing can allow golfers with most spine injuries to resume play. Awareness of lightning safety can be a lifesaver.

REFERENCES

Adams M, Hutton WC. The relevance of torsion to the mechanical derangement of the lumbar spine. *Spine*. 1981;6:241–248.

Batt ME. A survey of golf injuries in amateur golfers. *Br J Sports Med*. 1992;26:63–65.

Bishop AT, Beckenbaugh RD. Fracture of the hamate hook. *J Hand Surg [Am]*. 1988;13:135–139.

Boyer MI, Hastings H. Lateral tennis elbow: "Is there any science out there?" *J Shoulder Elbow Surg*. 1999;8:481–491.

Cahalan TD, Cooney WP, Tamai K, et al. Biomechanics of the golf swing in players with pathologic conditions of the forearm, wrist and hand. *Am J Sports Med*. 1991;19:288–293.

Cherington M. Lightning injuries in sports. *Sports Med*. 2001;31:301–308.

Christensen BV, Iuhl IU, Vilbek H, et al. Acupuncture treatment of severe knee osteoarthrosis. A long-term study. *Acta Anaesthesiol Scand*. 1992;36:519–525.

Fink M, Wolkenstein E, Karst M, Gehrke A. Acupuncture in chronic epicondylitis: a randomized controlled trial. *Rheumatology (Oxford)*. 2002;41:205–209.

Galer BS, Dworkin RH, eds. *A Clinical Guide to Neuropathic Pain*. Minneapolis: McGraw-Hill; 2000.

Gatt CJ, Pavol MJ, Parker RD, et al. Three-dimensional knee joint kinetics during a golf swing: Influences of skill level and footwear. *Am J Sports Med*. 1998;26:285–294.

Grimshaw PN, Burden AM. Case report: Reduction of low back pain in a professional golfer. *Med Sci Sports Exerc*. 2000;32:1667–1673.

Guten GN. Knee injuries in golf. *Clin Sports Med*. 1996;15:111–128.

Haher TR, O'Brien MO, Kauffman C, et al. Biomechanics of the spine in sports. *Clin Sports Med*. 1993;12:449–464.

Hogan B. *Five Lessons: The Modern Fundamentals of Golf.* New York: Simon & Schuster; 1957.

Hosea TM, Gatt CJ. Back pain in golf. *Clin Sports Med.* 1996;15:37–53.

Jensen MC, Brant-Zawadzki MN, Obuchowski N, et al. Magnetic resonance imaging of the lumbar spine in people without back pain. *N Engl J Med.* 1994;331:69–73.

Jobe FW, Moynes DR, Antonelli DJ. Rotator cuff function during a golf swing. *Am J Sports Med.* 1986a;14:388–392.

Jobe F, Moynes D. *30 Exercises for Better Golf.* Inglewood, CA: Champion Press; 1986b.

Jobe FW, Pink MM. Shoulder pain and golf. *Clin Sports Med.* 1996;15:55–63.

Kelly EG. Major injuries occurring during use of a golf cart. *Orthopedics.* 1996;19:519–521.

Kohn HS. Prevention and treatment of elbow injuries in golf. *Clin Sports Med.* 1996;15:65–83.

Lord MJ, Ha KI, Song KS. Stress fractures of the ribs in golfers. *Am J Sports Med.* 1996;24:118–122.

Mallon WJ, Liebelt RA, Mason JB. Total joint replacement and golf. *Clin Sports Med.* 1996;15:179–190.

McArdle WD, Katch FI, Katch VL. *Exercise Physiology: Energy, Nutrition, and Human Performance,* 3d ed. Malvern, PA: Lea & Febiger; 1991.

McCarroll JR, Gioe TJ. Professional golfers and the price they pay. *Phys Sports Med.* 1982;10:54–70.

McCarroll JR. The frequency of golf injuries. *Clin Sports Med.* 1996;15:1–7.

McGuffie AC, Fitzpatrick MO, Hull D. Golf related head injuries in children: The Little Tigers. *Scot Med J.* 1998;43:139–140.

Mulvihill A, O'Sullivan J, Logan P. Penetrating eye injury caused by a golf tee. *Br J Ophthalmol.* 1997;81:91.

Murray PM, Cooney WP. Golf-induced injuries of the wrist. *Clin Sports Med.* 1996;15:85–109.

Nicklaus JN, Bowden K. *Golf My Way.* New York: Simon & Schuster; 1998.

Oegema TR. Biochemistry of the intervertebral disk. *Clin Sports Med.* 1993;12:419–439.

Parkkari J, Natri A, Kannus P, et al. A controlled trial of the health benefits of regular walking on golf course. *Am J Med.* 2000;109:102–108.

Pink M, Jobe FW, Perry J. Electromyographic analysis of the shoulder during the golf swing. *Am J Sports Med.* 1990;18:137–140.

Pollack JS, Mieler WF, Mittra RA. Golf-related ocular injuries. *Curr Opin Ophthalmol.* 1997;8:15–18.

Sherman CA, Finch CF. Preventing injuries to competitive and recreational adult golfers: What is the evidence? *J Sci Med Sport.* 2000;3:65–68.

Skolnick AA. "Golfer's wrist" can be a tough break to diagnose. *JAMA.* 1998;279:571–522.

Smith S. Links for life. *Golf Digest.* October 1999.

Spinner RJ, Speer KP, Mallon WJ. Avulsion injury to the conjoined tendons of the latissimus dorsi and teres major muscles. *Am J Sports Med.* 1998;26:847–849.

Travell JG, Simons DG. *Myofascial Pain and Dysfunction: The Trigger Point Manual.* Baltimore: Williams & Wilkins; 1982.

Watkins RG. Lumbar disc injury in the athlete. *Clin Sports Med.* 2002;21:147–165.

44 | Strength Training and Weight Lifting

Laurie Donaldson and William W. Dexter

INTRODUCTION

Lifting weights to increase muscle size and strength has been pursued since the 6th century BC when the six-time Olympian Milo of Crotona pioneered progressive resistance training by using a growing calf to build muscle by lifting it onto his shoulders daily until the calf was fully grown. Since then, athletes have used resistance exercise to achieve success from the circus arena to the Olympics. Power lifting, Olympic weight lifting, and body-building are three disciplines that encompass the growing sport of weight training. Competitive athletes from all sports also incorporate weight lifting into their training routines. In the general population, about one in five US adults participate in weight training activities monthly.

Power lifting and Olympic weight lifting are popular international sports. Power lifting consists of three maximal lifts for competition: the bench press, squat, and dead lift. The bench press is performed with the lifter lying supine on a bench and the bar racked horizontally above his head. The bar is gripped, then lowered down to the chest, and finally returned to the rack by extending the arms. The squat is performed with the weighted bar held horizontally across the shoulders. The body is lowered by bending at the knees until the top surface of the legs at the hip joint is lower than the tops of the knees. The athlete must then recover to a knees-locked standing position and re-rack the bar. The dead lift is performed with the bar laid horizontally in front of the lifter's feet. The competitor bends down to grip the bar with both hands, and then lifts the bar to the standing position. Power lifting is a test of pure strength. There are many federations for power lifting, thus there may be multiple "world champions" each year. There is currently a petition to the International Olympic Committee to include power lifting as an official event in future Olympics.

Weight lifting has been a sport included in men's Olympic competitions since the 1896 start of the modern games held in Athens, Greece, but women's Olympic participation was not sanctioned until the 2000 Sydney Games. The International Weight Lifting Federation comprises 167 nations and approximately 10,000 weight lifters compete annually. Olympic lifting has two lifts. The first is the snatch, in which the barbell is lifted from the floor to an overhead position in one explosive continuous movement. The second is the clean and jerk, in which the barbell is lifted from the floor to shoulder level and then jerked overhead to finish the lift with a second movement. The best lifters can lift nearly 600 pounds in the clean and jerk.

Body builders use weight lifting exercises to build strength and sculpt their muscles for appearance to compete for such titles as Mr. or Ms. Universe. This group is notorious for use of anabolic steroids and other muscle-enhancing substances. There are "clean" competitions that require athletes to abstain from using these substances and physicians should encourage natural competitions.

In the past 25 years weight training has grown in popularity, involving more than 45 million Americans on a regular basis. Most men and women in the gym today lift weights for overall physical fitness and conditioning. Strength training is often a means to enhance performance in a specific sport and to prevent injuries. It also serves to improve many basic functions in daily activities. Cardiovascularly, weight training may serve to decrease blood pressure and improve lipid profiles. In addition, weight training benefits weight loss programs, increases lean body mass and bone mineral density, and improves balance in the elderly. Weight training has the potential to build bones and prevent osteoporosis and fractures associated with aging by providing the skeletal load needed to stimulate bone mineralization. A recent study that used resistive back strengthening exercises performed for 2 years in a group of women compared to a sedentary control group demonstrated fewer vertebral fractures in the exercise group in a 10-year follow-up. In addition to physical enhancement, resistance training may reduce anxiety and depression and may result in improved self-confidence and overall psychological well-being.

The scientific principles of strength training are discussed in Chapter 9. This chapter will discuss resistance training guidelines for healthy adults, special populations, and common injuries encountered within the sport.

GUIDELINES FOR HEALTHY ADULTS

Many health organizations have published research and recommendations for strength training in healthy and special populations. The American College of Sports Medicine developed guidelines for healthy, sedentary, low-risk populations as follows: a minimum of one exercise set per major muscle group (eg, chest press, shoulder press, triceps extension, biceps curl, pull-down) (upper back), lower back extension, abdominal crunch/curl-up, quadriceps extension, leg curls (hamstrings), and calf raise. Participants should do 8–12 repetitions 2–3 days per week.

These recommendations are based on the time constraints and compliance of patients, although research does support that more benefits may be achieved with 3 sets on a 3-day-per-week schedule. In general, a rest period of 48 hours between sessions is recommended to allow for muscle recuperation and development. Too much rest between training sessions will result in detraining. Existing literature states that for the first 3–4 months of training, single-set programs are equally effective as multiple set programs in improving muscular strength in previously untrained subjects, again supporting better compliance in the beginner. Those who are more advanced and have been following a program beyond this time period will need to increase the number of sets to see further benefits, although benefits gained will be maintained with the one-set-per-workout routine. As training progresses, repetitions should be modified based on perceived exertion. When one can comfortably lift a specific weight 12 times using good form and perceive it to be light to somewhat hard, 5–10% should be added to the next training session to continue strength increases. To maximize strength gains, the participant lifts for 10–12 repetitions and should not be able complete another repetition beyond this number with good form. Progression to higher weight should occur every 1–2 weeks. If the weight cannot be lifted for more than eight repetitions, it should be reduced for the next training session.

SPECIAL POPULATIONS

Certain populations have special considerations for participating in strength training. Older, younger, female, and pregnant athletes will be discussed. The physician prescribing a resistance exercise program should be familiar with the contraindications to weight lifting. The older healthy athlete, considered in studies to be age 60 and above, should be encouraged to participate because increased strength is beneficial to longevity. Studies have shown that older men displayed strength gains that were, relative to initial levels, similar to strength gains for younger subjects if the training level was the same. Many studies have shown similar results in increased strength and muscle mass in women who do regular resistance training. Improvement in muscle mass, strength, ability to perform daily tasks, and decreased falls are substantial benefits of strength training in the elderly. The increase in muscle mass promotes greater insulin sensitivity and glucose tolerance. Overall improvement in body composition is helpful with management of co-morbidities associated with obesity such as coronary artery disease, hypertension, and type II diabetes mellitus. The ACSM guidelines mentioned previously can be extended to the elderly with the following exceptions: (1) exercises should start at a low intensity and progress more gradually because of the increased potential for orthopedic injury, and (2) resistance machines may also prove safer and enhance compliance in this older population.

A few female athletes utilized resistance training exercises in the 1950s and 1960s, principally to improve performance in track and field. Since the passage of Title IX in 1972, the number of female athletes has grown exponentially and that increase has spawned a growth in strength training. Female athletes historically avoided weight training because of the misconception that training would cause them to become larger and heavier, and that women should only perform low-weight, high-repetition workouts to avoid muscle bulk. In reality the outcome of resistance training for women and girls is reduced body fat, increased lean weight, significant increases in strength, unchanged or decreased lower body girth, and a very small increase in upper body girth. Many female athletes have noted significant improvements in their sport with the addition of a strength training program. Women need to train at or above the intensity recommended by the general ACSM guidelines to gain maximum benefit and will benefit from 2002 ACSM guidelines for more sport-specific and intense training.

Strength training during pregnancy may offer relief from many of the undesirable side effects associated with pregnancy and the benefits include improved circulation and decreased edema, relief of low back pain, reduced muscle cramps, and potential for more rapid postpartum recovery. Training during pregnancy, however, should be aimed at maintaining abilities rather than increasing performance. The American College of Obstetricians and Gynecologists has revised guidelines (2001) for exercise in pregnancy that apply to strength training and weight lifting. Of note, pregnant women are discouraged from exercising in the supine position due to the possiblity of compromised fetal blood flow. For the same reason proper breathing technique during strength training should be stressed.

Studies have demonstrated that weight training can increase strength in preadolescents and adolescents when the program is properly structured with regard to frequency, mode, intensity, and duration. In preadolescents, this increased strength is likely due to neuromuscular "learning" with increases in the number of motor neurons firing with each muscle contraction. Adolescents in puberty and beyond have increased androgen levels and will experience muscle hypertrophy along with neuromuscular learning. The American Academy of Pediatrics published a guide for physicians counseling younger athletes that acknowledges that strength training can be safe and effective if safety precautions are followed. However, they recommend that preadolescents and adolescents should avoid competitive weight lifting, power lifting, body building, and maximal lifts until they are physically and skeletally mature to reduce the risk of growth plate injury. Preparticipation clearance by a physician should be completed prior to starting a weight training program in this age group. Aerobic conditioning is an important adjunct to youth strength training programs and each workout should include a warm-up and cool-down. Exercises should be learned without resistance and loads added in small increments when 12–15 repetitions can be completed at a given weight with good form. All major muscle groups should be addressed and full range of motion should be used with each exercise. Finally, the AAP reccommends that any sign of illness or injury should be evaluated prior to continuing a strength training program, which is appropriate advice for all age groups.

WEIGHT TRAINING INJURIES

Injuries associated with weight training occur with technical errors, skeletal immaturity, and anabolic steroid use. Serious injuries are rare, and only 56,400 of 5.4 million emergency room visits for all sports were attributed to weight training injuries in 1995. A range of both acute and chronic overuse injuries are common to the sport and have increased along with the popularity of weight training. An emergency department retrospective study looking at visits from 1978 through 1998 found that there were 980,173 patients treated for injuries related to weight training or weight training equipment, and the number of visits increased 35% from 1978 to 1998. One in four of the injuries studied were related to misuse or abuse of weight training equipment. The 15–24 age group had the highest injury rate. Hands were most often injured, followed by the upper trunk, head, lower trunk, and foot. The most common diagnosis was soft tissue injury followed by laceration and fracture/dislocation. Only 2.3% of injuries studied during this time period were serious enough to warrant hospital admission. However, there were 34 deaths related to weight training injury. Most of the fatal injuries occurred in men with a mean age of 21 who had head or neck trauma using free weights and were due to suffocation by strangulation from the bar across the neck. This emphasizes the importance of supervision and spotting during weight lifting sessions. Physicians should be aware of the risks, injuries, and safety precautions associated with this sport.

Several of the more common musculoskeletal and medical conditions associated with weight training will be discussed below.

Musculoskeletal Injuries

Lumbar Spine

Effective weight is amplified three times through the lumbar spine and excessive hyperextension of the lumbar spine worsens the damaging effects. Heavy lifting, especially with improper technique, puts the lumbar spine at increased risk. Squats, military presses, and bench presses are often improperly performed using excessive lumbar extension. Spondylolysis or stress fracture of the pars interarticularis has been detected in 36% of competitive weight lifters compared with 5% of the general population. These patients may be asymptomatic or present with chronic, often unilateral lumbar pain.

Spondylolisthesis is the anterior slip of a vertebral body in relation to the one below. Neurologic symptoms may be associated with this slippage and may be an indication for surgery. Evaluation and treatment is discussed in Chapter 16. Physicians who care for young athletes should maintain a high index of suspicison for both spondylolysis and spondylolisthesis in skeletally immature athletes who present with low back pain. Patients should be taught to protect the spine while lifting by contracting the abdominal muscles while maintaining neutral position of the spine.

Upper Extremity

The muscles and tendons of the shoulder rotator cuff can be excessively stressed during weight lifting maneuvers like the military press and upright row. Muscle imbalances that arise with neglect of the scapular stabilizers lead to increased stress and inflammation in the rotator cuff. Posture correction, scapular stabilizer strengthening, anterior chest wall stretching, and proper technique will improve muscle balance and can be used both to treat and prevent rotator cuff pathology associated with weight lifting.

Anterior shoulder instability is common in long-time weight lifters who use improper technique. The shoulder capsule is over-stretched with shoulder hyperextension during bench presses, military presses, and lattisimus dorsi pull-downs performed behind the neck. Lifters report vague shoulder symptoms, often with a sensation of looseness or instability. Treatment requires aggressive rehabilitation to strengthen the muscle supports for the anterior capsule.

Distal clavicle osteolysis is seen in weight lifters from repetitive strain on the acromioclavicular joint during the bench press, mainly from hyperextension of the shoulders. Lifters report a gradual onset of aching pain in the area of the acromioclavicular joint that worsens with exercises involving horizontal adduction and overhead motions. Radiographs will show the osteolysis and the bone scan will be positive. Treatment is rest and improvement of lifting technique. Corticosteroid injections may relieve pain, but if the pain persists, surgical excision of the distal clavicle will cure the problem.

Elbow dislocations may occur during weight lifting, especially at the competitive level. These more commonly occur during the overhead press or snatch and involve a medial dislocation of the ulnar olecranon from the humerus. Radiographs should be taken to assess for coexisting fractures. A thorough neurovascular exam should always be performed before and after reduction. Ideally, immediate reduction will decrease tissue and neurologic damage.

Although uncommon, weight lifting injuries include biceps ruptures from an excessive load or rapid stress on the tendon. Anabolic steroid use may often be an associated risk factor. It is paramount to differentiate between a proximal versus distal biceps rupture as management of the latter often requires surgical repair. Athletes with a rupture of the proximal biceps often report an acute onset of sharp anterior shoulder pain that can be associated with an audible pop or snapping sensation. Some present only with a visible or palpable mass between the elbow and shoulder and a Popeye-type muscle. Distal ruptures present in a similar fashion with symptoms and findings located closer to the elbow and the distal biceps tendon will not be palpable at its attachment.

Overuse about the elbow occurs with microtrauma and both medial and lateral epicondylitis are common. Treatment is conservative with rest, stretching, and focused strengthening. The athlete should also avoid aggravating lifting maneuvers until there is clinical improvement.

Similar to the stress placed on the lower extremities during long-distance running, the upper extremity withstands tremendous repetitive microtrauma when lifting weights. Stress fractures have been reported to develop in the ulna, humerus, and sternum. Symptoms are chronic, progressive pain in the area of the stress fracture with tenderness on palpation. Treatment is with removal from the inciting activity for 6–8 weeks.

Lower Extremity

Hamstring strains are common acute injuries associated with weight training, often as a consequence of strength imbalance between the hamstrings and quadriceps, and the hamstring tightness that is so common in this population. During forceful contraction of the hamstring, the patient will report the sudden onset of searing or tearing pain. On examination, hamstring tenderness with decreased range of motion will be present, and with grade III tears, a step-off can be palpated in the muscle belly. Strength should be relatively preserved when the musculotendinous unit is still intact. Treatment is conservative with rest, ice, and compression, progressing to strength and flexibility training.

Osteoarthritis of the patellofemoral compartment is present in 31% of former competitive weight lifters compared to 14% of former competitive runners. Improper weight lifting technique induces repetitive shearing forces on the cartilage and accelerates the degenerative changes when standing squats are performed with heavy weight and the thighs descend beyond parallel to the floor. Acute injuries also occur about the knee during weight training and competitions, including MCL and LCL sprains, meniscal tears, and patellar tendon ruptures.

MEDICAL CONDITIONS

Several interesting medical conditions are associated with weight training. Weight lifter's headache or weight lifter's cephalgia is a headache of sudden onset during training with posterior head and neck pain described as burning or boring. The headache may be of brief duration or last days to weeks. The mechanism of onset is unknown, but it is most likely related to improper technique and cervical strain. Treatment involves temporary avoidance of weight training, cervical range of motion and stretching, and medication for pain. After pain resolution, lifting technique should be reviewed to identify potential errors.

Weight lifter's heart is the enlargement of the ventricular septum in relation to the free ventricular wall due to adaptation of the myocardium to the stress load of lifting. This is a normal finding, not to be confused with hypertrophic cardiomyopathy, the leading cause of sudden cardiac death in young athletes.

Blood pressure elevations as high as 480/350 have been recorded during weight lifting. These elevations may contribute to vascular injury. Weight trainers should be advised to exhale slowly during the concentric phase of the lift and avoid Valsalva maneuvers during the lifts to reduce blood pressure elevation and potential vascular compromise during the lifts.

Compartment syndrome should be suspected in weight lifters when there is the report of progressive severe muscle pain in any of the extremities during or immediately following strenuous lifting. Pain may be out of proportion to physical examination findings; pain with passive stretching of the involved muscle, paresis, paresthesias, and pulselessness may or may not be evident unless examined while symptoms are present. A high index of suspicion should be maintained, and when suspected, compartment pressures should be measured before and after exercise. Immediate fasciotomy is the treatment for acute compartment syndrome to prevent permanent nerve and muscle damage.

Rhabdomyolysis can occur with high-intensity lifting and is also associated with compartment syndrome. It can potentially lead to acute renal failure. Intravenous hydration, urine alkalinization, and diuretics are the treatment for this life-threatening complication.

CONCLUSION

Strength training is a growing sport and an effective method for gaining strength, power, and muscular endurance while maintaining or improving one's health. These positive health effects are equally effective for men, women, the young, and the old. An individualized program can be developed to optimize health status, training, and personal goals. Physicians need to have an understanding of the demands and potential injuries that these athletes may encounter. Treatment of strength training injuries should be paired with instruction on proper form and education to prevent future injuries. From exercise prescription for the elderly to treatment of the Olympic weight lifting competitor, this can be a gratifying field of knowledge that all physicians should pursue.

REFERENCES

American Academy of Pediatrics. Strength training by children and adolescents. Policy statement. *Pediatrics*. 2001;107:1470–1472.

American College of Sports Medicine Position Stand. Progression models in resistance training for healthy adults. *Med Sci Sports Exerc*. 2002;34:364–380.

American College of Sports Medicine. The recommended quantity and quality of exercise for developing and maintaining cardiorespiratory and muscular fitness and flexibility in healthy adults. *Med Sci Sports Exerc*. 1998;30:975–991.

Deschenes MR, Kraemer WJ. Performance and physiologic adaptations to resistance training. *Am J Phys Med Rehabil*. 2002;81(Suppl):S3–S16.

Ebben WP. Strength training for women: debunking myths that block opportunity. *Phys Sports Med*. 1998;26:86–88, 91–92, 97.

Feigenbaum MS. Prescription of resistance training for health and disease [Clinical Sciences: Symposium: Resistance Training for Health and Disease.] *Med Sci Sports Exerc*. 1999;31:38–45.

Jones CS, Christensen C, Young M. Weight training injury trends: A 20 year survey. *Physician Sports Med*. 2000;28:61–62, 65–66, 71–72.

Kuhala UM, Kettunen J, Paananen H. Knee osteoarthritis in former runners, soccer players, weight lifters, and shooters. *Arthritis Rheum*. 1995;38:539–546.

MacDougall JD, McKelvie RS, Moroz DE, et al. Factors affecting blood pressure during heavy weight lifting and static contractions. *J Appl Physiol*. 1992;73:1590–1597.

National Strength and Conditioning Association. Position Paper: Health Aspects of Resistance Exercise and Training. National Strength and Conditioning Association, Colorado Springs, 2000.

Namey TC, Carek JC. Power lifting, weight lifting, and body building. In: Fu FH, Stone DA, eds. *Sports Injuries: Mechanisms, Prevention, Treatment*. Baltimore: Williams & Wilkins; 1994;519–529.

Petranick K, Berg K. The effects of weight training on bone density of premenopausal, postmenopausal and elderly women: a review. *J Strength Conditioning Res.* 1997;11:200–208.

Reeves KR, Laskowski ER, Smith J. Weight training injuries: Part 1: Diagnosing and managing acute conditions. *Physician Sports Med.* 1998;26:67–83.

Sinaki M, Itoi E, Wahner HW, et al. Stronger back muscles reduce the incidence of vertebral fractures: A prospective 10 year follow-up of postmenopausal women. *Bone.* 2002;30:836–841.

45 | Lacrosse

Barry Bartlett, Doreen Cress, R. Charles Bull, and William O. Roberts

Lacrosse is North America's oldest sport and is officially Canada's national sport. The game originated with the Native Americans as a method of training warriors and may have had some religious significance. It was first recorded in 1636 by the Jesuit priests. Games could last for 2 or 3 days and were quite violent. The modern game is played in an enclosed rink as box lacrosse and on open spaces as field lacrosse. Men and women have different sets of rules governing play.

THE GAME

Men's Field Lacrosse

Field lacrosse is a contact-collision sport usually played outdoors on a 110 yard by 60-yard field divided into offensive and defensive zones by a center line. The goal is 6 feet square and is surrounded by a 9-foot radius crease. There are 10 players on the field: 3 attack, 3 mid fielders, 3 defense, and a goalkeeper. Substitutions are done on the fly, with some restrictive substitution rules, and are generally made for mid fielders. Play begins with a face off and the main theme of the game is ball control. Teams try to set up plays and work for the high percentage shot. There is no time requirement to take a shot, so the team can maintain control of the ball.

Stick

The sticks used by field players usually have a plastic head with a wooden shaft. The minimum length for any stick is 40 inches and the maximum is 72 inches. Attack and midfielders play with short sticks, and defensive players use long sticks. The minimum width for a stick head is 4 inches. Goalkeepers have no limit on the length of stick used.

Shoes

Players may use rubber-soled boots or shoes with cleats or studs. A larger number of cleats shorter in length help decrease the chance of injury found with shoes with longer and fewer cleats. Shoes should include the following: a sturdy heel counter, medial arch support, a flexible forefoot, and shock-absorbing qualities.

Padding

Players wear gloves, testicle cup, and kidney, shoulder, rib, and elbow pads. Goalkeepers also wear leg protectors, padded pants, and chestpads. The leg guards cannot have any felt or other material extending past the shin protectors. No modifications can be made to a goalkeeper's gloves, so it is important to obtain the correct glove the first time around. It is suggested that goalkeepers wear hockey gloves instead of lacrosse gloves because they offer better protection. Blocking pads and trappers are not allowed.

Helmets

Helmets are specifically designed for field lacrosse. The helmets have a brim to help shield the face from the sun, are tied in the back to ensure a good

741

fit, and have a four-point chinstrap to keep the helmet in place. An approved face mask is required for all players, and a throat protector is mandatory for goalkeepers.

Protective Devices

Protective devices are permitted on the field. Casts and splints require the appropriate padding.

On-Field Injury Care

Medical help must be called onto the field by the referee. If play is stopped for an injury, the injured player must leave the playing field for the game to resume. No blood-soaked clothing or open wounds are permitted in any form of lacrosse.

Women's Field Lacrosse

Women's lacrosse is essentially a noncontact sport played outdoors in all kinds of weather and varying field conditions. The stick has a shallow pocket (not deeper than the diameter of the ball). Players must stand when the whistle is blown, except following a goal, and play resumes on the whistle. The goal is 6 feet square, surrounded by a crease of 2.6 meters (7 feet). There is also an 11-meter (33-foot) working area and 15-meter (40-foot) fan area for attacking and defensive players. The officials are two or three umpires, and dangerous stick-checking results in a "free position" for the fouled player. High-sticking around the player's head is a major foul.

Stick

Sticks are made of wood, plastic, or fiberglass, with a nylon, leather, rubber, or gut basket. Only the handle is allowed to be aluminum or graphite. The length of the stick must be between 0.9 and 1.1 meters in length and cannot exceed 567 grams in weight. A goalkeeper's stick must measure between 0.9 and 1.22 meters in length, and it cannot exceed 733 grams in weight. The pockets of the stick cannot be mesh but must be made of four to five vertical thongs supported by cross-lacing. The pocket must be no deeper than the diameter of the ball.

Shoes

Players may use rubber-soled boots or shoes with cleats or studs similar to those worn in the men's game.

Padding and Protective Equipment

It is mandatory for the goalkeeper to wear a helmet and a throat protector. Other players are not permitted to wear headgear, helmets, or face masks. Nose- and eyeguards and close-fitting gloves are permitted. Protective eyewear is strongly recommended for field players, and is now required for high school players in the United States. Mouthguards are mandatory for all players. The goalkeeper can wear a chest or body pad, leg pads, arm pads, and gloves. The goalkeeper's gloves are tight-fitting at the wrist without webbing between the fingers. The pads worn cannot exceed 3 centimeters in thickness at any point. Jewelry cannot be worn by any player unless it is for medical reasons, and then it is required to tape the piece down to the skin.

Protective Devices

Protective devices must be padded. The umpire has the final ruling if they may be worn during play, with the concern being that the device might present a hazard to other players.

On-Field Injury Care

An umpire must call medical help onto the field. Incapacitated players have 2 minutes, whereas goalkeepers have 5 minutes in which an assessment must be made as to whether they can continue play. After the appropriate time limit, the game will restart without the player. The player may return to play as long as she is able to, no substitutions were made for her, and the umpire agrees.

Box Lacrosse

Box lacrosse is a fast-paced, high-intensity game that originated in the 1930s and is played by people of all ages in indoor hockey arenas or outdoor boxes. A team can roster 20 players including two goalkeepers, and five players plus a goalkeeper are on the floor at one time. There is a 10-second limit on moving the ball past the center line and a 30-second limit on shots on the opposition's goal. Slashing and cross-checking from behind are not permitted, and players are penalized for their actions.

Competition begins during the spring and ends in late summer when hockey rinks are often idle. The major skills required in box lacrosse are passing, catching, and shooting, skills that must be developed early in a player's career. Unlike hockey, there is no offside rule, which adds to the speed and scoring.

Stick

The player's stick has to be between 42 and 46 inches in overall length. The width of the inside frame is a minimum of 4 inches and a maximum of 8 inches. The goalkeeper's stick can be of any length suitable to the player, but the maximum width for the inside frame cannot exceed 15 inches. Sticks can be made of wood or plastic.

Shoes

Cross-training or basketball shoes with a sturdy heel counter, medial arch support, flexible forefoot, and shock-absorbing capabilities work well. High-cut shoes can give good stability to the ankle joint. Goalkeepers should also consider wearing shoes with hard rubber toes for protection against shots.

Padding

The player's padding can include kidney pads, protective cup, rib pads, spine guards, shoulder pads, elbow pads, and gloves. Equipment must be checked regularly for wear and replaced or repaired to ensure proper protection is given. Many players cut out the palms of their gloves for better contact with the stick, but this drastically reduces the protection offered for their hands and fingers. Players often add padding to the upper arms by taping extra pads over the lateral aspect of the upper arm. This aids in deflecting and absorbing cross-checks and slashes.

Goalkeepers wear leg protectors, padded pants, chestpads, kidney pads, rib pads, shoulder pads, elbow pads, and gloves. The leg guards cannot have any felt or other material extending past the shin protectors. No modifications can be made to a goalkeeper's gloves, so it is important to obtain the correct glove the first time around. It is suggested that goalkeepers wear hockey gloves instead of lacrosse gloves, because they offer better protection. Blocking and trappers are not allowed.

If further padding is required over the rest of the body, it is best to use dense foam for absorption and a plastic piece over the top of the foam for deflection. The most common areas to pad for goalkeepers are between the neck and shoulder cap, over the shoulders and upper arms, and inside of the glove hand. Goalkeeper's pads must conform to the player's body and may not be thicker than 3 inches on any part of the body.

Helmets

All members of a team wear the same colored helmet with an approved wire mask. Cutting bars out of the mask is illegal and can lead to serious injury if the ball penetrates the face mask. Mouthguards are mandatory in some leagues and are highly recommended. To help prevent concussions, helmets must be secured appropriately with straps done up. Throat protectors are mandatory for goalkeepers and are usually suspended about 1 inch below the bottom of the face mask by string or leather.

Protective Devices

Players on the floor may wear protective devices. Any cast or splintlike material must be appropriately padded.

On-Field Injury Care

Medical help must be called onto the floor by the referee. Any player other than the goalkeeper must leave the playing surface after being tended to.

Inter-Lacrosse

This is a co-ed game played in elementary and secondary schools. There is no stick or body contact permitted, and protective equipment is not required. The stick is made of flexible plastic. This game can be played indoors or outdoors. The number of players on the team can be adapted, but five is recommended for indoor play. Goals can be hockey nets, hoops, pylons, or even a target on the wall. A goalkeeper may or may not by used.

Because of the simplicity and flexibility of inter-lacrosse, it is adaptable to just about any situation. There are four basic rules: possession is limited to 5 seconds, players must run with the ball, no physical contact is allowed, and covering a loose ball with the stick results in immediate possession.

Younger Players

Many lacrosse players start at an early age; therefore, it is important not to forget the prepubescent players and their particular circumstances. With younger players there are different rules and contact is limited. Their skill level is lower. Their diminished speed, size, and strength decreases the probability of sustaining some of the more serious injuries. They are, however, more prone to other injuries that need to be kept in mind. As younger bodies develop, their muscles, tendons, and ligaments are stronger than their bones, thus predisposing them to Salter fractures. Particular attention should be paid to severe sprains that occur where growth plates exist. Growth plate fractures are often misdiagnosed as sprains. This missed diagnosis can lead to the closing of the growth plate prematurely. The most common fractures are Colles fracture of the ulna and radius and the clavicle. Osgood-Schlatter's disease and jumper's knee are common in the younger player group. They are three times more common in males, especially between the ages of 10 and 15, although they do occur in females between the ages of 8 and 13 years. The younger players are typically developing their coordination at this age and tend to trip, fall, and run into each other habitually, predisposing them to contusions, lacerations, and fractures.

COMMON LACROSSE INJURIES

Owing to the contact nature of lacrosse, it is important to remember that anything is possible with regard to injury. This section reviews the injuries unique to lacrosse and the most common injuries with suggestions for prevention and treatment. It is important to remember that other injuries are not foreign to lacrosse; the reader may find information about them elsewhere in this volume.

Heat Conditions

Heat problems are common in box lacrosse, when it is played in poorly ventilated arenas where the temperatures can rise to dangerous levels. Field lacrosse players are also susceptible to heat conditions during the hot weather and in direct sunlight. Goalies are especially vulnerable owing to the excessive protective equipment they wear and their inability to drink during the periods.

Prevention Tips

- Provide buckets of ice water on the bench with towels in them to help the players cool down between shifts and periods.
- Monitor the temperatures and players closely with an eye toward cancelling when the heat stress is in the higher-risk zones to ensure that players do not get exertional heat stroke.
- Ensure that there are plenty of fluids on the bench and allow the players to drink regularly during the practice or game.

Treatment Tips

Players showing signs of heat exhaustion or heat-stroke should be removed and evaluated. Get the player to a cooler area and start immediate treatment with wet towels and cold drinks.

Concussion

Concussion is caused by a direct or indirect blow to the head. An appropriate, well-fitted helmet with straps properly done up and a mouthguard with superior absorption qualities decreases the amount of force transmitted to the brain. However, a lacrosse helmet is quite different from a hockey or football helmet. It is loosely fitted, vented, and much more flexible. It is effective in deflecting blows with the stick, but it is relatively ineffective in high-speed collisions and contact with the floor.

Whiplash

A quick jarring of the cervical or lumbar spine from an unexpected cross-check or body check can cause acute and prolonged pain from forced extension and then rapid flexion with slight rotation, similar to the mechanism of injury in a rear end motor vehicle accident. Prevention is most important and lacrosse players must develop strong cervical, abdominal, lumbar erector spinae, and quadratus lumborum muscles to protect against this injury. Look for signs of concussion and neurologic signs and symptoms after a whiplash.

Lumbar Back Pain

This can be caused by pounding on the hard, unforgiving floor in box lacrosse or the uneven terrain of the field in field lacrosse. Rapid acceleration and deceleration and rotation with a pivot or fake move can strain the lumbar, psoas, hamstring, or adductor muscles. Prevention involves intensive conditioning and core strengthening with appropriate fast-twitch dexterity drills. Shoes with sufficient shock-absorbing qualities are important. Back problems are hard to diagnose on the field, and although they are more apt to be associated with muscle spasm, a serious back problem cannot be ruled out. A player with serious back injury must be removed from the game on the back board and full precautions taken, as with a serious neck injury.

Hamstring Strains

Hamstring strains are caused by overstretching or overcontracting the muscle, especially if fatigued. This is usually an overtraining, overuse, repetitive strain injury. Decreased traction due to moisture on the floor in box lacrosse or wet grass can result in splits and groin pulls. In addition to hamstring, quadriceps, and abductor/adductor strengthening, stretching the quads, hams, and adductors before and after practices and games seems to reduce risk. A player with a moderately pulled groin should be taken out of the game because the problem will become more severe soon after the game.

Hip Pointer

A direct blow to an inadequately protected iliac crest by a helmet, stick, or the floor may cause a contusion associated with a hematoma of the tissue adjacent to and beneath the periosteum covering the crest. This is a very painful injury with immediate muscle spasm and immobility. The patient is unable to rotate the trunk or flex the thigh without pain. Most comfort is obtained by trunk flexion, leaning forward and toward the side of the injury. A fractured pelvis should be ruled out with radiographic imaging. The majority of cases respond to the PRICE regimen (protection, rest, ice, compression, and elevation).

Contusions

The lacrosse ball is made of a dense rubber compound, weighs roughly 170 grams, and can travel over 100 miles per hour, so the possibility of contusions occurring anywhere on the body is enormous. Although the rules discourage slashing on places such as the quads, it is not uncommon to receive blows from the stick on the forearms, deltoids, hands, lower legs, and back.

Bodychecking is encouraged in men's lacrosse. If a player continuously gets contusions in the same area, a piece of permanent, custom padding may be used to protect the injury from recurring.

Blocker's Exostosis

Repeated blows to the deltoid insertion, especially from cross-checking, may result in blocker's exostosis. This can be prevented by using a deltoid cup to protect the deltoid insertion from repeated blows. Reassess regularly for myositis ossificans, especially with players who are offensive specialists. Add an extra pad, taped on, to help disperse the force.

Medial and Lateral Epicondylitis

Medial and lateral epicondylitis occur because lacrosse requires the ball carrier to cradle the stick. This requires a rapid rotation, flexion, and extension motion of the wrist in order to maintain control and possession of the ball. This rapid repetitive flexion and extension motion can lead to tendinitis (Fig. 45-1). This injury can be prevented and treated with stretching programs, and forearm braces should be used to reduce time lost from play.

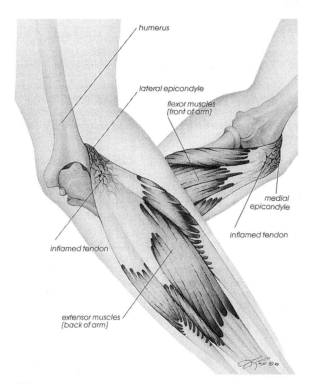

humerus

lateral epicondyle

flexor muscles (front of arm)

medial epicondyle

inflamed tendon

inflamed tendon

extensor muscles (back of arm)

FIG 45-1 Tennis elbow/golfer's elbow. This condition plagues lacrosse players, both amateur and professional. It is basically a tendinopathy of the origins of the muscles attached to the epicondyles in the elbow area.

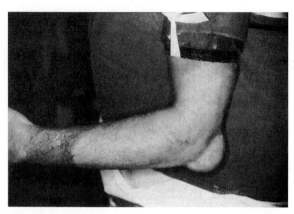

FIG 45-2 Olecranon bursitis should be prevented by more satisfactory elbow pads. Once it reaches this stage surgery is mandatory. The players say they have "bone chips" in their elbow, but the particles in the bursa are fibrous and unrelated to the elbow joint.

Olecranon Bursitis

This commonly occurs from falls on a hard floor or field. The player can wear lightweight shoulder and elbow pads, but they do not offer much protection and players are not required to wear them. Figure 45-2 illustrates a large chronic olecranon bursitis in the operating room, just prior to surgery.

Fractures of the Forearm

These often occur from direct stick contact, a cross-check, or a slash. These are legal checks. The offensive player will hold the stick and ball in one hand and place the opposite arm in a protective fashion to ward off the opponent's blows, resulting in an isolated ulnar shaft fracture, or less commonly a fracture of both bones occurs. Arm pads are not always used.

Hand Injuries

Dislocated metacarpal, phalangeal, and interphalangeal joints are common, and these are best handled at the time of the accident by traction (pulling the finger into the normal anatomical position) and reduction. This is often difficult in the case of a thumb dislocated at the metacarpophalangeal joint because the tendons from the adductor pollicis often catch around the neck of the metacarpal in a fashion similar to that of the neck reins of a horse. This prevents the reduction and often makes it difficult, even under general anesthesia (Fig. 45-3).

Fracture of the hook of hamate is often missed. It is caused by repeated impact from the handle of the lacrosse stick on the heel of the hand. In some cases this fracture may require surgery. Protective padding over the heel of the hand in the glove can be an effective prevention strategy, but may limit technique. Encourage the player to carry the stick up closer to the metacarpophalangeal joints.

Gamekeeper's thumb or skier's thumb occurs when a player falls and the thumb is trapped by the stick and forced into hyperextension. This tears the

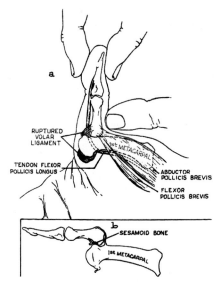

FIG 45-3   A dislocated thumb may be impossible to reduce due to the adductor tendons catching around the neck of the metacarpal.

ulnar collateral ligament or fractures a small piece of bone from the proximal phalanx (Stener lesion). Defensive specialists are susceptible owing to their technique of cross-checking, which is completely legal and can be done forcefully and repetitively. These injuries are treated with a hand-based thumb spica cast or open reduction and immediate repair of the ligaments. Bennett's fracture of the first metacarpal usually requires immediate open reduction and K-wire fixation.

Hands are injured by a stick slash, contact with an opponent's equipment, and being stepped on. Lacrosse gloves provide satisfactory protection, but players often cut out the palms to get a better feel of the stick. This leaves the hands partially unprotected, and injuries occur when the hands slip out of the gloves. Prevention is simply not allowing players to cut any of the palm out of their gloves.

Ankle Sprains

There is a high incidence of ankle sprains associated with running required by the sport particularly at the lower levels with poor quality fields, and stepping into divots on the uneven terrain. Landing on someone's foot, similar to basketball, is a frequent problem. Twisting when the foot has been fixed in place and decelerating and rolling the foot into inversion is the most common mechanism.

Turf Toe

The turf shoe sticking to the artificial turf and stopping abruptly while the player's momentum continues forward results in turf toe. This causes the first metatarsal joint to be driven into hyperextension and an inflammatory condition commonly results. This problem can be prevented by proper shoe fit with a little space left in the front of the shoe for toe and forefoot movement. A larger toe box is also suggested. A wrap using a turf toe support technique that limits hyperextension of the first metatarsal phalangeal joint helps to reduce excessive motion and usually provides enough splinting to allow comfortable return to play.

On-Field Emergencies

Laryngeal fractures can present a life-threatening situation. Symptoms are loss of airway, hemoptysis, crepitus, and loss of the Adam's apple prominence. The necessity of a cricothyrotomy or tracheotomy has to be considered. Treatment consists of rest, humidification, and no contact for 6–12 weeks. It is basically impossible to protect against this injury. The incidence of cross-checking over the neck or garroting from behind should be controlled by proper enforcement of the rules.

Mouthguards are mandatory in most leagues, and the custom mouthguard made by the player's dentist is the only one that is truly satisfactory. If a player's tooth is broken, take the player and the broken tooth or its pieces to the dentist immediately. Do not clean or wash the root.

Fractured ribs are common because of cross-checking and little, if any, protective equipment for the rib cage in many players. A quilted kidney protector is allowed. Fractured ribs obviously have to be immobilized initially with a Velcro strap that replaces the old style of rib taping. Some players with fractured ribs can play within 10 days of the injury if they wear a flak jacket. Watch for injuries to the spleen or liver that can be associated with rib fractures.

Pneumothorax

Pneumothorax can occur spontaneously from a rupture of a bleb or from direct trauma. A player in this condition must be taken to the hospital immediately. If cyanosis or hypotension is noted, a large-bore needle can be placed in the second intercostal space 2 inches (5 centimeters) from the sternal border. The finger of a glove with a hole in the tip can be taped to the needle to act as a one-way valve.

Abdominal Injuries

Blows to the solar (celiac) plexus will "knock the wind out" of a player. This problem is usually transient, and the player can later re-enter the game.

Lacerations of the liver and spleen can occur and go unrecognized. A subscapular hematoma can occur in the spleen, and the patient can be ambulatory and seem well until the capsule suddenly ruptures. Be very careful with players who have received abdominal injuries and transport suspicious injuries to the hospital immediately. This type of abdominal injury has to be thoroughly investigated in a hospital setting. Any player with blood in the urine should be investigated prior to return to lacrosse.

CONCLUSIONS

The lacrosse medical team should be prepared, be on time, be visible, and be alert. Watch the game closely. Be aware of any potential problem. Examine athletes before a game. Be careful not to allow any long-term damage.

Be available between periods or quarters and check the dressing room and opposing team's dressing room after the game. Be cautious. Send any doubtful case to the hospital and follow it up with further investigation when necessary. Be sure that players have reached 100% of their capability before they return to sport after an injury.

Acknowledgment

Illustrations, unless otherwise attributed, are taken from Schneider RC, Kennedy JC, Plant ML, eds. *Sports Injuries: Mechanisms, Prevention and Treatment*. Baltimore: Williams & Wilkins; 1985.

IV | APPENDICES: TEAM PHYSICIAN CONSENSUS CONFERENCE STATEMENTS

A | Team Physician Consensus Statement

DEFINITION

The team physician must have an unrestricted medical license and be an MD or DO who is responsible for treating and coordinating the medical care of athletic team members. The principal responsibility of the team physician is to provide for the well-being of individual athletes, enabling each to realize his or her full potential. The team physician should possess special proficiency in the care of musculoskeletal injuries and medical conditions encountered in sports. The team physician also must actively integrate medical expertise with other healthcare providers, including medical specialists, athletic trainers, and allied health professionals. The team physician must ultimately assume responsibility within the team structure for making medical decisions that affect the athlete's safe participation.

QUALIFICATIONS

The primary concern of the team physician is to provide the best medical care for athletes at all levels of participation. To this end, the following qualifications are necessary for all team physicians:

- Have an MD or DO in good standing, with an unrestricted license to practice medicine.
- Possess a fundamental knowledge of emergency care regarding sporting events.
- Be trained in CPR.
- Have a working knowledge of trauma, musculoskeletal injuries, and medical conditions affecting the athlete.

In addition, it is desirable for team physicians to have clinical training/experience and administrative skills in some or all of the following:

- Specialty Board certification
- Continuing medical education in sports medicine
- Formal training in sports medicine (fellowship training, board recognized subspecialty in sports medicine [formerly known as a Certificate of Added Qualification in Sports Medicine])
- Additional training in sports medicine
- Fifty percent or more of practice involving sports medicine
- Membership and participation in a sports medicine society
- Involvement in teaching, research, and publications relating to sports medicine
- Training in advanced cardiac life support
- Knowledge of medical/legal, disability, and workers' compensation issues
- Media skills training

DUTIES OF A TEAM PHYSICIAN

The team physician must be willing to commit the necessary time and effort to provide care to the athlete and team. In addition, the team physician must develop and maintain a current, appropriate knowledge base of the sport(s) for which he or she is accepting responsibility. The duties for which the team physician has ultimate responsibility include the following.

Medical Management of the Athlete

- Coordinate pre-participation screening, examination, and evaluation.
- Manage injuries on the field.
- Provide for medical management of injury and illness.
- Coordinate rehabilitation and return to participation.
- Provide for proper preparation for safe return to participation after an illness or injury.
- Integrate medical expertise with other healthcare providers, including medical specialists, athletic trainers, and allied health professionals.
- Provide for appropriate education and counseling regarding
  - Nutrition.
  - Strength and conditioning.
  - Ergogenic aids.
  - Substance abuse.
  - Other medical problems that could affect the athlete.
- Provide for proper documentation and medical record keeping.

Administrative and Logistical Duties

- Establish and define the relationships of all involved parties.
- Educate athletes, parents, administrators, coaches, and other necessary parties of concerns regarding the athletes.
- Develop a chain of command.
- Plan and train for emergencies during competition and practice.
- Address equipment and supply issues.
- Provide for proper event coverage.
- Assess environmental concerns and playing conditions.

EDUCATION

Ongoing education pertinent to the team physician is essential. Currently, there are several state, regional, and national stand-alone courses for team physician education. There are also many other resources available. Information regarding team physician-specific educational opportunities can be obtained from the following organizations.

American Academy of Family Physicians (AAFP)
8880 Ward Parkway
Kansas City, MO 64114
816-333-9700

American Academy of Orthopaedic Surgeons (AAOS)
6300 North River Road
Rosemont, IL 60018
847-823-7186

American College of Sports Medicine (ACSM)
401 West Michigan Street
Indianapolis, IN 46202
317-637-9200

American Medical Society for Sports Medicine (AMSSM)
11639 Earnshaw
Overland Park, KS 66210
610-662-1000

American Orthopaedic Society for Sports Medicine (AOSSM)
6300 North River Road Suite 200
Rosemont, IL 60018
847-292-4900

American Osteopathic Academy of Sports Medicine (AOASM)
7611 Elmwood Avenue Suite 201
Middleton, WI 53562
608-831-4400

Team physician education is also available from other sources such as sport-specific (e.g., National Football League Team Physician's Society) or level-specific (e.g., United States Olympic Committee) meetings; National Governing Bodies' (NGB) meetings; state and/or county medical societies meetings; professional journals; and other relevant electronic media (web sites, CD-ROMs).

CONCLUSION

This Consensus Statement establishes a definition of the team physician and outlines a team physician's qualifications, duties, and responsibilities. It also contains strategies for the continuing education of team physicians. Ultimately, this statement provides guidelines that best serve the health care needs of athletes and teams.

EXPERT PANEL

Stanley A. Herring, MD, Chair, Seattle, Washington
John Bergfeld, MD, Cleveland, Ohio
Joel Boyd, MD, Edina, Minnesota
Per Gunnar Brolinson, DO, Toledo, Ohio
Timothy Duffey, DO, Columbus, Ohio
David Glover, MD, Warrensburg, Missouri
William A. Grana, MD, Oklahoma City, Oklahoma
Brian C. Halpern, MD, Marlboro, New Jersey
Peter Indelicato, MD, Gainesville, Florida
W. Ben Kibler, MD, Lexington, Kentucky
E. Lee Rice, DO, San Diego, California
William O. Roberts, MD, White Bear Lake, Minnesota

B | Sideline Preparedness for the Team Physician

DEFINITION

Sideline preparedness is the identification of and planning for medical services to promote the safety of the athlete, limit injury, and provide medical care at the site of practice or competition.

GOAL

The safety and on-site medical care of the athlete is the goal of sideline preparedness. To accomplish this goal, the team physician should be actively involved in developing an integrated medical system that includes

- Pre-season planning
- Game-day planning
- Post-season evaluation

PRE-SEASON PLANNING

Pre-season planning promotes safety and minimizes problems associated with athletic participation at the site of practice or competition. The team physician should coordinate

- Development of policy to address pre-season planning and the pre-participation evaluation of athletes.
- Participation of the administration and other key personnel in medical issues.
- Implementation strategies.

Medical Protocol Development

It is essential that

- Prospective athletes complete a pre-participation evaluation.

In addition, it is desirable that

- The pre-participation evaluation be performed by an MD or DO in good standing with an unrestricted license to practice medicine.
- A comprehensive pre-participation evaluation form be used (e.g., the form found in the current edition of *Preparticipation Physical Evaluation,* 1997).
- The team physician has access to all pre-participation evaluation forms.
- The team physician review all pre-participation evaluation forms and determine eligibility of the athlete to participate.
- Timely pre-participation evaluations be performed to permit the identification and treatment of injuries and medical conditions.

Administrative Protocol Development

It is essential for the team physician to coordinate

- Development of a chain of command that establishes and defines the responsibilities of all parties involved.
- Establishment of an emergency response plan for practice and competition.

759

- Compliance with Occupational Safety and Health Association standards relevant to the medical care of the athlete.
- Establishment of a policy to assess environmental concerns and playing conditions for modification or suspension of practice or competition.
- Compliance with all local, state, and Federal regulations regarding storing and dispensing pharmaceuticals.
- Establishment of a plan to provide for proper documentation and medical record keeping.

In addition, it is desirable for the team physician to coordinate

- Regular rehearsal of the emergency response plan.
- Establishment of a network with other health care providers, including medical specialists, athletic trainers, and allied health professionals.
- Establishment of a policy that includes the team physician in the dissemination of any information regarding the athlete's health.
- Preparation of a letter of understanding between the team physician and the administration that defines the obligations and responsibilities of the team physician.

GAME-DAY PLANNING

Game-day planning optimizes medical care for injured or ill athletes. The team physician should coordinate

- Game-day medical operations.
- Game-day administrative medical policies.
- Preparation of the sideline medical bag and sideline medical supplies.

Medical Protocol

It is essential for the team physician to coordinate

- Determination of final clearance status of injured or ill athletes on game-day prior to competition.
- Assessment and management of game-day injuries and medical problems.
- Determination of athletes' same-game return to participation after injury or illness.
- Follow-up care and instructions for athletes who require treatment during or after competition.
- Notifying the appropriate parties about an athlete's injury or illness.
- Close observation of the game by the medical team from an appropriate location.
- Provision for proper documentation and medical record keeping.

In addition, is it desirable for the team physician to coordinate

- Monitoring of equipment safety and fit.
- Monitoring of post-game referral care of injured or ill athletes.

Administrative Protocol

It is essential for the team physician to coordinate

- Assessment of environmental concerns and playing conditions.
- Presence of medical personnel at the competition site with sufficient time for all pre-game preparations.

- Planning with the medical staff of the opposing team for medical care of the athletes.
- Introductions of the medical team to game officials.
- Review of the emergency medical response plan.
- Checking and confirmation of communication equipment.
- Identification of examination and treatment sites.

In addition, it is desirable for the team physician to coordinate

- Arrangements for the medical staff to have convenient access to the competition site.
- A post-game review and make necessary modifications of medical and administrative protocols.

On-Site Medical Supplies

The team physician should have a game-day sideline medical bag and sideline medical supplies. The following is a list of medical bag items and medical supplies for contact/collision and high-risk sports.

It Is Highly Desirable for the Medical Bag to Include

General

- Alcohol swabs and povidone iodine swabs
- Bandage scissors
- Bandages, sterile/nonsterile, band-aids
- D-50%-W
- Disinfectant
- Gloves, sterile/nonsterile
- Large-bore angiocath for tension pneumothorax (14–16 gauge)
- Local anesthetic/syringes/needles
- Paper
- Pen
- Sharps box and red bag
- Suture set/Steri-strips
- Wound irrigation materials (sterile normal saline, 10–50 cc syringe)

Cardiopulmonary

- Airway
- Blood pressure cuff
- Cricothyrotomy kit
- Epinephrine 1:1000 in a prepackaged unit
- Mouth-to-mouth mask
- Short-acting beta agonist inhaler
- Stethoscope

Head and Neck/Neurologic

- Dental kit (cyanoacrylate, Hank's solution)
- Eye kit (blue light, fluorescein stain strips, eye patch pads, cotton tip applicators, ocular anesthetic and antibiotics, contact remover, mirror)
- Flashlight
- Pin or other sharp object for sensory testing
- Reflex hammer

It Is Highly Desirable for Sideline Medical Supplies to Include

General

- Access to a telephone
- Extremity splints
- Ice
- Oral fluid replacement
- Plastic bags
- Sling

Head and Neck/Neurologic

- Face mask removal tool (for sports with helmets)
- Semi-rigid cervical collar
- Spine board and attachments

In Addition, It Is Desirable for the Medical Bag to Include

General

- Benzoin
- Blister care materials
- Contact lens case and solution
- 30% Ferric subsulfate solution (e.g., Monsel's, for cauterizing abrasions and cuts)
- Injury and illness care instruction sheets for the patient
- List of emergency phone numbers
- Nail clippers
- Nasal packing material
- Oto-ophthalmoscope
- Paper bags for treatment of hyperventilation
- Prescription pad
- Razor and shaving cream
- Rectal thermometer
- Scalpel
- Skin lubricant
- Skin staple applicator
- Small mirror
- Supplemental oral and parenteral medications
- Tongue depressors
- Topical antibiotics

Cardiopulmonary

- Advanced Cardiac Life Support (ACLS) drugs and equipment
- IV fluids and administration set
- Tourniquet

In Addition, It Is Desirable for Sideline Medical Supplies to Include

General

- Blanket
- Crutches
- Mouth guards
- Sling psychrometer and temperature/humidity activity risk chart
- Tape cutter

Cardiopulmonary

- Automated external defibrillator

Head and Neck/Neurologic

- A sideline concussion assessment protocol

There are many different sports, levels of competition, and available medical resources that must all be considered when determining the on-site medical bag and sideline medical supplies.

POST-SEASON EVALUATION

Post-season evaluation of sideline coverage optimizes the medical care of injured or ill athletes and promotes continued improvement of medical services for future seasons. The team physician should coordinate

- Summarization of injuries and illnesses that occurred during the season.
- The improvement of the medical and administrative protocols.
- Implementation strategies to improve sideline preparedness.

Medical Protocol

It is essential for the team physician to coordinate

- A post-season meeting with appropriate team personnel and administration to review the season.
- Identification of athletes who require post-season care of injury or illness and encourage follow up.

In addition, it is desirable for the team physician to coordinate

- Monitoring of the health status of the injured or ill athlete.
- Post-season physicals.
- An off-season conditioning program.

Administrative Protocol

It is essential for the team physician to coordinate

- Review and modification of current medical and administrative protocols.

In addition, it is desirable for the team physician to coordinate

- Compilation of injury and illness data.

CONCLUSION

This Consensus Statement outlines the essential and desirable components of sideline preparedness for the team physician to promote the safety of the athlete, to limit injury, and to provide medical care at the site of practice or competition. This statement was developed by the collaboration of six major professional associations concerned about clinical sports medicine issues: the American Academy of Family Physicians, the American Academy of Orthopaedic Surgeons, the American College of Sports Medicine, the American Medical Society for Sports Medicine, the American Orthopaedic Society for Sports Medicine, and the American Osteopathic Academy of Sports Medicine.

CONTINUING EDUCATION

Ongoing education pertinent to the team physician is essential. Information regarding team physician specific educational opportunities can be obtained from the six participating organizations:

American Academy of Family Physicians
11400 Tomahawk Creek Parkway
Leawood, KS 66211-2672
1-800-274-2237
www.aafp.org

American Academy of Orthopaedic Surgeons
6300 North River Road
Rosemont, IL 60018
1-800-346-AAOS
www.aaos.org

American College of Sports Medicine
401 West Michigan Street
Indianapolis, IN 46202
317-637-9200
www.acsm.org

American Medical Society for Sports Medicine
11639 Earnshaw
Overland Park, KS 66210
913-327-1415
www.amssm.org

American Orthopaedic Society for Sports Medicine
6300 North River Road Suite 200
Rosemont, IL 60018
(847) 292-4900
www.sportsmed.org

American Osteopathic Academy of Sports Medicine
7611 Elmwood Avenue Suite 201
Middleton, WI 53562
608-831-4400
www.aoasm.org

REFERENCE

Preparticipation Physical Evaluation, 2nd edition. New York: McGraw-Hill; 1997.

C | The Team Physician and Conditioning of Athletes for Sports

SUMMARY

The objective of this Consensus Statement is to provide physicians who are responsible for the healthcare of teams with guidelines regarding conditioning for sports. This statement specifically addresses the role of exercise in conditioning. Nutrition and supplements are outside the scope of this statement. It is not intended as a standard of care, and should not be interpreted as such. This statement is only a guide, and as such, is of a general nature, consistent with reasonable, objective practice of the healthcare professional. Individual conditioning issues will depend on the specific facts and circumstances presented to the physician.

Adequate insurance should be in place to help protect the athlete, the sponsoring organization, and the physician.

This Statement was developed by a collaboration of six major professional associations concerned with clinical sports medicine issues; they have committed to forming an ongoing project-based alliance to bring together sports medicine organizations to best serve active people and athletes. The organizations are the American Academy of Family Physicians, the American Academy of Orthopaedic Surgeons, the American College of Sports Medicine, the American Medical Society for Sports Medicine, the American Orthopaedic Society for Sports Medicine, and the American Osteopathic Academy of Sports Medicine.

EXPERT PANEL

Stanley A. Herring, MD, Chair, Seattle, Washington
John A. Bergfeld, MD, Cleveland, Ohio
Joel L. Boyd, MD, Edina, Minnesota
Per Gunnar Brolinson, DO, Toledo, Ohio
Cindy J. Chang, MD, Berkeley, California
David W. Glover, MD, Warrensburg, Missouri
William A. Grana, MD, Tucson, Arizona
Peter Indelicato, MD, Gainesville, Florida
Robert J. Johnson, MD, Minneapolis, Minnesota
W. Ben Kibler, MD, Lexington, Kentucky
William J. Kraemer, PhD, CSCS, Muncie, Indiana
Joseph P. McNerney, DO, Vallejo, California
Robert M. Pallay, MD, Hillsborough, New Jersey
Jeffrey L. Tanji, MD, Sacramento, California

DEFINITION

Conditioning is a process in which stimuli are created by an exercise program performed by the athlete to produce a higher level of function.

GOAL

The goal of conditioning is to optimize the performance of the athlete and minimize the risk of injury and illness. To accomplish this goal, the team physician should have knowledge of and be involved with

- General conditioning principles
- Pre-season issues
- In-season issues
- Off-season issues
- Available resources

General Conditioning Principles

Specificity

Training adaptations are specific to the nature of the exercise stimulus (e.g., muscle contraction type, mechanics, metabolic demand). Athletes are subject to specific demands in the performance of sport. Therefore, performance is dependent upon the individual athlete's ability to meet those demands.

Progressive Overload

A conditioning program should begin at a tolerable level of exercise and progress in intensity and volume toward a targeted goal for the individual athlete.

- *Intensity* is the percent of the maximal functional capacity of the exercise mode (e.g., percent of maximal heart rate, percent of one repetition maximum).
- *Volume* is the total amount of exercise performed in specific periods of time (e.g., total distance run, total amount of weight lifted).

Prioritization

Priorities should be developed according to the individual's capabilities and sport-specific demands, because not all elements of a conditioning program can be optimized at the same time, rate, or magnitude.

Periodization

Periodized training is planned variation in the total amount of exercise performed in a given period of time (intensity and volume of exercise.) All periodization terminology describes either a certain type of training, a certain portion of a training cycle, or a certain length of time within a training cycle. Research supports periodization as an important corollary to the principle of progressive overload, because this type of planned variation is key to optimal physical development. Periodized training has shown greater improvements compared to low-volume, single-set training. Such training programs have been shown to be very effective during both short- and long-term training cycles, while reducing the risk of overtraining. Several combinations of variables may be manipulated to produce an adaptation specific to training goals.

Periodization Cycles

- *Macrocycle:* an entire training year. For athletes it is normally thought of as beginning and ending after the last competition of a season.
- *Mesocycle:* a training period lasting 3–6 months.
- *Microcycle:* a training period lasting 1 week or 7 days (can also relate to a training cycle of up to 4 weeks in length depending upon the program design).

Types of Periodization Programs

Strength Training

- *Linear Programs:* Linear programs address conditioning for sports with a limited number of competitions in-season and a well-defined off-season. Classic periodization methods utilize a progressive increase in the intensity and a decrease in the volume of exercise with small variations in each micro-cycle. The linear method is based on developing neuromuscular function and muscle hypertrophy with concomitant improvements in strength and power. The linear method is repeated with each mesocycle as progress is made in the program. Rest between the training cycles (active recovery phase) allows for the needed recovery so that overtraining problems are reduced.
- *Nonlinear (Undulating) Periodized Programs:* Nonlinear programs address conditioning for sports with long competitive seasons, multiple competitions, and year-round practice. The nonlinear program allows for variation in the intensity and volume within each 7- to 10-day cycle by rotating different protocols over the course of the training program. Typically, 3-month cycles are used before an active recovery phase. Nonlinear methods attempt to train the various components of the neuromuscular system within the same 7- to 10-day cycle. However, during a single workout only one feature is trained on that day (e.g., high-force strength, power, local muscular endurance).

  Linear and nonlinear programs have been shown to accomplish similar training effects. Both are superior to constant intensity and volume training programs. The key to workout success is variation. Different approaches can be used during the macrocycle to accomplish this training need.

Program Variables Several variables may be periodized to alter the resistance-training stimulus to achieve the conditioning goal. Different combinations of these variables will create different workouts.

- *Exercise Order:* the sequence in which exercises are performed during a training session (e.g., large muscles before smaller ones and multi-joint exercises performed before single joint exercises).
- *Exercise Selection:* for example, open and closed-chain exercises, free weights, machines.
- *Frequency:* the number of training sessions performed during a specific period of time.
- *Intensity:* the percent of the maximal functional capacity of the exercise as it relates to strength training.
- *Load:* the amount of weight lifted per repetition or set as it relates to strength training.
- *Muscle Action:* concentric, eccentric, or isometric.
- *Repetition Speed:* varying resistive training speed from slow (strength development) to fast (power development) while utilizing the appropriate load.
- *Rest Periods:* the amount of rest taken between sets, exercises, and/or repetitions.
- *Volume:* the total number of repetitions performed during a training session as it relates to strength training.

Aerobic Conditioning Aerobic conditioning can be achieved with a multi-tude of programs (e.g., interval training, continuous training) and modes of exercise (e.g., running, cycling, swimming). It is important that the aerobic conditioning be specific to the sport. Conditioning should be progressive, periodized, prioritized, and compatible with other elements of the conditioning program and the practice sessions.

SPORT-SPECIFIC CONDITIONING

Sport-specific conditioning is the preparation of the athlete for unique physiologic and biomechanical demands and the injury risks inherent in each sport.

- Physiologic demands (e.g., anaerobic/aerobic, environmental)
- Biomechanical demands (e.g., throwing, running)
- Injury risks (e.g., site-specific, traumatic, overload, age- and gender-specific)

Objectives of a Sport-Specific Conditioning Program

Performance

Sports conditioning can be described as a pyramid of fitness and skills:

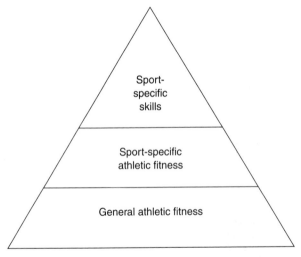

- *General athletic fitness* serves as a base for sport-specific fitness and includes total body flexibility, total body muscular strength and power, cardiorespiratory endurance, and body type, size and structure.
- *Sport-specific athletic fitness* addresses physiologic parameters, biomechanical actions, anatomic sites, and muscle activation patterns common or essential to the individual sport. These components are addressed through specific flexibility, strength balance, power/work, and aerobic/concentric training.
- *Sport-specific skill* is the ultimate goal. Optimal performance demands a refinement of unique training and skill acquisition.

Injury and Illness Prevention

Conditioning may decrease injury and illness by influencing sport-specific risk parameters (e.g., acclimatization, site-specific flexibility, strength, balance, force production of muscle).

Components of a Sport-Specific Conditioning Program

- An individualized *preconditioning evaluation* to determine a fitness profile for the purpose of entering a conditioning program. This includes both a general and a sport-specific athletic fitness evaluation.
- A *periodized protocol* for the individual athlete that addresses the unique demands of that sport.
- An *evaluation process* to determine efficacy of the conditioning program.

Conditioning Modifications

In certain populations, conditioning programs may need to be modified to optimize performance and minimize the risk of injury.

Youth

Physiologic and biomechanical capabilities in young athletes are different from those of adults. Conditioning injuries in this population include physeal, apophyseal, joint injury, overload tendinitis, and unique susceptibility to environmental stressors.

Strength. Strength training programs are important for the young athlete. Strength gains in this population will be due to increases in recruitment and synchronization of muscle activation patterns. *Strength training modifications for youth, particularly during periods of rapid growth, focus on proper supervision, and lower intensity and volume.* As the athlete matures, gains in muscle mass will play a more significant role in strength increases.

Flexibility. Flexibility is traditionally included as a component of conditioning for youth; however, its benefit is unclear in this population.

Aerobics. Aerobic gains in this population are obtainable but young athletes do not respond so effectively as adults.

Female Athletes

There are gender-related differences in muscle performance, particularly in the upper body. However, female athletes can obtain strength gains and aerobic gains in the same proportion as male athletes in a comparable training program. All female athletes should participate in a total body conditioning program. The lower extremity and shoulder are frequent areas of injury in the female athlete. Strength deficits in these areas are more closely associated with injury in females than in males. In the female athlete's total body resistance conditioning program, the upper body should always be emphasized. In addition, the female athlete at risk of unique sport-related injuries (e.g., anterior cruciate ligament [ACL], ankle sprains) should participate in specific resistance conditioning programs. Proper conditioning programs to decrease ACL injuries particularly demonstrate these principles.

Multi-Sport Athletes

With overlapping seasons, multi-sport athletes have unique conditioning challenges. Multi-sport athletes need to maintain their general athletic fitness base and focus their sport-specific conditioning toward their current sport. There is a distinct need for recovery between seasons; therefore, including an active recovery phase into the athletic participation and conditioning cycle is of particular importance to multi-sport athletes. Conditioning injuries may occur when an athlete tries to prepare simultaneously for two different sports.

Athletes Who Are Physically Challenged

Athletes who are physically challenged benefit from a conditioning program. Their program should be modified depending on the specific type of impairment and associated disability. Medical conditions in this population such as temperature regulation, skin problems, cardiovascular function, and entrapment neuropathies can affect or be affected by the conditioning process. A conditioning program for this population must also accommodate such unique concerns as access and equipment.

PRE-SEASON ISSUES

Network

The team physician should be involved in the network that integrates expertise regarding conditioning matters with certified strength and conditioning specialists, the coaches, and other healthcare providers (who may include certified athletic trainers, physical therapists, and medical specialists).

Education

Education of athletes and coaches about conditioning provides a framework for understanding the importance of such training for sports, and will optimize sports performance and minimize the risk of injury and illness.

It Is Essential That

- Instruction about the goals and content of the periodized pre-season, in-season, and off-season conditioning programs.
- Instruction about needs for modification of the conditioning program.
- Medical information that affects the conditioning program.

It Is Desirable For

- The entire network, including the team physician, to understand the goals and content of the periodized conditioning program.
- The entire network, including the team physician, to be involved in the educational process.

Conditioning Programs

It Is Essential For

- The network to implement the proper periodized sport-specific conditioning programs.
- Medical information that affects the conditioning program to be made available to allow for appropriate program modification.

It Is Desirable For

- The entire network, including the team physician, to monitor the conditioning program.
- The entire network, including the team physician, to be available to address concerns about the conditioning program.

- There to be an adequate facility for the conditioning program.
- The network to provide for proper documentation of individual conditioning programs.

IN-SEASON ISSUES

Network

The network should continue to integrate expertise regarding the conditioning program during the in-season.

Implementation of the In-Season Conditioning Program

It Is Essential For

- The network to implement the periodized in-season sport-specific conditioning program.

It Is Desirable For

- The entire network, including the team physician, to monitor the in-season conditioning program.
- The entire network, including the team physician, to be available to address concerns about the in-season conditioning program.
- There to be an adequate facility for the in-season conditioning program.
- The network to provide proper documentation of individual conditioning programs.
- The team physician to observe the conditioning program.

Management and Rehabilitation of Injuries That Impact or Are a Result of Conditioning

The coordination of management and rehabilitation of injuries affecting conditioning is the duty of the team physician (as detailed in the Team Physician Consensus Statement, 82000).

It Is Essential For the Team Physician To

- Be familiar with conditioning matters and the injuries that occur with conditioning.
- Coordinate the modification or cessation of a high risk activity once identified.
- Coordinate the medical management of injury and illness.
- Coordinate rehabilitation of any conditioning injury or illness, focusing on return to conditioning with any modifications and return to play.

It Is Desirable For

- The entire network, including the team physician, to be available to review conditioning matters.
- The entire network, including the team physician, to participate in the design of the reporting system for conditioning injuries.
- The entire network, including the team physician, to participate in injury surveillance to help identify practices that may be leading to increased rates of injury.
- The entire network, including the team physician, to develop proper documentation to identify and report conditioning injuries.

OFF-SEASON ISSUES

Review of Network and Conditioning Program

Off-season evaluation of the network and conditioning program established in the pre-season promotes continued effectiveness. A timely meeting of the network should be held to review and modify the network and the conditioning program.

It Is Essential For the Team Physician To

• Coordinate the evaluation of the possible role of the conditioning program in prevention or production of injuries.

It Is Desirable For the Network To

• Determine whether the conditioning program met the network's goals.
• Coordinate the development of an off-season conditioning program.
• Document and evaluate the sport-specific fitness level of each athlete.

Implementation of the Off-Season Conditioning Program

The network should implement an active recovery phase followed by the proper, periodized, sport-specific off-season conditioning program.

AVAILABLE RESOURCES

Ongoing education pertinent to the team physician is essential. Information regarding team physician-specific educational opportunities is available from the six participating organizations:

American Academy of Family Physicians (AAFP)
11400 Tomahawk Creek Parkway
Leawood, KS 66211
800-274-2237
www.aafp.org

American Academy of Orthopaedic Surgeons (AAOS)
6300 North River Road
Rosemont, IL 60018
800-346-AAOS
www.aaos.org

American College of Sports Medicine (ACSM)
401 West Michigan Street
Indianapolis, IN 46202
317-637-9200
www.acsm.org

American Medical Society for Sports Medicine (AMSSM)
11639 Earnshaw
Overland Park, KS 66210
913-327-1415
www.amssm.org

American Orthopaedic Society for Sports Medicine (AOSSM)
6300 North River Road Suite 200
Rosemont, IL 60018
847-292-4900
www.sportsmed.org

American Osteopathic Academy of Sports Medicine (AOASM)
7611 Elmwood Avenue Suite 201
Middleton, WI 53562
608-831-4400
www.aoasm.org

Also, specific information and education regarding conditioning issues is available from:

National Strength and Conditioning Association
PO Box 9908
Colorado Springs, CO 80932
800-815-6826
www.nsca-lift.org

SUGGESTED RESOURCES

Baechle TR, Earle RW, eds. *Essentials of Strength Training and Conditioning.* 2nd ed. Champaign, Ill: Human Kinetics; 2000.

Chandler TJ, Kibler WB. Muscle training in injury prevention. In *IOC Encyclopedia of Sports Medicine—Sports Injuries.* London: Blackwell; 1993;252–261.

Faigenbaum AD, Kraemer WJ, Cahil B, et al. Youth resistance training: Position statement paper and literature review (NSCA). *Strength and Conditioning.* 1996;18:62–75.

Fleck SJ, Kraemer WJ. *Designing Resistance Training Programs.* 2nd ed. Champaign, Ill: Human Kinetics; 1997.

Kibler WB, Chandler J. Sport specific conditioning. *Am J Sports Med.* 1994;22:424–432.

Kibler WB, Livingston B. Closed-chain rehabilitation for upper and lower extremity. *J Am Acad Orthop Surg.* 2001;9:412–421.

Komi PV. *Strength and Power and Sport.* Oxford: Blackwell; 1992.

Kraemer WJ, Faigenbaum AD, Bush JA, Nindl BC. Resistance training and youth: Enhancing muscle fitness. In Rippe JM, ed. *Lifestyle Medicine.* Mass: Blackwell; 2000;626–637.

Kraemer WJ, Fleck SJ. *Strength Training for Young Athletes.* Champaign, Ill: Human Kinetics; 1993.

Kraemer WJ, Hakkinen K, eds. *Strength Training for Athletes.* Oxford: Blackwell; IOC Medical Commission; in press.

Kraemer WJ, Newton RU. In: Young J, ed. *Training for Muscular Power: Clinics in Sports Medicine.* Philadelphia: Saunders; 2000;341–368.

Kraemer WJ, Ratamess NA. Physiology of resistance training: Current issues. In: Hughes, C, ed. *Orthopaedic Physical Therapy Clinics of North America.* Philadelphia: Saunders; 2000;467–513.

Kraemer WJ, Ratamess NA, Rubin MR. Basic principles of resistance training. In: *Nutrition and the Strength Athlete.* Boca Raton, Fla: CRC Press; 2000;1–29.

Kreider R, O'Toole M, Fry AC. *Overtraining in Sport.* Champaign, Ill: Human Kinetics; 1998.

Zatsiorsky V. *Science and Practice of Strength Training.* Champaign, Ill: Human Kinetics; 1995.

SUGGESTED JOURNAL RESOURCES

Strength and Conditioning Journal. National Strength and Conditioning Association, Colorado Springs, CO (bimonthly)

Journal of Strength and Conditioning Research. National Strength and Conditioning Association, Colorado Springs, CO (quarterly)

D | The Team Physician and Return-to-Play Issues

SUMMARY

The objective of this Consensus Statement is to provide physicians who are responsible for the healthcare of teams with a decision process for determining when to return an injured or ill athlete to practice or competition. This statement is not intended as a standard of care, and should not be interpreted as such. This statement is only a guide, and as such is of a general nature consistent with the reasonable and objective practice of the healthcare professional. Individual decisions regarding returning an injured or ill athlete to play will depend on the specific facts and circumstances presented to the physician.

Adequate insurance should be in place to help protect the athlete, the sponsoring organization, and the physician.

This statement was developed by the collaborative effort of six major professional associations concerned with clinical sports medicine issues; they have committed to forming an ongoing project-based alliance to bring together sports medicine organizations to best serve active people and athletes. The organizations are the American Academy of Family Physicians, the American Academy of Orthopaedic Surgeons, the American College of Sports Medicine, the American Medical Society for Sports Medicine, the American Orthopaedic Society for Sports Medicine, and the American Osteopathic Academy of Sports Medicine.

EXPERT PANEL

Stanley A. Herring, MD, Chair, Seattle, Washington
John A. Bergfeld, MD, Cleveland, Ohio
Joel L. Boyd, MD, Edina, Minnesota
Timothy Duffey, D.O., Columbus, Ohio
Karl B. Fields, MD, Greensboro, North Carolina
William A. Grana, MD, Tucson, Arizona
Peter Indelicato, MD, Gainesville, Florida
W. Ben Kibler, MD, Lexington, Kentucky
Robert Pallay, MD, Hillsborough, New Jersey
Margot Putukian, MD, University Park, Pennsylvania
Robert E. Sallis, MD, Alta Loma, California

DEFINITION

Return-to-play is the process of deciding when an injured or ill athlete may safely return to practice or competition.

GOAL

The goal is to return an injured or ill athlete to practice or competition without putting the individual or others at undue risk for injury or illness. To accomplish this goal, the team physician should have knowledge of and be involved with:

- Establishing a return-to-play process
- Evaluating injured or ill athletes
- Treating injured or ill athletes

- Rehabilitating injured or ill athletes
- Returning an injured or ill athlete to play

Establishing a Return-to-Play Process

Establishing a process for returning an athlete to play is an essential first step in deciding when an injured or ill athlete may safely return to practice or competition. It is essential for the team physician to coordinate

- Establishing a chain of command regarding decisions to return an injured or ill athlete to practice or competition.
- Communicating the return-to-play process to the player, family, certified athletic trainers coaches, administrators, and other healthcare providers.
- Establishing a system for documentation.
- Establishing protocols to release information regarding an athlete's ability to return to practice or competition following an injury or illness.

It is essential that the return-to-play process address the

- Safety of the athlete.
- Potential risk to the safety of other participants.
- Functional capabilities of the athlete.
- Functional requirements of the athlete's sport.
- Federal, state, local, school, and governing body regulations related to returning an injured or ill athlete to practice or competition.

Evaluating Injured or Ill Athletes

Evaluation of an injured or ill athlete establishes a diagnosis, directs treatment, and is the basis for deciding when an athlete may safely return to practice or competition. Repeated evaluations throughout the continuum of injury or illness management optimize medical care. It is essential that evaluation of an injured or ill athlete include

- A condition-specific medical history.
- A condition-specific physical examination.
- Appropriate medical tests and consultations.
- Psychosocial assessment.
- Documentation.
- Communication with the player, family, certified athletic trainer, coaches, and other healthcare providers.

In addition, it is desirable that

- The team physician coordinate evaluation of the injured or ill athlete.

Treating Injured or Ill Athletes

Treatment of an injured or ill athlete promotes the safe and timely return to practice or competition. It is essential that treatment of the injured or ill athlete

- Begin in a timely manner (see *Sideline Preparedness for the Team Physician: A Consensus Statement*, ©(2000).
- Follow an individualized plan, which may include consultations and referrals.
- Include a rehabilitation plan.
- Include equipment modification, bracing, and orthoses as necessary.

- Address psychosocial issues.
- Provide a realistic prognosis as to the safe and timely return to practice or competition.
- Include continued communication with the player, family, certified athletic trainer, coaches, and other healthcare providers.
- Include documentation.

In addition, it is desirable that

- The team physician coordinate the initial and ongoing treatment for the injured or ill athlete.

Rehabilitating Injured or Ill Athletes

Comprehensive treatment includes proper rehabilitation of an injured or ill athlete, which optimizes the safe and timely return to practice or competition. The team physician should be involved in a network that integrates expertise regarding rehabilitation. This network should include certified athletic trainers, physical therapists, medical specialists, and other healthcare providers. It is essential that the rehabilitation network

- Coordinate the development of a rehabilitation plan that is designed to
  - Restore function of the injured part.
  - Restore and promote musculoskeletal and cardiovascular function, as well as overall well-being of the injured or ill athlete.
  - Provide sport-specific assessment and training, which can serve as a basis for sport-specific conditioning (see *The Team Physician and Conditioning of Athletes for Sports: A Consensus Statement*, ©(2001).
  - Provide for continued equipment modification, bracing and orthoses.
- Continue communication with the player, family, rehabilitation network, and coaches concerning the athlete's progress.
- Include documentation.

In addition, it is desirable that

- The team physician coordinate the rehabilitation program for the injured or ill athlete.

Returning an Injured or Ill Athlete to Play

The decision for safe and timely return of an injured or ill athlete to practice or competition is the desired result of the process of evaluation, treatment, and rehabilitation. It is essential for return-to-play that the team physician confirm the following criteria:

- The status of anatomic and functional healing
- The status of recovery from acute illness and associated sequelae
- The status of chronic injury or illness
- That the athlete pose no undue risk to the safety of other participants
- Restoration of sport-specific skills
- Psychosocial readiness
- Ability to perform safely with equipment modification, bracing, and orthoses
- Compliance with applicable federal, state, local, school, and governing body regulations

Prior to return-to-play, these criteria should be confirmed at a satisfactory level.

CONCLUSION

Using the information in this document allows the team physician to make an informed decision as to whether an injured or ill athlete may safely return to practice or competition.

The return-to-play process should be under the direction of the team physician whenever possible. Although it is desirable that the team physician coordinate evaluating, treating, and rehabilitating the injured or ill athlete, it is essential that the team physician ultimately be responsible for the return-to-play decision.

Individual decisions regarding returning an injured or ill athlete to play will depend on the specific facts and circumstances presented to the team physician.

AVAILABLE RESOURCES

Ongoing education pertinent to the team physician is essential. Information regarding team physician-specific educational opportunities can be obtained from the six participating organizations:

American Academy of Family Physicians (AAFP)
11400 Tomahawk Creek Parkway
Leawood, KS 66211
800-274-2237
www.aafp.org

American Academy of Orthopaedic Surgeons (AAOS)
6300 North River Road
Rosemont, IL 60018
800-346-AAOS
www.aaos.org

American College of Sports Medicine (ACSM)
401 West Michigan Street
Indianapolis, IN 46202
317-637-9200
www.acsm.org

American Medical Society for Sports Medicine (AMSSM)
11639 Earnshaw
Overland Park, KS 66210
913-327-1415
www.amssm.org

American Orthopaedic Society for Sports Medicine (AOSSM)
6300 North River Road Suite 200
Rosemont, IL 60018
847-292-4900
www.sportsmed.org

American Osteopathic Academy of Sports Medicine (AOASM)
7611 Elmwood Avenue Suite 201
Middleton, WI 53562
608-831-4400
www.aoasm.org

SUGGESTED REFERENCES

AAFP, AAP, AMSSM, AOSSM, AOASM. Preparticipation physical evaluation. In *The Physician and Sportsmedicine.* 2nd ed. Minneapolis: McGraw-Hill Healthcare; 1997.

Adams BB. Transmission of cutaneous infections in athletes. *Br J Sports Med.* 2000;34:413–414.

American College of Sports Medicine, American College of Cardiology, 26th Bethesda Conference. Recommendations for competition in athletes with cardiovascular abnormalities. *Med Sci Sports Exerc.* 1994;26:5223–5283.

American Medical Society for Sports Medicine, American Academy of Sports Medicine. Human immunodeficiency virus and other blood-borne pathogens in sports (Joint position statement). *Clin J Sports Med.* 1995;5:199–204.

Cantu RC. Return-to-play guidelines after a head injury. *Clin J Sports Med.* 1998;17:45–60.

Cantu RC. Stingers, transient quadriplegia and cervical spinal stenosis: Return-to-play criteria. *Med Sci Sports Exerc.* 1997;29(7 suppl):S233–S235.

Committee on Sports Medicine and Fitness. Cardiac dysrhythmias and sports. *Pediatrics.* 1995;95:786–789.

Goodman R, Thacker S, Soloman S, et al. Infectious disease in competitive sports. *JAMA.* 1994;271:862–866.

Herring SA. Rehabilitation of muscle injuries. *Med Sci Sports Exerc.* 1990;22:453–456.

Kibler WB, Herring SA, Press JM. *Functional Rehabilitation of Sports and Musculoskeletal Injuries.* Aspen; 1998.

Kibler WB, Livingston BP. Closed-chain rehabilitation for upper and lower extremities. *J Am Acad Orthop Surg.* 2001;9:412–421.

Maron BJ. Cardiovascular risks to young persons on the athletic field. *Ann Intern Med.* 1998;129:379–386.

Mellion MB, Walsh WM, Madden C, et al, eds. *Team Physician's Handbook.* 3rd ed. Philadelphia: Hanley & Belfus; 2002.

Mitten MJ, Mitten RJ. Legal considerations in treating the injured athlete. *J Orthop Sports Phys Ther.* 1995;21:38–43.

E | Female Athlete Issues for the Team Physician

SUMMARY

This document provides an overview of select musculoskeletal and medical issues that are important to team physicians who are responsible for the medical care of female athletes. It is not intended as a standard of care, and should not be interpreted as such. This document is only a guide, and as such, is of a general nature, consistent with the reasonable, objective practice of the healthcare professional. Individual treatment will turn on the specific facts and circumstances presented to the physician.

Adequate insurance should be in place to help protect the physician, the athlete, and the sponsoring organization.

This statement was developed by a collaboration of six major professional associations concerned about clinical sports medicine issues; they have committed to forming an ongoing project-based alliance to bring together sports medicine organizations to best serve active people and athletes. The organizations are the American Academy of Family Physicians, the American Academy of Orthopaedic Surgeons, the American College of Sports Medicine, the American Medical Society for Sports Medicine, the American Orthopaedic Society for Sports Medicine, and the American Osteopathic Academy of Sports Medicine.

EXPERT PANEL

Stanley A. Herring, MD, Chair, Seattle, Washington
John A. Bergfeld, MD, Cleveland, Ohio
Lori A. Boyajian-O'Neill, DO, Kansas City, Missouri
Timothy Duffey, DO, Columbus, Ohio
Letha Yurko Griffin, MD, PhD, Atlanta, Georgia
Jo A. Hannafin, MD, PhD, New York, New York
Peter Indelicato, MD, Gainesville, Florida
Elizabeth A. Joy, MD, Salt Lake City, Utah
W. Ben Kibler, MD, Lexington, Kentucky
Constance M. Lebrun, MD, London, Ontario, Canada
Robert Pallay, MD, Hillsborough, New Jersey
Margot Putukian, MD, University Park, Pennsylvania

DEFINITION

Female athletes experience musculoskeletal injuries and medical problems, resulting from and/or impacting athletic activity. Team physicians must understand the gender-specific implications of these issues.

GOAL

The goal is to assist the team physician in providing optimal medical care for the female athlete.

THE FEMALE ATHLETE AND ANTERIOR CRUCIATE LIGAMENT INJURIES

It is essential that the team physician understand
• That the female is at increased risk of anterior cruciate ligament (ACL) injury in multiple sports and activities.

- The anatomy, biomechanics and mechanisms of injury of the ACL.
- Treatment strategies including surgical indications.

It is desirable that the team physician

- Understand current prevention strategies.
- Coordinate a network to identify risk factors and implement treatment.
- Understand the potential long-term sequelae of ACL injury.

Epidemiology

- Noncontact ACL injury rate is 2–10 times higher in female athletes than in their male counterparts.
- Examples of high-risk sports include basketball, field hockey, lacrosse, skiing, and soccer.

Physiology and Pathophysiology

- Causes of noncontact ACL injuries may be multifactorial; proposed risks include environmental, anatomic, hormonal, biomechanical, and neuromuscular factors.
- Noncontact ACL injuries occur commonly during deceleration, landing, or cutting. At-risk positions during these maneuvers include knee extension, flat foot, and off-balance body position.

Evaluation and Treatment

It is essential that the team physician

- Delineate the mechanism of the injury.
- Conduct a comprehensive physical examination of the knee, including ACL assessment.
- Know the indications for and utility of imaging techniques.
- Know the indications for surgical consideration.
- Facilitate early rehabilitation to improve strength, flexibility, and neuromuscular control.

It is desirable that the team physician:

- Review the results of imaging studies.
- Understand the principles of the surgical management of the ACL injury.

Prevention

It is essential that the team physician

- Understand that neuromuscular factors may contribute to increased risk of noncontact ACL injuries, and may be amenable to prevention with specific conditioning programs.
- Recognize that conditioning programs may need to be gender specific (see *The Team Physician and Conditioning of Athletes for Sports—A Consensus Statement* [2001]).

It is desirable that the team physician

- Identify proposed risk factors during the pre-participation evaluation.
- Coordinate a prevention program.

- Educate athletes, parents, coaches, and other healthcare providers, including information about at-risk positions and game situations that are associated with ACL injury.

THE FEMALE ATHLETE AND THE PATELLOFEMORAL JOINT

It is essential that the team physician understand

- The anatomy and biomechanics of the patellofemoral joint.
- The mechanisms of patellofemoral pain and dysfunction.

It is desirable that the team physician

- Coordinate the evaluation and treatment of athletes with patellofemoral problems.
- Understand the potential long-term sequelae of patellofemoral pain and dysfunction.

Epidemiology

- Patellofemoral problems occur frequently in female athletes.
- Patellofemoral pain and dysfunction result from macro- and micro-trauma.

Physiology and Pathophysiology

- Normal patellofemoral mechanics involve a balance between bone alignment, articular cartilage, soft tissue (ligaments, muscles, tendons, fascia), and coordinated neuromuscular activation.
- Patellofemoral pain and dysfunction are multifactorial, including malalignment, articular cartilage lesions, instability, soft tissue factors, and psychosocial issues.
- Patellofemoral pain may occur in what appears to be a normal knee joint.
- Risk factors include
  - Static and/or dynamic malalignment of the pelvis, hip, knee, ankle, and foot.
  - Muscle weakness and/or imbalance and inflexibility.
  - Altered patellar position and/or morphology.
  - Trauma, overuse, and/or training errors.

Evaluation and Treatment

It is essential that the team physician

- Delineate key points relating to the history of the patellofemoral problem.
- Conduct a specific examination for the patellofemoral problem.
- Know the indications for and utility of imaging techniques.
- Understand nonoperative management of patellofemoral problems, including patient education, activity modification, rehabilitation, bracing, orthoses, and medications.

It is desirable that the team physician

- Review the results of imaging studies.
- Understand the principles of and indications for surgical management.

Prevention

It is essential that the team physician

- Know the risk factors for patellofemoral problems.

It is desirable that the team physician

- Identify risk factors during the pre-participation evaluation.
- Implement a screening program for risk factors.
- Educate athletes, parents, coaches, administrators, and healthcare providers.

THE FEMALE ATHLETE AND SHOULDER CONDITIONS

It is essential that the team physician understand

- The anatomy and biomechanics of the shoulder.
- The mechanisms of shoulder injury and dysfunction.

It is desirable that the team physician

- Recognize that shoulder conditions may result from strength and flexibility imbalances or injuries elsewhere in the body.
- Identify risk factors associated with shoulder conditions.
- Coordinate the evaluation and treatment of shoulder conditions.

Epidemiology

- Examples of high-risk sports include diving, gymnastics, swimming, tennis, throwing sports, and volleyball.
- Shoulder conditions result from macro- and micro-trauma.

Physiology and Pathophysiology

- The integration of coordinated neuromuscular activation, capsular/ligament stiffness, and glenohumeral and scapulothoracic positioning is key to shoulder function.
- The female athlete's shoulder is at risk for injury due to increased biomechanical load, resulting from specific risk factors, including
  - Increased joint laxity (translation).
  - Increased muscle and joint flexibility (range of motion).
  - Decreased upper-body strength and poor posture.
  - Acquired internal rotation deficits.

Evaluation and Treatment

It is essential that the team physician

- Delineate key points relating to the history of the shoulder condition.
- Conduct a comprehensive examination for the shoulder condition, including assessment of range of motion, instability, rotator cuff pathology, and scapular dysfunction.
- Know the indications and utility of imaging techniques.
- Understand the principles of shoulder rehabilitation.

It is desirable that the team physician

- Evaluate strength and flexibility imbalances or injuries elsewhere in the body that may contribute to shoulder conditions.
- Review the results of imaging studies.
- Understand the principles of and indications for surgical management.

Prevention

It is essential that the team physician

- Know the risk factors for shoulder conditions.

It is desirable that the team physician

- Identify risk factors during the pre-participation evaluation.
- Implement a screening program for risk factors.
- Educate athletes, parents, coaches, administrators, and healthcare providers.

THE FEMALE ATHLETE AND STRESS FRACTURES

It is essential that the team physician understand

- A stress fracture in a female athlete can be an isolated injury, or may indicate underlying medical and psychosocial problems. Therefore, evaluation and treatment must take into account the etiology of the stress fracture.
- Certain stress fractures are at high risk for complications and long-term sequelae.

It is desirable that the team physician

- Coordinate, when necessary, multidisciplinary evaluation and treatment.

Epidemiology

- Stress fractures occur frequently in female athletes.
- Some studies suggest a higher incidence of stress fractures in women, but there is little evidence to support a gender difference in stress fractures among trained athletes.
- Common anatomic areas include the foot, tibia, fibula, femur, and pelvis.

Physiology and Pathophysiology

- Stress fractures occur when bone is subjected to repetitive loads beyond its physiologic capacity.
- An imbalance between bone resorption and deposition creates bone that may not withstand repetitive loads.
- Risk factors associated with stress fractures include
  - Extrinsic factors (exercise [type, volume, and intensity], footwear).
  - Intrinsic musculoskeletal factors (muscle strength and imbalance, limb alignment).
  - Medical factors (osteopenia, osteoporosis, menstrual dysfunction, poor nutrition, disordered eating and other psychosocial issues).

Evaluation and Treatment

It is essential that the team physician

- Delineate key points relating to the history of the stress fracture.
- Conduct a specific physical examination pertinent to the suspected stress fracture.
- Identify potential underlying risk factors.
- Know the indications for and utility of imaging techniques.
- Identify stress fractures at high risk of complication and long-term sequelae.
- Know the indications for surgical consideration.
- Understand nonoperative management and rehabilitation.

It is desirable that the team physician

- Review the results of the imaging studies.

- Understand the principles of and indications for surgical management.
- Coordinate, when necessary, a multi-disciplinary team approach to treatment.

Prevention

It is essential that the team physician

- Recognize there can be multiple risk factors for stress fractures.

It is desirable that the team physician

- Recognize risk factors during the pre-participation evaluation.
- Implement a screening program for risk factors.
- Educate athletes, parents, coaches, administrators, and healthcare providers.

THE FEMALE ATHLETE AND OSTEOPENIA AND OSTEOPOROSIS

It is essential that the team physician understand that

- Osteopenia and osteoporosis (as defined by the World Health Organization [WHO]) can exist in the young female athlete.
- These conditions have implications for athletic performance and long-term sequelae.
- Disordered eating and menstrual dysfunction are common risk factors.

It is desirable the team physician understand

- The evaluation and treatment of osteopenia and osteoporosis.
- The importance of educating athletes, parents, coaches, administrators, and healthcare providers.
- The value of prevention and early detection of osteopenia and osteoporosis.

Epidemiology

- The incidence of osteopenia and osteoporosis in the female athlete is unknown.
- Several studies have demonstrated osteopenia and osteoporosis in young female athletes with menstrual dysfunction and/or eating disorders.
- The major determinant of adult bone mineral density (BMD) is bone mass achieved during adolescence and young adulthood. Osteoporosis-related fractures in later life are associated with significant morbidity and mortality.

Physiology and Pathophysiology

- Bone mass depends on the overall balance between resorption and deposition.
- Ninety percent of total bone mineral content is accrued by the end of adolescence, creating a window of opportunity to maximize BMD.
- Eighty percent of variance in BMD is attributed to genetic factors. Lean body mass, estrogen, exercise, and calcium intake are other important influences.
- Tobacco use, excessive alcohol consumption, certain medical conditions (e.g., renal disease, hyperparathyroidism), and medications (e.g., glucocorticoids) can negatively affect bone density.
- Athletes involved in impact sports and/or strength training routinely have higher site-specific BMD than athletes in nonimpact sports and nonathletes.

- The effect of impact activities and/or strength training is most pronounced during puberty and dependent upon intensity and volume of conditioning (see *The Team Physician and Conditioning of Athletes for Sports—A Consensus Statement* [2001]).

Evaluation and Treatment

It is essential that the team physician

- Recognize risk factors for low BMD.
- Know the indications for and the utility of imaging techniques.
- Facilitate treatment for osteopenia and osteoporosis once identified.

It is desirable that the team physician

- Understand WHO criteria for osteopenia (1–2.5 standard deviations [SD] below young adult mean BMD) and osteoporosis (>2.5 SD below young adult mean BMD).
- Coordinate a screening process to identify athletes at risk.
- Coordinate a comprehensive evaluation including assessment of menstrual status, nutritional intake, measurement of BMD, and laboratory testing as necessary.
- Understand that multi-disciplinary treatment may include restoration of normal menstrual cycles, optimization of physical activity and nutrition, psychological therapy, and pharmacologic intervention.

Prevention

It is essential that the team physician understand

- That optimal BMD is achieved by maintaining physiologic estrogen levels, adequate nutrition, and load-bearing exercise.
- The importance of prevention and early detection of osteopenia and osteoporosis.

It is desirable that the team physician

- Identify risk factors during the pre-participation evaluation.
- Implement a screening program for risk factors, including information regarding strategies for maintaining optimal BMD and the effect of negative behaviors on BMD.
- Educate athletes, parents, coaches, administrators, and healthcare professionals.

THE FEMALE ATHLETE AND DISORDERED EATING

It is essential the team physician understand

- The importance of adequate nutrition in sports.
- The spectrum of disordered eating and how it affects the female athlete.
- That disordered eating can occur in any sport.

It is desirable that the team physician understand

- The evaluation and treatment of the athlete with disordered eating.
- The importance of educating athletes, coaches, parents, administrators, and other healthcare providers.
- The value of prevention and early detection of disordered eating.

Epidemiology

- Disordered eating occurs on a spectrum. This ranges from calorie, protein, and/or fat restriction and pathogenic weight control measures (e.g., diet pills, laxatives, excessive exercise, self-induced vomiting) to classic eating disorders (ED), such as anorexia nervosa (AN) and bulimia nervosa (BN).
- Athletes in sports involving aesthetics, endurance, and weight classifications are at particular risk for the spectrum of disordered eating.
- Fifteen to 62 percent of college female athletes report a history of disordered eating.
- ED are psychiatric disorders with distortion of body image, significant nutritional and medical complications, including a mortality rate of 12–18% for untreated AN.
- Female athletes are at higher risk for developing ED than the general population.

Physiology and Pathophysiology

- Nutritional and medical consequences of the spectrum of disordered eating include
  - Nutritional deficiencies and electrolyte disturbances.
  - Decreased BMD.
  - Gastrointestinal problems (e.g., bleeding, ulceration, bloating, constipation).
  - Cardiovascular abnormalities (e.g., arrhythmias, heart block).
  - Psychiatric problems (e.g., depression, anxiety, suicide).
- Risk factors include
  - Pressure to optimize performance and/or modify appearance.
  - Psychological factors, such as low self-esteem, poor coping skills, perceived loss of control, perfectionism, obsessive compulsive traits, depression, anxiety, and history of sexual/physical abuse.
  - Underlying chronic diseases related to caloric utilization (e.g., diabetes).

Evaluation and Treatment

It is essential that the team physician

- Recognize risk factors for the spectrum of disordered eating.
- Facilitate treatment once identified with a multidisciplinary approach as needed.
- Understand the necessity of mental health treatment for ED.

It is desirable that the team physician

- Coordinate a screening process to identify athletes at risk.
- Understand a comprehensive evaluation includes assessment of nutrition, exercise behaviors, pathogenic weight control measures, and psychosocial factors; additional laboratory and other diagnostic testing as necessary.
- Understand treatment may involve a multidisciplinary approach (medical, mental health, and nutritional management), including parents, coaches, Certified Athletic Trainers, physical therapists, and administrators.

Prevention

It is essential that the team physician understand

- The importance of prevention and early detection of the spectrum of disordered eating.

It is desirable that the team physician

- Identify risk factors during the pre-participation evaluation.
- Implement a screening program for risk factors, including information to dispel misconceptions about body weight, body composition, and athletic performance.
- Educate athletes, parents, coaches, administrators, and healthcare providers.

THE FEMALE ATHLETE AND SELECTED MENSTRUAL DYSFUNCTION

It is essential that the team physician understand

- The normal menstrual cycle and the spectrum of menstrual dysfunction.
- The consequences of menstrual dysfunction on bone density and fertility.

It is desirable that the team physician understand

- The evaluation and treatment of the athlete with menstrual dysfunction.
- The importance of educating athletes, parents, coaches, administrators, and healthcare providers.
- The value of prevention and early detection of menstrual dysfunction.

Epidemiology

- Menstrual dysfunction occurs in different forms:
  - *Delayed menarche*—onset of menstrual cycles after 16 years of age.
  - *Secondary amenorrhea*—absence of menses for 3 or more months after regular menses has been established.
  - *Oligomenorrhea*—6–9 cycles per year; cycle length greater than 35 days or less than 3 months.
  - *Anovulation*—absence of ovulation; may have regular menstrual bleeding.
  - *Luteal phase deficiency*—cycle length may be normal, but there are decreased progesterone levels.
- In the athlete, menstrual dysfunction is at least two to three times more common than in the nonathlete; 10–15% have amenorrhea or oligomenorrhea.

Physiology and Pathophysiology

- Normal menstrual cycle depends on intact hypothalamic-pituitary-ovarian (HPO) axis and normal pelvic organ function.
- The etiology of menstrual dysfunction is multifactorial, including body weight and composition, nutrition, training, previous menstrual function, and psychosocial factors.
- The *energy drain hypothesis* states that energy expenditure exceeds stored and consumed energy, leading to disruption of the HPO axis.
- Intense exercise alone does not necessarily cause menstrual dysfunction, provided there is adequate caloric intake for the energy needs.
- Consequences of menstrual dysfunction may include lower levels of estrogen and/or progesterone, lower BMD, higher incidence of stress fractures, and infertility.
- Effects of lower levels of estrogen on BMD are not completely reversible; therefore, early detection and treatment of menstrual dysfunction are important.

Evaluation and Treatment

It is essential that the team physician

- Understand menstrual dysfunction related solely to exercise is a diagnosis of exclusion.
- Recognize risk factors for and implications of menstrual dysfunction.
- Facilitate treatment of these conditions once identified, with a multidisciplinary approach as necessary.

It is desirable that the team physician

- Coordinate a screening program to identify athletes at risk.
- Understand that a comprehensive evaluation includes assessment for other causes of menstrual dysfunction; detailed menstrual, nutrition and medication history; laboratory testing and additional diagnostic testing as necessary.
- Understand that treatment may include increasing caloric intake, decreasing energy expenditure, hormone supplementation, and psychotherapy as necessary.

Prevention

It is essential that the team physician understand

- The importance of prevention and early detection of menstrual dysfunction.

It is desirable that the team physician

- Identify risk factors during the pre-participation evaluation.
- Implement a screening program for risk factors, including information about the importance of normal menstrual function.
- Educate athletes, parents, coaches, administrators, and healthcare providers.

THE FEMALE ATHLETE AND PREGNANCY AND CONTRACEPTION

The majority of team physicians do not provide obstetric care for female athletes, nor do they offer specific contraceptive counseling. Prenatal and postpartum care in the United States is generally carried out by an obstetrician/gynecologist and/or family medicine physician. Team physicians may defer to the specific expertise of the physician(s) providing primary obstetric care, but can coordinate and collaborate in the management of sports-related injuries and illnesses.

It is essential that the team physician

- Recognize the signs and symptoms of pregnancy.
- Understand that absolute and relative contraindications to exercise throughout pregnancy exist.
- Understand the importance of family planning and contraception.

It is desirable that the team physician understand

- Basic physiologic changes associated with pregnancy and the postpartum period.
- Sport-specific risks and benefits of exercise in pregnancy and exercise prescription.

- The effects of certain medications on maternal and fetal health.
- Medical and obstetric conditions affecting participation and performance.
- Specific considerations in the pregnant athlete, including nutritional needs, environmental risks, appropriate use of imaging, and contraindications for physical therapy modalities.
- Contraceptive methods and alternatives, at-risk behaviors for unplanned pregnancy, as well as sexually transmitted diseases (STDs).

Epidemiology

- Exercise throughout pregnancy is generally safe, but must be carefully monitored and limitations applied as necessary.
- Benefits of exercise throughout pregnancy include
  - Avoidance of excessive weight gain, improved balance, and decreased back pain.
  - Improved well-being, energy levels, and sleep patterns.
  - Improved labor symptoms and facilitation of postpartum recovery.
- Risks include environmental exposure, dehydration, hypoxia, and uterine trauma.
- Contraceptive methods have different efficacies, potential side effects, and risks for STDs.
  - In certain populations, there may be a positive association between oral contraceptive use and BMD.
  - Use of injectable depot medroxyprogesterone acetate may lead to amenorrhea, lower estrogen levels, and decreased BMD.
- Unplanned pregnancy and/or presence of STDs indicates high-risk behavior.

Physiology and Pathophysiology

- Physiologic changes that may affect exercise throughout pregnancy include
  - Musculoskeletal changes including weight gain.
  - Medical changes including increased heart rate, cardiac output, blood volume, and respiratory rate.
- The goals of exercise throughout pregnancy are to maintain or improve preexisting levels of maternal fitness without undue risk to the mother or the developing fetus.
- Pregnancy increases nutritional needs for calories, iron, calcium, and folic acid.
- Exercise in the supine position after 16 weeks should be avoided due to potential great vessel compression.

Evaluation and Treatment

It is essential that the team physician understand that

- There are specific issues of the female athlete in terms of pregnancy and contraception.

It is desirable that the team physician

- Facilitate obstetric care and treatment, including referral.
- Understand evaluation includes a medical examination, nutritional assessment, and ongoing assessment of absolute and relative contraindications to exercise throughout pregnancy and the postpartum period.

- Understand treatment may include the limitation of physical activity as pregnancy progresses and that discussion with others (healthcare providers, parents, coaches, and Certified Athletic Trainers) may be necessary.

Prevention

It is essential that the team physician understand

- The importance of family planning and contraceptive options for the athlete.
- The implications of pregnancy and the postpartum period for training and competition.

It is desirable that the team physician

- Implement a screening and education program for athletes at risk for pregnancy, including information regarding safe sexual practices, family planning, and contraceptive options.
- Educate athletes, parents, coaches, administrators, and healthcare providers as to the benefits and risks of exercise throughout pregnancy and the postpartum period.

REFERENCES

ACL

Anderson AF, Dome DC, Gautam S, Awh MH, Rennirt GW. Correlation of anthropometric measurements, strength, anterior cruciate ligament size, and intercondylar notch characteristics to sex differences in anterior cruciate ligament tear rates. *Am J Sports Med.* 2001;29:58–66.

Arendt E, Dick R. Knee injury patterns among men and women in collegiate basketball and soccer: NCAA data and review of the literature. *Am J Sports Med.* 1995;23:694–701.

Aune AK, Holm I, Risberg MA, Jensen HK, Steen H. Four-strand hamstring tendon autograft compared with patellar tendon-bone autograft for anterior cruciate ligament reconstruction: A randomized study with two-year follow-up. *Am J Sports Med.* 2001;29:722–728.

Chappell JD, Yu B, Kirkendall DT, Garrett WE. A comparison of knee kinetics between male and female recreational athletes in stop-jump tasks. *Am J Sports Med.* 2002;30:261–267.

Griffin LY, Agel J, Albohm MJ, et al. Noncontact anterior cruciate ligament injuries: Risk factors and prevention strategies. *J Am Acad Orthop Surg.* 2000;8:142–150.

Hewett T, Lindenfeld TN, Riccobene JV, Noyes FR. The effect of neuromuscular training on the incidence of knee injury in female athletes: A prospective study. *Am J Sports Med.* 1999;27:699–706.

Huston L, Wojtys EM. Neuromuscular performance characteristics in elite female athletes. *Am J Sports Med.* 1996;24:427–436.

Myklebust G, Maehlum S, Engebretsen L, Strand T, Solheim E. Registration of cruciate ligament injuries in Norwegian top level team handball: A prospective study covering two seasons. *Scand J Med Sci Sports.* 1997;7:289–292.

Pinczewski LA, Deehan DJ, Salmon LJ, Russell VJ, Clineleffer A. A five-year comparison of patellar tendon versus four-strand hamstring tendon autograft for arthroscopic reconstruction of the anterior cruciate ligament. *Am J Sports Med.* 2002;30:523–536.

Rozzi SL, Lephart SM, Gear WS, Fu FH. Knee joint laxity and neuromuscular characteristics of male and female soccer and basketball players. *Am J Sports Med.* 1999;27:312–319.

Wilk K, et al. Prevention of anterior cruciate ligament injuries in female athletes. *Sports Medicine Update Med Sci Sports Exercise.* 2002;16:21–25.

Wojtys EM, Huston LJ, Boynton MD, Spindler KP, Lindenfeld TN. The effect of the menstrual cycle on anterior cruciate ligament injuries in women as determined by hormone levels. *Am J Sports Med.* 2002;30:182–188.

Patellofemoral

Arroll B, Ellis-Pelger E, Edwards A, et al.: Patellofemoral pain syndrome: A critical review of the clinical trials on non-operative therapy. *Am J Sports Med.* 1997;25:207–212.

Baker MM, Juhn MS. Patellofemoral pain syndrome in the female athlete. In: Harmon K, Agostini R, eds. The Athletic Woman. *Clin Sports Med.* 2000;19:315–320.

Bockrath K, Wooden C, Worrell T, et al. Effects of patella taping on patella position and perceived pain. *Med Sci Sports Exerc.* 1993;25:989–992.

Fairbank JCT, Pynsent PB, Van Poortvliet JA, et al. Mechanical factors in the incidence of knee pain in adolescents and young adults. *J Bone Joint Surg.* 1984;66:685–693.

Fulkerson JP, Hungerford DS, eds. *Disorders of the Patellofemoral Joint.* 2nd ed. Baltimore: Williams & Wilkins; 1990;117–119.

Kowall MG, Kolk G, Nuber GW, et al. Patellar taping in the treatment of patellofemoral pain: a prospective randomized study. *Am J Sports Med.* 1996;24:61–66.

Natri A, Kannus P, Jarvinen M. Which factors predict the long term outcome in chronic patellofemoral pain syndrome? A prospective follow-up study. *Med Sci Sports Exerc.* 1998;30:1572–1577.

Shoulder

Chandler TJ, Kibler WB, Uhl TL, Wooten B, Kiser A, Stone E. Flexibility findings in elite tennis players. *Am J Sports Med.* 1990;18:134–136.

Griffin LY. The female athlete. In: Renstrom P, ed. *The IOC Book on Sports Injuries—Principles of Prevention and Care.* London: Blackwell; 1993.

Hannafin JA. Upper extremity injuries—shoulder. In: Garrett WE, ed. *Women's Health in Sports and Exercise.* Rosemont Ill: AAOS; 2001.

Kibler WB. Rehabilitation of shoulder and knee injuries. In Garrett WE, ed. *Women's Health in Sports and Exercise.* Rosemont Ill: AAOS; 2001.

Kibler WB, Chandler TJ, et al. A musculoskeletal approach to the preparticipation physical examination. Preventing injury and improving performance. *Am J Sports Med.* 1989;17:525–531.

Stress Fractures

Barrow GW, Saha S. Menstrual irregularity and stress fractures in collegiate female distance runners. *Am J Sports Med.* 1998;16:209–216.

Bennell KL, Malcolm SA, Thomas SA, et al. Risk factors for stress fractures in track and field athletes: A twelve-month prospective study. *Am J Sports Med.* 1996;24:810–818

Boden BP, Osbahr DC, Jimenez C. Low-risk stress fractures. *Am J Sports Med.* 2001;29:100–111.

Myburgh KH, Hutchins J, Fataar AB, Hough SF, Noakes TC. Low bone density in an etiologic factor for stress fractures in athletes. *Ann Intern Med.* 1990;113:754–759.

Nattiv A, Armsey TD Jr. Stress injury to bone in the female athlete. *Clin Sports Med.* 1997;16:197–224.

Disordered Eating

Beals KA, Manore MM. Disorders of the female athlete triad among collegiate female athletes. *Int J Sport Nutr.* 2002;12:281–293.

Biller BMK, Saxe V, Herzog DB, Rosenthal DI, Holzman S, Klibanski A. Mechanisms of osteoporosis in adult and adolescent women with anorexia nervosa. *J Clin Endocrinol Metab*. 1989;68:548–554.

Rigotti NA, Neer RM, Skates SJ, et al. The clinical course of osteoporosis in anorexia nervosa. *JAMA*. 1991;265:1133–1138.

Rosenblum J, Forman S. Evidence-based treatment of eating disorders. *Pediatrics*. 2002;14:379–383.

Sundgot-Borgen J. Risk and trigger factors for the development of eating disorders in female elite athletes. *Med Sci Sports Exerc*. 1994;26:414–419.

Sundgot-Borgen J. Eating disorders. In: Drinkwater B, ed. *Women in Sport*. London: Blackwell Science; 2000;364–376.

Walsh JME, Wheat ME, Freund K. Detection, evaluation and treatment of eating disorders: The role of the primary care physician. *J Gen Intern Med*. 2000;15:577–590.

Menstrual Dysfunction

ACSM Position Stand on the female athlete triad. *Med Sci Sports Exerc*. 1997;29:1–9.

Drinkwater BL, Bruemmer B, Chestnut CH III. Menstrual history as a determinant of current bone density in young athletes. *JAMA*. 1990;263:545.

Drinkwater BL, Nilson K, Chestnut CH III, et al. Bone mineral content of amenorrheic and eumenorrheic athletes. *New Engl J Med*. 1984;311:277–281.

Drinkwater BL, Nilson K, Ott S, et al. Bone mineral density after resumption of menses in amenorrheic athletes. *JAMA*. 1986;256:380–382.

Loucks AB, Verdun M, Heath EM, et al. Low energy availability, not the stress of exercise, alters LH pulsatility in exercising women. *J Appl Phys*. 1998;84:37.

Medical Concerns in the Female Athlete. American Academy of Pediatrics Committee on Sports Medicine and Fitness, 1999–2000. *Pediatrics*.

Zanker CL, Swaine. The relationship between serum oestradiol concentration and energy balance in young women distance runners. *Int J Sports Med*. 1998;19:104–108.

Bone Issues

Gibson J. Osteoporosis. In: Drinkwater B, ed. *Women in Sport*. London: Blackwell; 2000;391–406.

Hawker GA, Jamal SA, Ridout R, et al: A clinical prediction rule to identify premenopausal women with low bone mass. *Osteoporosis Int*. 2002;13:400–406.

Kanis JA. Diagnosis of osteoporosis. Osteoporos Int 1997;7:S108–S116.

Kanis JA, Melton LJ, Christiansen C, Johnston CC, Khaltaev N. The diagnosis of osteoporosis. *J Bone Miner Res*. 1994;9:1137–1141.

Khan K, McKay H, Kannus P, Bailey D, Wark J, Bennell K. *Physical Activity and Bone Health*. Champaign, Ill: Human Kinetics; 2001.

Lindsay R, Meunier. Osteoporosis: Review of the evidence for prevention, diagnosis and treatment and cost-effectiveness analysis status report. *Osteoporos Int*. 1998;4(Suppl):S1–S88.

Modlesky CM, Lewis RD. Does exercise during growth have a long-term effect on bone health? *Exerc Sport Sci Rev*. 2002;30:171–176.

Myburgh KH, Bachrach LK, Lewis B, et al. Low bone mineral density at axial and appendicular sites in amenorrheic athletes. *Med Sci Sports Exerc*. 1993;25:1197–1202.

Recker RR, Davies KM, Hinders SM, Heaney RP, Stegman MR, Kimmel DB. Bone gain in young adult women. *JAMA*. 1992;268:2403–2408.

Rencken M, Chesnut CH, Drinkwater BL. Decreased bone density at multiple skeletal sites in amenorrheic athletes. *JAMA*. 1996;276:238–240.

Scholes D, Lacroix AX, Ott SM, Ichikawa LE, Barlow WE. Bone mineral density in women using depot medroxyprogesterone acetate for contraception. *Obstet Gynecol*. 1999;93:233–238.

World Health Organization. Assessment of fracture risk and its application to screening for postmenopausal osteoporosis. Technical report series 843. Geneva: WHO; 1994.

World Health Organization. Assessment of fracture risk and its application to screening for postmenopausal osteoporosis: Technical report series 843. Geneva: WHO; 1994.

Pregnancy and Contraception

Artal R, O'Toole M. Guidelines of the American College of Obstetricians and Gynecologists for exercise during pregnancy and the postpartum period. *Br J Sports Med.* 2003;37:6–12.

Index